Clinical Pain Management

Clinical Pain Management

Edited by Pam Kellner

hayle
medical

New York

Hayle Medical,
750 Third Avenue, 9th Floor,
New York, NY 10017, USA

Visit us on the World Wide Web at:
www.haylemedical.com

ISBN: 978-1-63241-436-6

The publisher's policy is to use permanent paper from mills that operate a sustainable forestry policy. Furthermore, the publisher ensures that the text paper and cover boards used have met acceptable environmental accreditation standards.

Printed in China.

Cataloging-in-Publication Data

Clinical pain management / edited by Pam Kellner.
p. cm.
Includes bibliographical references and index.
ISBN 978-1-63241-436-6
1. Pain. 2. Pain--Treatment. 3. Pain--Physiological aspects. 4. Pain medicine. I. Kellner, Pam.
RB127 .C55 2017
616.047 2--dc23

Table of Contents

Preface

Pain management is defined as the science of easing chronic pain and improving quality of life. This book on clinical pain management discusses pain intensity and the effectiveness of technology to assist in physiotherapy. Those experiencing chronic pain go through intense emotional and physical stress. Pain management techniques involve cognitive behavioural therapy, interventional procedures like injections, etc. This book strives to provide a fair idea about this discipline and to help develop a better understanding of the latest advances within this field. Most of the topics introduced in this text cover new techniques and applications of pain management. This book will be a great help to those in the fields of anaesthesia, physiotherapy and musculoskeletal sciences.

This book unites the global concepts and researches in an organized manner for a comprehensive understanding of the subject. It is a ripe text for all researchers, students, scientists or anyone else who is interested in acquiring a better knowledge of this dynamic field.

I extend my sincere thanks to the contributors for such eloquent research chapters. Finally, I thank my family for being a source of support and help.

Editor

1

Statins Do Not Alter the Incidence of Mesothelioma in Asbestos Exposed Mice or Humans

Cleo Robinson[1,2]*, Helman Alfonso[3], Samantha Woo[1], Amy Walsh[1], Nola Olsen[4], Arthur W. Musk[1,5], Bruce W. S. Robinson[1], Anna K. Nowak[1], Richard A. Lake[1]

1 National Centre for Asbestos Related Diseases, School of Medicine and Pharmacology, University of Western Australia, Harry Perkins Institute for Medical Research, Nedlands, Perth, Western Australia, Australia, **2** Anatomical Pathology, PathWest, Perth, Western Australia, Australia, **3** School of Public Health, Curtin University, Perth, Western Australia, Australia, **4** Occupational Respiratory Epidemiology, School of Population Health, University of Western Australia, Perth, Western Australia, Australia, **5** Department of Respiratory Medicine, Sir Charles Gairdner Hospital, Perth, Western Australia, Australia

Abstract

Mesothelioma is principally caused by asbestos and may be preventable because there is a long latent period between exposure and disease development. The most at-risk are a relatively well-defined population who were exposed as a consequence of their occupations. Although preventative agents investigated so far have not been promising, discovery of such an agent would have a significant benefit world-wide on healthcare costs and personal suffering. Statins are widely used for management of hypercholesterolemia and cardiovascular risk; they can induce apoptosis in mesothelioma cells and epidemiological data has linked their use to a lower incidence of cancer. We hypothesised that statins would inhibit the development of asbestos-induced mesothelioma in mice and humans. An autochthonous murine model of asbestos-induced mesothelioma was used to test this by providing atorvastatin daily in the feed at 100 mg/kg, 200 mg/kg and 400 mg/kg. Continuous administration of atorvastatin did not alter the rate of disease development nor increase the length of time that mice survived. Latency to first symptoms of disease and disease progression were also unaffected. In a parallel study, the relationship between the use of statins and development of mesothelioma was investigated in asbestos-exposed humans. In a cohort of 1,738 asbestos exposed people living or working at a crocidolite mine site in Wittenoom, Western Australia, individuals who reported use of statins did not have a lower incidence of mesothelioma (HR = 1.01; 95% CI = 0.44–2.29, p = 0.99). Some individuals reported use of both statins and non-steroidal anti-inflammatory drugs or COX-2 inhibitors, and these people also did not have an altered risk of mesothelioma development (HR = 1.01; 95% CI = 0.61–1.67, p = 0.97). We conclude that statins do not moderate the rate of development of mesothelioma in either a mouse model or a human cohort exposed to asbestos.

Editor: Sumitra Deb, Virginia Commonwealth University, United States of America

Funding: This work was funded by NHMRC Centre for Research Excellence grant ID 1001020 and a grant from Insurance Commission of Western Australia. Funding received by CR, BWSR, AKN, RAL. The funders had no role in study design, data collection and analysis, decision to publish, or preparation of the manuscript.

Competing Interests: The authors have declared that no competing interests exist.

* Email: cleo.robinson@uwa.edu.au

Introduction

Mesothelioma is a cancer of the pleural and peritoneal cavities, caused predominantly by asbestos exposure [1]. Following its widespread use in multiple industries, millions of people are living with known asbestos exposure and preventative measures against mesothelioma would have a global impact. Whilst asbestos use and mining have been banned in many countries, they are still permitted in some regions and safe disposal of the asbestos already in use remains a considerable hazard [2]. Thus, mesothelioma is an ongoing concern and its incidence continues to rise in industrialized and developing nations: asbestos related diseases are predicted to remain a substantial economic and human burden across the world for the foreseeable future [1].

Epidemiological data indicating beneficial correlations between cancer incidence and dietary intake of vitamins, minerals and commonly used drugs has intensified interest in finding cancer prevention strategies and instigated many randomised controlled trials and animal studies [3–6]. An understanding of cancer mechanisms and biological activities of such compounds has supported their potential for cancer prevention. Although mesothelioma does not usually feature in the epidemiological studies because of its relative rarity, it is a good candidate for targeted prevention because the carcinogen is known, and the 'at risk' population can be readily identified.

Asbestos triggers chronic inflammation and production of reactive oxygen and nitrogen species. These are both carcinogenic mechanisms that are recognised hallmarks of cancer which could be targeted by preventative agents to inhibit mesothelioma development [7]. The long-term persistence of asbestos fibres lodged within the body and the long latency between asbestos exposure and disease development suggests that an agent that is safe for long-term use would be appropriate. Anti-oxidants and anti-inflammatories have been investigated for their ability to prevent cancer in different models with a range of effectiveness, from none, to a substantial reduction in cancer development [8].

Despite a strong rationale, the antioxidants, vitamins A, E, D and selenium were found to be ineffective in preventing mesothelioma [9,10]. This is consistent with the finding that in humans beta carotene and retinoic acid forms of vitamin A do not affect mesothelioma incidence [11]. We have also investigated the use of aspirin and cyclooxygenase-2 inhibitors (COX-2i), again finding no benefit in either the mouse model or a human cohort [12,13]. Here the search for a prevention strategy was extended to investigate the ability of statins to inhibit mesothelioma development in asbestos exposed mouse and human populations.

Statins inhibit the enzyme 3-hydroxy-3-methylglutaryl coenzyme A (HMG-CoA) reductase, which is key to the production of endogenous cholesterol, a fundamental structural component of cell membranes and essential for cell proliferation. Statins are widely used, often with long term regularity and at a known dosage, thus enabling large epidemiological studies. These studies have suggested an association between statin use and a reduced incidence of cancers including lung, breast, prostate, colon and bowel [14]. However, this finding conflicts with a meta-analysis of 27 randomised controlled trials that did not show protective effects [15]. Animal models and cell line studies demonstrate the role of statins in many cellular mechanisms (proliferation, apoptosis, angiogenesis, cell migration and inflammation), supporting the rationale for its preventative action on cancer growth or development [16–18]. In mesothelioma, lovastatin induces apoptosis in vitro [19] and was effective in vivo when combined with doxorubicin chemotherapy, possibly by reversing doxorubicin resistance of the cells [20].

A combination of chemoprevention agents could be more effective by repression of a wider range of the mechanisms involved in tumorigenesis. Furthermore, this strategy may also result in improved efficacy of safer and lower doses of drugs such as aspirin and statins, which have potential toxicities associated with long-term use.

In this study the effect of high, medium and low doses of statin on the survival rate of asbestos-induced mesothelioma is investigated in the MexTAg mouse model of asbestos-induced mesothelioma, which is highly suited to testing potential cancer prevention agents [12]. Alongside this investigation human epidemiological data has been analysed from the Wittenoom cohort, consisting of people who lived or worked in Wittenoom while asbestos mining was taking place. Participants were recruited from a cancer surveillance project for which significant asbestos exposure was the key inclusion criterion [21]. Participants reported use of statins at a defined time point in the recruitment questionnaire and were followed up until 2011. We hypothesised that use of statins would be associated with lower incidence of mesothelioma, and that the combined use of both non-steroidal anti-inflammatory drugs (NSAIDs) or COX-2i and statins would have an additional benefit.

Materials and Methods

Transgenic mice

MexTAg 299h transgenic mice were generated by insertion of a 2,148-bp of SV40 TAg open reading frame cloned downstream of 1,850 bp of the mesothelin promoter as described previously [22]. Groups of experimental mice were matched for age and gender.

Asbestos-induced mesothelioma

Asbestos fibres (IUCC reference sample of Wittenoom Gorge crocidolite, Western Australia) were suspended in PBS (6 mg/ml) and passed through a 23-gauge needle several times. MexTAg 299 h mice were injected in the peritoneum with two doses of 3 mg asbestos, 1 month apart. Mice were monitored and the animals were euthanized when ascites became evident or sickness, distress or loss of condition was noticed (endpoint). A standardized-system of criteria was used to define the first signs of disease and this was taken as the diagnosis date [12]. All experiments had University of Western Australia Animal Ethics Committee approval (#RA5/100/1075) and were carried out in strict accordance with National Health and Medical Research Council guidelines.

Animal diets

Diets were made by Specialty Feeds, Glen Forest, Western Australia. The base diet was AIN93 and was used for control groups. Atorvastatin was added to AIN93 at 100, 200 and 400 mg/kg at source and provided ad libitum.

Human study population

Former workers and residents of Wittenoom have been followed up since 1975. In 1989 all ex-residents and/or ex workers were invited to participate in the "Vitamin A programme" which began accepting participants in July 1990 [23]. On acceptance for the trial participants completed a questionnaire, which included their current use of medication. The statins reported as used were simvastatin, atorvastatin, pravastatin, rosuvastatin or fluvastatin. There was no indication of dosage, frequency of use or duration of use. Out of 2,363 participants in the Vitamin A programme, 1,738 provided information on medication use.

Incident cases of cancer were obtained from the West Australian Cancer Registry, the Western Australia Mesothelioma Registry, and the Registrar General's Office for WA. The date of an incident cancer was taken as the first relevant diagnostic pathological specimen. Participants were followed up until diagnosis of mesothelioma or death, or were censored at 30th June 2012. There were 107 mesothelioma cases during this follow up period.

Statistical Analysis

Animal studies

Kaplan Meier survival curves were compared by log rank test for survival. The one-way ANOVA test for variance was used to analyse latency time and survival time data from three or more test groups. The non-parametric, unpaired, two-tailed t test was used to compare data from two test groups.

Human cohort

Baseline descriptive data were shown as mean and standard deviations (SD), or percentages (%). On average participants were followed up for 11.94 years (SD 6.28, IQR = 6.67–17.80). Cox regression modelling was applied to examine the association (as hazard ratios and their 95% CI) between each main exposure (statins, alone or in combination with COX-2i or NSAIDs) and mesothelioma. Analyses were adjusted for age, sex, body mass index, smoking and intensity of asbestos exposure. The assumption of proportionality was examined by plotting the Schoenfeld residuals. Alpha was set at 5% and all statistical tests were two-tailed. The statistical package Stata version 12.1 (StataCorp, College Station, Texas, USA) was used.

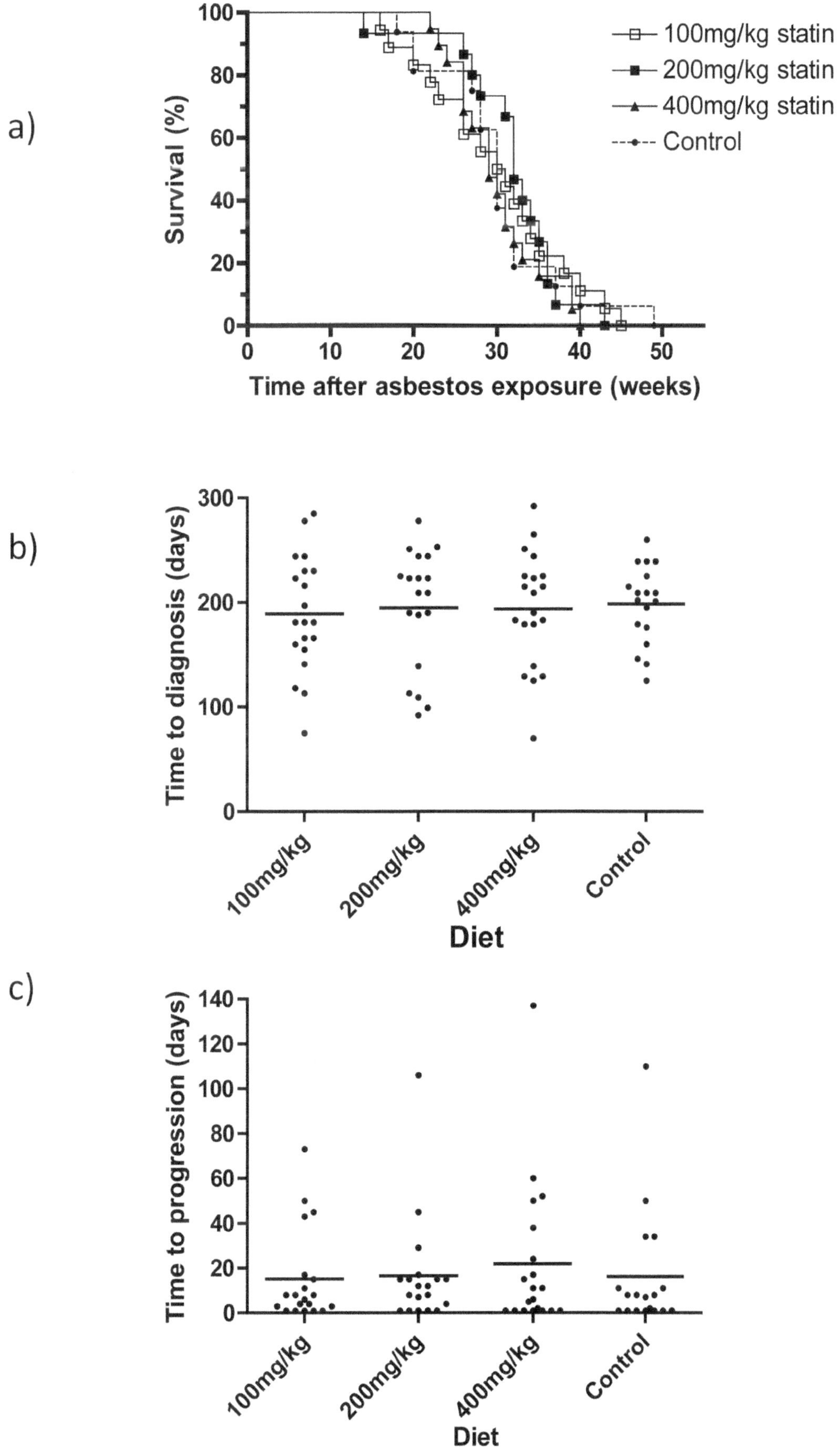
a)
100
80
60
40
20
0
Survival (%)
0
10
20
30
40
50
Time after asbestos exposure (weeks)
100mg/kg statin
200mg/kg statin
400mg/kg statin
Control
b)
300
200
100
0
Time to diagnosis (days)
100mg/kg
200mg/kg
400mg/kg
Control
Diet
c)
140
120
100
80
60
40
20
0
Time to progression (days)
100mg/kg
200mg/kg
400mg/kg
Control
Diet

Figure 1. Statin supplementation does not affect mouse survival from asbestos-induced mesothelioma. Diets containing 0 (base diet AIN93), 100, 200 or 400 mg/kg of atorvastatin were provided 2 weeks prior to asbestos exposure and for the duration of the experiment. (a) Kaplan Meier survival curve for mice receiving the test diets or base diet (n = 20, log rank test for survival, p = 0.84). (b) Latency time to first diagnosis. One-way analysis of variance across all groups: p = 0.96. (c) Disease progression, defined as survival after diagnosis, one-way analysis of variance across all groups: p = 0.87.

Results

Statins do not alter survival of asbestos-induced mesothelioma

Provision of atorvastatin in mouse diets from 2 weeks prior to disease induction at a range of doses did not alter incidence of or survival with mesothelioma (Fig 1a, p = 0.84). The latency from asbestos exposure to first diagnosis of disease was not significantly different between groups (Fig 1b) and nor was disease progression from first diagnosis (Fig 1c). Thus, in this model, continued use of low to high levels of statins did not affect the rate of mesothelioma development or tumour growth rate once a tumour had arisen.

Characteristics of the Wittenoom cohort

Participants reporting taking statin or statin in combination with NSAIDs or COX-2i were significantly older than those who did not (p<0.001, Table 1). Use of a statin alone was not different between genders, but reported use of a combination of the drugs was less frequent in females than in males (p<0.001, Table 1). Overweight and obese people reported using a statin or a combination of the drugs more frequently than people with a normal body mass index (BMI). Use of statins was not consistently related to smoking habits. Those subjects working directly in the mines reported significantly higher statin use (alone or in combination with NSAIDs or COX-2i), compared to those who resided in the town but did not work in the mines. However, there was no correlation between the cumulative asbestos exposure and statin use (Table 1).

Statin use in the asbestos exposed Wittenoom subjects

554 people reported taking statins, with simvastatin and atorvostatin being most frequently used (Table 2). 346 people reported taking statins plus any NSAID and 54 reported using statin with a COX-2i. 1,200 people reported not using statin and 798 reported using none of these medications.

Statin use is not associated with an altered risk of mesothelioma

At the end of study date (June 2012) mesothelioma had been diagnosed in 107 people. Participants taking statins alone were no less likely to develop mesothelioma than those not taking the medication (adjusted HR 1.01, 95% CI = 0.44, 2.29; p = 0.99) and nor were those taking statins in combination with NSAIDs or COX-2i (HR 0.91; 95%CI = 0.50–1.66, p = 0.77; Table 3 and Figure 2a)

Survival from the date of first exposure was also not different for the statin users compared to non-users (HR, 0.81, 95%CI: 0.35–

Table 1. Demographic and exposure characteristics of the Wittenoom cohort.

Variable	Whole cohortn = 1754	Statins alone n = 154	NSAIDS/COX-2i alone n = 402	Statins and NSAID or COX-2i n = 400	None n = 798	p value
Age (at questionnaire)						<0.001
Yrs, mean (SD)	58.75 (12.13)	62.5 (8.6)	59.6 (10.6)	66.0 (8.3)	54.0 (12.8)	
Sex, n (%)						<0.001
male	1235 (70.4)	110 (71.4)	288 (71.6)	316 (79.0)	521 (65.3)	
female	519 (29.6)	44 (28.6)	114 (28.4)	84 (21.0)	277 (34.7)	
BMI, n(%)						<0.001
<25, (normal)	343 (19.6)	19 (12.3)	74 (18.4)	53 (13.3)	197 (24.7)	
25–29.9 (overweight)	689 (39.3)	74 (48.1)	159 (39.6)	171 (42.8)	285 (35.7)	
>30 (obese)	468 (26.7)	50 (32.5)	104 (25.9)	145 (36.3)	169 (21.2)	
Smoking, n(%)						<0.001
never	573 (32.7)	54 (35.1)	113 (28.1)	124 (31.0)	282 (35.3)	
past	804 (45.8)	71 (46.1)	219 (54.5)	205 (51.3)	309 (38.7)	
current	373 (21.3)	29 (18.8)	70 (17.4)	69 (17.3)	205 (25.7)	
Occupation, n(%)						<0.001
workers	1011 (57.6)	95 (61.7)	237 (59.0)	269 (67.3)	410 (51.4)	
Ex-residents	743 (42.4)	59 (38.3)	165 (41.0)	131 (32.8)	388 (48.6)	
Cumulative asbestos exposure (f/ml.y)						0.247
<4.85(p50), n(%)	823 (46.9)	74 (48.1)	168 (41.8)	186 (46.5)	395 (49.5)	
4.85–12.98 (p50–p75)	422 (24.1)	32 (20.8)	105 (26.1)	93 (23.3)	192 (24.1)	
>12.98	442 (25.2)	41 (26.6)	114 (28.4)	102 (25.5)	185 (23.2)	

*p-values obtained using Pearson chi-square for categorical variables and one-way analysis of variance for continuous variables (age) across the 4 groups. F/ml.y: fibre per millilitre.year.

Table 2. Statin and NSAID usage.

Drug name	Number of people using drug	Percent of cohort using drug (n = 1,754)
Simvastatin	225	12.8%
Atorvastatin	200	11.4%
Pravastatin	85	4.8%
Rosuvastatin	32	1.8%
Fluvastatin	11	0.6%
Cerivastatin	1	0.06%
No statins	1,200	68%
Any statin alone	154	8.8%
Any statin plus any NSAID	346	20%
Any statin plus any COX-2i	54	37.7%
Statin, plus NSAID or COX2i	400	22.8%
Statin, NSAID and COX2i	0	0%
No NSAID, COX2i or statin	798	45.5%

1.83, p = 0.61. Those reporting use of statin plus any NSAID or COX-2i had a lower hazard ratio of 0.67 (95%CI 0.37–1.22), however this was not significant (p = 0.19; Table 3, Figure 2b).

Discussion

Despite a sound biological rationale for our hypothesis, we found that the use of statins did not alter the rate of development or incidence of mesothelioma in asbestos-exposed mice or people. An analysis of data from the Wittenoom cohort of asbestos-exposed individuals who have been closely monitored for decades found no link between mesothelioma risk and reported use of statins or statins plus either a NSAID or a COX-2i. Similarly, low, medium or high doses of atorvastatin provided to mice from two weeks prior to disease induction with asbestos did not have a significant effect on survival, latency, rate of tumor progression, nor on macroscopic tumor burden.

The MexTAg asbestos-induced model and the Wittenoom cohort of asbestos-exposed individuals are appropriate companion studies because in both cases exposure was to the same type of asbestos, crocidolite, which is considered as more carcinogenic than the more common form, chrysotile [24]. Furthermore, MexTAg tumor pathogenesis is similar to human mesothelioma in terms of many factors including histology, latency, inflammatory response, localization and the response to cytotoxic chemotherapy [12].

In the mouse study the statin was provided starting two weeks prior to asbestos exposure to give maximum chance of detecting an effect. It was continued throughout the experiment, inclusive of the latency and disease progression periods. By comparison, the questionnaire upon which the use of statins and other drugs in the human cohort is based was conducted 24 years after the closure of the Wittenoom mine. Thus, given that human mesothelioma development occurs 40+ years after exposure to asbestos, these data indicate that the drug usage occurred within the latency period; however usage was not restricted to that time. As statins are predominantly administered on a long-term basis to lower cholesterol levels and treat cardiovascular disease, the individuals who reported usage in 1990, are most likely to have continued to do so for the duration of the study. At the time of the questionnaire, statins were new drugs; the first listing of lovastatin was in 1987 and clinical use began in the mid to late 1980s. Statin use in Australia has since escalated due to wider clinical availability [25]. Together with the fact that statin use correlates with age, the number of people taking statins since the start of the questionnaire is anticipated to have increased. This could result in misclassification bias, as some individuals in the control group may have an undisclosed subsequent statin use during the later latency phase. This is a limitation of the data, and as the adjusted hazard ratio between users and non-users was 1.01 (95%CI 0.44–2.29), it is feasible this could significantly affect the results. However, a recent review of multiple randomised controlled trials found no preventative benefit for statins, so it is more likely that this lack of benefit in the prevention of mesothelioma correct. [15].

Within the human cohort there is a diverse genetic background and variation in environmental factors such as lifestyle, diet, smoking, age, as well as levels of asbestos exposure. This is reflected in the variance in latency and survival times [26]. In contrast, in the mouse experiments, these factors are consistent across all study groups, i.e. the mice were genetically identical, lived under the same conditions, had the same base feed and the amount of asbestos received was equivalent. This makes the mouse model an ideal system to investigate the potential of statins to prevent asbestos-induced mesothelioma, and supports the validity of the epidemiological data.

There is excellent concordance in results from our studies of mice and humans not only in this study, but also in our previous work investigating potential preventive agents for mesothelioma. Our two previous investigations addressed vitamin A and non-steroidal anti-inflammatory drug usage and mesothelioma incidence [9,11]. In the vitamin A trials in both the Wittenoom cohort and the MexTAg mice, the supplementation level was fixed and controlled, and both trials demonstrated no benefit in vitamin A supplementation, despite a strong rationale for a preventative effect. This suggests that comparisons between these sets of mouse and human data are valid. Because we are able to induce mouse mesotheliomas using the same carcinogen as in human mesothelioma, with much the same pathological changes and clinical behaviour, we have an ideal situation to study preventative and therapeutic agents. Such a situation is very rare in the field of animal models of cancer.

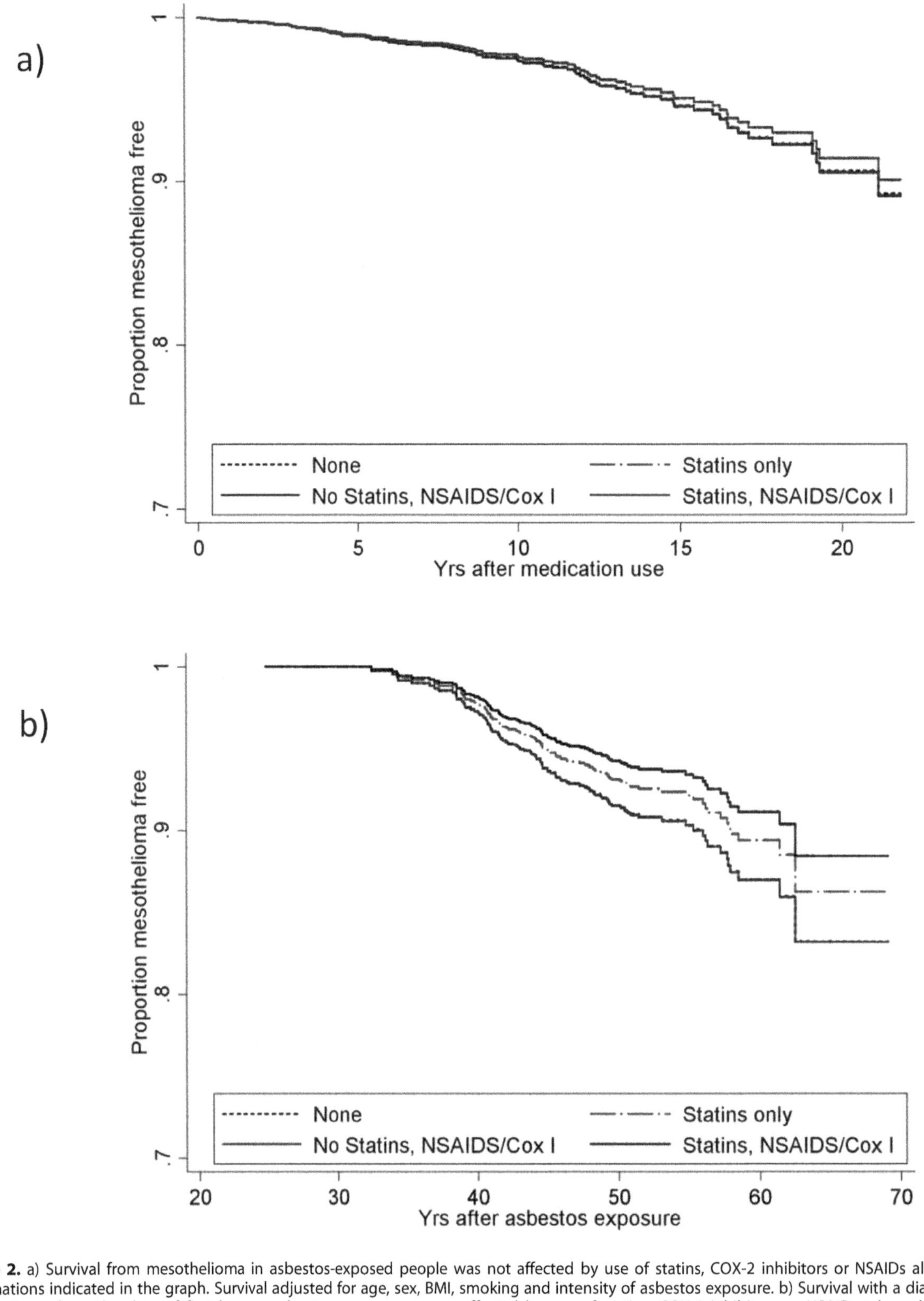

Figure 2. a) Survival from mesothelioma in asbestos-exposed people was not affected by use of statins, COX-2 inhibitors or NSAIDs alone or in combinations indicated in the graph. Survival adjusted for age, sex, BMI, smoking and intensity of asbestos exposure. b) Survival with a diagnosis of mesothelioma from the date of first known asbestos exposure was unaffected by use of statins, COX-2 inhibitors or NSAIDs taken alone or in combination. Adjusted for age, sex, BMI and smoking.

There are many examples of negative randomised controlled trials of putative cancer prevention strategies, which were not concordant with previous animal model studies. In some instances a detrimental effect has led to early termination of human clinical trials [27,28]. However, the key difference between these studies and the one we describe here is that in most murine models the

Table 3. Association of medication use and development of mesothelioma in the Wittenoom cohort.

Medication used	No mesothelioma n (%)	Mesothelioma n (%)	Unadjusted HR (95%CI) p-value	Adjusted* since start of study HR (95%CI) p-value	Adjusted** since first asbestos exposure HR (95%CI) p-value
Neither drug	747 (93.6)	51 (6.4)	[1]	[1]	[1]
Statins alone	146 (94.8)	8 (5.2)	1.19 (0.56,2.52) 0.65	1.01 (0.44,2.29) 0.99	0.81 (0.35,1.83) 0.61
No statin plus any NSAIDS or COX-2i	375 (93.3)	27 (6.7)	1.00 (0.63,1.60) 0.99	1.01 (0.61,1.67) 0.97	1.00 (0.61,1.66) 0.99
Both	379 (94.8)	21 (5.3)	1.17 (0.70,1.96) 0.55	0.91 (0.50,1.66) 0.77	0.67 (0.37,1.22) 0.19

*Adjusted for age, bmi, sex, smoking status and asbestos exposure category (worker or ex-resident at Wittenoom).
**Additional adjustment for time since asbestos exposure.

identical carcinogen that causes the human cancer is unable to induce an equivalent mouse cancer, either because the carcinogen is unknown or induces a different tumour or is non-carcinogenic in animals.

The potential benefits from statin use are more complex than might be expected from lowering cholesterol levels alone [29]. Statins have a pleiotropic effect on a number of key pathways, many of which have a role in cancer development, including cell proliferation, angiogenesis, apoptosis, metastasis and inflammation: mechanisms that are relevant to mesothelioma development [30]. For example, statins effectively induce apoptosis and enhance chemosensitivity in mesothelioma cell lines [19,20]. However, while there have been many proposals for a preventative action of statins, particularly in cohort studies and in vitro cancer cell line data, it is noted that many of these investigations contain caveats [30]. A lack of accord amongst cancer prevention studies in general is common [16]. In the case of statins, this could in part be because the data has mostly arisen from trials that were designed to investigate statin use in the treatment of cardiovascular disease; thus cancer prevention was explored in secondary analyses. In complete conflict, low cholesterol has even been associated with a higher cancer incidence [31]. A recent and comprehensive meta-analysis of randomised controlled trials proposes a lack of effect for statins [15]. Thus, this investigation is in accordance with the findings for the majority of studies.

In the human cohort there was a non-significant trend towards a benefit for combined use of statins and NSAIDs or COX-2i, suggesting the potential for concurrent use of multiple preventative agents to target inhibition of inflammation and other tumorigenic cellular mechanisms. Similarly, people using both NSAIDs and COX-2i compared to use of either drug type individually, also had a trend towards a lower risk of mesothelioma development, albeit non-significant [13]. The number of people using both types of drugs was very small. Thus, despite a hazard ratio that implied a benefit, it did not reach statistical significance. This combinatorial approach could be followed up in the mouse model, but given no effect with the single agents, and the minor improvement in survival associated with multiple drug use in the human cohort, it unlikely that a benefit would be detectable unless very large numbers of mice were used. Nevertheless a combinatorial approach to cancer prevention and more specifically use of statins together with NSAIDs is under investigation [32] and outcomes seem to be dependent on cancer type [33,34]. While this combination was not found to be inhibitory for mesothelioma development in this investigation, these drugs, which have a strong biological rationale for use in mesothelioma, could potentially be useful in combination with chemotherapy. Combining chemoprevention drugs with cytotoxic chemotherapies is being investigated for other cancers [35] and statins did enhance the efficacy of doxorubicin in mesothelioma cell lines [20].

In conclusion, although statins can induce apoptosis in mesothelioma cells [19] and epidemiological data has linked their use to a lower incidence of cancer, our data show that they do not alter the incidence of mesothelioma in asbestos exposed mice or humans. The long latency between asbestos exposure and presentation of mesothelioma suggests multiple events occur during carcinogenesis and more understanding of this could lead to a more informed approach to cancer prevention. Many people have a known exposure to asbestos and thus any effective prevention agent would immediately benefit this population. The MexTAg model is a good system for testing potential prevention agents because the disease is pathogenically the same as in humans and induced by the same carcinogen, with the distinct advantage that the mice have fewer variables to confound the data. Thus, although statin use did not prevent mesothelioma development, this approach of studying preventative agents in a uniquely relevant animal model plus a relevant patient cohort offers the prospect that other preventative agents, or combinations of such agents, could be evaluated.

Acknowledgments

Rob Mina and Jan Sleith are acknowledged for their contribution to the cohort questionnaire.

Author Contributions

Conceived and designed the experiments: CR AWM BWSR AKN RAL. Performed the experiments: CR HA SW NO AW. Contributed reagents/materials/analysis tools: CR HA AWM NO. Contributed to the writing of the manuscript: CR HA AKN RAL.

References

1. Robinson BW, Lake RA (2005) Advances in malignant mesothelioma. N Engl J Med 353(15): 1591–1603.
2. Olsen NJ, Franklin PJ, Reid A, de Klerk NH, Threlfall TJ, et al. (2011) Increasing incidence of malignant mesothelioma after exposure to asbestos during home maintenance and renovation. Med J Aust 195(5): 271–274.
3. Gonzalez CA (2006) Nutrition and cancer: the current epidemiological evidence. Br J Nutr 96 Suppl 1: S42–45.
4. Poynter JN, Gruber SB, Higgins PD, Almog R, Bonner JD, et al. (2005) Statins and the risk of colorectal cancer. N Engl J Med 352(21): 2184–2192.
5. Mamede AC, Tavares SD, Abrantes AM, Trindade J, Maia JM, et al. (2011) The role of vitamins in cancer: a review. Nutr Cancer 63(4): 479–494.
6. Algra AM, Rothwell PM (2012) Effects of regular aspirin on long-term cancer incidence and metastasis: a systematic comparison of evidence from observational studies versus randomised trials. Lancet Oncol 13(5): 518–527.

7. Hanahan D, Weinberg RA (2011) Hallmarks of cancer: the next generation. Cell 144(5): 646–674.
8. Shureiqi I, Reddy P, Brenner DE (2000) Chemoprevention: general perspective. Crit Rev Oncol Hematol 33(3): 157–167.
9. Robinson C, Woo S, Walsh A, Nowak AK, Lake RA (2012) The antioxidants vitamins A and E and selenium do not reduce the incidence of asbestos-induced disease in a mouse model of mesothelioma. Nutr Cancer 64(2): 315–322.
10. Robinson C, Woo S, Nowak AK, Lake RA (2014) Dietary Vitamin D Supplementation Does Not Reduce the Incidence or Severity of Asbestos-Induced Mesothelioma in a Mouse Model. Nutr Cancer.
11. Alfonso HS, Reid A, de Klerk NH, Olsen N, Mina R, et al. (2010) Retinol supplementation and mesothelioma incidence in workers earlier exposed to blue asbestos (Crocidolite) at Wittenoom, Western Australia. Eur J Cancer Prev 19(5): 355–359.
12. Robinson C, Walsh A, Larma I, O'Halloran S, Nowak AK, et al. (2011) MexTAg mice exposed to asbestos develop cancer that faithfully replicates key features of the pathogenesis of human mesothelioma. Eur J Cancer 47(1): 151–161.
13. Robinson C, Alfonso H, Woo S, Olsen N, Musk AW, et al. (2014) NSAIDS and COX-2 inhibitors do not reduce the incidence nor severity of asbestos-induced mesothelioma: evidence from an animal model and a human cohort. submitted.
14. Nielsen SF, Nordestgaard BG, Bojesen SE (2012) Statin use and reduced cancer-related mortality. N Engl J Med 367(19): 1792–1802.
15. Emberson JR, Kearney PM, Blackwell L, Newman C, Reith C, et al. (2012) Lack of effect of lowering LDL cholesterol on cancer: meta-analysis of individual data from 175,000 people in 27 randomised trials of statin therapy. PLoS One 7(1): e29849.
16. Demierre MF, Higgins PD, Gruber SB, Hawk E, Lippman SM (2005) Statins and cancer prevention. Nat Rev Cancer 5(12): 930–942.
17. Hoque A, Chen H, Xu XC (2008) Statin induces apoptosis and cell growth arrest in prostate cancer cells. Cancer Epidemiol Biomarkers Prev 17(1): 88–94.
18. Bu DX, Griffin G, Lichtman AH (2011) Mechanisms for the anti-inflammatory effects of statins. Curr Opin Lipidol 22(3): 165–170.
19. Rubins JB, Greatens T, Kratzke RA, Tan AT, Polunovsky VA, et al. (1998) Lovastatin induces apoptosis in malignant mesothelioma cells. Am J Respir Crit Care Med 157(5 Pt 1): 1616–1622.
20. Riganti C, Orecchia S, Pescarmona G, Betta PG, Ghigo D, et al. (2006) Statins revert doxorubicin resistance via nitric oxide in malignant mesothelioma. Int J Cancer 119(1): 17–27.
21. de Klerk NH, Musk AW, Ambrosini GL, Eccles JL, Hansen J, et al. (1998) Vitamin A and cancer prevention II: comparison of the effects of retinol and beta-carotene. Int J Cancer 75(3): 362–367.
22. Robinson C, van Bruggen I, Segal A, Dunham M, Sherwood A, et al. (2006) A novel SV40 TAg transgenic model of asbestos-induced mesothelioma: malignant transformation is dose dependent. Cancer Res 66(22): 10786–10794.
23. Musk AW, de Klerk NH, Ambrosini GL, Eccles JL, Hansen J, et al. (1998) Vitamin A and cancer prevention I: observations in workers previously exposed to asbestos at Wittenoom, Western Australia. Int J Cancer 75(3): 355–361.
24. Nicholson WJ, Raffn E (1995) Recent data on cancer due to asbestos in the U.S.A. and Denmark. Med Lav 86(5): 393–410.
25. Mant A, Lowinger J, Hall W, Whicker S, Ringland C, et al. (2007) Statins down under. Br J Clin Pharmacol 63(1): 125–127.
26. Musk AW, Olsen N, Alfonso H, Reid A, Mina R, et al. (2011) Predicting survival in malignant mesothelioma. Eur Respir J 38(6): 1420–1424.
27. Lippman SM, Klein EA, Goodman PJ, Lucia MS, Thompson IM, et al. (2009) Effect of selenium and vitamin E on risk of prostate cancer and other cancers: the Selenium and Vitamin E Cancer Prevention Trial (SELECT). Jama 301(1): 39–51.
28. The Alpha-Tocopherol BCCPSG (1994) The effect of vitamin E and beta carotene on the incidence of lung cancer and other cancers in male smokers. N Engl J Med 330(15): 1029–1035.
29. Liao JK, Laufs U (2005) Pleiotropic effects of statins. Annu Rev Pharmacol Toxicol 45: 89–118.
30. Graaf MR, Richel DJ, van Noorden CJ, Guchelaar HJ (2004) Effects of statins and farnesyltransferase inhibitors on the development and progression of cancer. Cancer Treat Rev 30(7): 609–641.
31. Strohmaier S, Edlinger M, Manjer J, Stocks T, Bjorge T, et al. (2013) Total serum cholesterol and cancer incidence in the Metabolic syndrome and Cancer Project (Me-Can). PLoS One 8(1): e54242.
32. Xiao H, Yang CS (2008) Combination regimen with statins and NSAIDs: a promising strategy for cancer chemoprevention. Int J Cancer 123(5): 983–990.
33. Beales IL, Vardi I, Dearman L (2012) Regular statin and aspirin use in patients with Barrett's oesophagus is associated with a reduced incidence of oesophageal adenocarcinoma. Eur J Gastroenterol Hepatol 24(8): 917–923.
34. Coogan PF, Kelly JP, Strom BL, Rosenberg L (2010) Statin and NSAID use and prostate cancer risk. Pharmacoepidemiol Drug Saf 19(7): 752–755.
35. Zhou P, Cheng SW, Yang R, Wang B, Liu J (2012) Combination chemoprevention: future direction of colorectal cancer prevention. Eur J Cancer Prev 21(3): 231–240.

2

TLR9 Ligands Induce S100A8 in Macrophages via a STAT3-Dependent Pathway which Requires IL-10 and PGE_2

Kenneth Hsu*, Yuen Ming Chung, Yasumi Endoh¤, Carolyn L. Geczy

Inflammation and Infection Research Centre, School of Medical Sciences, University of New South Wales, Sydney, New South Wales, Australia

Abstract

S100A8 and S100A9 are highly-expressed calcium-binding proteins in neutrophils and monocytes, and in subsets of macrophages in inflammatory lesions. Unmethylated CpG motifs found in bacterial and viral DNA are potent activators of innate immunity via Toll-like receptor 9 (TLR9). S100A8, but not S100A9, mRNA and protein was directly induced by CpG-DNA in murine and human macrophages. Induction in murine macrophages peaked at 16 h. CpG-DNA-induced S100A8 required *de novo* protein synthesis; IL-10 and Prostaglandin E_2 (PGE_2) synergistically enhanced expression and promoted earlier gene induction. Inhibitors of endogenous IL-10, PGE_2, and the E prostanoid (EP) 4 receptor strongly suppressed S100A8 expression, particularly when combined. Thus, S100A8 induction by *E. coli* DNA required both IL-10 and PGE_2/EP4 signaling. The MAPKs, PI3K and JAK pathways were essential, whereas ERK1/2 appeared to play a direct role. S100A8 induction by CpG-DNA was controlled at the transcriptional level. The promoter region responsible for activation, either directly, or indirectly via IL-10 and PGE_2, was located within a −178 to −34-bp region and required STAT3 binding. Because of the robust links connecting IL-10 and PGE_2 with an anti-inflammatory macrophage phenotype, the induction profile of S100A8 strongly indicates a role for this protein in resolution of inflammation.

Editor: Taishin Akiyama, University of Tokyo, Japan

Funding: This work was supported by project grants #455406 and #455307 from the National Health and Medical Research Council (NHMRC) Australia (http://www.nhmrc.gov.au/grants). The funder had no role in study design, data collection and analysis, decision to publish, or preparation of the manuscript.

Competing Interests: The authors have declared that no competing interests exist.

* Email: k.hsu@unsw.edu.au

¤ Current address: Department of Internal Medicine, Division of Cardiology, Nippon Medical School Tama-Nagayama Hospital, Tama-shi, Tokyo, Japan

Introduction

Responses in the innate immune system in vertebrates rely on germline-encoded pattern recognition receptors (PRRs), including the Toll-like receptor (TLR) family, to sense pathogen-associated molecular patterns (PAMPs) on microbial pathogens. Macrophages are crucial mediators in this process, producing proinflammatory cytokines, chemokines and antimicrobial proteins in response to PRR signaling [1]. Response genes in activated macrophages can be fundamentally divided into primary (0.5–2 h, e.g. TNFα) and secondary response genes (2–8 h, e.g. IL-10) (reviewed in [2]) that may display differences in their chromatin architecture (e.g. presence of CpG islands) and/or their regulation by different categories of transcription factors [3]. Secondary genes induced by LPS generally require *de novo* synthesis and further chromatin remodelling that regulates subsequent waves of late gene expression over a prolonged period, thus determining the fate of activated macrophages. However, mechanisms involved in generation of late-phase responses by secondary response genes are poorly defined.

Bacterial and viral DNAs are PAMPs, distinct from their vertebrate counterparts, containing unmethylated CpG motifs that are generally absent, and mostly methylated in eukaryotic DNA [4]. The 2′-deoxyribose sugar backbone of DNA is also critical for recognition of oligodeoxynucleotides on naturally-formed phosphodiester backbones [5]. Bacterial and viral CpG-containing DNA (CpG-DNA) motifs, which can be mimicked by synthetic CpG-containing oligodeoxynucleotides (CpG-ODN), are recognized by TLR9 [6] and used as an adjuvant for treating infectious diseases, cancer, and allergies. TLR9 is most abundant in plasmacytoid dendritic cells and B cells and to lesser extent in monocytes, macrophages and neutrophils [7–9]. Like other nucleic-sensing TLRs, the intracellular localization and proteolytic maturation of TLR9 may reduce recognition of self-DNA [10].

CpG-DNA activation normally skews the host's immune system to Th1-type responses *via* the MyD88-dependent pathway. In macrophages, bacterial DNA induces TNFα, IL-1, IL-6, IL-12, IFN-α/β, IFN-γ, and inducible nitric oxide synthase (iNOS) within hours, in pathways that may be direct or *via* other mediators [4]. For example, CpG-DNA directly induces IFN-β which promotes STAT1 phosphorylation and CXCL-10 (IP-10) production through the IFN-α/β receptor in an autocrine manner [11]. TLRs 3, 4 and 9 can also directly control expression of the anti-inflammatory cytokine IL-10 *via* the tumour necrosis factor receptor-associated factor 3 (TRAF3) pathway, indicating the importance of TLR signaling in restoration of immunological homeostasis [12]. Mechanisms restricting prolonged inflammation and limiting its damaging effects are just beginning to be unravelled and IL-10 signaling integrates several regulatory pathways [13].

S100 is a multigene family of 21 members of highly-conserved calcium-binding proteins [14]; S100A8 (also known as MRP8 or Calgranulin A) forms a stable complex with S100A9 (MRP9 or Calgranulin B) and these comprise the major calcium-binding proteins constitutively expressed in neutrophils and monocytes. Subsets of macrophages at inflammatory sites, but not normal tissue macrophages [15,16] express the proteins and are regarded as a major source of S100A8 and S100A9 [17]. The S100A8/A9 complex (known as calprotectin) is antimicrobial and strongly expressed in lesions, and systemically, in patients with a variety of infections, and inhibits invasion and growth of a range of bacteria and fungi [18].

S100A8 is not always co-expressed with S100A9, particularly in elicited murine macrophages stimulated by LPS, Poly I:C, IFNγ or TNF [19] [20]. This, together with its chemotactic properties, which can cause mild transient leukocyte infiltration when injected into mice [21], originally suggested a proinflammatory role. However, corticosteroids [22], IL-10 and cAMP/PGE$_2$ modulate LPS-induced mS100A8 expression [23] and S100A8 induction in response to TLR3 activation by Poly I:C or viral RNA, and to TLR4 by LPS, is IL-10-dependent [20]. Moreover, S100A8/A9 suppresses differentiation, antigen presentation, and release of inflammatory mediators such as IL-6, IL-12 and iNOS in dendritic cells [24]. This pattern of gene regulation in macrophages, and effects on dendritic cells, indicates anti-inflammatory properties. In keeping with this, we found that S100A8 scavenges oxidants, particularly peroxide, and hypochlorite (HOCl/OCl$^-$) generated by the myeloperoxidase system [25] and may modulate redox in chronic inflammatory lesions such as in human atheroma [26] and human asthma [27]. Moreover, S100A8 is readily S-nitrosylated and this form suppresses leukocyte transmigration triggered by mast cell activation in the microcirculation [28]. Furthermore, suppression of ROS required for IgE-mediated signaling of antigen-sensitized mast cells may mediate the suppression of symptoms in acute asthma seen following S100A8 administration to murine lung [29]. S100A8 also reduces phosphorylation of p38 MAPK provoked by S100A9, and may modulate S100A9-associated phagocyte transmigration [30].

This is the first study to report the strong upregulation of an S100 protein by CpG-DNA in macrophages. S100A8 expression was dependent on two secondary gene products, IL-10 and PGE$_2$ at the transcriptional level and involved multiple pathways, including MAPKs, PI3K, and JAK-STAT signaling. On the other hand, ERK1/2 activation, independent of IL-10 and PGE$_2$, was apparently required for direct S100A8 induction by CpG-DNA. The −178 to −34-bp region in the S100A8 promoter contained important *cis*-elements, STAT3, C/EBP, AP-1, Ets, and NF-1 binding sites that may contribute to its transcriptional activation. The induction pattern of S100A8 supports the proposal that S100A8 may regulate the magnitude of inflammatory responses and contribute to resolution.

Materials and Methods

Ethics statement

All protocols involving the use of human and murine macrophages were approved by the Human Research Ethics Committee and the Animal Care and Ethics Committee of the University of New South Wales, respectively. All participants provided their written informed consent to participate in this study. This consent procedure was approved by the Human Research Ethics Committee of the University of New South Wales.

Materials

LPS was from *E. coli* O55:B5 (Sigma). Synthetic oligodeoxynucleotides (ODNs) were from Invitrogen and were resuspended in endotoxin-free Tris-EDTA buffer. The sequences of ODNs for positive activation of TLR9 at the indicated concentrations are: murine-specific CpG ODN 5′-TCCATGACGTTCCTGACGTT-3′ (CpG-1826, also referred to as CpG if not specifically indicated by types), human-specific CpG ODN 2216 5′-ggGGGACGATCGTCgggggg-3′ (CpG-2216, lowercase letters represent phosphorothioate linkage; capitals, phosphodiester linkage 3′ of the base). The sequence for non-nCpG control ODN 1982: 5′-TCCAGGACTTCTCTCAGGTT-3′ (nCpG). To prevent TLR9 and CpG colocalization in endosomal vesicles, thereby inhibiting TLR9 activation by its agonist, we pretreated cells with the inhibitory iCpG ODN 2088: 5′-TCCTGGCGGGGAAGT-3′ (iCpG) at the indicated concentrations for 30 min prior to stimulation with agonists. IL-10 and anti-mouse IL-10 mAb were from R&D systems. Cycloheximide (CHX), SB202190, U0126, JNK inhibitor II, LY294002, AG490, prostaglandin E$_2$ (PGE$_2$), indomethacin (Indo), and NS398 were from Calbiochem. Ruxolitinib was obtained from Selleck Chemicals. EP receptor antagonists SC-19220, AH-6809, and AH-2348 were from Sigma. PhosphoPlus Stat3 (Tyr705) antibody kit, including anti-phospho-Stat3 Ab, anti-Stat3 Ab, and untreated and IFNα-treated HeLa cell extracts, was from Cell Signaling.

Macrophage culture

Culture media and reagents, including RPMI-1640 and Hank's balanced salt solution, were either liquid or prepared from powder (Invitrogen) using Baxter water and filtered through 0.2 μm Zetapore filters (Cuno) to remove traces of endotoxin. Medium and mediators were only used if endotoxin levels were <20 pg/ml (chromogenic Limulus amebocyte assay; Associates of Cape Cod). Bovine calf serum (HyClone) was pretested for endotoxin content before purchase.

The murine macrophage-like cell line RAW 264.7 (ATCC, referred as RAW cells) was used within 15 passages after retrieval from frozen storage, and cultured at 37°C in a humidified atmosphere of 5% CO_2 in air in RPMI-1640 supplemented with 100 U/ml penicillin, 100 μg/ml streptomycin (Invitrogen), and 10% heated (56°C, 30 min) bovine calf serum, referred to as complete medium (CM). RAW cells were passaged twice weekly in a 1:40 split on Petri dishes (Falcon). Thioglycollate (TG)-elicited murine macrophages were obtained as described and cultured in RPMI 1640 with antibiotics supplemented with 2% BCS [23]. For mRNA measurements and protein analysis, macrophages were seeded into 24-well tissue culture plates (Nunc) at 1.5×10^5 in 500 μl CM and cultured overnight before stimulation.

Human monocyte-derived macrophages were prepared as described [31]. Briefly, PBMCs isolated from peripheral blood of health subjects using Ficol-paque plus (GE Healthcare) were dispensed into 24-well Costar plates (2.5×10^6/well) in RPMI-1640 containing 10% heated (56°C, 30 min) autologous serum, 2 mM L-glutamine, penicillin/streptomycin, and 10 ng/ml M-CSF and incubated at 37°C in 5% CO_2 in air for 3 days. Non-adherent cells were gently rinsed off with warm RPMI-1640 and adherent cells cultured in RPMI-1640 with 10% autologous serum and antibiotics for another 4 days. For experiments using pathway inhibitors, cells were pretreated with inhibitors for 20 min, then untreated or stimulated for the indicated time.

DNA manipulation

E. coli DNA, *M. luteus* DNA, and human placental DNAs (Sigma) were further purified by two-step CsCl ultracentrifugation

[32]. DNA digestion was performed using RNase-free Turbo DNase (Ambion) at 2 U/µg DNA in buffer supplied with the enzyme, for 2 h at 37°C. Endotoxin levels in all DNA preparations were <2 pg/µg DNA, assayed by the *Limulus* amebocyte lysate assay.

RNA isolation and quantitative RT-PCR analysis

RNA preparation and real time RT-PCR were performed essentially as described [14]. Briefly, 1.0 µg was treated with Turbo DNase to eliminate DNA and then converted to cDNA using SuperScript VILO cDNA Synthesis Kit (Life technology) according to the manufacturer's instructions. Real-time PCR was performed with LightCycler 480 SYBR Green I Master (Roche) on a LightCycler 480 Real-Time PCR System (Roche) under standard cycle conditions. Relative quantities of mRNA in duplicate samples were obtained using the LightCycler 480 Software 1.5 and the Efficiency-Method and normalized against hypoxanthine-guanine phosphoribosyltransferase (HPRT) or β-actin as endogenous controls, there is no difference in terms of fold changes using either endogenous controls. Unless otherwise stated, data represent the fold changes of mRNA relative to unstimulated samples; means ± SD of 3 separate experiments are given. The PCR primer sequences used for S100A8, S100A9 and HPRT were as described [14]. Other primer sequences were IL-10 (forward: GGTTGCCAAGCCTTATCGGA, reverse: ACCTGCTCCACTGCCTTGCT), COX-2 (forward: TGAGCAACTATTCCAAACCAGC, reverse: GCACGTAGTCTTCGATCACTATC), C/EBPβ (forward: TGATGCAATCCGGATCAA, reverse: ACACGTGTGTTGCGTAGTCC) and β-actin (forward: AGTGTGACGTTGACATCCGTA, reverse: GCCAGAGCAGTAATCTCCTTCT).

S100A8 and IL-10 measurements

S100A8 levels in culture supernates from untreated or stimulated RAW 264.7 cells were quantified by ELISA as described [20]. IL-10 was quantitated using the IL-10-specific DuoSet ELISA kit (R&D Systems; Minneapolis) according to manufacturer's instructions.

Western blotting

RAW cells were incubated in CM ± CpG-1826 or IL-10 for the indicated times. Following lysis (M-PER Extraction Reagent, Pierce Biotechnology), total protein content was determined by the Bradford assay (Bio-Rad). Protein (30 µg) was separated by 10% SDS-PAGE, and resolved proteins transferred to PVDF membranes (Millipore). Blots were probed with anti-phospho-Stat3 (Tyr 705) or -Stat3 Abs, detected with HRP-conjugated anti-rabbit Ab and visualized by ECL (Millipore). Lysates of HeLa cells treated with IFNα (5 min) were used as a positive control for detection of phosphorylated STAT3.

Luciferase reporter gene assays

Constructs of S100A8 luciferase reporter plasmids and transient transfection of RAW cells were described elsewhere [23]. Briefly, cells were seeded into 24 well plates (Nunc, 0.3×10^5 per well) 2 days before transfection. S100 promoter luciferase reporter constructs or pGL-basic and pGL-promoter control plasmids (Promega, 0.3 µg) and 0.05 µg reference plasmid (pRL-TK; Promega) were co-transfected in the presence of 300 µg/ml DEAE-dextran (Sigma-Aldrich). For Stat3 plasmid co-transfection, cells were transfected with 0.2 µg S100A8 promoter construct (−178/465) in combination with 0.8 µg vector pcDNA3.1 (Invitrogen) or the dominant-positive Stat-3C cloned into pcDNA3.1, or vector pIRES-EGFP, or the dominant-negative Stat-3β cloned into pIRES-EGFP, which are previously described [33]. All Stat3 and control vectors were kindly provided by Dr. Hua Yu (Beckman Research Institute, City of Hope, California, USA). After recovery for 24 h, fresh medium was replaced and cells stimulated for 20 h with the agents indicated, then firefly and *Renella* luciferase activities analysed using the dual luciferase assay kit (Promega). Results are expressed as means ± SD of luciferase activities from 3 separate experiments.

Chromatin immunoprecipitation (ChIP) assays

RAW cells (2×10^6) in 3 ml CM in 6-well plates were cultured for 24 h before stimulation. Assays were performed essentially as described [20]. Anti-STAT3 polyclonal IgG and control IgG (Santa Cruz Biotechnology) were used at 2 µg for each reaction.

Statistical analysis

Data for statistical analyses are expressed as means ± SD of at least 3 independent experiments. Statistical comparisons between groups were assessed by Student's *t*-test, or between multiple groups by one-way ANOVA with post-analysis. Statistical significance was defined as $p<0.05$.

Results

CpG motifs in bacterial DNA induce S100A8, but not S100A9

The TLR4 ligand, LPS, strongly induces S100A8, but not S100A9, in murine macrophages [34]. Because human S100A8 and S100A9 are considered markers of specific types of human inflammatory macrophages [16], and because CpG-containing DNA activates macrophages via TLR9 ligation, we tested whether the S100 genes were induced. RAW 264.7 macrophages were exposed to various DNA products ± a predetermined subthreshold concentration of LPS (0.3 ng/ml). *E. coli* DNA directly induced S100A8 mRNA ~400-fold above basal levels compared to the ~700-fold induction by an optimized dose of LPS (100 ng/ml; Fig. 1A). DNA from the Gram-positive organism *M. luteus* increased S100A8 mRNA 50-fold. Simultaneous treatment with *E. coli* DNA and a suboptimal LPS (0.3 ng/ml) dose used to identify synergy, only increased S100A8 induction <1.4-fold. In contrast to the bacterial DNAs, placental DNA, which contains highly methylated CpG dinucleotides, did not induce S100A8 mRNA either alone, or with subthreshold levels of LPS, confirming that activation was dependent upon non-methylated CpG motifs. This was confirmed using the synthetic non-methylated CpG-containing murine-specific ODN 1826, or the human-oriented ODN 2006, although mRNA levels were lower (Fig. 1B), again with little synergy with LPS.

In contrast to the immune-reactive ODNs, non-CpG-containing ODN 1982 did not influence S100A8 gene expression (Fig. 1B). Importantly, when bacterial DNA was treated with DNase (Fig. 1A) or CpG-ODN co-incubated with inhibitory iCpG (Fig. 1C), responses were ablated. Conversely, iCpG did not affect LPS-induced responses, confirming the specificities of each interaction. S100A9 is co-expressed with S100A8 in neutrophils and in human monocytes, but was below the detection limit when cells were stimulated with CpG-containing DNA (table S1, bone marrow cells were used as positive controls).

E. coli DNA also induced S100A8 mRNA in elicited murine macrophages in a dose-dependent manner whereas human placental DNA had no effect (Fig. 1D). In human monocyte-derived macrophages, S100A8 induction by type A CpG-OND (2216), but not by nGpG, confirming a specific response to the

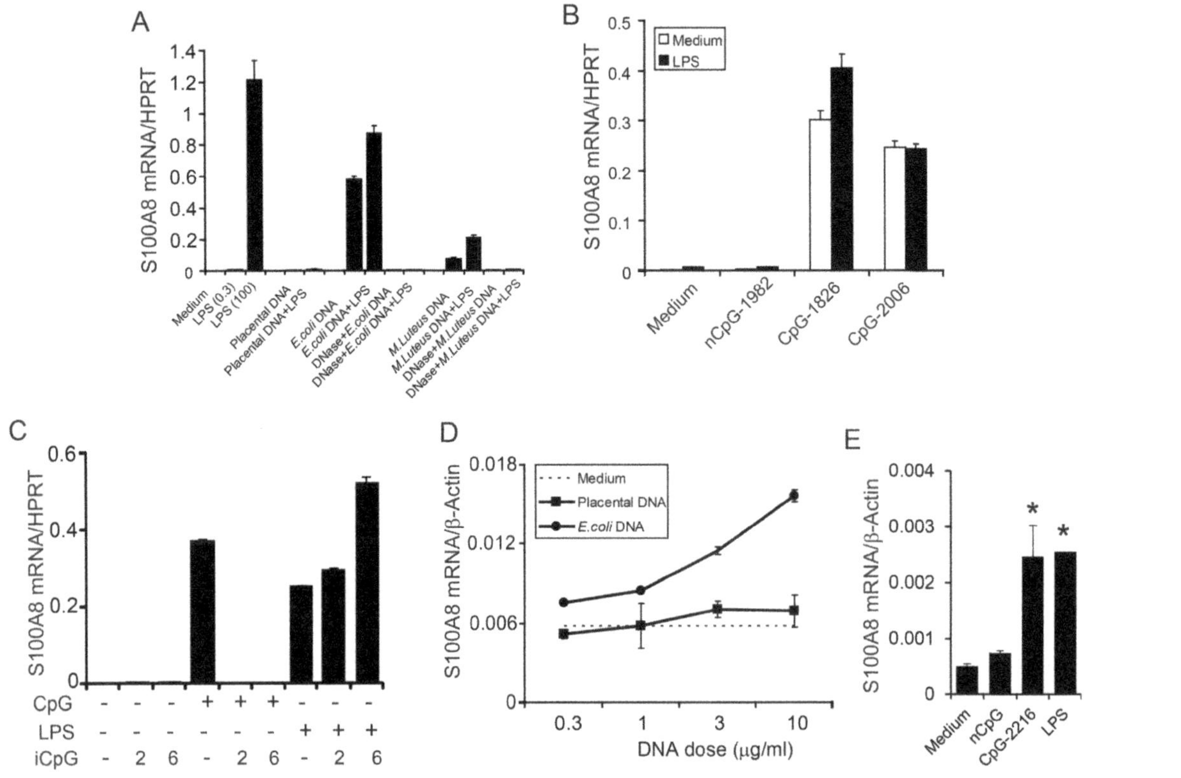

Figure 1. Induction of S100A8 mRNA in macrophages by *E. coli* DNA, *M. luteus* DNA, and synthetic CpG-ONDs. (A) RAW 264.7 macrophages were incubated with *E. coli* DNA (3 μg/ml) or *M. luteus* DNA (3 μg/ml) ±0.3 ng/ml LPS. Controls include placental DNA (3 μg/ml) ± LPS (0.3 ng/ml), Turbo DNase-treated *E. coli* DNA or *M. luteus* DNA ± LPS (0.3 ng/ml). RAW cells were also stimulated with two doses of LPS alone as positive controls (0.3 or 100 ng/ml). (B) RAW cells were untreated (medium) or treated with a synthetic non-CpG-containing OND 1982 (nCpG), a murine-oriented CpG-containing ODN (CpG-1826), or a human-oriented CpG-containing ODN (CpG-2006) (all 3 μM final concentration) ± LPS (0.3 ng/ml). (C) medium control, CpG-1826 (3 μM) or LPS (20 ng/ml) were co-stimulated with inhibitory CpG ODN 2088 (iCpG) 2 or 6 μM. (D) Elicited murine macrophages were untreated or stimulated with human placental DNA or *E. coli* DNA at the indicated concentrations. (E) Human monocyte-derived macrophages stimulated with 3 μM of nCpG or CpG-2216; LPS (20 ng/ml) was positive control. Combined data from 3 independent experiments are presented as the mean ± SD (*, $p<0.05$). All treatments were for 24 h before cell harvest. Total RNAs were extracted and S100A8 mRNA quantitated by real-time RT-PCR and normalized to the house-keeping genes (murine HPRT was used as endogenous control for A, B and C; murine β-actin for D; human β-actin for E). All data, except E, are represented as means (relative to the HPRT or actin mRNA levels) ± SD of duplicate measurements and are representative of at least 3 experiments.

type A CpG motif, and was similar to levels generated with a pre-optimized dose of 10 ng LPS.

S100A8 mRNA induction by *E. coli* DNA was dose-dependent between 0.3–3 μg/ml, with little increase with higher doses; LPS only slightly increased mRNA levels over the entire dose range (Fig. 2A). Neither DNase-treated DNA (Fig. 2A) nor human DNA (not shown) was active at these doses. S100A8 is secreted by stimulated macrophages [23]. Fig. 2B shows that S100A8 increased from 57.9±16 pg/ml/10^6 cells stimulated with 0.3 μg/ml *E. coli* DNA to 808.9±61 pg/ml/10^6 cells with 3 μg/ml DNA; LPS only slightly (1.4-fold) increased amounts. Consistent with mRNA expression, neither human DNA nor DNase-treated *E. coli* DNA generated S100A8 (not shown). Supernates from RAW cells treated with 10 μg/ml CpG-containing ODN 1826 contained high amounts of S100A8 whereas control ODN 1982 failed to generate detectable secreted protein (Fig. 2C). These experiments confirmed that DNA-containing CpG-dinucleotides strongly induced S100A8 in a dose-dependent manner.

Induction of S100A8 by *E. coli* DNA requires IL-10 and PGE_2

CpG-DNA induces IL-10 and COX-2, an inducible rate-limiting enzyme that converts arachidonic acid to PGE_2. We compared kinetics of expression of these genes, with S100A8 induction. Fig. 3A shows that *E. coli* DNA, but not placental DNA, increased S100A8 mRNA levels from 8 h, was optimal at 16–24 h, and declined to 15% of peak levels by 48 h. Similarly, S100A8 mRNA induction by LPS was maximal at ~24 h, but relatively stable over 48 h [23]. In contrast, induction of IL-10 (Fig. 3B) and COX-2 (Fig. 3C) mRNAs by *E. coli* DNA was more rapid, peaking at 8 h and 4 h respectively, returning to baseline by 24 h. Placental DNA induced neither gene.

Cycloheximide (CHX) pretreatment completely blocked S100A8 mRNA induction in RAW cells treated with *E. coli* DNA, CpG-1826 or LPS (Fig. 3D), confirming a secondary event dependent on new protein(s) synthesis. IL-10 and PGE_2 generally inhibit induction of proinflammatory mediators. These do not directly induce S100A8 in murine macrophages, but potentiate its induction by LPS [23]. Both mediators enhanced induction by *E. coli* DNA (Fig. 3E) and promoted earlier S100A8 mRNA induction. At 8 h, IL-10 increased S100A8 mRNA levels 6-fold

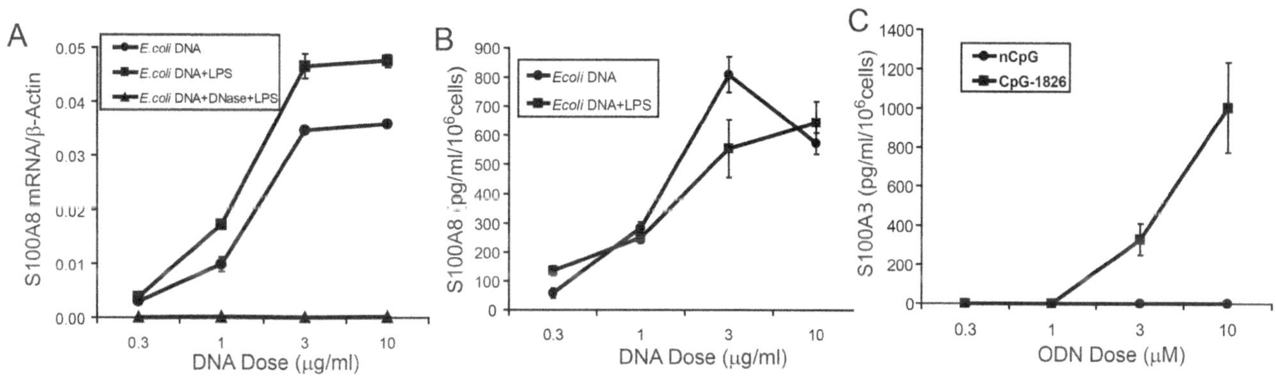

Figure 2. Induction of S100A8 by CpG-DNA is dose-dependent. (A) RAW 264.7 macrophages were incubated with *E. coli* DNA at the indicated concentrations ±0.3 ng/ml LPS for 24 h before harvesting and (A) mRNAs quantitated by qRT-PCR with different doses of DNase-treated *E. coli* DNA ± LPS (0.3 ng/ml) as control. (B) S100A8 levels in culture supernates from (A) were quantitated by ELISA. Other controls included various concentrations of placental DNA ± LPS (0.3 ng/ml) or DNase-treated *E. coli* DNA, but mRNA levels were same as control and proteins were below the detectable level (not shown). (C) S100A8 in supernates from RAW cells treated with synthetic nCpG-1982 or CpG-1826 at the indicated concentrations was quantitated. QRT-PCR data represent means (relative to the γ-actin mRNA levels) ± SD of duplicates and are representative of 3 experiments. ELISA data are means ± SD of duplicate samples from 2 separate experiments.

and at 12 h, ~4-fold. PGE_2 increased S100A8 mRNA ~2-fold at these time points.

The requirement for IL-10 in S100A8 induction, was confirmed using a neutralizing anti-IL-10 mAb which decreased CpG-DNA-induced S100A8 mRNA by 65% (Fig. 4A), and protein levels by 94% (Fig. 4B); 10-fold more mAb only marginally increased inhibition. The specific COX-2 inhibitor (NS389) suppressed S100A8 mRNA induction to the same extent (Fig. 4A), although suppression of protein production required a higher dose to achieve 83% reduction (Fig. 4B). Indomethacin, a general COX-1 and COX-2 inhibitor, also inhibited S100A8 protein production (Fig. 4B). Importantly, effects of IL-10 and COX-2 inhibitors were synergistic, and when combined, S100A8 mRNA levels decreased almost to baseline (Fig. 4A), with no secreted S100A8 detected (Fig. 4B). Thus, IL-10 and/or PGE_2 generated by TLR9 ligation may act together or independently to promote S100A8 induction in macrophages.

PGE_2 exerts its action through G protein-coupled E prostanoid (EP) receptors 1–4. Using antagonists for EP1, 2 and 4 at two doses, we found that the EP4 antagonist (AH-2348; 10 μM)

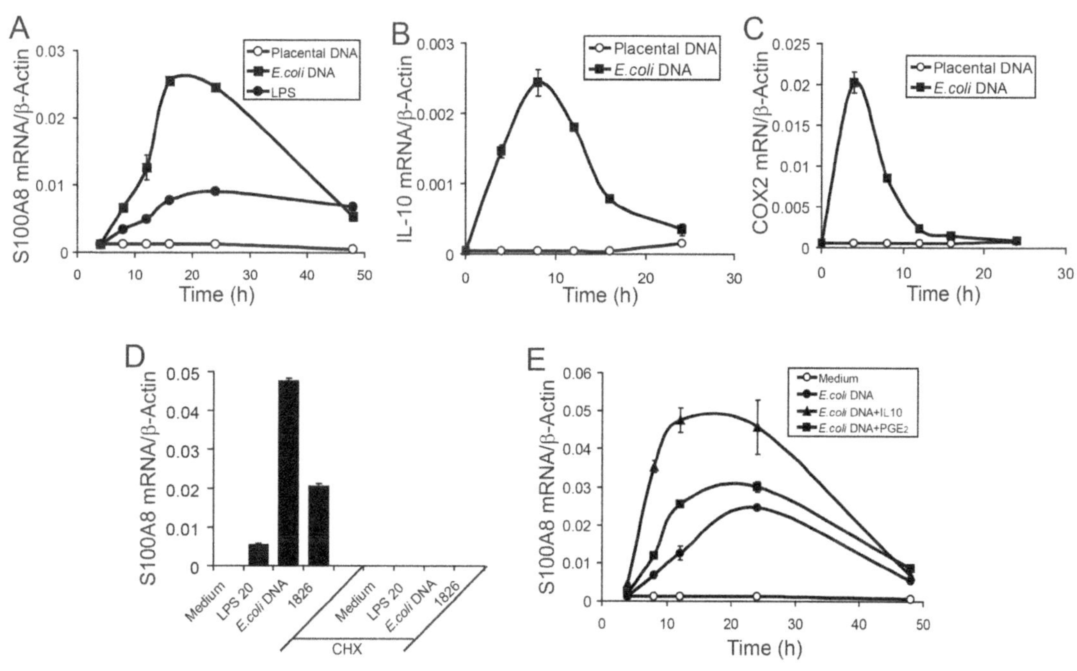

Figure 3. Induction of S100A8 in macrophages by *E. coli* DNA is late and requires newly synthesis proteins. (A–C) RAW264.7 macrophages were treated with 3 μg/ml placental DNA, 3 μg/ml *E. coli* DNA, or 20 ng/ml LPS for the indicated times. S100A8 (A), IL-10 (B), or COX-2 (C) mRNAs quantitated by qRT-PCR. (D) Effects of CHX (2 μg/ml) on LPS (20 ng/ml), *E. coli* DNA (3 μg/ml), or CpG-containing ODN (1826, 3 μM)-induced S100A8 mRNA expression. (E) Cells incubated with *E. coli* DNA (3 μg/ml) ± IL-10 (2 ng/ml) or ± PGE_2 (10 μM), harvested at the indicated time points and mRNAs quantitated. Data represent means ± SD of duplicates and representative of 3 experiments.

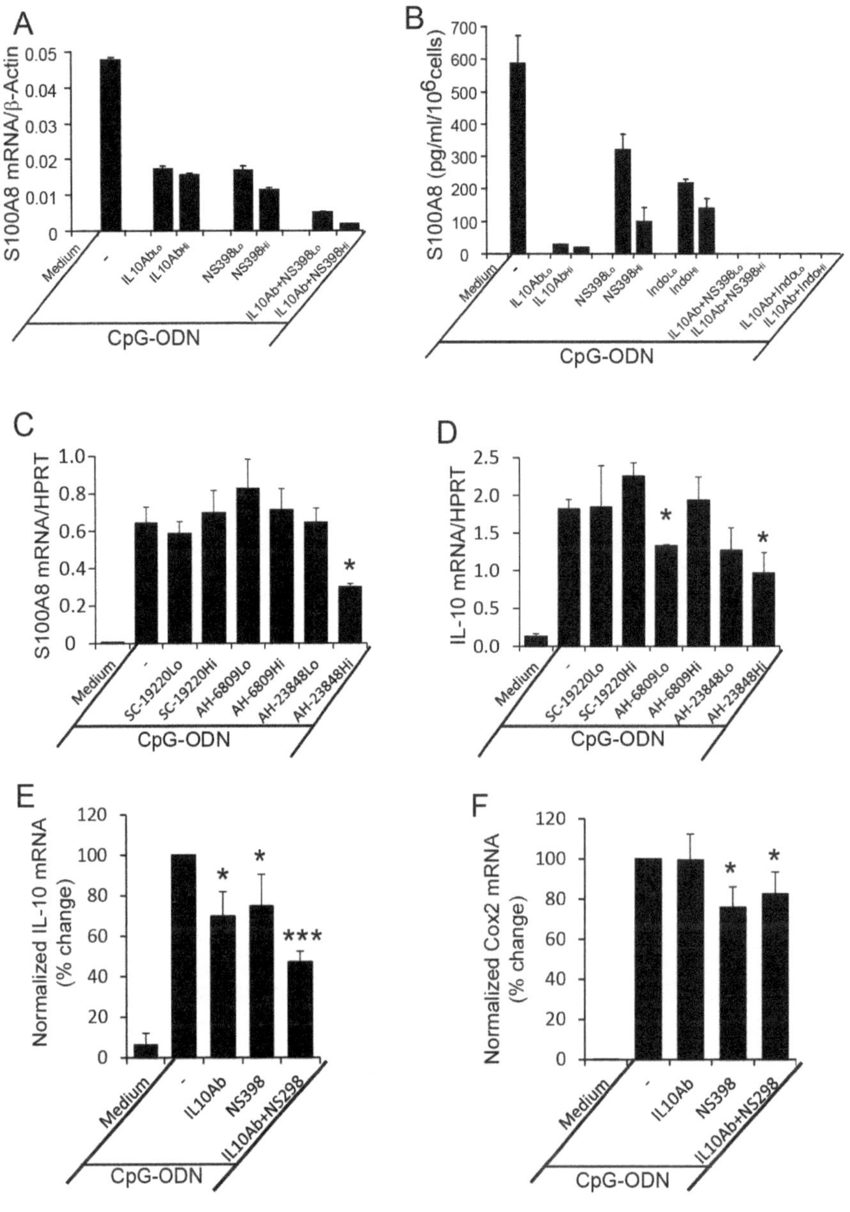

Figure 4. Induction of S100A8 in macrophages by CpG-ODN requires both IL-10 and PGE_2/EP4 dual signaling pathways. (A and B) RAW cells were incubated with CpG-ODN (3 μM) for 20 h in the presence/absence of two doses (Lo: low, 1 ng/ml; Hi: high, 10 ng/ml) of IL-10 Ab and/or COX inhibitors (NS389: Lo, 5 μM, Hi, 50 μM; Indomethacin (Indo): Lo, 2 μM; Hi, 20 μM). Cells and supernates were harvested, and S100A8 mRNA (A) or protein (B) quantitated. Data represent means ± SD of duplicates and representative of 3 experiments. (C and D) RAW cells were incubated with CpG-ODN (3 μM) in the presence/absence of two doses (Lo, 1 μM; Hi, 10 μM) of antagonists for EP1 (SC-19220), EP2 (AH-6809), and EP4 (AH-23848) for 8 (C) and 20 h (D). IL-10 (C) and S100A8 mRNA (D) quantitated by qRT-PCR. (E and F) RAW cells were untreated or treated with CpG-ODN (3 μM) for 6 h in the presence/absence of anti-IL-10 Ab (5 ng/ml) and/or NS389 (25 μM), and IL-10 (E) and Cox2 (F) mRNA quantitated by qRT-PCR, For C–F, data represent means ± SD of −5 separate experiments. *$P<0.05$, ***$P<0.001$ of differences between samples treated with CpG-ODN alone and CpG-ODN plus various inhibitors.

significantly suppressed S100A8 mRNA induction by CpG-ODN by 54% (Fig. 4C). Interestingly, IL-10 mRNA induction at 8 h was also suppressed by 48%. The EP2 antagonist also significantly inhibited IL-10 mRNA by 28% (Fig. 4D). Taken together, S100A8 mRNA induction in macrophages by TLR9 ligands required IL-10 and PGE_2 activation via the IL-10 receptor and EP4, respectively.

We also examined the cross regulation between IL-10 and PGE_2 pathways. Similar to S100A8 induction, inhibition of IL-10 or COX-2 pathways reduced IL-10 mRNA expression by ~25%, and more evident suppression (43%) was observed when both pathways were inhibited (Fig. 4E). CpG-DNA induced COX-2 mRNA was also self-regulated, but not by IL-10 production (Fig. 4F). Results indicate self- and/or cross-regulations of IL-10 and PGE_2 pathways, and further complicate the late induction of S100A8.

Role of MAPKs, PI3K and JAK2 in CpG-DNA-mediated S100A8 induction

In RAW 264.7 cells, CpG-DNA activates the three MAPK pathways: ERK, p38, and JNK [35]. Using the concentrations shown to specifically inhibit particular MAPKs in these cells [35], we found that these MAPK pathways were involved in S100A8 induction. U0126, SB202190, and JNK inhibitor II (inhibit ERK, p38, and JNK respectively) all abolished *E. coli* DNA-induced S100A8 mRNA by >95% when measured at the time of maximal expression (20 h). These inhibitors did not affect baseline S100A8 mRNA levels seen with vehicle (DMSO) in the absence of CpG-DNA (Fig. 5A). Effects of these inhibitors on IL-10 and COX-2 mRNA induction at 4 h, when both genes were strongly induced (Figs 5B, 5C), and secreted IL-10 protein at 20 h (Fig. 5D) indicated involvement of ERK and JNK in induction of both genes. p38 was significantly involved in IL-10 protein induction, but at mRNA levels, indicating its post-transcriptional role. Unlike S100A8, suppressions of IL-10 or COX-2 were only partial (compare Fig. 5B, 5C with 5A).

PI3K is also involved in TLR-mediated activation [36]. LY294002, a specific PI3K inhibitor, totally abolished S100A8 mRNA induction by CpG-DNA (Fig. 5A) and significantly reduced IL-10 and COX-2 mRNAs by 76% and 48%, respectively (Fig. 5B and 5C). Activation by IL-10 receptors (but not TLR) involves the JAK-STAT pathway. AG490, a JAK-2 inhibitor, reduced CpG-DNA- induced S100A8 mRNA by 97% (Fig. 5A) and IL-10 mRNA by ~53% (Fig. 5B), but did not affect COX-2 mRNA levels (Fig. 5C). Similarly, using recently developed, more specific JAK-2 inhibitor Ruxolitinib (Rux), CpG-DNA-induced S100A8 and IL-10 mRNAs were suppressed by 93% and 62% respectively (fig. S1C and 1A), with no significant reduction in COX-2 mRNA (fig. S1B). Thus, S100A8 induction by CpG-DNA appears complex, requiring multiple pathways, including MAPKs, PI3K, and JAK-STAT activation.

As S100A8 induction by CpG-DNA was indirectly modulated by IL-10 and COX-2-mediated events via the MAPK and PI3K pathways, we examined whether exogenous IL-10 or PGE_2 or their combination, facilitated S100A8 production in the presence of inhibitors. Fig. 5E shows that PGE_2 and IL-10 increased CpG-DNA-induced S100A8 mRNA 1.6- and 2.3-fold respectively; a 3.5-fold increase was apparent when combined. S100A8 mRNA was suppressed by >95% with the P38, JNK, PI3K, and JAK2 inhibitors (Figs 5A and 5E). Exogenous IL-10 or PGE_2 only marginally increased S100A8 mRNA levels generated in the presence of inhibitors, compared to CpG-DNA stimulation in the absence of inhibitors. However when combined, IL-10 and PGE_2 completely rescued S100A8 mRNA induction (1.3, 2.2, 2.7, and 1.6-fold above CpG-DNA-treated control, in cells treated with SB202190, JNK inhibitor II, LY209002, or AG490, respectively). Combined addition of IL-10 and PGE_2 also significantly induced S100A8 mRNA compared to individual components when JAK

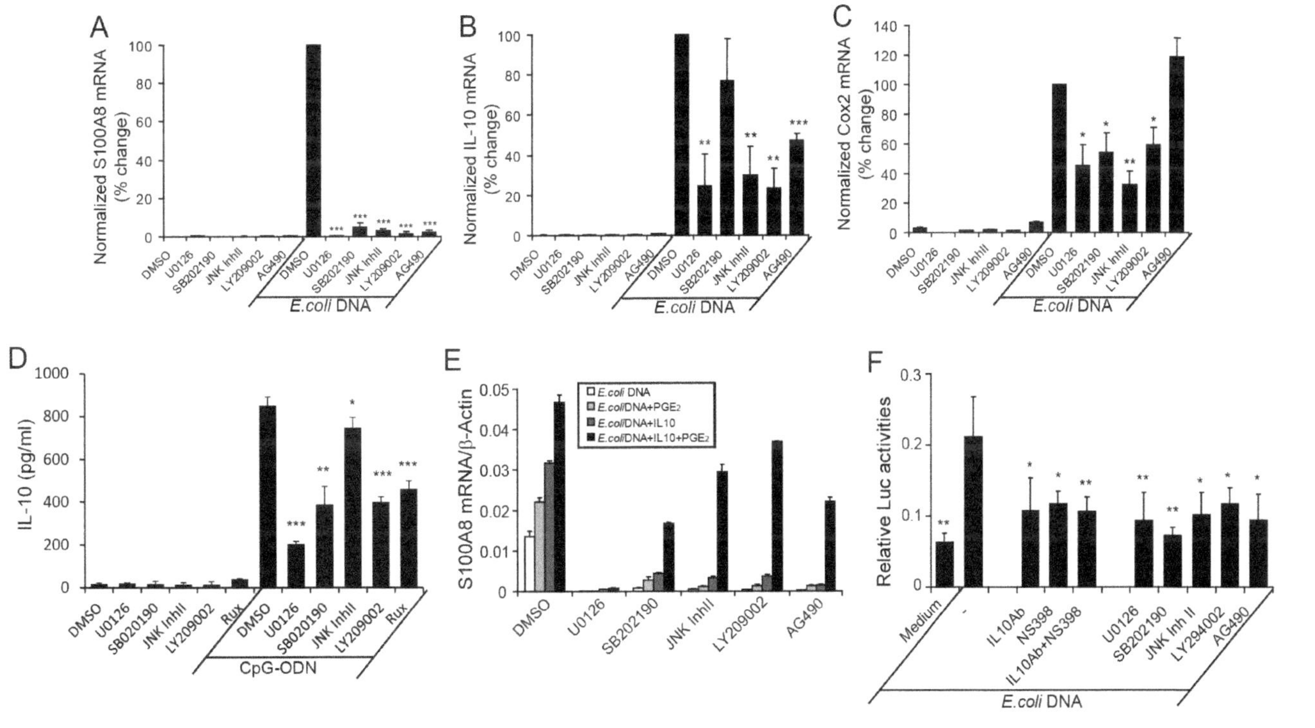

Figure 5. Contribution of MAPKs, PI3K, and JAK2 to *E. coli*-DNA-mediated S100A8, IL-10 and COX-2 mRNA induction. (A–C) RAW 264.7 cells were pretreated with DMSO (vehicle control), U0126 (2.5 μM), SB202190 (2.5 μM), JNK inhibitor (5 μM), LY209002 (10 μM), or AG490 (20 ng/ml) for 20 min then untreated or stimulated with *E. coli* DNA (3 μg/ml) for 20 h (A), or 4 h (B, C). mRNA for S100A8 (A), IL-10 (B) or COX-2 (C) was quantitated using qRT-PCR. (D) RAW cells were treated using same conditions as in (A), except that AG490 was replaced by Ruxolitinib (0.5 μM); IL-10 in supernatants were quantitated by ELISA. (E) RAW cells were treated with inhibitors for 20 min, stimulated with *E. coli* DNA for 30 min, and then ± PGE_2 (10 μM) or IL-10 (5 ng/ml) added and cells cultured for 20 h. S100A8 mRNA levels were quantitated; endogenous control was γ-actin. Data represent % S100A8 mRNA relative to *E. coli* DNA-stimulated samples without inhibitors ± SD of 3 separate experiments. (F) RAW 264.7 cells were transiently co-transfected with the S100A8 promoter (−178/465 bp) luciferase reporter construct and pRL-TK-luciferase control plasmid and pretreated with various MAPK and COX-2 inhibitors, or anti-IL-10 mAb for 20 min before adding *E. coli* DNA (3 μg/ml) for 16 h. Normalized S100A8 promoter-driven luciferase activities in cell extracts were analysed. Except for (E), data represent means ± SD of 3–4 separate experiments. *$P<0.05$, **$P<0.01$, ***$P<0.001$ of differences between *E. coli* DNA treatment alone and samples treated with *E. coli* DNA plus various inhibitors.

pathway was specifically inhibited by Rux (fig. S1C). Thus, suppression of S100A8 production by these inhibitors may be a direct consequence of reduced IL-10 and/or PGE_2 production by inhibitor-treated cells. In marked contrast, the ERK inhibitor (U0126) strongly suppressed S100A8 mRNA induction but this was not influenced by IL-10 or PGE_2 addition (Fig. 5E). Thus ERK1/2 activation appeared to be directly involved in S100A8 induction by CpG-DNA, independent of IL-10 and PGE_2.

Using the smallest construct identified in luciferase reporter assays (Fig. 6A and discussed below) that preserved the full response to CpG-DNA (−178/465), we next analysed the dependence of transcriptional regulation of S100A8 on IL-10 and PGE_2 via the MAPK, PI3K, and JAK pathways. Anti-IL-10 mAb or the COX-2 inhibitor reduced relative CpG-DNA-induced luciferase activities by ~50% (Fig. 5F), confirming their involvement at the transcriptional level, in a region largely confined to the −178 to −34 bp region of S100A8 promoter. P38, JNK, PI3K, and JAK inhibitors also significantly reduced luciferase activities driven by this region in response to CpG-DNA. The ERK1/2 pathway inhibitor U0126 reduced luciferase activity by 56%, indicating that this region of the promoter also contributed to direct transcription of the S100A8 gene via ERK1/2 activation (Fig. 5F).

Taken together, we propose that CpG-DNA induction of S100A8 at the transcriptional level is dependent on generation of IL-10 and COX-2/PGE_2 via p38, JNK, PI3K and JAK-STAT pathways, together with direct signaling through ERK1/2.

STAT3 mediates induction of S100A8 by CpG-DNA

Gene induction by CpG-DNA involves alteration of transcriptional activities and/or transcript stability [6]. To confirm S100A8 induction at the transcriptional level; and to locate likely response elements in the promoter region 5′ to the transcription start site of the gene, a series of 5′ deletion fragments linked to a luciferase reporter gene were transiently transfected into RAW cells. A region ~1.4 kb 5′ flanking the translation start site of the murine S100A8 gene, including a 917 bp 5′ region flanking the transcription start site, untranslated first exon and intron, and the untranslated region of the second exon, served as the full-length promoter (−917/465). Fig. 6A shows that CpG-DNA increased the activity of this full-length reporter ~6-fold above basal levels. Luciferase activities of a series of 5′ deletions from −917 bp to −178 bp (constructs −665/465, −317/465, −229/465, and −178/465) were similarly elevated, confirming induction at transcription; the region −917 bp to −178 bp did not contribute substantially. Further deletion of 84-bp from the 5′ end of −178/465 (construct −94/465), a region containing one Ets, two STAT, and three C/EBP binding sites (TRANSFAC database), reduced CpG-DNA-induced S100A8 promoter-luciferase activity by ~47%. These C/EBP binding sites are highly conserved between murine and human (Fig. 6B) and C/EBPβ mRNA was rapidly induced by CpG-DNA or PGE_2 at 1 h and sustained to 6 h (Fig. 6F), indicating the critical role of this transcription factor in S100A8 induction. Deletion of an additional 60 bp (−34/465), removing an NF-1 and an Ets site, but retaining the TATA box, completely abolished reporter activity (Fig. 6A). Thus, the −178 to −34-bp region in the S100A8 promoter contained important *cis*-elements, including C/EBP, STAT, Ets, and NF-1 binding sites that may contribute to S100A8 gene induction by CpG-DNA.

IL-10 signaling is dependent on STAT3 to mediate anti-inflammatory responses [37]; STAT3 is also involved in transcription of S100A8 and S100A9 in myeloid-derived suppressor cells (MDSC) [38] but precise mechanisms are unclear. We next tested whether STAT3 contributed to transcriptional activation of the defined promoter region. By searching for potential binding sites with the consensus sequences for STAT3, TT(N4)AA or TT(N5)AA [39], we identified a perfect candidate at position −117 upstream of the transcription initiation site in the murine S100A8 promoter, which is 100% conserved in the human S100A8 promoter. This site closely resembles a previously-defined STAT3-binding site within the VEGF and Jab1 promoters [33,40] (Fig. 6B). Functionally-active phospho-STAT3 was generated 4 h after stimulating RAW cells with CpG-ODN, with strong phosphorylation evident at 8 h. In contrast, IL-10 promoted STAT3 phosphorylation within 30 min and as expected, stimulation with IFNα promoted rapid STAT3 phosphorylation in HeLa cells within 5 min (Fig. 6C). Thus, the late activation of STAT3 in response to CpG-DNA may be a consequence of IL-10 production (mRNA levels peaked at 8 h, Fig. 4B).

Expression of a constitutively-active STAT3 mutant, STAT3C, in RAW cells potentiated luciferase expression driven by the S100A8 promoter (−178/465) without stimulation, and this significantly increased in response to CpG-ODN when compared to empty vector (pcDNA3) (1.43 and 1.85 fold respectively). In contrast, forced expression of dominant-negative STAT3β abolished the luciferase response to CpG-ODN, compared with the 2.2-fold induction by the corresponding empty vector pIRES-EGFP (Fig. 6D). To determine if STAT3 protein could directly bind to the putative −117 STAT3 binding site, ChIP assays were performed using primers flanking the region. STAT3 interacted with the defined promoter region in a time-dependent manner, with optimal interaction at 8 h that was maintained over 16 h (Fig. 6E). These results have identified a functional STAT3 binding site within the immediate promoter region of S100A8 in response to a TLR9 ligand.

Discussion

This study shows strong S100A8 induction in macrophages by TLR9 ligands. S100A8 was directly induced by bacterial DNA or CpG-containing ODNs but not by human placental DNA; activation was negated by DNase treatment, or by an inhibitory CpG. This finding was replicated in primary murine peritoneal exudate macrophages and human M-CSF-differentiated macrophages. S100A9, which is co-expressed with S100A8 in high amounts in neutrophils, was not induced in murine macrophages, indicating distinct functions for S100A8 independent of the heterocomplex.

The S100A8/A9 complex is elevated in acute and chronic inflammatory lesions in humans, and systemic levels can indicate the extent of inflammation [41]. Mediators that dampen inflammation are generally induced later in macrophages [42] and in inflamed tissues, macrophages may comprise different activation states depending on the environmental stimuli. Macrophage deactivation by IL-10, TGF-β, glucocorticoid receptors, and cAMP via protein kinase A (PKA), generally promotes tissue repair and suppresses inflammation (reviewed in [43] and [2]). In macrophages, CpG-DNA-induced PGE_2 and IL-10 inhibit IFN-γ [44] and IL-12 [35] responses respectively, thereby dampening Th1-responses. S100A8 induced by CpG-DNA required new protein synthesis, with kinetics much later than required for IL-10 or COX-2 mRNA expression and its induction was mediated in part by the secondary response gene products, IL-10 and PGE_2 in an autocrine manner.

Although neither IL-10 nor PGE_2 directly induced murine S100A8, they are also essential for its induction by LPS [23] and corticosteroids [22]; TGFβ and cAMP [19] also strongly synergize

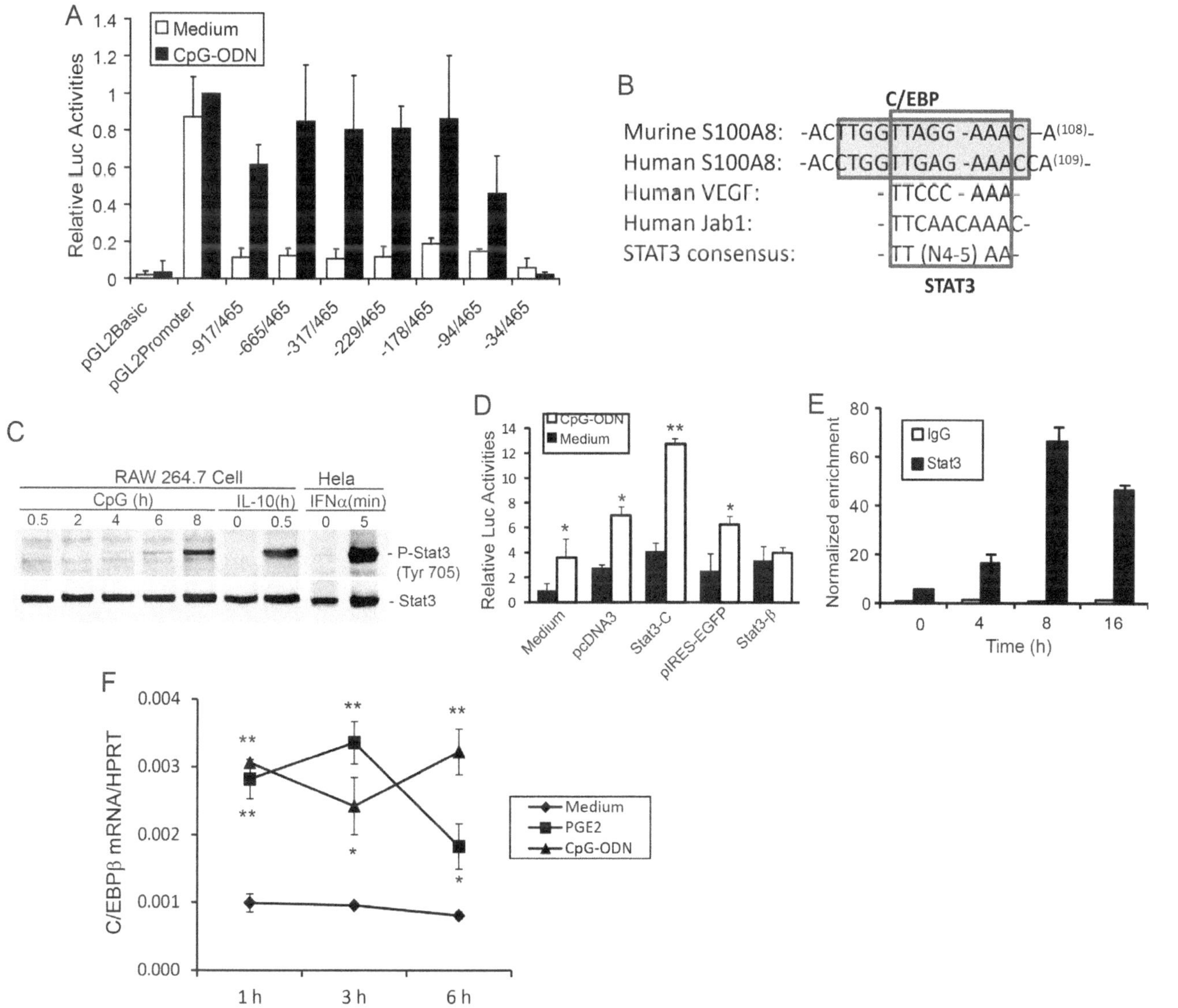

Figure 6. STAT3 is a critical transcription factor in CpG-DNA-induced S100A8 expression. (A) RAW 264.7 cells were transiently co-transfected with pRL-TK-luciferase and full-length (−917/465) or a series of 5′-deleted S100A8 promoter-luciferase reporters for 24 h. pGL-basic and pGL-promoter plasmids were transfected as controls. Transfected cells were either left untreated (open bars) or stimulated with CpG-ODN (3 μM, solid bars) for 16 h. Luciferase activities in cell extracts were analysed; data represent means (% luciferase activity of pGL-promoter luciferase reporter in cells stimulated with CpG-ODN) ± SD of 3 separate experiments. (B) A potential STAT3-binding element overlaps the C/EBP binding site in both murine and human S100A8 promoter (shaded). The matched bases of STAT3 binding sites are compared with verified binding sites in the VEGF and Jab1 promoters. (C) RAW cells were treated with CpG-ODN (3 μM) for the indicated times (h) before harvest, then proteins in lysates separated by SDS-PAGE. Western blotting used a phosphor-specific anti-STAT3 antibody; stripped blots were re-probed with anti-STAT3 antibody. RAW cells treated with IL-10 for 30 min or IFNα-treated Hela (5 min) were positive controls. Results are representative of 3 experiments. (D) RAW 264.7 cells were transiently co-transfected with the S100A8 promoter (−178/465 bp) luciferase reporter construct and pRL-TK-luciferase control plasmid, with either empty vectors, dominant-positive (Stat3-C), or dominant-negative (Stat3-β) STAT3 constructs for 24 h. Cells were then stimulated with (□) or without (■) CpG-ODN (3 μM) for 16 h prior to performing dual-luciferase assays. Results are mean ± SD of 3 independent experiments. *$P<0.05$ or **$P<0.01$ of differences with or without CpG-ODN treatments. (E) Time course of ChIP assays indicated binding of STAT3 to the S100A8 promoter in RAW cells stimulated with CpG-ODN (3 μM) (■). The same region was not enriched by IgG control (□). (F) RAW cells were untreated or treated with 10 μM PGE_2 or 3 μM CpG-ODN for the indicated time and C/EBPβ mRNA quantitated by qRT-PCR. Results are means ± SD of 3 independent experiments. *$P<0.05$ or **$P<0.01$ of differences compared to medium control.

with LPS to increase expression. The critical role for IL-10 was confirmed earlier using macrophages from IL-10$^{-/-}$ mice which failed to express S100A8 in response to LPS [23] or Poly I:C [20] although mechanisms are largely undefined. IL-10 has potent anti-inflammatory properties that suppress cytokine and chemokine production to limit host immune responses. Consistent with this, its suppressive effects are potentiated by its ability to induce other immunosuppressive products such as cytokine receptor antagonists [45]. Interestingly, like S100A8, induction of the IL-1 receptor antagonist, IL-1Ra by LPS in RAW 264.7 cells is enhanced by IL-10 although IL-10 had no direct effect [46].

PGE2 is also an important modulator of homeostasis and chronic inflammation (reviewed in [47]) with varying effects, depending on expression of particular PGE_2 receptor (EP) subtypes, and through these, exerts pro- or anti-inflammatory functions. EP2 and EP4 receptors activate adenylate cyclase, increasing cAMP levels and PKA signaling [48]. In late/chronic inflammation, PGE2 has specialized anti-inflammatory properties by controlling potentially harmful over-activation of neutrophils, macrophages and lymphocytes, particularly Th1 cells producing IFNγ [49]. CpG DNA induces COX-2, promoting PGE_2 production in RAW 264.7 macrophages [44,50] and we found a requirement for this pathway in S100A8 induction. IL-10 or PGE_2 enhanced CpG-induced S100A8 mRNA levels and shortened its maximal induction time by 12 h. Effects of IL-10 and COX-2 inhibitors on S100A8 and IL-10 were synergistic; S100A8 mRNA/protein expression was partially reduced by anti-IL-10, but when combined with a COX-2 inhibitor, mRNA levels were reduced by 96% and no secreted S100A8 was detected. PGE_2 mediated effects were mainly through EP2 whereas IL-10 induction by PGE_2 involved EP2 and EP4 (Fig. 4D). The COX2-PGE_2-PKA pathway is also important for LPS, but not for poly I:C-induced S100A8 expression in macrophages [20] although mechanisms were unclear. RAW 264.7 cells express high levels of EP2 but this is much lower on peritoneal macrophages [51] and may explain the modest S100A8 induction observed with these (Fig. 1E). Furthermore, when p38, JNK, PI3K and JAK-dependent signaling required for S100A8 gene induction was inhibited, the response was only restored with IL-10 and PGE_2 together, but not individually. PGE2 induces cAMP which promotes synergistic PKA- and p38-dependent IL-10 production in RAW 264.7 cells [52] and this pathway likely contributed to S100A8 induction in our study. CpG-DNA activates ERK, JNK, and p38 in RAW 264.7 cells to generate IL-10 [35]. Although the IL-10 and PGE_2 pathways were both essential, they were not sufficient for CpG-DNA-mediated S100A8 induction. Neither substituted for CpG-DNA and did not directly induce S100A8 alone or combined [23], implicating additional pathways, possibly mediated by ERK1/2 activation (Fig. 5D). We are currently investigating this pathway. Notwithstanding, PGE_2 activation of EP receptors initiates IL-10 gene induction and can also reprogram macrophages to an anti-inflammatory phenotype, indicating potentially important connections between PGE_2, IL-10 (reviewed in [48]) and S100A8.

A small region (−178 to −34 bp from the transcription start site) was responsible for CpG-DNA-induced transcriptional activation of the S100A8 gene. NF-κB is implicated in IL-10 and COX-2 induction in murine macrophages [53,54] but there is no NF-κB motif in this region and the NF-κB inhibitor (Bay 11-7082) did not inhibit the S100A8 luciferase response to CpG-DNA (data not shown), although the possibility that NF-κB may indirectly mediate S100A8 transcription by being required for generation of secondary mediators cannot be ruled out. CCAAT/enhancer binding protein β (C/EBPβ) is a cAMP-responsive transcription factor important for IL-10 induction in macrophages [55]. The essential promoter region of the murine S100A8 gene contains several C/EBPβ binding sites that are conserved in the human gene [14]. C/EBPβ is induced by CpG-DNA or PGE_2 at early time, which involved in TLR3-mediated S100A8 induction in murine macrophages [20] and the human S100A8 promoter is activated by C/EBPβ [56]. IL-10 signaling also requires C/EBP proteins to promote its anti-inflammatory and immunomodulatory actions, including reduced IL-6 production in IL-10-treated human intestinal epithelial cells [57] and suppression of HIV-1 transcription in macrophages [58].

CpG-DNA-induced S100A8 did not totally overlap with S100A8 induction by LPS [20], or by Poly I:C [20]. Compared to LPS, the optimal time for S100A8 mRNA induction by CpG-DNA was earlier and less sustained. Moreover, the −94/465 reporter construct does not respond to LPS [23], but this generated a partial response to CpG-DNA (Fig. 6A). An NF-1 motif located −58 bp from the transcription start site is essential for synergy of LPS and glucocorticoids [22], but not for induction by LPS. The contribution of NF-1 to the CpG-DNA response requires further examination.

IL-10 regulates a large range of genes induced by LPS by dependent STAT3-dependent pathways [37] and the IL-10-JAK-STAT axis is critical for both acute and chronic inflammation [59]. Phospho-STAT3 was generated 8 h post-stimulation of RAW 267 cells with CpG, significantly later than phosphorylation induced by IL-10. We confirmed the importance of STAT3 recruitment using a luciferase expression system (Fig. 6) and demonstrated STAT3 binding to the defined promoter region, that was optimal at 8 h post-stimulation. Together, these results confirm a secondary response mediated by STAT3. We also located multiple C/EBP binding sites surrounding a unique STAT3 site in the essential promoter region of S100A8, similar to that identified in the neutrophil gelatinase-associated lipocalin promoter in macrophages that allowed its maximal induction by IL-10 [60]. The possibility that these transcription factors form complexes by binding different C/EBP binding sites in response to different stimuli, and potential interactions between STAT3 and C/EBP, or putative complex formation, warrant further investigation.

The combination of two stimuli, one a TLR ligand, to suppress macrophage cytokine induction is reported. A similar "strength of signal" model is proposed for IL-10 production itself, in T cells and macrophages [61,62]. In this model, macrophage activation by a strong TLR agonist can induce pro-inflammatory cytokines, but is insufficient to produce high amounts of IL-10 and a second stimulus provides sufficient signaling strength for its production. In a manner similar to that reported here for S100A8, secondary modulators including adenosine, apoptotic cells, cAMP analogues, TGF-β, PGE2, and IL-10 can alter the balance to favour anti-inflammatory cytokine production, generated by so-called "regulatory macrophages" [62]. The main function of this macrophage type is to limit tissue damage. Despite the accepted role of S100A8 as a DAMP that propagates inflammation via interactions with TLR4 [63] or RAGE [64], the types of mediators involved in its induction in macrophages in response to TLR3, TLR4 and TLR9 ligands strongly implicate an immunomodulatory role. S100A8 down-regulates leukocyte adhesion and negatively regulates phagocyte transmigration [65], suppresses mast cell activation by scavenging ROS essential for signaling and inhibits acute murine asthma [29]. In addition, i.v. injection of S100A8/A9 into endotoxemic mice reduced neutrophil infiltration into organs and increased survival rates [66]. S100A8 is exquisitely sensitive to oxidation and may be critical in antioxidant defence in acute and chronic inflammation (reviewed in [67]). Indeed, we recently confirmed its ability to scavenge hypohalous acid oxidants in human asthma [27], and S-nitrosylated S100A8 inhibits leukocyte transmigration triggered by mast cell degranulation in the microcirculation [28]. Importantly, in cooperation with IL-10, S100A8 suppressed acute lung injury by suppressing mast-cell activation and leukocyte recruitment [68]. We propose that S100A8 contributes to anti-oxidant defence, particularly during the resolution phase of inflammation that is modulated by IL-10 and PGE2.

Supporting Information

Figure S1 Effects of selective JAK inhibitor Ruxolitinib on IL-10, Cox2 and S100A8 mRNA induction in RAW 264.7 cells. RAW 264.7 cells were pretreated with DMSO (vehicle control) or Ruxolitinib (0.5 μg/ml) for 30 min then untreated or stimulated with CpG-ODN (3 μM) for 6 h (A and B), or 20 h (C). PGE_2 (10 μM) and/or IL-10 (5 ng/ml) were added just before CpG-OND stimulation in (C). mRNA for IL-10 (A), COX-2 (B) or S100A8 (C) was quantitated using qRT-PCR. Results are means ± SD of 3 independent experiments. *P<0.05 or **P<0.01 of differences compared to CpG-ODN treatment along. Ns, not significant.
(TIF)

Table S1 Ct values obtained by qRT-PCR assessment of murine S100A8, S100A9, and HPRT in macrophages and bone marrow cells. RAW 264.7 cells were untreated (Med) or stimulated with CpG-ODN (CpG, 3 μM), LPS (20 ng/ml) or Poly I/C (pIC, 5 μM) for 20 h before harvesting. Bone marrow cells (BM) were obtained by flushing mouse femurs. mRNAs for S100A9, S100A8 or HPRT were quantitated using qRT-PCR. Ct values are presented in duplicate measurements of two separate samples. NAC, non-amplification control; UD, undetectable.
(DOCX)

Author Contributions

Conceived and designed the experiments: KH CLG. Performed the experiments: KH YMC YE. Analyzed the data: KH YMC YE. Wrote the paper: KH CLG.

References

1. Takeuchi O, Akira S (2010) Pattern recognition receptors and inflammation. Cell 140: 805–820.
2. Medzhitov R, Horng T (2009) Transcriptional control of the inflammatory response. Nat Rev Immunol 9: 692–703.
3. Smale ST (2010) Selective transcription in response to an inflammatory stimulus. Cell 140: 833–844.
4. Krieg AM (2002) CpG motifs in bacterial DNA and their immune effects. Annu Rev Immunol 20: 709–760.
5. Haas T, Metzger J, Schmitz F, Heit A, Muller T, et al. (2008) The DNA sugar backbone 2′ deoxyribose determines toll-like receptor 9 activation. Immunity 28: 315–323.
6. Kawai T, Akira S (2006) TLR signaling. Cell Death Differ 13: 816–825.
7. Hornung V, Rothenfusser S, Britsch S, Krug A, Jahrsdorfer B, et al. (2002) Quantitative expression of toll-like receptor 1–10 mRNA in cellular subsets of human peripheral blood mononuclear cells and sensitivity to CpG oligodeoxynucleotides. J Immunol 168: 4531–4537.
8. Jozsef L, Khreiss T, El Kebir D, Filep JG (2006) Activation of TLR-9 induces IL-8 secretion through peroxynitrite signaling in human neutrophils. J Immunol 176: 1195–1202.
9. Kadowaki N, Ho S, Antonenko S, Malefyt RW, Kastelein RA, et al. (2001) Subsets of human dendritic cell precursors express different toll-like receptors and respond to different microbial antigens. J Exp Med 194: 863–869.
10. Barton GM, Kagan JC, Medzhitov R (2006) Intracellular localization of Toll-like receptor 9 prevents recognition of self DNA but facilitates access to viral DNA. Nat Immunol 7: 49–56.
11. Hoshino K, Kaisho T, Iwabe T, Takeuchi O, Akira S (2002) Differential involvement of IFN-beta in Toll-like receptor-stimulated dendritic cell activation. Int Immunol 14: 1225–1231.
12. Hacker H, Redecke V, Blagoev B, Kratchmarova I, Hsu LC, et al. (2006) Specificity in Toll-like receptor signalling through distinct effector functions of TRAF3 and TRAF6. Nature 439: 204–207.
13. Murray PJ, Smale ST (2012) Restraint of inflammatory signaling by interdependent strata of negative regulatory pathways. Nat Immunol 13: 916–924.
14. Ravasi T, Hsu K, Goyette J, Schroder K, Yang Z, et al. (2004) Probing the S100 protein family through genomic and functional analysis. Genomics 84: 10–22.
15. Odink K, Cerletti N, Bruggen J, Clerc J, Tarcsay L, et al. (1987) Two calcium-binding proteins ininfiltrate macrophages of rheumatoid arthritus. Nature 330: 80–82.
16. Zwadlo G, Bruggen J, Gerhards G, Schlegel R, Sorg C (1988) Two calcium-binding proteins associated with specific stages of myeloid cell differentiation are expressed by subsets of macrophages in inflammatory tissues. Clin exp Immunol 72: 510–515.
17. Aochi S, Tsuji K, Sakaguchi M, Huh N, Tsuda T, et al. (2011) Markedly elevated serum levels of calcium-binding S100A8/A9 proteins in psoriatic arthritis are due to activated monocytes/macrophages. Journal of the American Academy of Dermatology 64: 879–887.
18. Hsu K, Champaiboon C, Guenther BD, Sorenson BS, Khammanivong A, et al. (2009) Anti-Infective Protective Properties of S100 Calgranulins. Antiinflamm Antiallergy Agents Med Chem 8: 290–305.
19. Xu K, Geczy CL (2000) IFN-gamma and TNF regulate macrophage expression of the chemotactic S100 protein S100A8. J Immunol 164: 4916–4923.
20. Endoh Y, Chung YM, Clark IA, Geczy CL, Hsu K (2009) IL-10-dependent S100A8 gene induction in monocytes/macrophages by double-stranded RNA. J Immunol 182: 2258–2268.
21. Cornish CJ, Devery JM, Poronnik P, Lackmann M, Cook DI, et al. (1996) S100 protein CP-10 stimulates myeloid cell chemotaxis without activation. J Cell Physiol 166: 427–437.
22. Hsu K, Passey RJ, Endoh Y, Rahimi F, Youssef P, et al. (2005) Regulation of S100A8 by glucocorticoids. J Immunol 174: 2318–2326.
23. Xu K, Yen T, Geczy CL (2001) IL-10 up-regulates macrophage expression of the S100 protein S100A8. J Immunol 166: 6358–6366.
24. Averill MM, Barnhart S, Becker L, Li X, Heinecke JW, et al. (2011) S100A9 differentially modifies phenotypic states of neutrophils, macrophages, and dendritic cells: implications for atherosclerosis and adipose tissue inflammation. Circulation 123: 1216–1226.
25. Harrison CA, Raftery MJ, Walsh J, Alewood P, Iismaa SE, et al. (1999) Oxidation regulates the inflammatory properties of the murine S100 protein S100A8. J Biol Chem 274: 8561–8569.
26. McCormick MM, Rahimi F, Bobryshev YV, Gaus K, Zreiqat H, et al. (2005) S100A8 and S100A9 in human arterial wall. Implications for atherogenesis. J Biol Chem 280: 41521–41529.
27. Gomes LH, Raftery MJ, Xing Yan W, Goyette JD, Thomas PS, et al. (2012) S100A8 and S100A9 - Oxidant scavengers in inflammation. Free Radic Biol Med 58: 170–186.
28. Lim SY, Raftery M, Cai H, Hsu K, Yan WX, et al. (2008) S-nitrosylated S100A8: novel anti-inflammatory properties. J Immunol 181: 5627–5636.
29. Zhao J, Endoh I, Hsu K, Tedla N, Endoh Y, et al. (2011) S100A8 modulates mast cell function and suppresses eosinophil migration in acute asthma. Antioxid Redox Signal 14: 1589–1600.
30. Vogl T, Ludwig S, Goebeler M, Strey A, Thorey IS, et al. (2004) MRP8 and MRP14 control microtubule reorganization during transendothelial migration of phagocytes. Blood 104: 4260–4268.
31. Goyette J, Yan WX, Yamen E, Chung YM, Lim SY, et al. (2009) Pleiotropic roles of S100A12 in coronary atherosclerotic plaque formation and rupture. J Immunol 183: 593–603.
32. Gao JJ, Xue Q, Papasian CJ, Morrison DC (2001) Bacterial DNA and lipopolysaccharide induce synergistic production of TNF-alpha through a post-transcriptional mechanism. J Immunol 166: 6855–6860.
33. Niu G, Wright KL, Huang M, Song L, Haura E, et al. (2002) Constitutive Stat3 activity up-regulates VEGF expression and tumor angiogenesis. Oncogene 21: 2000–2008.
34. Hu SP, Harrison C, Xu K, Cornish CJ, Geczy CL (1996) Induction of the chemotactic S100 protein, CP-10, in monocyte/macrophages by lipopolysaccharide. Blood 87: 3919–3928.
35. Yi AK, Yoon JG, Yeo SJ, Hong SC, English BK, et al. (2002) Role of mitogen-activated protein kinases in CpG DNA-mediated IL-10 and IL-12 production: central role of extracellular signal-regulated kinase in the negative feedback loop of the CpG DNA-mediated Th1 response. J Immunol 168: 4711–4720.
36. Ishii KJ, Takeshita F, Gursel I, Gursel M, Conover J, et al. (2002) Potential role of phosphatidylinositol 3 kinase, rather than DNA-dependent protein kinase, in CpG DNA-induced immune activation. J Exp Med 196: 269–274.
37. Murray PJ (2006) Understanding and exploiting the endogenous interleukin-10/STAT3-mediated anti-inflammatory response. Curr Opin Pharmacol 6: 379–386.
38. Cheng P, Corzo CA, Luetteke N, Yu B, Nagaraj S, et al. (2008) Inhibition of dendritic cell differentiation and accumulation of myeloid-derived suppressor cells in cancer is regulated by S100A9 protein. J Exp Med 205: 2235–2249.
39. Seidel HM, Milocco LH, Lamb P, Darnell JE, Jr., Stein RB, et al. (1995) Spacing of palindromic half sites as a determinant of selective STAT (signal transducers and activators of transcription) DNA binding and transcriptional activity. Proc Natl Acad Sci U S A 92: 3041–3045.
40. Shackleford TJ, Zhang Q, Tian L, Vu TT, Korapati AL, et al. (2011) Stat3 and CCAAT/enhancer binding protein beta (C/EBP-beta) regulate Jab1/CSN5 expression in mammary carcinoma cells. Breast Cancer Res 13: R65.

41. Nacken W, Roth J, Sorg C, Kerkhoff C (2003) S100A9/S100A8: Myeloid representatives of the S100 protein family as prominent players in innate immunity. Microsc Res Tech 60: 569–580.
42. Nathan C (2002) Points of control in inflammation. Nature 420: 846–852.
43. Gordon S, Taylor PR (2005) Monocyte and macrophage heterogeneity. Nat Rev Immunol 5: 953–964.
44. Chen Y, Zhang J, Moore SA, Ballas ZK, Portanova JP, et al. (2001) CpG DNA induces cyclooxygenase-2 expression and prostaglandin production. Int Immunol 13: 1013–1020.
45. Cassatella MA, Meda L, Gasperini S, Calzetti F, Bonora S (1994) Interleukin 10 (IL-10) upregulates IL-1 receptor antagonist production from lipopolysaccharide-stimulated human polymorphonuclear leukocytes by delaying mRNA degradation. J Exp Med 179: 1695–1699.
46. Carl VS, Gautam JK, Comeau LD, Smith MF, Jr. (2004) Role of endogenous IL-10 in LPS-induced STAT3 activation and IL-1 receptor antagonist gene expression. J Leukoc Biol 76: 735–742.
47. Kalinski P (2012) Regulation of immune responses by prostaglandin E2. J Immunol 188: 21–28.
48. Rodriguez M, Domingo E, Municio C, Alvarez Y, Hugo E, et al. (2014) Polarization of the Innate Immune Response by Prostaglandin E2: A Puzzle of Receptors and Signals. Mol Pharmacol 85: 187–197.
49. Harris SG, Padilla J, Koumas L, Ray D, Phipps RP (2002) Prostaglandins as modulators of immunity. Trends Immunol 23: 144–150.
50. Yeo SJ, Gravis D, Yoon JG, Yi AK (2003) Myeloid differentiation factor 88-dependent transcriptional regulation of cyclooxygenase-2 expression by CpG DNA: role of NF-kappaB and p38. J Biol Chem 278: 22563–22573.
51. Akaogi J, Yamada H, Kuroda Y, Nacionales DC, Reeves WH, et al. (2004) Prostaglandin E2 receptors EP2 and EP4 are up-regulated in peritoneal macrophages and joints of pristane-treated mice and modulate TNF-alpha and IL-6 production. J Leukoc Biol 76: 227–236.
52. Goldsmith M, Avni D, Ernst O, Glucksam Y, Levy-Rimler G, et al. (2009) Synergistic IL-10 induction by LPS and the ceramide-1-phosphate analog PCERA-1 is mediated by the cAMP and p38 MAP kinase pathways. Mol Immunol 46: 1979–1987.
53. Liu YW, Chen CC, Tseng HP, Chang WC (2006) Lipopolysaccharide-induced transcriptional activation of interleukin-10 is mediated by MAPK- and NF-kappaB-induced CCAAT/enhancer-binding protein delta in mouse macrophages. Cell Signal 18: 1492–1500.
54. Yeo SJ, Yoon JG, Hong SC, Yi AK (2003) CpG DNA induces self and cross-hyporesponsiveness of RAW264.7 cells in response to CpG DNA and lipopolysaccharide: alterations in IL-1 receptor-associated kinase expression. J Immunol 170: 1052–1061.
55. Csoka B, Nemeth ZH, Virag L, Gergely P, Leibovich SJ, et al. (2007) A2A adenosine receptors and C/EBPbeta are crucially required for IL-10 production by macrophages exposed to Escherichia coli. Blood 110: 2685–2695.
56. DiSepio D, Malhotra M, Chandraratna RA, Nagpal S (1997) Retinoic acid receptor-nuclear factor-interleukin 6 antagonism. A novel mechanism of retinoid-dependent inhibition of a keratinocyte hyperproliferative differentiation marker. J Biol Chem 272: 25555–25559.
57. Robb BW, Hershko DD, Paxton JH, Luo GJ, Hasselgren PO (2002) Interleukin-10 activates the transcription factor C/EBP and the interleukin-6 gene promoter in human intestinal epithelial cells. Surgery 132: 226–231.
58. Tanaka N, Hoshino Y, Gold J, Hoshino S, Martiniuk F, et al. (2005) Interleukin-10 induces inhibitory C/EBPbeta through STAT-3 and represses HIV-1 transcription in macrophages. Am J Respir Cell Mol Biol 33: 406–411.
59. Mosser DM, Zhang X (2008) Interleukin-10: new perspectives on an old cytokine. Immunological Reviews 226: 205–218.
60. Jung M, Weigert A, Tausendschon M, Mora J, Oren B, et al. (2012) Interleukin-10-induced neutrophil gelatinase-associated lipocalin production in macrophages with consequences for tumor growth. Mol Cell Biol 32: 3938–3948.
61. Saraiva M, O'Garra A (2010) The regulation of IL-10 production by immune cells. Nat Rev Immunol 10: 170–181.
62. Fleming BD, Mosser DM (2011) Regulatory macrophages: setting the threshold for therapy. Eur J Immunol 41: 2498–2502.
63. Vogl T, Tenbrock K, Ludwig S, Leukert N, Ehrhardt C, et al. (2007) Mrp8 and Mrp14 are endogenous activators of Toll-like receptor 4, promoting lethal, endotoxin-induced shock. Nat Med 13: 1042–1049.
64. Turovskaya O, Foell D, Sinha P, Vogl T, Newlin R, et al. (2008) RAGE, carboxylated glycans and S100A8/A9 play essential roles in colitis-associated carcinogenesis. Carcinogenesis 29: 2035–2043.
65. Newton RA, Hogg N (1998) The human S100 protein MRP-14 is a novel activator of the beta 2 integrin Mac-1 on neutrophils. J Immunol 160: 1427–1435.
66. Sun Y, Lu Y, Engeland CG, Gordon SC, Sroussi HY (2013) The anti-oxidative, anti-inflammatory, and protective effect of S100A8 in endotoxemic mice. Mol Immunol 53: 443–449.
67. Lim SY, Raftery MJ, Geczy CL (2011) Oxidative modifications of DAMPs suppress inflammation: the case for S100A8 and S100A9. Antioxid Redox Signal 15: 2235–2248.
68. Hiroshima Y, Hsu K, Tedla N, Chung YM, Chow S, et al. (2014) S100A8 induces IL-10 and protects against acute lung injury. J Immunol 192: 2800–2811.

Delta-Opioid Receptor Analgesia Is Independent of Microglial Activation in a Rat Model of Neuropathic Pain

Joanna Mika*[⁹], Katarzyna Popiolek-Barczyk[⁹], Ewelina Rojewska, Wioletta Makuch, Katarzyna Starowicz, Barbara Przewlocka*

Department of Pain Pharmacology, Institute of Pharmacology, Polish Academy of Sciences, Krakow, Poland

Abstract

The analgesic effect of delta-opioid receptor (DOR) ligands in neuropathic pain is not diminished in contrast to other opioid receptor ligands, which lose their effectiveness as analgesics. In this study, we examine whether this effect is related to nerve injury-induced microglial activation. We therefore investigated the influence of minocycline-induced inhibition of microglial activation on the analgesic effects of opioid receptor agonists: morphine, DAMGO, U50,488H, DPDPE, Deltorphin II and SNC80 after chronic constriction injury (CCI) to the sciatic nerve in rats. Pre-emptive and repeated administration of minocycline (30 mg/kg, i.p.) over 7 days significantly reduced allodynia and hyperalgesia as measured on day 7 after CCI. The antiallodynic and antihyperalgesic effects of intrathecally (i.t.) administered morphine (10–20 μg), DAMGO (1–2 μg) and U50,488H (25–50 μg) were significantly potentiated in rats after minocycline, but no such changes were observed after DPDPE (10–20 μg), deltorphin II (1.5–15 μg) and SNC80 (10–20 μg) administration. Additionally, nerve injury-induced down-regulation of all types of opioid receptors in the spinal cord and dorsal root ganglia was not influenced by minocycline, which indicates that the effects of opioid ligands are dependent on other changes, presumably neuroimmune interactions. Our study of rat primary microglial cell culture using qRT-PCR, Western blotting and immunocytochemistry confirmed the presence of mu-opioid receptors (MOR) and kappa-opioid receptors (KOR), further we provide the first evidence for the lack of DOR on microglial cells. In summary, DOR analgesia is different from analgesia induced by MOR and KOR receptors because it does not dependent on injury-induced microglial activation. DOR agonists appear to be the best candidates for new drugs to treat neuropathic pain.

Editor: Bradley Taylor, University of Kentucky Medical Center, United States of America

Funding: This work was supported by MNiSzW/NCN grant NN405375937, grant OPUS NCN 2011/03/B/NZ4/00042, grant PRELUDIUM NCN 2012/07/N/NZ3/00379, grant MAESTRO NCN 2012/06/A/NZ4/00028 and statutory funds. Katarzyna Popiolek-Barczyk is a Ph.D. student and has a scholarship from the KNOW sponsored by the Ministry of Science and Higher Education, Republic of Poland. The funders had no role in study design, data collection and analysis, decision to publish, or preparation of the manuscript.

Competing Interests: The authors have declared that no competing interests exist.

* Email: przebar@if-pan.krakow.pl (BP); joamika@if-pan.krakow.pl (JM)

⁹ These authors contributed equally to this work.

Introduction

Neuropathic pain has been shown in clinical and animal studies to be resistant to alleviation by morphine [1,2,3,4,5], but the mechanism of this effect is unclear. The classical opioid system modulates nociception through three G-protein-coupled receptors: delta-opioid receptors (DOR) [6,7] kappa-opioid receptors (KOR) [8,9] and mu-opioid receptors (MOR) [8]. Opioid receptors do not necessarily function independently and can exist as heterodimers that modulate their pharmacology [10,11,12]. Several experimental studies have emphasised that the effects of DOR agonists are distinctively more potent than those of MOR and KOR receptors [13,14,15] in neuropathic pain. The field of DOR analgesia has been widely studied [16,17,18] and the DOR agonists seems to be a good drugs that would be effective in neuropathic pain, but still some of the aspects of DOR ligands interactions have to be clarified.

Reduction of morphine antinociceptive potency has been postulated to be a consequence of changes in the activity of opioid systems or opioid-specific signalling [3,19]. Although a reduction in the number of receptors may be a major factor in the reduced efficacy of opioids, it has become clear that many other factors affect the efficacy of morphine. Such factors include heterologous desensitisation between opioid and proinflammatory chemokine receptors via shared G-protein-coupled systems [20], down-regulation of glutamate transporters in glial cells [21] or release of such substances as NO, ATP, excitatory amino acids, prostaglandins, and proinflammatory cytokines from activated glia [22,23,24,25,26,27]. In a previous study, we used minocycline, which is a tetracycline derivative with pleiotropic biological effects, to clarify whether the analgesic opioid effect is associated with the activation of microglia. Minocycline is a potent inhibitor of the microglial activation [22,28,29,30] that impairs microglial viability and migration [31,32]. Minocycline also up-regulates a tissue inhibitors of matrix metalloproteinases (TIMPs) [33], inhibits MMP-9 [34] and has been shown in many studies to have neuroprotective effects [35,36]. Some authors have suggested that minocycline may also reduce pain by inhibiting Ca^{2+} and Na^{+} currents in sensory neurons in DRG [35,37]. It was shown that pain after nerve injury depended on activation of the p38 MAPK signalling pathway in the spinal cord and p38 MAPK was co-localized with activated microglia [38,39]. It was shown [40,41,42] that the level of phospho-p38 MAPK in microglia was reduced after minocycline treatment, which suggests that this kinase is a minocycline target. Little is known about its influence on neurons, but some authors suggest its neuroprotective effects in dopaminergic and glutamatergic neurons [43,44]. We demonstrated in our previous study that chronic administration of minocycline attenuated the development of neuropathic pain and enhanced morphine analgesia [45,46,47]. Filipovic and Zecevic [48] demonstrated in *in vitro* studies that minocycline protects neurons from LPS-induced inflammation by inhibiting the activation of microglia. Activated microglia may weaken morphine analgesia by releasing pronociceptive factors, and the administration of minocycline antagonises this weakening [23,46,47].

The aim of the present study was to determine the extent to which the activation of microglia induced by injury to the sciatic nerve (by chronic constriction injury, CCI) in rats changes the analgesic effect of opioid receptors agonists. Minocycline, a well characterized drug for inhibiting microglial activity [49], was intraperitoneally (i.p.) administered pre-emptively and repeatedly to CCI-exposed rats, subsequently its influence on allodynia and hyperalgesia was measured. On day 7 after CCI, vehicle-treated and minocycline-treated rats received the opioid receptor agonists morphine, DAMGO, U50,488H, DPDPE, deltorphin II and SNC80 intrathecally. We conducted behavioural experiments and simultaneously analysed molecular changes in the transcription of *MOR*, *KOR*, and *DOR* mRNA in the dorsal horn of the lumbar spinal cord and in DRG (L4–L6) at day 7 after injury in CCI-exposed rats after minocycline or vehicle administration. We also analysed the presence of MOR, KOR and DOR in rat primary microglial cell cultures by using qRT-PCR, Western blotting and immunocytochemistry.

Methods

Animals

Male Wistar rats (200–350 g) were housed in cages that were lined with sawdust under a standard 12/12 h light/dark cycle (lights on at 08:00 h), with food and water available *ad lib*. Care was taken to reduce the number of animals used, and all experiments were performed according to the recommendations of IASP [50] and the NIH Guide for the Care and Use of Laboratory Animals and were approved by the II Local Bioethics Committee branch of the National Ethics Committee for Experiments on Animals based at the Institute of Pharmacology, Polish Academy of Sciences (Cracow, Poland).

Surgical preparations

Chronic constriction injury (CCI) was produced in rats by tying four ligatures around the sciatic nerve under sodium pentobarbital anaesthesia (60 mg/kg; i.p.). The *biceps femoris* and the *gluteus superficialis* were separated, and the right sciatic nerve was exposed. The ligatures (4/0 silk) were tied loosely around the nerve distal to the sciatic notch with 1-mm spacing until they elicited a brief twitch in the respective hind limb. The procedure has been described in detail by Bennett and Xie, [51]. After the surgery, all rats developed long-lasting neuropathic pain symptoms such as allodynia and hyperalgesia. Because we have shown in earlier studies that there are no differences between the nociceptive responses of naïve and sham rats [52], we used naïve animals for the behavioural experiments in the present study.

Intrathecal (i.t.) injection

Rats were prepared for intrathecal (i.t.) injection by implanting catheters under pentobarbital anaesthesia (60 mg/kg i.p.). The intrathecal catheter consisted of polyethylene tubing that was 12 cm long (PE 10, Intramedic; Clay Adams, Parsippany, NJ) with an outside diameter of 0.4 mm and a dead space of 10 µl that had been sterilised by immersion in 70% (v/v) ethanol and fully flushed with sterile water before insertion. Rats were placed on a stereotaxic table (David Kopf Instruments, Tujunga, CA), and an incision was made in the atlanto-occipital membrane. The catheter (7.8 cm of its length) was carefully introduced into the subarachnoid space at the rostral level of the spinal cord lumbar enlargement (L4–L5) according to the method of Yaksh and Rudy [53]. After the implantation, the first injection of 10 µl of water was performed slowly and the catheter was tightened. One day after catheter implantation, the rats were monitored for physical impairments. Those showing motor deficits were excluded from further study. Animals were allowed a minimum 1 week of recovery after the surgery before the experiment began. Water for injection or respective drugs were delivered slowly (1–2 min) in a volume of 5 µl through the i.t. catheter and were followed by 10 µl of water for injection, which flushed the catheter.

Behavioural tests

Tactile allodynia (von Frey test). Allodynia was measured in rats subjected to CCI by the use of an automatic von Frey apparatus (Dynamic Plantar Aesthesiometer Cat. No. 37400, Ugo Basile Italy). Rats were placed in plastic cages with a wire net floor 5 min before the experiment. The von Frey filament was applied to the midplantar surface of the hind foot, and measurements were taken automatically [23]. The strength of the von Frey stimuli ranged from 0.5 to 26 g in rats.

Cold hyperalgesia (cold plate test). Hyperalgesia was assessed using the cold plate test (Cold/Hot Plate Analgesia Meter No. 05044 Columbus Instruments, USA) as has been described previously [23,45]. The temperature of the cold plate was maintained at 5°C, and the cut-off latency was 30 s. The rats were placed on the cold plate, and the time until lifting of the hind foot was recorded. The injured foot was the first to react in every case.

Drug administration

The chemicals used in this study and their sources were as follows: morphine hydrochloride – Polfa (Kutno, Poland); DAMGO (Sigma-Aldrich, USA), Deltorphin II (Sigma-Aldrich, USA), DPDPE (Sigma-Aldrich, USA), U50,488H (Tocris, UK), SNC80 (Sigma-Aldrich, USA) and minocycline hydrochloride (Sigma-Aldrich, USA). Minocycline (MC; 30 mg/kg; i.p.) was dissolved in sterile water and pre-emptively administered intraperitoneally 16 h and 1 h before CCI and then twice daily for 7 days. This method of minocycline administration was used throughout the work and is referred to in the text as "repeated administration". The control groups received a vehicle (water for injection) according to the same schedule. One hour after the last morning of minocycline or vehicle administration on day 7 after CCI, morphine (M; 20; 40 µg; 62.3 nM; 124.6 nM), DAMGO (MOR selective ligand; 1; 2 µg; 1.94 nM; 3.9 nM), U50,488H (KOR selective ligand; 25; 50 µg; 61.6 nM; 123.2 nM), DPDPE (DOR I selective ligand; 10; 20 µg; 15.48 nM; 30.96 nM), deltorphin II (del II; DOR II selective ligand; 1.5; 15 µg; 1.9 nM; 19 nM), SNC80 (10; 20 µg; 22.24 nM; 44.48 nM) or a vehicle was intrathecally injected. The von Frey test (25 and 45 min later) and cold plate tests (30 and 50 min later) were

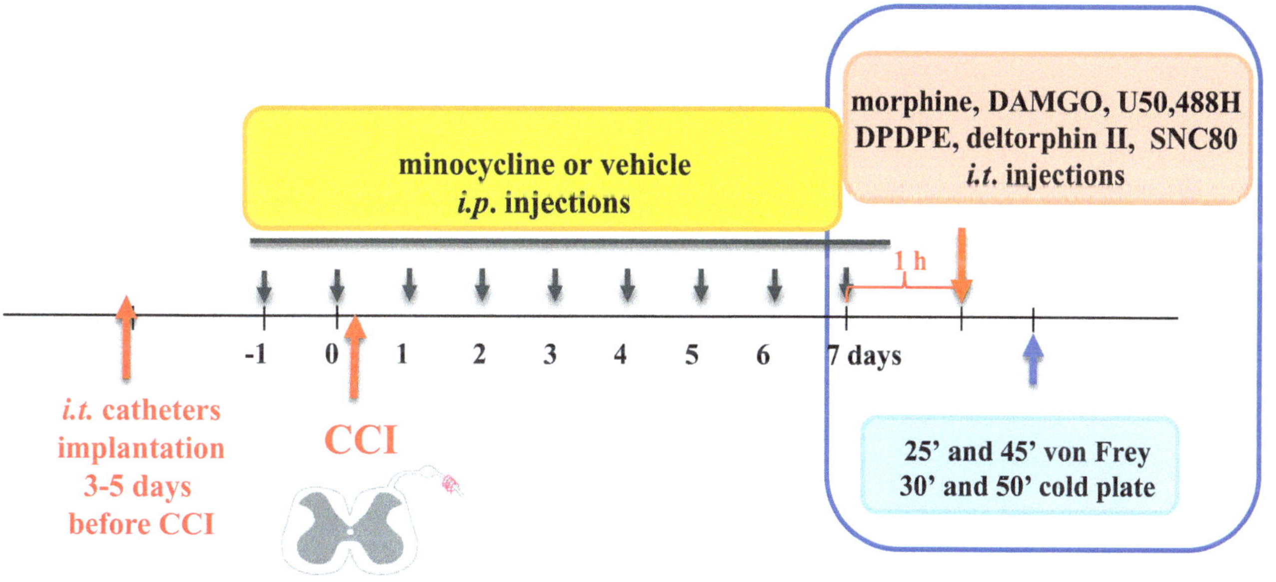

Figure 1. Drug administration.

carried out after vehicle or opioid agonist administration (Figure 1).

Microglial cell cultures and treatments

Primary cultures of microglial cells were prepared from 1-day-old Wistar rat pups as has been previously described [54] Briefly, cells were isolated from the rats' cerebral cortices and were plated at a density of 3×10^5 cells/cm^2 in a culture medium that consisted of DMEM/Glutamax/high glucose (Gibco, USA) supplemented with heat-inactivated 10% foetal bovine serum (Gibco, USA), 100 U/ml penicillin, and 0.1 mg/ml streptomycin (Gibco, USA) on poly-L-lysine coated 75 cm^2 culture flasks and were maintained at 37°C and 5% CO_2. The culture medium was changed after 4 days. The loosely adherent microglial cells were recovered after 9 days by mild shaking and centrifugation. Microglial cells were suspended in a culture medium and plated at a final density of 2×10^5 cells onto 24 well plates and 1.2×10^6 cells onto 6 well plates. Adherent cells were incubated for 48 h in a culture medium before being used for the analyses. Cell specificity was determined using an antibody to OX-42 (microglial marker) in cultures of primary microglia. Levels of mRNA for *C1q* (a microglial marker) and *GFAP* (an astroglial marker) were also investigated. Cultured primary microglia were more than 95% positive for OX-42 and C1q.

We have also analyzed the level of MOR, DOR and KOR mRNA level after LPS-stimulation (data not shown). Cells were prepared as described above and then incubated for 6 h with LPS [100 ng/ml] [55] or vehicle (PBS). We have not observed any significant changes in expression of MOR and KOR transcripts in comparison with vehicle-treated cells. In the LPS-stimulated microglial cells the presence of *DOR* mRNA also haven't been detected. Lipopolysaccharides from *Escherichia coli* 0111:B4 (Sigma-Aldrich, USA).

qRT-PCR analysis of gene expression

Total RNA was extracted according to the method Chomczynski and Sacchi [56] using the TRIzol reagent (Invitrogen) as previously described [57]. The RNA concentration was measured using a NanoDrop ND-1000 Spectrometer (NanoDrop Technologies). Reverse transcription was performed on 500 ng (from cell cultures) or 1000 ng (from tissue) of total RNA using Omniscript reverse transcriptase (Qiagen Inc.) at 37°C for 60 min. cDNA was diluted 1:10 with H_2O. qRT-PCR was performed using Assay-On-Demand TaqMan probes according to the manufacturer's protocol (Applied Biosystems) and run on a Real-Time PCR iCycler device (BioRad, Hercules, CA, USA). Rn00561699_m1 (*Oprd1*), Rn01430371_m1 (*Oprm1*), and Rn00567737_m1 (*Oprk1*) were used as TaqMan primers and probes. The expression of HPRT (a housekeeping gene) was quantified to control for variation in cDNA amounts. Cycle threshold values were calculated automatically by iCycler IQ 3.0 software with default parameters. Abundance of RNA was calculated as $2^{-(\text{threshold cycle})}$.

Western blot analysis

Cell lysates were collected in a RIPA buffer with a protease inhibitor cocktail and cleared by centrifugation (14000×g for 30 min, 4°C). Samples containing 20 µg of protein were heated in a loading buffer (50 mM Tris–HCl, 2% SDS, 2% β-mercaptoethanol, 4% glycerol and 0.1% bromophenol blue) for 5 min at 70°C and resolved by SDS–PAGE on 12% polyacrylamide gels. Following gel electrophoresis, the proteins were electrophoretically transferred to Immune-Blot PVDF membranes (Bio-Rad). The blots were blocked for 30 min using 5% non-fat dry milk (Bio-Rad) in Tris-buffered saline with 0.1% Tween 20 (TBST). The blots were incubated with primary antibodies (rabbit polyclonal anti-MOR, 1:500 [58]; rabbit polyclonal anti-DOR, 1:500 [59]; rabbit polyclonal anti-KOR 1:500, Abcam [58] that had been diluted in a SignalBoost Immunoreaction Enhancer Kit (Merck Millipore) for 24 h at 4°C and then incubated with a goat polyclonal antibody that had been conjugated to horseradish peroxidase (goat anti-rabbit IgG, BioRad) at a dilution of 1:1000 for 1 h at room temperature. After four 5-minute washes in TBST, immunocomplexes were detected using a Lumi-Light Western Blotting Kit and visualised using a Fujifilm LAS-4000 fluorimager system. The blots were washed 4 times for 5 minutes each in TBST and reprobed with a mouse antibody against GAPDH (1:5000, Millipore) as a loading control. The relative levels of immunoreactivity were quantified using Fujifilm Image Gauge software.

Immunocytochemical analysis

We used commercially available specific anti-MOR, anti-KOR and anti-OX/42 antibodies. Cells were fixed for 20 minutes in 4% paraformaldehyde in a 0.1 M phosphate buffer (pH 7.4) and incubated with primary antibodies (rabbit anti-MOR, 1:400 [60], rabbit anti-KOR, 1:400 [61], rabbit anti-DOR, 1:400, [62] Neuromics; mouse anti-OX/42, 1:500, Serotec) for 2 days at 4°C. After three washes in PB, double immunofluorescence was revealed by incubation for 2 h in the appropriate fluorochrome-conjugated secondary antibody, Alexa Fluor546 donkey anti-rabbit and Alexa Fluor488 donkey anti-mouse, diluted 1:500 in 5% NDS. Sections were then washed with PB and coverslipped with an Aquatex mounting medium (Merck, Darmstadt, Germany). Sections without primary antibodies were used as negative controls.

Data analysis

The behavioural data are presented as the mean ± S.E.M of 8–16 rats per group. The results of the experiments were statistically evaluated using one-way analysis of variance (ANOVA). All of the differences between the treatment groups were further analysed with Bonferroni's post-hoc tests. Significant differences in comparisons with vehicle-treated CCI-exposed rats are indicated by *P (<0.05), **P (<0.01) and ***P (<0.001). Significant differences between vehicle-treated CCI-exposed rats that had received a single dose of opioid receptor ligands and minocycline-treated CCI-exposed rats that had received a single dose of opioid receptor ligands are indicated by #P (<0.05), ##P (<0.01) and ###P (<0.001).

The qRT-PCR analyses were performed in three groups: naïve, CCI-exposed and minocycline-treated CCI-exposed rats. The results are presented as fold changes compared with the naïve rats in the ipsilateral dorsal lumbar spinal cord and DRG. The qRT-PCR data are presented as the mean ± S.E.M and represent the normalised averages that were derived from the threshold qRT-PCR cycles from four to eight samples for each group. Intergroup differences were analysed using ANOVAs followed by Bonferroni's multiple comparison tests. Significant differences resulting from comparison with naïve rats are indicated by *P (<0.05), **P (<0.01) and ***P (<0.001). The data from 3 to 10 cell cultures are presented.

Results

Repeated administration of minocycline significantly diminished allodynia and hyperalgesia in neuropathic pain in rats

All vehicle-treated CCI rats exhibited neuropathic pain symptoms in the behavioral tests. The rats exhibited strong allodynia on the seventh day after ligation as measured by the von Frey test (11.6 g±0.6 vs. 25.8 g±0.2 for naïve rats) (Fig. 2A,C,E; 3A,C,E) and potent hyperalgesia as measured by the cold plate test (7.6 s±0.9 vs. 29.7 s±0.3 for naïve rats) (Fig. 2B,D,F; 3B,D,F). Repeated administration of minocycline (MC; 30 mg/kg; i.p.) attenuated allodynia (17.4 g±0.5 vs. 11.6 g±0.6 for the vehicle-treated CCI rats) (Fig. 2A,C,E; 3A,C,E) and also hyperalgesia (12.1 s±0.9 vs. 7.6 s±0.9 for the vehicle-treated CCI rats) (Fig. 2B,D,F; 3B,D,F) to a similar extent at both time points.

Repeated administration of minocycline significantly influenced the effects of morphine in neuropathic pain in rats

The doses of morphine effective in neuropathic pain (M; 20 and 40 µg; i.t.) were used. Morphine was injected one hour after the last morning dose of minocycline (30 mg/kg; i.p. repeatedly) or vehicle, and allodynia and hyperalgesia were measured (see Figure 1). Morphine at a dose of 20 µg significantly diminished allodynia 25 and 45 minutes after injection compared with vehicle-treated animals (18.60 g±0.4 vs. 11.6 g±0.6 and 17.57 g±0.39 vs. 11.9 g±0.5, respectively; Fig. 2A). In minocycline-treated animals, the antiallodynic effect of morphine at a dose of 20 µg was potentiated by minocycline at both times as shown in the von Frey test (25 minutes: 22.04 g±0.52 vs. 18.60 g±0.4 for morphine-treated rats, 45 minutes: 22.3 g±0.34 vs. 17.57 g±0.39 for morphine-treated rats; Fig. 2A). Morphine at a dose of 20 µg did not influence thermal hyperalgesia but in the group which was injected repeatedly with minocycline, the antihyperalgesic effect of morphine was demonstrated (30 minutes: 18.30 s±1.6 vs. 11.3 g±0.8 for morphine-treated rats, 50 minutes: 22.5 s±1.7 vs. 13.5 s±1.5 for morphine-treated rats; Fig. 2B). A higher dose of morphine (40 µg) was effective in reducing mechanical allodynia 25 and 45 minutes after injection compared with vehicle-treated animals (25 minutes: 21.1 g±0.48 vs. 11.6 g±0.6, 45 minutes: 23.9 g±0.6 vs. 11.9 g±0.5; Fig. 2A). In minocycline-treated rats, the antiallodynic effect of morphine at a dose of 40 µg was potentiated at both times (25 minutes: 24.84 g±0.27 vs. 21.1 g±0.48, 45 minutes: 23.98 g±0.51 vs. 20.25 g±0.6; Fig. 2A). In opposite to the lower dose, morphine at a dose of 40 µg showed antihyperalgesic effect at both time points (30 minutes: 16.5 s±1.9 vs. 7.6 s±0.9, 50 minutes: 19.1 s±2.2 vs. 8.2 s±0.8; Fig. 2B). The increased effect of morphine at a dose of 40 µg in minocycline-treated group was observed at both time points, however, this effect was more significant after 50 minutes (25.8 s±1.0 vs. 19.1 s±2.2; Fig. 2B).

Repeated administration of minocycline significantly influenced the effects of MOR (DAMGO) and KOR (U50,488H) agonists in neuropathic pain in rats

DAMGO at a dose of 1 µg significantly diminished allodynia 25 and 45 minutes after injection compared with vehicle-treated animals (25 minutes: 20.4 g±0.5 vs. 11.6 g±0.6, 45 minutes: 18.7 g±0.4 vs. 11.9 g±0.5; Fig. 2C). In minocycline-treated animals, the antiallodynic effect of DAMGO (1 µg) was potentiated at both times as shown in the von Frey test (25 min: 22.6 g±0.7 vs. 20.4 g±0.5 for DAMGO-treated rats, 45 min: 21. 4 g±1.0 vs. 18.7 g±0.4 for DAMGO-treated rats; Fig. 2C). DAMGO at a dose of 1 µg did not influence thermal hyperalgesia but in minocycline- and DAMGO-treated group the antyhiperalgesic effect occurred at both time points but the better effect we observed 50 min after injection (21.2 s±1.8 vs. 16.4 s±1.7 for DAMGO-treated rats; Fig. 2D). The higher dose of DAMGO (2 µg) was effective in reducing mechanical allodynia 25 and 45 minutes after injection compared with vehicle-treated animals (25 min: 21.3 g±0.9 vs. 11.6 g±0.6, 45 min: 20.6 g±1.1 vs. 11.9 g±0.5; Fig. 2C). As shown in the von Frey test, repeated minocycline administration potentiated effect of DAMGO at a dose of 2 µg at both times, but a better effect was present after 45 minutes (24.9 g±0.5 vs. 20.6 g±1.1; Fig. 2C). In opposite to the lower dose, DAMGO at a dose of 2 µg showed antihyperalgesic effect at both time points (30 min: 18.0 s±2.9 vs. 7.6 s±0.9, 50 min: 16.9 s±1.5 vs. 8.2 s±0.8; Fig. 2D). We also observed increased effect of DAMGO in minocycline-treated

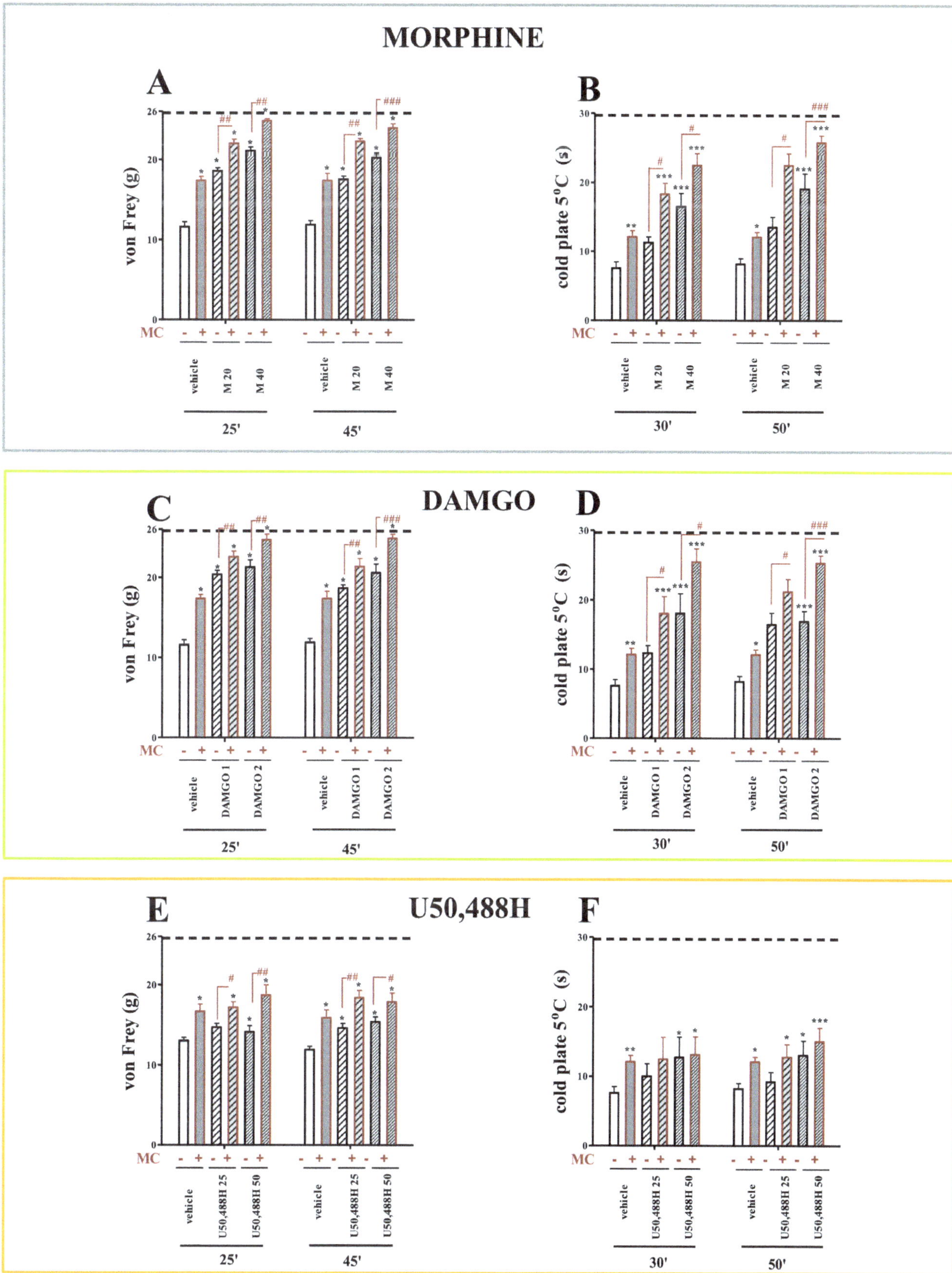

Figure 2. The effects of morphine, DAMGO and U50,488H on vehicle- and minocycline-treated CCI-exposed rats. The response to morphine, DAMGO and U50,488H was measured 25 and 45 minutes after administration by the von Frey test (A, C, E) and 30 and 50 minutes after

administration by the cold plate test (B, D, F). Minocycline (MC; 30 mg/kg; i.p.) was administered intraperitoneally pre-emptively 16 h and 1 h before CCI, and then repeatedly twice daily for 7 days. Vehicle-treated and minocycline-treated rats received intrathecal morphine (M; 20; 40 µg/5 µl), DAMGO (1; 2 µg/5 µl) or U50,488H (25; 50 µg/5 µl) one hour after the last morning administration on day 7 after CCI. The data are presented as the mean response ± S.E.M. (8–16 rats per group). The results of the experiments were statistically evaluated using One-way Analyses of Variance (ANOVA). The differences between the treatment groups throughout the study were further analysed with Bonferroni's *post-hoc* tests. *$P<0.05$, **$P<0.01$ and ***$P<0.001$ indicate significant differences compared with vehicle-treated CCI-exposed rats; #$P<0.05$, ##$P<0.01$ and ###$P<0.001$ indicate significant differences between vehicle-treated CCI-exposed rats that received a single dose of morphine and minocycline-treated CCI-exposed rats that received a single dose of morphine, DAMGO or U50,488H. Dotted line is a value for naïve animals (for von Frey test 25.8 g; for cold plate test 29.7 s).

group 30 minutes after opioid injection, however, this effect was more significant after 50 minutes (25.3 s±1.1 vs.16.9 s±1.5; Fig. 2D).

During neuropathy, the antiallodynic effect of U50,488H appeared after doses of 25 µg i.t. only 45 minutes after injection (14.6 g±0.6 vs. 11.9 g±0.5; Fig. 2E). The effect of this dose of U50,488H was potentiated in minocycline-treated group as shown in the von Frey test at both times, but at 45 minutes after injection the effect was more pronounced (18.4 g±0.9 vs. 14.6 g±0.6; Fig. 2E). U50,488H at a dose of 25 µg did not influence hyperalgesia and minocycline did not change this action (Fig. 2F). The higher dose (50 µg; i.t.) diminished allodynia at both times (25 min: 14.1 g±0.8 vs. 11.6 g±0.6, 45 min: 15.4 g±0.6 vs. 11.9 g±0.5; Fig. 2E). In minocycline-treated rats, the antiallodynic effect of U50,488H at a dose of 50 µg was potentiated at both times, but it potentiation was higher after 25 minutes (18.7 g±1.3 vs. 14.1 g±0.8; Fig. 2E). This dose of U50,488H slightly diminished hyperalgesia at 30 (12.7 s±2.9 vs. 7.6 s±0.9; Fig. 2F) and 50 (13.0 s±2.1 vs. 8.2 s±0.8; Fig. 2F) minutes after injection. Repeated minocycline administration did not change the action of U50,488H at a dose of 50 µg (Fig. 2F).

Repeated administration of minocycline did not influence the effects of DOR agonists (DPDPE, Deltorphin II and SNC80) in neuropathic pain in rats

DPDPE at a dose of 10 µg diminished allodynia 25 and 45 minutes after injection compared with vehicle-treated animals (25 min: 19.8 g±2.1 vs. 11.6 g±0.6, 45 min: 16.6 g±2.4 vs. 11.9 g±0.5; Fig. 3A) and minocycline treatment did not change this effect (Fig. 3A). Higher dose of DPDPE (20 µg) was effective in reducing mechanical allodynia only 25 minutes after injection compared with vehicle-treated animals (20.3 g±1.9 vs. 11.6 g±0.6, Fig. 3A) and this antiallodynic effect was not changed by minocycline (Fig. 3A). As shown in the cold plate test, DPDPE significantly diminished thermal hyperalgesia after both doses of 10 and 20 µg (30 min: 16.1 s±2.3 vs. 7.6 s±0.9; 50 min: 17.50 s±1.9 vs. 8.2 s±0.8 and 30 min: 20.3 s±1.9 vs. 7.6 s±0.9; 50 min: 23.6 s±1.7 8.2 s±0.8; respectively; Fig. 3B) and minocycline did not modulate this action (Fig. 3B).

Deltorphin II at a dose of 1.5 µg slightly diminished allodynia 25 and 45 minutes after injection compared with vehicle-treated animals (25 min: 17.7±1.7 vs. 11.6 g±0.6, 45 min: 17.4 g±1.4 vs. 11.9 g±0.5; Fig. 3C) and no changes in deltorphin II action in minocycline-treated group were observed (Fig. 3C). The higher dose of Deltorphin II (15 µg) was effective in reducing mechanical allodynia 25 (17.8 g±1.5 vs. 11.6 g±0.6; Fig. 3C) and 45 (17.2 g±2.1 vs. 11.9 g±0.5; Fig. 3C) minutes after injection compared with vehicle-treated animals. Repeated minocycline injection did not change the antiallodynic effect of deltorphin II (Fig. 3D). Deltorphin II at a dose of 1.5 µg did not influence hyperalgesia in CCI-exposed rats and minocycline also did not change this effect (Fig. 3D). As shown in the cold plate test, deltorphin II at a dose of 15 µg diminished thermal hyperalgesia only 50 minutes after injection (11.3 s±2.8 vs. 8.2 s±0.8; Fig. 3D) and minocycline did not change the antihyperalgesic action of the higher dose of Deltorphin II (Fig. 3D).

SNC80 at a dose of 10 µg slightly diminished allodynia 25 and 45 minutes after injection compared with vehicle-treated animals (25 min: 16.4 g±0.8 vs. 11.6 g±0.6, 45 min: 17.9 g±1.7 vs. 11.9 g±0.5; Fig. 3E). The higher dose of SNC80 (20 µg) was effective in reducing mechanical allodynia 25 (19.9 g±0.6 vs. 11.6 g±0.6; Fig. 3E) and 45 (19.0 g±1.2 vs. 11.9 g±0.5; Fig. 3E) minutes after injection compared with vehicle-treated animals. Repeated minocycline injection did not change the antiallodynic effect of both doses of SNC80 (Fig. 3E). As shown in the cold plate test, SNC80 at a dose of 10 µg influenced hyperalgesia in CCI-exposed rats (30 min: 19.5 s±2.8 vs. 7.6 s±0.9; 50 min: 13.0 s±2.3 vs. 8.2 s±0.8; Fig. 3F) SNC80 at a dose of 20 µg diminished thermal hyperalgesia 30 (24.2 s±2 vs. 7.6 s±0.9; Fig. 3F) and 50 (20.8 s±4.0 vs. 8.2 s±0.8; Fig. 3F) minutes after injection. Minocycline did not change the antihyperalgesic action of both doses of SNC80 (Fig. 3F).

Repeated administration of minocycline did not influence *MOR*, *DOR* and *KOR* mRNAs during neuropathic pain in rats

In the spinal cord the downregulation of *MOR* mRNA from 1±0.05 to 0.7±0.07 (Fig. 4A) and in the DRG from 1±0.03 to 0.5±0.06 (Fig. 4B) was observed compared to the naïve rats. Minocycline not influence the level of *MOR* mRNA in the spinal cord and in the DRG (Fig. 4A and B, respectively).

In the spinal cord the downregulation of *KOR* mRNA from 1±0.06 to 0.8±0.05 (Fig. 4C) and in the DRG from 1±0.06 to 0.6±0.04 (Fig. 4D) was observed compared to the naïve rats. Minocycline not influence the level of *KOR* mRNA in the spinal cord and in the DRG (Fig. 4C and D, respectively).

In the spinal cord the downregulation of *DOR* mRNA from 1±0.1 to 0.67±0.05 (Fig. 4E) and in the DRG from 1±0.1 to 0.3±0.07 (Fig. 4F) was observed compared to the naïve rats. Minocycline not influence the level of *KOR* mRNA in the spinal cord and in the DRG (Fig. 4E and F, respectively).

Opioid receptor expression in primary microglial cell cultures

Using a reverse transcriptase-polymerase chain reaction, we found that mRNA for *MOR* and *KOR*, but not for *DOR*, is expressed in rat primary microglial cell cultures (Fig. 5A). In the Western blot analysis, we found that protein for MOR and KOR is present in microglia (Fig. 5B). The protein for DOR was undetectable (Fig. 5B). The expression of MOR and KOR, but not DOR, in microglial cells was confirmed by immunocytochemistry (Fig. 5C).

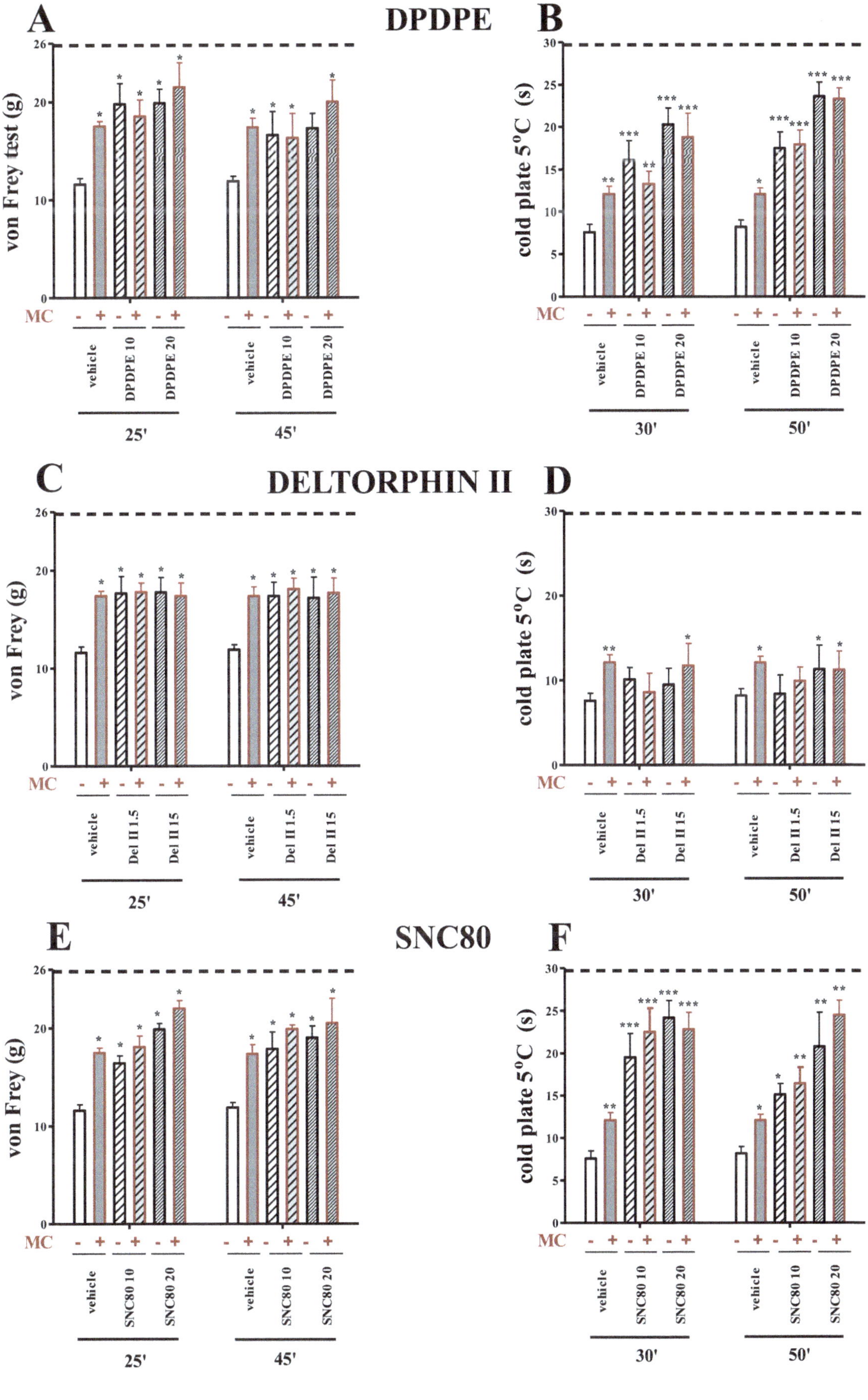
A
DPDPE
B
von Frey test (g)
cold plate 5°C (s)
MC
vehicle
DPDPE 10
DPDPE 20
25'
45'
30'
50'
C
DELTORPHIN II
D
von Frey (g)
Del II 1.5
Del II 15
E
SNC80
F
SNC80 10
SNC80 20

Figure 3. The effects of DPDPE, deltorphin II and SNC80 on vehicle- and minocycline-treated CCI-exposed rats. The response to DPDPE, deltorphin II and SNC80 was measured 25 and 45 minutes after administration by the von Frey test (A, C, E) and 30 and 50 minutes after administration by the cold plate test (B, D, F). Minocycline (MC; 30 mg/kg; i.p.) was administered intraperitoneally pre-emptively 16 h and 1 h before CCI, and then repeatedly twice daily for 7 days. Vehicle-treated and minocycline-treated rats received intrathecal DPDPE (10; 20 μg/5 μl), deltorphin II (del II; 1.5; 15 μg/5 μl) or SNC80 (10; 20 μg/5 μl) one hour after the last morning administration on day 7 after CCI. The data are presented as the mean response ± S.E.M. (8–16 rats per group). The results of the experiments were statistically evaluated using ANOVAs. The differences between the treatment groups throughout the study were further analysed with Bonferroni's *post-hoc* tests. *$P<0.05$, **$P<0.01$ and ***$P<0.001$ indicate significant differences compared with vehicle-treated CCI-exposed rats. Dotted line is a value for naïve animals (for von Frey test 25.8 g; for cold plate test 29.7 s).

Discussion

Opioids are fundamental to the treatment of pain, but their efficacy is limited by side effects, including tolerance and hyperalgesia [63]. Some authors suggest that reduced sensitivity to opioids and the increases in their dosages that are necessary to obtain adequate analgesia heighten the risk of side effects [4,5,64]. It remains unclear why morphine is a less potent analgesic in clinical [65,66] and experimental [15,46,67] studies of neuropathic pain in contrast to inflammatory pain [15,67]. In many studies it was shown that selective DOR agonists do not lose their effectiveness in the treatment of neuropathic pain [13,15,68]. It has been suggested that the lesser effects of morphine on neuropathic pain are due to the reduced number of presynaptic opioid receptors that results from nerve damage-induced degeneration of primary afferent neurons [64,69] besides other effects, like upregulation of the anti-opioid system CCK, and the NMDA receptor-dependent central sensitization, between others. Obara *et al.* [15] used ED_{50} analysis to demonstrate in 2009 that much higher doses of MOR and KOR agonists injected intraplantarly are required to produce antinociception in neuropathic than in inflammatory pain. However, it remains unclear why the ED_{50} of DOR agonists, but not those of MOR and KOR agonists, is comparable in both neuropathic and inflammatory pain [15]. Our study showed that the expression of all types of opioid receptor mRNA in the spinal cord and DRG was decreased in neuropathic pain. Also Stone *et al.* [70], using three animals models of peripheral nerve injury (CCI, SNL and SNT), observed decreases in spinal DOR expression at day 10th after operations at the side of injury. Herradon *et al.* [71] compared two strains of rats, Fischer 344 and Lewis rats, in neuropathic pain model and found significant down-regulation of DOR mRNA 28 days after CCI in the DRG of Lewis rats and the same trend was observed in F344 rats. Those data correspond well with our results obtained at day 7th after CCI in Wistar rats. In the study of Obara *et al.* [15] biochemical experiments were conducted at 3rd and 14th day (but not day 7th) after CCI and showed a non-significant, downward trend in the expression of mRNA for *MOR*, *DOR* and *KOR* at the spinal cord level. At the DRG level of neuropathic rats these authors observed down-regulation of mRNA level for *MOR* in L4–L5 DRGs (at day 3rd) and in L5 DRG (at day 14th), for *DOR* in L5 DRG (at both days) and for *KOR* in L4 and L5 DRGs (at day 3rd) and in L5 DRG (at day 14th) in comparison with naive animals. Those data correspond well with our results obtained at day 7th after CCI, however, in our experiments we pooled L4–L6 DRGs [15]. In the paper of Kabli and Cahill [68] the up-regulation of DOR protein was observed 14 days after sciatic nerve injury at the DRG level. The authors suggest that the increase in DOR protein is correlated with DOR trafficking to the site of injury, which may explain the lower level of mRNA as shown by our results. Should be noted, however, that in some papers no decrease in opioid receptor expression was observed [71,72]. Those discrepant data may result from different animal species used in experiments or time of the tissue collection after injury as it is shown in the mentioned works.

However, minocycline does not affect the reduced levels of all opioid receptor mRNAs, although it potentiates analgesia after such opioid agonists as morphine, DAMGO and U50,488H. Therefore, we should consider other mechanisms of weakened analgesia in neuropathic pain that can be restored by minocycline administration. These mechanisms may be important for sustained analgesia after administration of DOR ligands.

Several studies have suggested that the activation of glia and the enhancement of proinflammatory cytokine levels in the spinal cord and DRG are responsible for the development of both neuropathic pain and morphine tolerance [73,74,75]. We have previously observed an attenuation of the development of neuropathic pain when we administered minocycline, which is a substance that inhibits microglial activation in CCI-exposed rats [45,46]. Although minocycline can influence some neuronal functions, its ability to reduce microglial activation [76] as well as its selectivity of the action has been recently demonstrated [49]. We show in the present paper that the antiallodynic and antihyperalgesic effects of morphine, DAMGO and U50,488H, but not of DPDPE, deltorphin II or SNC80, were significantly potentiated with minocycline in CCI-subjected rats. In many studies we may found pharmacological evidence of distinct subtypes of DOR [77]. It is known that DOR_1 is activated by DPDPE, DOR_2 by deltorphin II and SNC80 is a a highly selective agonist for DOR. We had demonstrated in our previous studies the occurrence of strong antiallodynic and antihyperalgesic effects of DOR_1 and DOR_2 agonists after their acute and chronic i.t. administration in a rat neuropathic pain model [13]. Analgesic effects of i.t. injected SNC80 was also shown in many pain models [77,78,79]. In the present paper we have shown that the effectiveness of DPDPE, deltorphin II and SNC80 is not enhanced by minocycline treatment. Our results suggest that DOR analgesia is not dependent on injury-induced microglial activation. DORs are therefore a promising target for the development of analgesics. Indeed as previously reported by Holdridge *et al.* [80,81] the prolonged morphine treatment-induced incensement in microglial cell size was not functionally relevant in DOR analgesia, which confirms our research concerning the presence of DOR on microglia.

In the *in vitro* study, we used qRT-PCR, Western blot and immunocytochemistry assays to confirm the presence of MOR and KOR in microglia, and we have shown for the first time that those microglial cells do not express DOR. Our results are in agreement with other studies that have shown that microglia express MOR and KOR [82,83,84]. Chao *et al.* [85] first reported in 1996 that KOR was present in human microglia using qRT-PCR and a ligand-binding assay. The expression of KOR in microglial cells was also confirmed by the membrane binding of selective ligand [^{3}H]U69,593. Additionally, Chao *et al.* 1997 [86] have shown that morphine and DAMGO suppressed human microglia chemotaxis in a dose-dependent fashion and this effect is significantly attenuated by β-funaltrexamine (a MOR selective

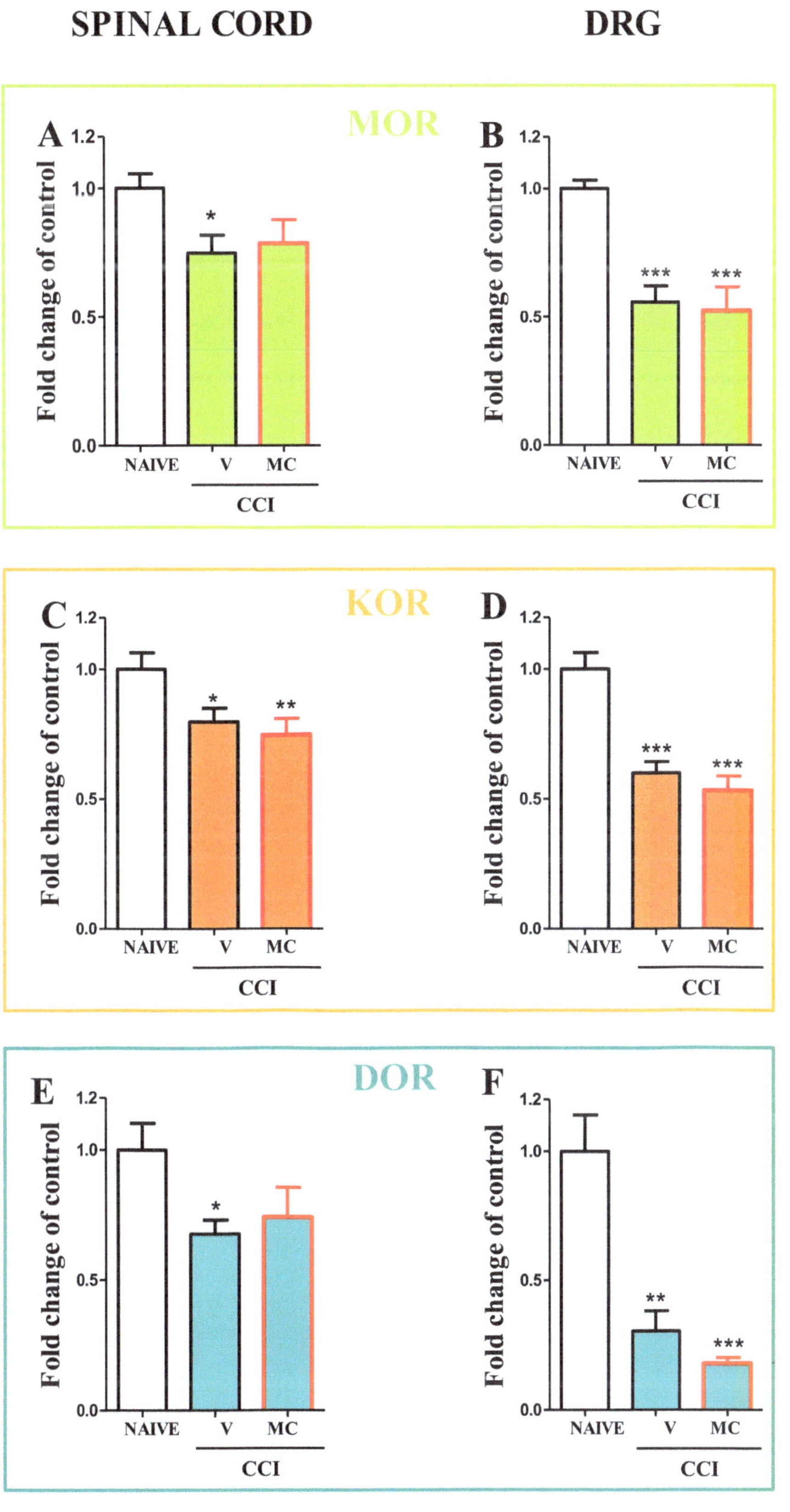

Figure 4. *MOR, DOR, KOR* mRNAs in spinal cord and DRGs in vehicle- and minocycline-treated CCI-exposed rats. Minocycline (MC; 30 mg/kg; i.p.) was administered intraperitoneally pre-emptively 16 h and 1 h before CCI, and then repeatedly twice daily for 7 days. On the seventh day, spinal cords (L4–L6) and DRG were collected for the qRT-PCR analysis of *MOR* (A, B), *KOR* (C, D) and *DOR* (E, F) gene expression. The data are presented as the means ± SEM and represent the normalised averages derived from the threshold qRT-PCR cycles from four to eight samples for each group. Intergroup differences were analysed using ANOVAs followed by Bonferroni's multiple comparison tests. *$P<0.05$; **$P<0.01$; ***$P<0.001$ indicate significant differences compared with naïve rats.

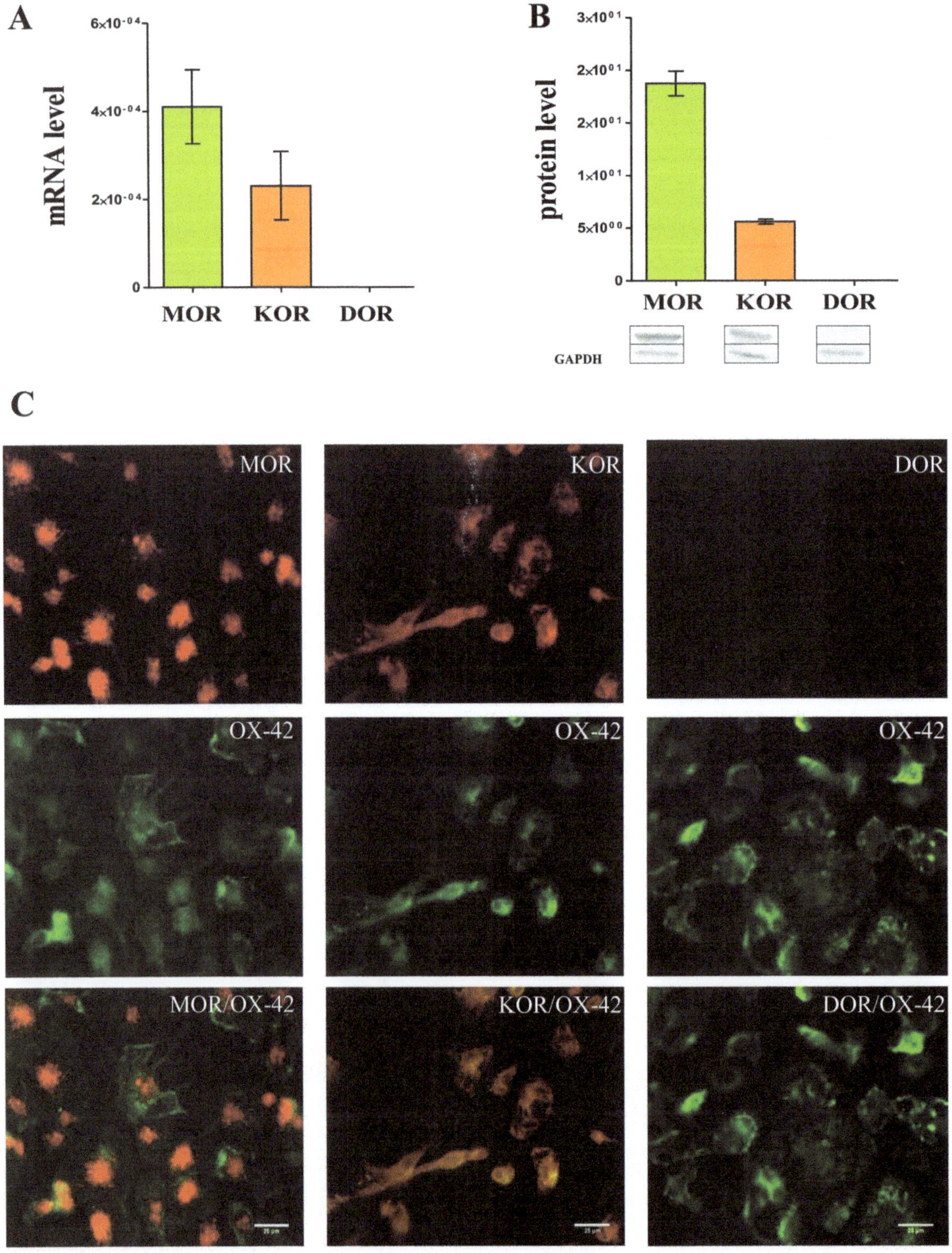

Figure 5. The presence of opioid receptors on microglia cells - *in vitro* studies. We analysed the presence of opioid receptors in primary microglial cell cultures. Using reverse transcriptase-polymerase chain reaction, we found that mRNA for *MOR* and *KOR*, but not *DOR*, is expressed in rat primary microglial cells cultures (A). Western blot analysis (B) detected proteins for MOR and KOR, but not DOR, in microglia. The presence of MOR and KOR, but not DOR, were confirmed by immunocytochemistry (C), and we show the colocalisation of MOR (left panel) and KOR (middle panel) antibodies (red) with OX/42 antibodies (green). The scale bar for all microphotographs is 25 μm. The data from 3–10 cell cultures are presented.

antagonist), which is consistent with our confirmation of the presence of MOR in microglial cells. The occurrence of DOR in microglial cells is still controversial. Our results strongly suggest that there is no DOR in rat primary microglial cells, although the studies of Turchan-Chlewo *et al.* [87] suggest their presence. However, Turchan-Chlewo *et al.* [87] used the PCR method (Sybr

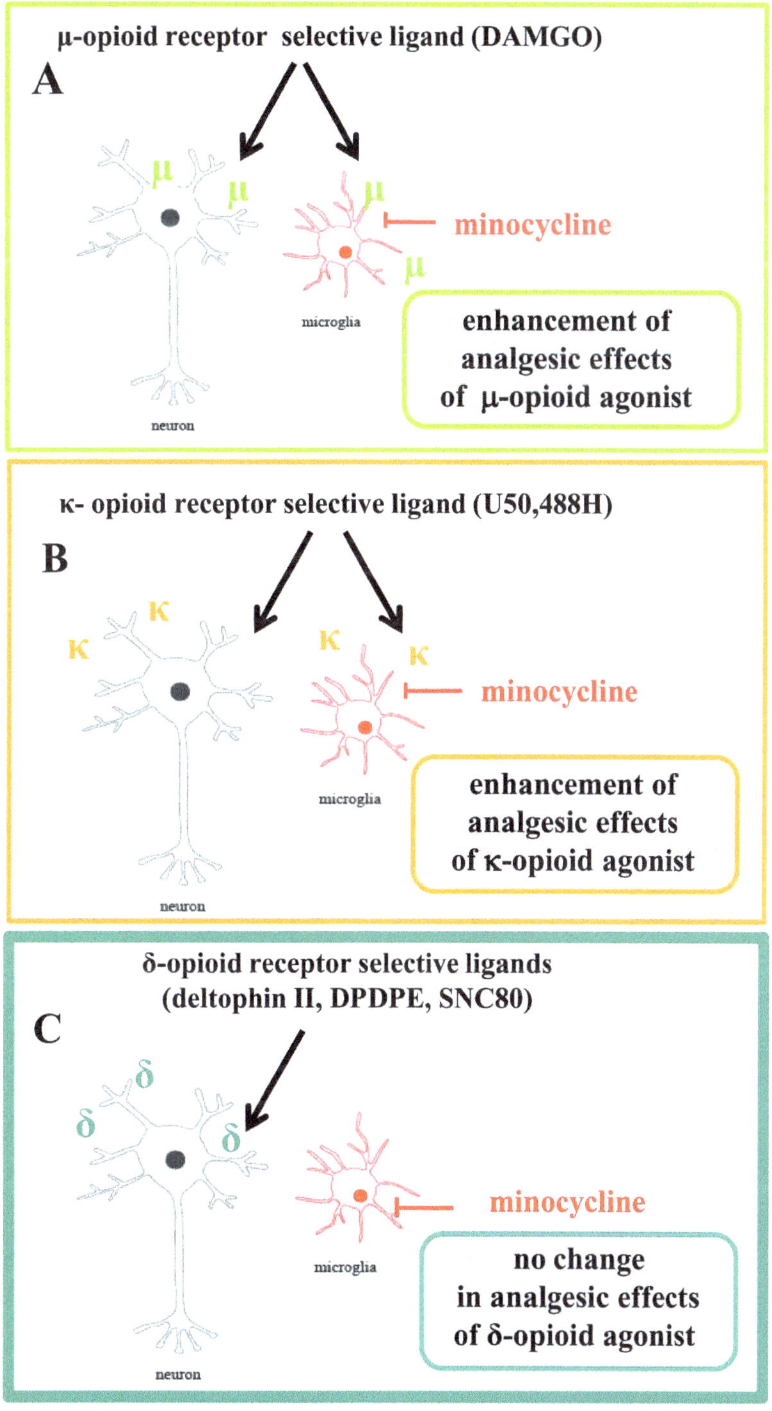

Figure 6. The possible influence of minocycline on analgesia after opioid receptors ligands. In our opinion, activated spinal microglia are key factors in the development of neuropathic pain and play a major role in the antagonizing of some opioids effectiveness. The results of our paper show for the first time that that DOR, in contrast to MOR and KOR, is not present in microglial cells. This phenomenon might be responsible for the different analgesic effects of MOR, KOR and DOR ligands (Fig. 2 and 3). We provide evidence that minocycline (a potent inhibitor of microglial activation and proliferation) enhances the effects of selective MOR (DAMGO; Fig. 2C,D) and selective KOR (U50,488H; Fig. 2E,F) agonists by inhibition of microglial cell activation. The effectiveness of DOR agonists (DPDPE, deltorphin II and SNC80) is not changed by minocycline (Fig. 3A–F). Our results indicate that an important element of the effectiveness of opioid drugs in neuropathic pain is the activation of microglia. The lack of DOR receptors in these cells causes that DOR receptor-mediated analgesia is not weaker under neuropathic pain, in which there is a strong activation of microglia. Earlier inhibition of microglial activation by minocycline administration therefore did not influence the effect of DOR selective agonists. The above results indicate not only that minocycline potentiates analgesia after MOR and KOR agonists but also that DOR is a potentially important target in the search for new drugs that would be effective against neuropathic pain.

Green), which is not sufficiently selective and can give false positive results. The TaqMan assay that we used is standardised and highly specific, and we confirmed the lack of DOR in microglia cell cultures by using Western blot and immunocytochemistry, therefore, our results are not consistent with those that were obtained by immunostaining by Turchan-Cholewo *et al.* [87] and Thorlin *et al.* [88]. Moreover studies by Turchan-Cholewo *et al.* [87] used commercial antibodies against DOR, which are no longer recommended for such studies. Due to the lack of selective DOR antibody a unique genetic mouse model was developed in order to investigate the distribution of DOR in the nervous system [16,89]. Opioid receptors have high degrees of homology, and antibodies may recognise other subtypes within the same family. DOR expression has also been observed on glial-like cells in the dentate gyrus [90] and rat cervical spinal cord [91], but none of these authors distinguished between astrocytes and microglia. Our results concerning the absence of DOR in microglia are consistent with recently published results of pharmacological studies that were conducted by Merighi *et al.* [84]. These authors have shown in primary microglia cell cultures that DPDPE, a DOR agonist, does not change the level of protein for PKC after LPS stimulation, while morphine and DAMGO up-regulate this kinase. The ineffectiveness of DPDPE in this study may be explained by the lack of DOR receptors in microglial cells. Horvath and DeLeo, [92] showed that selective agonists of DOR_1 DPDPE had no effect on microglial migration, which confirms our results that DOR, in contrast to MOR and KOR, is not present in microglial cells. DOR shows a functional profile that is distinct from that of MOR or KOR [93] and plays an important role in chronic pain, for example DOR knockout mice showed augmented neuropathic pain [94,95]. DOR agonists are poor analgesics in acute pain [96], but are highly effective following inflammatory or neuropathic pain [13,96,97,98,99].

Happel *et al.* [100] suggested in 2008 that morphine and DAMGO influence the immune system. For example, opioids alter macrophage functions and they modulate cytokine production and chemokine and chemokine receptor expression. Activation of proinflammatory chemokine receptors is known to down-regulate the analgesic functions of opioid receptors, and this enhances the perception of pain [101]. Horvath *et al.* [102] showed that morphine increases microglial migration by means of an interaction between *MOR* and $P2X_4$ receptors. This interaction is dependent on PI3K/Akt pathway activation [102]. Under neuropathic pain, the phosphorylation of p38 MAPK in microglia results in increased synthesis of the proinflammatory cytokines IL-1β, IL-6, and TNF-α. Spinal blockade of these cytokines is known to attenuate neuropathic pain and morphine tolerance [74,103]. Therefore, in cases where MOR and KOR agonists target microglial signalling by inhibiting the actions of chemokines (fractalkine, CCL2), ATP receptors (P2X4, P2X7), MMP-9, p38 MAPK, or/and proinflammatory cytokines (IL-1β, IL-6, and TNF-α) improve their effectiveness. However, this is not the case with DOR agonists. This difference deserves future exploration.

MOR agonists, especially morphine, still remain the drugs of choice for the treatment of neuropathic pain, despite the side effects and limited efficacy. It was shown that DOR agonists were effective in persistent pain [13,68,81,104,105] and the mechanisms underlying this analgesic action was probably linked with trafficking to the cell membrane or better receptor coupling to signalling effectors [104]. Nadal *et al.* [95] demonstrated that neuropathic pain was enhanced in delta-opioid receptor knockout mice. Some authors suggest a delta opioid agonists as a promising alternative to mu analgesics in the treatment of chronic pain [13,95,104,106]. Currently, research is being conducted on analgesic effects of new DOR ligands [107] and some of these substances are being tested in clinical trials [108].

The results of the present study document for the first time that DOR, in contrast to MOR and KOR, are not present in microglial cells (Figure 6). In conclusion, we provide evidence that minocycline not only diminishes neuropathic pain-related behaviour but also enhances the effectiveness of morphine and selective MOR and KOR opioid ligands under neuropathic pain conditions. Our findings lend support to the view that neuroimmunological changes in the spinal cord and DRG are important for opioid effectiveness in neuropathic pain. In our opinion, activated spinal microglia are key factors in not only the development of neuropathic pain but also in the different efficacies of opioid analgesics. Our results also suggest that DOR analgesia is not dependent on injury-induced microglial activation. We therefore suggest that DOR is an interesting target for the development of new drugs that would be effective against neuropathic pain.

Acknowledgments

This work was supported by MNiSzW/NCN grant NN405375937, grant OPUS NCN 2011/03/B/NZ4/00042, grant PRELUDIUM NCN 2012/07/N/NZ3/00379, grant MAESTRO NCN 2012/06/A/NZ4/00028 and statutory funds. Katarzyna Popiolek-Barczyk, is a Ph.D. student and has a scholarship from the KNOW sponsored by the Ministry of Science and Higher Education, Republic of Poland.

Author Contributions

Conceived and designed the experiments: JM KP-B ER KS BP. Performed the experiments: JM KP-B ER WM KS BP. Analyzed the data: JM KP-B ER WM KS BP. Contributed reagents/materials/analysis tools: JM KP-B ER WM KS BP. Wrote the paper: JM KP-B ER KS BP.

References

1. Hirsch SJ, Dickenson AH (2014) Morphine sensitivity of spinal neurons in the chronic constriction injury neuropathic rat pain model. Neurosci Lett 562: 97–101.
2. Przewlocki R, Przewlocka B (2001) Opioids in chronic pain. Eur J Pharmacol 429:79–91.
3. Przewlocki R, Przewlocka B (2005) Opioids in neuropathic pain. Curr Pharm Des 11: 3013–3025.
4. Eisenberg E, McNicol ED, Carr DB (2005) Efficacy and safety of opioid agonists in the treatment of neuropathic pain of non- malignant origin: Systematic review and meta-analysis of randomized controlled trials. JAMA; 293:3043–3052.
5. McQuay HJ (2002) Neuropathic pain: evidence matters. Eur J Pain.;6:11–8.
6. Evans CJ, Keith DE Jr, Morrison H, Magendzo K, Edwards RH (1992) Cloning of a delta opioid receptor by functional expression. Science 258: 1952–1955.
7. Kieffer BL, Befort K, Gavériaux-Ruff C, Hirth CG (1992) The delta-opioid receptor: isolation of a cDNA by expression cloning and pharmacological characterization. Proc Natl Acad Sci U S A 89: 12048–12052.
8. Chen Y, Mestek A, Liu J, Yu L (1993) Molecular cloning of a rat kappa opioid receptor reveals sequence similarities to the mu and delta opioid receptors. Biochem J 295: 625–628.
9. Minami M, Hosoi Y, Toya T, Katao Y, Maekawa K, et al. (1993) In situ hybridization study of kappa-opioid receptor mRNA in the rat brain. Neurosci Lett 162: 161–164.
10. George SR, Fan T, Xie Z, Tse R, Tam V, et al. (2000) Oligomerization of mu- and delta-opioid receptors. Generation of novel functional properties. J Biol Chem 275: 26128–26135.
11. Gomes I, Jordan BA, Gupta A, Trapaidze N, Nagy V, et al. (2000) Heterodimerization of mu and delta opioid receptors: a role in opiate synergy. J Neurosci 20: RC110.
12. Gomes I, Gupta A, Filipovska J, Szeto HH, Pintar JE, et al. (2004) A role for heterodimerization of mu and delta opiate receptors in enhancing morphine analgesia. Proc Natl Acad Sci USA 101: 5135–5139.
13. Mika J, Przewlocki R, Przewłocka B (2001) The role of delta-opioid receptor subtypes in neuropathic pain. Eur J Pharmacol 415: 31–37.

14. Nozaki C, Le Bourdonnec B, Reiss D, Windh RT, Little PJ, et al. (2012) δ-Opioid mechanisms for ADL5747 and ADL5859 effects in mice: analgesia, locomotion, and receptor internalization. J Pharmacol Exp Ther 342: 799–807.
15. Obara I, Parkitna JR, Korostynski M, Makuch W, Kaminska D, et al. (2009) Local peripheral opioid effects and expression of opioid genes in the spinal cord and dorsal root ganglia in neuropathic and inflammatory pain. Pain 141: 283–291.
16. Gavériaux-Ruff C, Kieffer BL (2011) Delta opioid receptor analgesia: recent contributions from pharmacology and molecular approaches. Behav Pharmacol 22: 405–414.
17. Fenalti G, Giguere PM, Katritch V, Huang XP, Thompson AA, et al. (2014) Molecular control of δ-opioid receptor signalling. Nature 506: 191–196.
18. Somvanshi RK, Kumar U (2014) δ-Opioid Receptor and Somatostatin Receptor-4 Heterodimerization: Possible Implications in Modulation of Pain Associated Signaling. PLoS One 9: e85193.
19. Lee YW, Chaplan SR, Yaksh TL (1995) Systemic and supraspinal, but not spinal, opiates suppress allodynia in a rat neuropathic pain model. Neurosci Lett 199: 111–114.
20. Steele AD, Szabo I, Bednar F, Rogers TJ (2002) Interactions between opioid and chemokine receptors: heterologous desensitization. Cytokine Growth Factor Rev 13: 209–222.
21. Osikowicz M, Mika J, Przewlocka B (2013) The glutamatergic system as a target for neuropathic pain relief. Exp Physiol 98: 372–384.
22. Cui Y, Liao XX, Liu W (2008) A novel role of minocycline: attenuating morphine antinociceptive tolerance by inhibition of p38 MAPK in the activated spinal microglia. Brain Behav Immun 22: 114–123.
23. Makuch W, Mika J, Rojewska E, Zychowska M, Przewlocka B (2013) Effects of selective and non-selective inhibitors of nitric oxide synthase on morphine- and endomorphin-1-induced analgesia in acute and neuropathic pain in rats. Neuropharmacology 75: 445–447.
24. Mika J, Rojewska E, Makuch W, Przewlocka B (2010) Minocycline reduces the injury-induced expression of prodynorphin and pronociceptin in the dorsal root ganglion in a rat model of neuropathic pain. Neuroscience 165: 1420–1428.
25. Mika J, Zychowska M, Popiolek-Barczyk K, Rojewska E, Przewlocka B (2013) Importance of glial activation in neuropathic pain. Eur J Pharmacol 716: 106–119.
26. Watkins LR, Maier SF (2003) Glia: a novel drug discovery target for clinical pain. Nat Rev Drug Discov 2: 973–985.
27. Wieseler-Frank J, Maier SF, Watkins LR (2005) Central proinflammatory cytokines and pain enhancement. Neurosignals 14: 166–174.
28. Amin AR, Attur MG, Thakker GD (1996) A novel mechanism of action of tetracyclines: effects on nitric oxide synthases. Proc Natl Acad Sci U S A 93: 14014–14019.
29. Colovic M, Caccia S (2003) Liquid chromatographic determination of minocycline in brain-to-plasma distribution studies in the rat. Life Sci 791: 337–343.
30. Ledeboer A, Sloane EM, Milligan ED, Frank MG, Mahony JH, et al. (2005) Minocycline attenuates mechanical allodynia and proinflammatory cytokine expression in rat models of pain facilitation. Pain 115: 71–83.
31. Pinkernelle J, Fansa H, Ebmeyer U, Keilhoff G (2013) Prolonged minocycline treatment impairs motor neuronal survival and glial function in organotypic rat spinal cord cultures. PLoS One 8: e73422.
32. Tikka T, Fiebich BL, Goldsteins G, Keinanen R, Koistinaho J (2001) Minocycline, a tetracycline derivative, is neuroprotective against excitotoxicity by inhibiting activation and proliferation of microglia. J Neurosci 21: 2580–2508.
33. Niimi N, Kohyama K, Matsumoto Y (2013) Minocycline suppresses experimental autoimmune encephalomyelitis by increasing tissue inhibitors of metalloproteinases. Neuropathology 33: 612–616.
34. Machado LS, Kozak A, Ergul A, Hess DC, Borlongan CV, et al. (2006) Delayed minocycline inhibits ischemia-activated matrix metalloproteinases 2 and 9 after experimental stroke. BMC Neurosci 7: 56.
35. Liu X, Su H, Chu TH, Guo A, Wu W (2013) Minocycline inhibited the pro-apoptotic effect of microglia on neural progenitor cells and protected their neuronal differentiation in vitro. Neurosci Lett 542: 30–36.
36. Garcia-Martinez EM, Sanz-Blasco S, Karachitos A, Bandez MJ, Fernandez-Gomez FJ, et al. (2010) Mitochondria and calcium flux as targets of neuroprotection caused by minocycline in cerebellar granule cells. Biochem Pharmacol 79: 239–250.
37. Kim TH, Kim HI, Kim J, Park M, Song JH (2011) Effects of minocycline on Na+ currents in rat dorsal root ganglion neurons. Brain Res 1370: 34–42.
38. Jin SX, Zhuang ZY, Woolf CJ, Ji RR (2003) p38 mitogen-activated protein kinase is activated after a spinal nerve ligation in spinal cord microglia and dorsal root ganglion neurons and contributes to the generation of neuropathic pain. J Neurosci 23: 4017–4022.
39. Zhuang ZY, Wen YR, Zhang DR, Borsello T, Bonny C, et al. (2006) A peptide c-Jun N-terminal kinase (JNK) inhibitor blocks mechanical allodynia after spinal nerve ligation: respective roles of JNK activation in primary sensory neurons and spinal astrocytes for neuropathic pain development and maintenance. J Neurosci 26: 3551–3560.
40. Chang YW, Waxman SG (2010) Minocycline attenuates mechanical allodynia and central sensitization following peripheral second-degree burn injury. J Pain 11: 1146–1154.
41. Hains BC, Waxman SG (2006) Activated microglia contribute to the maintenance of chronic pain after spinal cord injury. J Neurosci 26: 4308–4317.
42. Hua XY, Svensson CI, Matsui T, Fitzsimmons B, Yaksh TL, et al. (2005) Intrathecal minocycline attenuates peripheral inflammation-induced hyperalgesia by inhibiting p38 MAPK in spinal microglia. Eur J Neurosci 22: 2431–2440.
43. Radad K, Moldzio R, Rausch WD (2010) Minocycline protects dopaminergic neurons against long-term rotenone toxicity. Can J Neurol Sci 37: 81–85
44. González JC, Egea J, Del Carmen Godino M, Fernandez-Gomez FJ, Sánchez-Prieto J, et al. (2007) Neuroprotectant minocycline depresses glutamatergic neurotransmission and Ca(2+) signalling in hippocampal neurons. Eur J Neurosci 26: 2481–2495.
45. Mika J, Osikowicz M, Makuch W, Przewlocka B (2007) Minocycline and pentoxifylline attenuate allodynia and hyperalgesia and potentiate the effects of morphine in rat and mouse models of neuropathic pain. Eur J Pharmacol 560: 142–149.
46. Mika J, Wawrzczak-Bargiela A, Osikowicz M, Makuch W, Przewlocka B (2009) Attenuation of morphine tolerance by minocycline and pentoxifylline in naive and neuropathic mice. Brain Behav Immun 23: 75–84.
47. Zychowska M, Rojewska E, Kreiner G, Nalepa I, Przewlocka B, et al. (2013) Minocycline influences the anti-inflammatory interleukins and enhances the effectiveness of morphine under mice diabetic neuropathy. J Neuroimmunol 262: 35–45.
48. Filipovic R, Zecevic N (2008) Neuroprotective role of minocycline in co-cultures of human fetal neurons and microglia. Exp Neurol 211: 41–51.
49. Kobayashi K, Imagama S, Ohgomori T, Hirano K, Uchimura K, et al. (2013) Minocycline selectively inhibits M1 polarization of microglia. Cell Death Dis 4: e525.
50. Zimmermann M (1983) Ethical guidelines for investigations of experimental pain in conscious animals. Pain 16: 109–110.
51. Bennett GJ, Xie Y (1988) A peripheral mononeuropathy in rat that produces disorders of pain sensation like those seen in man. Pain 33: 87–107.
52. Osikowicz M, Mika J, Makuch W, Przewlocka B (2008) Glutamate receptor ligands attenuate allodynia and hyperalgesia and potentiate morphine effects in a mouse model of neuropathic pain. Pain 139: 117–126.
53. Yaksh TL, Rudy TA (1976) Chronic catheterization of the spinal subarachnoid space. Physiol. Behav 17: 1031–10.
54. Zawadzka M, Kaminska B (2005) A novel mechanism of FK506-mediated neuroprotection: downregulation of cytokine expression in glial cells. Glia 49: 36–51.
55. Przanowski P, Dabrowski M, Ellert-Miklaszewska A, Kloss M, Mieczkowski J, et al. (2014) The signal transducers Stat1 and Stat3 and their novel target Jmjd3 drive the expression of inflammatory genes in microglia. J Mol Med (Berl) 92: 239–254.
56. Chomczynski P, Sacchi N (1987) Single-step method of RNA isolation by acid guanidinium thiocyanate-phenol-chloroform extraction. Anal Biochem 162: 156–159.
57. Mika J, Obara I, Przewlocka B (2011) The role of nociceptin and dynorphin in chronic pain: implications of neuro-glial interaction. Neuropeptides 45: 247–261.
58. Kerros C, Brood I, Sola B, Jauzac P, Allouche S (2010) Reduction of cell proliferation and potentiation of Fas-induced apoptosis by the selective kappa-opioid receptor agonist U50 488 in the multiple myeloma LP-1 cells. J Neuroimmunol 220: 69–78.
59. Abcam website. Available: http://www.abcam.com/delta-opioid-receptor-antibody-ab66317.html. Accessed 2014 May 20.
60. Neuromics website. Available: http://www.neuromics.com/ittrium/visit/A1x66x1y1x85b1x1x9cy1x6217x1x96y1x4fax1x82y1x510x1x7f. Accessed 2014 May 20.
61. Mansson E, Bare L, Yang D (1994) Isolation of a human kappa opioid receptor cDNA from placenta. Biochem Biophys Res Commun 202: 1431–1437.
62. Ko JL, Arvidsson U, Williams FG, Law PY, Elde R, et al. (1999) Visualization of time-dependent redistribution of delta-opioid receptors in neuronal cells during prolonged agonist exposure. Brain Res Mol Brain Res 69: 171–185.
63. Mayer DJ, Mao J, Holt J, Price DD (1999) Cellular mechanisms of neuropathic pain, morphine tolerance, and their interactions. Proc Natl Acad Sci U S A 96: 7731–7736.
64. Ossipov MH, Lopez Y, Nichols ML, Bian D, Porreca F (1995) The loss of antinociceptive efficacy of spinal morphine in rats with nerve ligation injury is prevented by reducing spinal afferent drive. Neurosci Lett 199: 87–90.
65. Rowbotham MC, Twilling L, Davies PS, Reisner L, Taylor K, et al. (2003) Oral opioid therapy for chronic peripheral and central neuropathic pain. N Engl J Med 13: 1223–1232.
66. Gilron I, Bailey JM, Dongsheng Tu ME, Holden RR, et al. (2005) Morphine, Gabapentin, or Their Combination for Neuropathic Pain. N Engl J Med 13: 1324–1334.
67. Przewlocka B, Mika J, Labuz D, Toth G, Przewlocki R (1999) Spinal analgesic action of endomorphins in acute, inflammatory and neuropathic pain in rats. Eur J Pharmacol 367: 189–196.
68. Kabli N, Cahill CM (2007) Anti-allodynic effects of peripheral delta opioid receptors in neuropathic pain. Pain 127: 84–93.

69. Porreca F, Tang QB, Bian D, Riedl M, Elde R, et al. (1998) Spinal opioid mu receptor expression in lumbar spinal cord of rats following nerve injury. Brain Res 795: 197–203.
70. Stone LS, Vulchanova L, Riedl MS, Williams FG, Wilcox GL, et al. (2004) Effects of peripheral nerve injury on delta opioid receptor (DOR) immunoreactivity in the rat spinal cord. Neurosci Lett 361: 208–211.
71. Herradon G, Ezquerra L, Nguyen T, Wang C, Siso A, et al. (2008) Noradrenergic and opioidergic alterations in neuropathy in different rat strains. Neurosci Lett 438: 186–189.
72. Pol O, Murtra P, Caracuel L, Valverde O, Puig MM, et al. (2006) Expression of opioid receptors and c-fos in CB1 knockout mice exposed to neuropathic pain. Neuropharmacology 50: 123–132.
73. Raghavendra V, Tanga F, Rutkowski MD, DeLeo JA (2003) Anti-hyperalgesic and morphine-sparing actions of propentofylline following peripheral nerve injury in rats: mechanistic implications of spinal glia and proinflammatory cytokines. Pain 104: 655–664.
74. Raghavendra V, Rutkowski MD, DeLeo JA (2002) The role of spinal neuroimmune activation in morphine tolerance/hyperalgesia in neuropathic and sham-operated rats. J Neurosci 22: 9980–9989.
75. Mika J, Korostynski M, Kaminska D, Wawrzczak-Bargiela A, Osikowicz M, et al. (2008) Interleukin-1alpha has antiallodynic and antihyperalgesic activities in a rat neuropathic pain model. Pain 13: 587–597.
76. Cunningham CL, Martínez-Cerdeño V, Noctor SC (2013) Microglia regulate the number of neural precursor cells in the developing cerebral cortex. J Neurosci 33: 4216–4233.
77. Quock RM, Burkey TH, Varga E, Hosohata Y, Hosohata K, et al. (1999) The delta-opioid receptor: molecular pharmacology, signal transduction, and the determination of drug efficacy. Pharmacol Rev 51: 503–532.
78. Scherrer G, Imamachi N, Cao YQ, Contet C, Mennicken F, et al. (2009) Dissociation of the opioid receptor mechanisms that control mechanical and heat pain. Cell 137: 1148–1159.
79. Sluka KA, Rohlwing JJ, Bussey RA, Eikenberry SA, Wilken JM (2002) Chronic muscle pain induced by repeated acid Injection is reversed by spinally administered mu- and delta-, but not kappa-, opioid receptor agonists. J Pharmacol Exp Ther 302: 1146–1150.
80. Holdridge SV, Cahill CM (2007a) Spinal administration of a delta opioid receptor agonist attenuates hyperalgesia and allodynia in a rat model of neuropathic pain. Eur J Pain 11: 685–693.
81. Holdridge SV, Armstrong SA, Taylor AM, Cahill CM (2007b) Behavioural and morphological evidence for the involvement of glial cell activation in delta opioid receptor function: implications for the development of opioid tolerance. Mol Pain 3: 7.
82. Chang AC, Chao CC, Takemori AE, Gekker G, Hu S, et al. (1996) Arylacetamide-derived fluorescent probes: synthesis, biological evaluation, and direct fluorescent labeling of kappa opioid receptors in mouse microglial cells. J Med Chem 39: 1729–1735.
83. El-Hage N, Dever SM, Podhaizer EM, Arnatt CK, Zhang Y, et al. (2013) A novel bivalent HIV-1 entry inhibitor reveals fundamental differences in CCR5-μ-opioid receptor interactions between human astroglia and microglia. AIDS 27: 2181–2190.
84. Merighi S, Gessi S, Varani K, Fazzi D, Stefanelli A, et al. (2013) Morphine mediates a proinflammatory phenotype via μ-opioid receptor-PKCε-Akt-ERK1/2 signaling pathway in activated microglial cells. Biochem Pharmacol 86: 487–496.
85. Chao CC, Gekker G, Hu S, Sheng WS, Shark KB, et al. (1996) Kappa opioid receptors in human microglia downregulate human immunodeficiency virus 1 expression. Proc Natl Acad Sci U S A 93: 8051–8056.
86. Chao CC, Hu S, Shark KB, Sheng WS, Gekker G, et al. (1997) Activation of mu opioid receptors inhibits microglial cell chemotaxis. J Pharmacol Exp Ther 281: 998–1004.
87. Turchan-Cholewo J, Dimayuga FO, Ding Q, Keller JN, Hauser KF, et al. (2008) Cell-specific actions of HIV-Tat and morphine on opioid receptor expression in glia. J Neurosci Res 86: 2100–2110.
88. Thorlin T, Persson PA, Eriksson PS, Hansson E, Rönnbäck L (1999) Delta-opioid receptor immunoreactivity on astrocytes is upregulated during mitosis. Glia 25: 370–378.
89. Scherrer G, Tryoen-Tóth P, Filliol D, Matifas A, Laustriat D, et al. (2006) Knockin mice expressing fluorescent delta-opioid receptors uncover G protein-coupled receptor dynamics in vivo. Proc Natl Acad Sci U S A 103: 9691–9696.
90. Commons KG, Milner TA (1996) Cellular and subcellular localization of delta opioid receptor immunoreactivity in the rat dentate gyrus. Brain Res 738: 181–195.
91. Cheng PY, Liu-Chen LY, Pickel VM (1997) Dual ultrastructural immunocytochemical labeling of mu and delta opioid receptors in the superficial layers of the rat cervical spinal cord. Brain Res 778: 367–380.
92. Horvath RJ, DeLeo JA (2009) Morphine enhances microglial migration through modulation of P2X4 receptor signaling. J Neurosci 29: 998–1005.
93. Kieffer BL, Gavériaux-Ruff C (2002) Exploring the opioid system by gene knockout. Prog Neurobiol 66: 285–306.
94. Gavériaux-Ruff C, Karchewski LA, Hever X, Matifas A, Kieffer BL (2008) Inflammatory pain is enhanced in delta opioid receptor-knockout mice. Eur J Neurosci 27: 2558–2567.
95. Nadal X, Baños JE, Kieffer BL, Maldonado R (2006) Neuropathic pain is enhanced in delta-opioid receptor knockout mice. Eur J Neurosci 23: 830–834.
96. Gallantine EL, Meert TF (2005) A comparison of the antinociceptive and adverse effects of the mu-opioid agonist morphine and the delta-opioid agonist SNC80. Basic Clin Pharmacol Toxicol 97: 39–51.
97. Cahill CM, Morinville A, Hoffert C, O'Donnell D, Beaudet A (2003) Up-regulation and trafficking of delta opioid receptor in a model of chronic inflammation: implications for pain control. Pain 101: 199–208.
98. Fraser GL, Gaudreau GA, Clarke PB, Ménard DP, Perkins MN (2000) Antihyperalgesic effects of delta opioid agonists in a rat model of chronic inflammation. Br J Pharmacol 129: 1668–1672.
99. Hurley RW, Hammond DL (2000) The analgesic effects of supraspinal mu and delta opioid receptor agonists are potentiated during persistent inflammation. J Neurosci 20: 1249–1259.
100. Happel C, Steele AD, Finley MJ, Kutzler MA, Rogers TJ (2008) DAMGO-induced expression of chemokines and chemokine receptors: the role of TGF-beta1. J Leukoc Biol 83: 956–963.
101. Szabo I, Chen XH, Xin L, Adler MW, Howard OM, et al. (2002) Heterologous desensitization of opioid receptors by chemokines inhibits chemotaxis and enhances the perception of pain. Proc Natl Acad Sci U S A 99: 10276–10281.
102. Horvath RJ, Romero-Sandoval EA, De Leo JA (2010b) Inhibition of microglial P2X4 receptors attenuates morphine tolerance, Iba1, GFAP and μ opioid receptor protein expression while enhancing perivascular microglial ED2. Pain 150: 401–413.
103. Hutchinson MR, Coats BD, Lewis SS, Zhang Y, Sprunger DB, et al. (2008) Proinflammatory cytokines oppose opioid-induced acute and chronic analgesia. Brain Behav Immun 22: 1178–1189.
104. Cahill CM, Holdridge SV, Morinville A (2007) Trafficking of delta-opioid receptors and other G-protein-coupled receptors: implications for pain and analgesia. Trends Pharmacol Sci 28: 23–31.
105. Bie B, Pan ZZ (2007) Trafficking of central opioid receptors and descending pain inhibition. Mol Pain 3: 37.
106. Zhang X, Bao L, Guan JS (2006) Role of delivery and trafficking of delta-opioid peptide receptors in opioid analgesia and tolerance. Trends Pharmacol Sci. 27:324–329.
107. Pradhan AA, Befort K, Nozaki C, Gavériaux-Ruff C, Kieffer BL (2011) The delta opioid receptor: anevolving target for the treatment of braindisorders. Trends Pharmacol Sci 32: 581–590.
108. Clinicaltrials website. Available: http://clinicaltrials.gov/ct2/results?term = delta+opioid&Search = Search. Accessed 2014 May 20.

Intraoperative and Anesthesia-Related Cardiac Arrest and Its Mortality in Older Patients: A 15-Year Survey in a Tertiary Teaching Hospital

Juscimar C. Nunes[1], Jose R. C. Braz[1], Thais S. Oliveira[1], Lidia R. de Carvalho[2], Yara M. M. Castiglia[1], Leandro G. Braz[1]*

1 Department of Anesthesiology, Botucatu Medical School, UNESP – Univ Estadual Paulista, Botucatu, São Paulo, Brazil, **2** Department of Biostatistics, Institute of Biosciences, UNESP – Univ Estadual Paulista, Botucatu, São Paulo, Brazil

Abstract

Background: Little information is known about factors that influence perioperative and anesthesia-related cardiac arrest (CA) in older patients. This study evaluated the incidence, causes and outcome of intraoperative and anesthesia-related CA in older patients in a Brazilian teaching hospital between 1996 and 2010.

Methods: During the study, older patients received 18,367 anesthetics. Data collected included patient characteristics, surgical procedures, American Society of Anesthesiologists (ASA) physical status, anesthesia type, medical specialty team and outcome. All CAs were categorized by cause into one of four groups: patient's disease/condition-related, surgery-related, totally anesthesia-related or partially anesthesia-related.

Results: All intraoperative CAs and deaths rates are shown per 10,000 anesthetics. There were 100 CAs (54.44; 95% confidence intervals [CI]: 44.68–64.20) and 68 deaths (37.02; 95% CI: 27.56–46.48). The majority of CAs were patient's disease-/condition-related (43.5; 95% CI: 13.44–73.68). There were six anesthesia-related CAs (3.26; 95% CI: 0.65–5.87) - 1 totally and 5 partially anesthesia-related, and three deaths, all partially anesthesia-related (1.63; 95% CI: 0.0–3.47). ASA I-II physical status patients presented no anesthesia-related CA. Anesthesia-related CA, absent in the last five years of the study, was due to medication-/airway-related causes. ASA physical status was the most important predictor of CA (odds ratio: 14.52; 95% CI: 4.48–47.08; $P<0.001$) followed by emergency surgery (odds ratio: 8.07; 95% CI: 5.14–12.68; $P<0.001$).

Conclusions: The study identified high incidence of intraoperative CAs with high mortality in older patients. The large majority of CAs were caused by factors not anesthesia-related. Anesthesia-related CA and mortality rates were 3.26 and 1.63 per 10,000 anesthetics, with no anesthesia-related CA in the last five years of the study. Major predictors of intraoperative CAs were poorer ASA physical status and emergency surgery. All anesthesia-related CAs were medication-related or airway-related, which is important for prevention strategies.

Editor: Giovanni Landoni, San Raffaele Scientific Institute, Italy

Funding: The authors have no funding or support to report.

Competing Interests: The authors have declared that no competing interests exist.

* Email: lbraz@fmb.unesp.br

Introduction

The global population is ageing. According to the World Health Organization, people ≥60 years old in developing countries, such as Brazil, are considered elderly [1]. A significant proportion of older people are living with chronic diseases, such as cardiovascular disease, cognitive impairments and a reduced physiological reserve, which remain a challenge for all areas of medicine [2].

Few studies on perioperative cardiac arrest (CA) and mortality carried out exclusively in geriatric patients undergoing all types of surgery have been published [3–6]. However, there are no studies on anesthesia-related CA and death exclusively in elderly patients. Therefore, little information is known about factors that influence intraoperative and anesthesia-related CA and death in older surgical patients.

A survey performed from 1996 to 2005 in a Brazilian general tertiary teaching hospital [7] and other studies that included patients of all age groups [8,9], found that the perioperative CA and mortality rates were higher in older adults than in young adults. Recognizing the importance of identification of high-risk patients to guide the planning, resourcing, and expert staffing required to enhance the safety and improve the anesthesia outcomes for older patients, our institution developed initiatives for the purpose of improving the care of surgical patients. This involved the organization of services for the care of older patients, including the operating room (OR) materials and equipments such as anesthesia workstations with ventilators to provide adequate ventilation and monitoring, and devices for temperature control, new drugs for anesthesia induction and increasing the number of adult intensive care beds.

The aim of this study was to evaluate the incidence, triggering factors, causes and outcome of intraoperative and anesthesia-related CA in older surgical patients over a 15-yr period in a Brazilian general tertiary teaching hospital.

Methods

The project was approved by the Human Research Ethics Committee of the Botucatu Medical School (Ref: 3694-2010), who waived the requirement for written informed consent. This survey analyzed all reported CA in 18,367 consecutive anesthetics given to all older patients at least 60 years of age requiring anesthesia services at the Hospital of the Botucatu Medical School, *Universidade Estadual Paulista* (UNESP), São Paulo State, Brazil, a public tertiary teaching hospital, from January 1, 1996 to December 31, 2010. The UNESP hospital is a 450-bed tertiary-care referral facility with a catchment of 2 million people that performs approximately 7,000 surgeries per year on people of all age groups. The hospital has a 33-bed adult intensive care unit.

The basic safety monitoring protocol in the OR during regional and neuroaxial anesthesia and sedation included electrocardiogram, automatic non-invasive blood pressure and pulse oximetry. For general anesthesia were measured the core temperature, ventilation parameters, capnography and oxygen concentration. After 2005 the delivered nitrous oxide and halogenated anesthetic vapour concentrations were also measured. Critically ill patients received invasive blood pressure and central venous pressure monitoring. The same basic monitoring described for the OR was also used in the postanesthesia care unit (PACU).

Cardiac arrests and deaths in older patients in the OR and PACU were identified through an anesthesia database developed from a quality assessment form that is part of the mandatory documentation for each anesthetic procedure. The forms were completed by the anesthesia staff responsible for each administration of anesthetic. The recorded data included the date and location; patient characteristics; American Society of Anesthesiologists (ASA) physical status classification; surgical procedures (elective, urgent or emergency surgery); medical specialty team; anesthesia type (general, regional or monitored and supportive anesthesia care associated or not with local anesthesia in critically ill patients); outcome; and a 95-item checklist of airway, respiratory, cardiocirculatory, neurological, renal and miscellaneous events related to the OR or PACU stay.

Cardiac arrest was defined as the cessation of cardiac mechanical activity with loss of effective circulation determined by the absence of a palpable central pulse. The resuscitation was performed according to the interventions and protocols for Advanced Cardiovascular Life Support (ACLS) guidelines.

The anesthetist responsible for each case of CA was asked to review the case and provide a written summary for peer review. The medical and anesthesia records, the written summary, and, when applicable, the necropsy report were analyzed by the Anesthesia Cardiac Arrest Study Commission, which was composed of three authors who are faculty members in the Department of Anesthesiology (YMMC, JRCB and LGB). The triggering factors of CA and death were retrospectively assigned to one of four groups: (1) totally related to the surgery when a technical surgical problem was the only or the major contributory factor, (2) totally related to an older patient's disease or condition, (3) totally related to anesthesia when anesthesia was the only or the major contributory factor or (4) partially related to anesthesia when an older patient's condition/disease or surgical procedure was a factor additional to anesthesia in the CA or death. Unanimity was reached on the triggering factors in the majority of the CAs and deaths. Disagreements among the three members were resolved by discussion, and agreement was reached in all cases when at least two of the three members agreed on the triggering factors.

Some of the CAs in the current study were likely included in our previous study that examined perioperative CAs in all age groups from April 1996 to March 2005, but did not evaluate CAs in older patients exclusively [7]. Thus, only some of these older patients who experienced intraoperative CA (48) are included in the numerator in the present study whereas all of the older patients (6,796 who received anesthesia) are included in the denominator.

Statistical analysis

The incidence (expressed per 10,000 anesthetics) and 95% confidence interval (CI) of intraoperative CA and mortality were calculated according to age, sex, ASA physical status, surgical procedures, anesthetic technique, surgical area and triggering factors. In these cases, the difference between rates were considered statistically significant if their respective 95% CIs did not overlap. Factors predicting intraoperative CA (age, sex, ASA physical status, surgical procedures and anesthesia technique) were analyzed with multivariate forward stepwise logistical regression with odds ratio and 95% CI reported. The conditional independence of all variables and stratifications was verified by the Cochran-Mantel-Haenszel test while the homogeneity of the odds ratio was validated by the Breslow-Day test. The statistical analysis was performed using the software Statistical Package for Social Sciences for Windows (version 17.1; SPSS Inc., Chicago, IL, USA). A P value<0.05 was considered statistically significant.

Results

Over the 15 years of the study, 18,367 older patients were anesthetized. One hundred CAs (54.44 per 10,000 anesthetics; 95% CI: 44.68–64.20) and 68 deaths (37.02 per 10,000 anesthetics; 95% CI: 27.56–46.48) were identified within the intraoperative period (OR and PACU). Thus, only 32% of the older patients who experienced intraoperative CA survived. The majority of CAs and deaths occurred in the OR (93% and 94.12%, respectively) compared with the PACU (7% and 5.88%, respectively).

The intraoperative CA and death incidence in older surgical patients increased with the ASA physical status classification, in emergency surgery (12:1 compared with elective surgery) (Table 1). General anesthesia (6.6:1 compared with neuroaxial anesthesia) and an older patient's disease/condition were important factors of intraoperative CA (13.4:1 compared with anesthesia and 5.7:1 compared with surgery) and death (Tables 2 and 3, respectively). Multiclinical (two or more surgical areas) per 10,000 anesthetics (1034; 95% CI: 706–1,362), cardiac (412; 95% CI: 158–665), vascular (124; 95% CI: 61–185), thoracic (58; 95% CI: 24–91) or gastroenterological surgery (56; 95% CI: 10–102) were also important CA factors.

Poorer ASA physical status (III–V), emergency surgery and general anesthesia were significant predictive factors of intraoperative CA and death in older patient (Tables 4 and 5, respectively). However, age and sex were not predictors of intraoperative CA or mortality (Tables 4 and 5, respectively).

Anesthesia-related CA was considered a contributing factor in 5 cases and a primary factor in 1 case. Furthermore, anesthesia was considered a contributing factor in all 3 anesthesia-related deaths

Table 1. Intraoperative cardiac arrest and death incidences among 18,367 anesthetics according to the characteristics of the older patients.

	Anesthetics	Cardiac Arrests			Deaths		
	n	*n*	Incidence per 10,000	95% CI	*n*	Incidence per 10,000	95% CI
Age, yr							
60–74	13,546	71	52.41	40.25–64.57	48	35.43	25.42–45.44
75–90	4,586	28	61.05	38.50–83.60	19	41.43	22.84–60.02
≥91	235	1	42.55	0.00–125.77	1	42.55	0.00–125.77
Sex							
Male	9,716	56	57.64	36.07–79.21	35	36.02	24.11–47.93
Female	8,651	44	50.86	28.42–73.30	33	38.15	25.16–51.14
ASA physical status							
I	1,836	1	5.45	0.00–20.66	1	5.45	0.00–16.13
II	8,975	2	2.22	0.00–6.87	1	1.11	0.00–3.29
III	5,754	23	39.97	17.10–62.84	16	27.80	14.20–41.40
IV	1,660	54	325.30	194.81–455.79	36	216.86	146.80–286.94
V	142	20	1408.45	650.88–2166.02	14	985.91	495.58–1476.24
Surgical procedures							
Elective	11,531	27	23.41	10.78–36.04	21	18.21	10.43–25.99
Urgent	4,610	10	21.69	1.72–41.66	5	10.84	1.34–20.34
Emergency	2,226	63	283.01	173.32–392.70	42	188.67	132.15–245.19

CI = confidence interval.

Table 2. Intraoperative cardiac arrest and death incidences among 18,367 anesthetics in older patients according to anesthesia technique.

Anesthesia technique	Anesthetics	Cardiac Arrests			Deaths		
	n	*n*	Incidence per 10,000	95% CI	*n*	Incidence per 10,000	95% CI
General anesthesia	10,541	86	81.58	56.70–106.48	57	54.07	40.07–68.07
Regional anesthesia							
- Epidural/spinal	6,520	8	12.27	0.04–24.50	5	7.66	0.95–14.39
- Plexus block	597	0	0.00	0.00–0.00	0	0.00	0.00–0.00
Sedation	488	0	0.00	0.00–0.00	0	0.00	0.00–0.00
Other#	221	6	271.49	10.54–532.44	6	271.49	57.22–485.76

CI = confidence interval;
#Monitored anesthesia and supportive care in ASA IV-V physical status patients.

(Table 3). With regard to the triggering factors, 50% of the older patients who experienced anesthesia-related CAs survived, compared with 28.6% in the cases of surgery-related CAs and 31.25% in those of patient condition-/disease-related CAs. All anesthesia-related CAs and deaths in older surgical patients occurred from 1996 to 2005 at rates of 5.42 (95% CI: 1.2–9.6) and 2.7 (95% CI: 0.0–5.7) per 10,000 anesthetics, respectively, against CA and mortality rates of zero per 10,000 anesthetics in the 2006–2010 period.

Additional information on the 94 intraoperative CAs and 65 deaths attributable to an older patient's disease/condition or surgery factors is provided in Table 6. Sepsis and multiple organ failure were the most common causes of CA, while a ruptured aneurysm was the most common cause of mortality.

Medication-related adverse events accounted for four (66.66%) anesthesia-related CAs, three of which were caused by cardiovascular collapse after neuroaxial anesthesia. Of these three patients, two ASA physical status IV older patients passed away in the OR during vascular surgery (lower limb amputation) while undergoing continuous epidural anesthesia. In the third patient, a 63-year-old male with an ASA physical status of III who suffered a femur fracture in a motor vehicle accident, and had multiple rib fractures, the CA occurred after the administration of a spinal anesthetic with hyperbaric bupivacaine (20 mg). Immediately after anesthesia induction, he developed hypotension and bradycardia, followed by cardiovascular collapse and CA. In this case, CA was attributed entirely to the anesthesia. Fortunately, the patient was successfully resuscitated and recovered completely. There was 1 case of fluid overload followed by acute pulmonary edema in the PACU after general anesthesia in a female patient with an ASA physical status of III and a medical history of chronic renal failure. This patient passed away.

Respiratory events accounted for two (33.33%) anesthesia-related CAs. In both cases, there was loss of airway and difficulty to intubate while the patients had significant underlying disease with an ASA physical status of III or IV. One patient with chronic obstructive pulmonary disease and *diabetes mellitus* had a cervical abscess and mediastinitis; intubation and ventilation were difficult after general anesthesia induction followed by hypoxemia, cardiovascular collapse and CA. The patient was successfully resuscitated and recovered. In another case, a patient, with atrial fibrillation after thoracoscopy to drain a pleural effusion, undergoing general anesthesia presented hypoventilation after tracheal extubation in the PACU followed by a difficult intubation, hypoxemia and CA. The patient was successfully resuscitated and recovered with myocardial infarction.

Discussion

The main findings in this study were: (i) older patients continued to present high incidence of intraoperative CA with high mortality; (ii) anesthesia-related CA and mortality rates were 3.26 and 1.63 per 10,000 anesthetics, respectively; (iii) there was no anesthesia-related CA in ASA I–II physical status patients; (iv) there were no anesthesia-related CA and deaths rates in the last five years of the study; (v) the large majority of CAs (94%) and deaths (95.5%) that occurred during anesthesia were caused by factors not anesthesia-related, and (vi) ASA physical status and emergency surgery, but not age and sex, were significant predictors of intraoperative CA and death in older patients.

A study conducted in Thailand in older surgical patients reported a 24-hour perioperative death rate of 39.33 per 10,000 anesthetics [5]. Another Thai study reported 24-hour perioperative CA and death rates of 40.42 and 31.44 per 10,000 anesthetics,

Table 3. Intraoperative cardiac arrest and death incidences among 18,367 anesthetics in older patients according to triggering factor.

	Cardiac Arrests			Deaths		
Triggering factor	**n**	**Incidence per 10,000**	**95% CI**	**n**	**Incidence per 10,000**	**95% CI**
Patient's disease/condition	80	43.55	13.44–73.60	55	29.94	22.05–37.85
Surgery	14	7.62	3.63–11.61	10	5.44	2.07–8.81
Anesthesia	6	3.26	0.65–5.87	3	1.63	0.00–3.4
- Totally-related	1	0.54	-	0	0.00	-
- Partially-related	5	2.72	-	3	1.63	-

CI = confidence interval.

respectively, in older patients who underwent non-cardiac surgery [3]. A previous survey of the perioperative CA rate in all age groups conducted at our institution revealed a higher incidence of perioperative CA in older patients of 70.62 per 10,000 anesthetics [7]. A few other studies conducted in developed countries in the last decade reported lower perioperative CA rates ranging from 10.73 to 16.08 per 10,000 anesthetics in older surgical patients [9,10]. A systematic review [11] and a meta-analysis [12] of the literature verified that perioperative mortality rates reported in surgical patients of all age groups were higher in developing than in developed countries.

It is difficult to compare the intraoperative CA and mortality rates in our study with the results of previous studies (Table 7) because of considerable differences in the methods and patient populations among studies [3,5–10,13–16]. There is no consensus in the literature regarding the definition of perioperative and anesthesia-related mortality [17].

Some perioperative CA studies excluded ASA V older patients [8], cardiac surgery [3,6,9,13,16] or trauma [9] and transplant surgeries [9,16]. Therefore, the inclusion of both all surgery types and poorer ASA physical status patients, resulting from certain pre-existing morbidities, certainly influenced our CA and death rates. Ninety-seven percent of the intraoperative CAs occurred in poorer ASA physical status (III–V) patients with sepsis and multiple organ failure being the most important causes (30.8%). Sepsis occurs at a high incidence in Brazil and other developing countries with high mortality [18].

The elderly are more predisposed to vascular disease than young persons. Thus, a ruptured aneurysm, or complications associated with cardiac surgery or intraoperative myocardial infarction were also important causes of intraoperative CA and death attributed to an older patient's disease/condition or surgical factors in the current study. Our study demonstrated that patients presenting a poorer ASA physical status (III–V) were more likely (14-fold) to suffer intraoperative CA than ASA I–II patients. Previous studies have shown a similar association of perioperative CA and mortality with poorer ASA physical status in the older individuals [3,5,6]. In our study, it was verified that many older patients arrived at the OR in poor health. Intraoperative CAs and deaths that occurred in some of these patients might have been

Table 4. Factors associated with intraoperative cardiac arrest in older patients.

Factors	Odds Ratio	95% CI	Estimated Coefficient	*P* value
Age, yr				
60–74	1.0 (Reference)			
75–90	0.89	0.57–1.42	−0.10	0.65
≥91	0.70	0.09–5.27	−0.35	0.73
Sex				
Male	1.0 (Reference)			
Female	1.01	0.67–1.52	0.10	0.96
ASA physical status				
I–II	1.0 (Reference)			
III–V	14.52	4.48–47.08	2.67	<0.001
Surgical procedures				
Nonemergency	1.0 (Reference)			
Emergency	8.07	5.14–12.68	2.09	<0.001
Anesthesia technique				
No general anesthesia	1.0 (Reference)			
General anesthesia	4.31	2.21–8.41	1.46	<0.001

ASA = American Society of Anesthesiologists; OR: odds ratio; CI = confidence interval.

Table 5. Factors associated with intraoperative mortality in older patients.

Factors	Odds Ratio	95% CI	Estimated Coefficient	*P* value
Age, yr				
60–74	1.0 (Reference)			
75–90	0.91	0.56–1.59	−0.09	0.75
≥91	1.07	0.14–8.16	0.07	0.97
Sex				
Male	1.0 (Reference)			
Female	0.858	0.52–1.40	−0.15	0.54
ASA physical status				
I–II	1.0 (Reference)			
III–V	13.34	3.15–56.47	2.59	<0.001
Surgical procedures				
Nonemergency	1.0 (Reference)			
Emergency	7.14	4.16–12.26	1.97	<0.001
Anesthesia technique				
No general anesthesia	1.0 (Reference)			
General anesthesia	4.06	1.86–8.85	1.40	<0.001

ASA = American Society of Anesthesiologists; OR: odds ratio; CI = confidence interval.

prevented by an adequate preoperative assessment. A study showed that perioperative death might have been prevented by anesthesia care in approximately 1 per 13,900 anesthetics [19]. These findings demonstrate a persistent need to improve the quantity and quality of resource utilization and access to healthcare, which are inadequate in Brazil and in other developing countries. In addition, it is necessary to adopt perioperative medical practices with demonstrable effectiveness, organize multidisciplinary discussion of adverse effects and implement of evidence-based safety protocols to improve perioperative patient care [20,21].

As demonstrated in our study and in others [3,5,6], the urgency of surgery is a well-established preoperative predictive factor for intraoperative CA and mortality in older patients. The risk of CA in emergency surgery is likely due to many factors, such as the impossibility of adequate evaluation and optimization of the patients before the surgery.

Despite the differences in methodology, studies [6–10,15] have suggested that anesthesia-related CA and mortality rates in older people are lower today than they were 40 years ago (35.91 per 10,000 anesthetics) [14]. Most studies performed in the last two decades in developed countries have reported in older patients anesthesia-related death rates ranging from 0.00 to 1.72 per 10,000 anesthetics [8,15,19], which represents an improvement of almost twenty-fold. Our study confirmed this trend (i.e., 1.63 anesthesia-related deaths per 10,000 anesthetics in its entire timeframe and zero per 10,000 anesthetics in its last five years in older patients). These data may be associated with the improvements achieved in the geriatric anesthesia safety in our institution in the recent years.

Table 6. Causes of intraoperative cardiac arrests and deaths attributed to an older patient's disease/condition or surgical factors.

	Cardiac arrests		Deaths		Mortality
Cause	*n*	%	*n*	%	%
Sepsis and multiple organ failure	29	30.85	14	21.53	48.27
Ruptured aneurysm: abdominal, thoracic or cerebral	21	22.34	19	29.23	90.48
Complications associated with cardiac surgery including inability to wean from cardiopulmonary bypass	19	20.22	15	23.08	78.95
Intraoperative myocardial infarction	6	6.38	4	6.15	66.66
Trauma: motor vehicle accident, gunshot wound or stab wound with exsanguinating hemorrhage	5	5.32	4	6.15	80.00
Exsanguinating hemorrhage during surgery associated with primary disease	5	5.32	3	4.62	60.00
Pulmonary embolus	3	3.19	3	4.62	100.0
Complications associated with radical cancer surgery	3	3.19	2	3.08	66.66
Technical surgical complications	3	3.19	1	1.54	33.34

Table 7. Previous studies of perioperative and anesthesia-related cardiac arrest and mortality in older patients.

Investigators and publication	Time period and data source	Number of patients Time of CA/ death	Age (yr)	CA incidence per 10,000 anesthetics		Mortality incidence per 10,000 anesthetics	
				Perioperative	Anesthesia-related	Perioperative	Anesthesia-related
Marx et al. [14]	1965–1969	4,176	**>60**	**NR**	**NR**	**514.84**	**35.91**
1973	Teaching hospital	Death within 7 days	61–70			442.02	20.40
	USA		71–80			679.86	34.23
			>81			821.91	684.93
Olsson & Hallen [13]]	1967–1984	NR	**>60**	**NR**	**7.1**	**NR**	**NR**
1988	Teaching hospital	CA and death in OR					
	Sweden	Excluded: cardiac surgery					
Aubas et al. [15]	1983–1987	34,633	**≥55**	**NR**	**4.33**	**NR**	**1.44**
1991	Teaching hospital	CA and deaths in OR and PACU	55–74		2.67		1.14
	France		75–84		8.86		2.95
			≥85		12.04		0
Kubota et al. [16]	1962–1992	15,351	**≥65**	**NR**	**0.65**	**NR**	**0**
1994	Teaching hospital	CA and death in OR	65–70		0		0
	Japan	Excluded: cardiac surgery	70–80		1.66		0
		transplant cases					
			80–90		0		0
			90–95		0		0
Biboulet et al. [8]	1989–1995	28,987	**≥55**	**NR**	**2.75**	**NR**	**1.72**
2001	Teaching hospital	CA and death within 12 h	55–74		1.86		0.46
	France	Excluded: ASA V patients	75–84		1.83		1.83
			>84		14.36		14.36
Kawashima et al. [10]]	1999	208,568	**≥66**	**10.73**	**NR**	**NR**	**0.33**
2002	Group of hospitals	CA and death within 7 days	66–85	11.02		6.56	0.25
	Japan		≥86	6.66		5.18	1.48
Braz et al. [7]	1996–2005	6,796	**≥65**	**70.62**	**5.88**	**NR**	**2.94**
2006	Teaching hospital	CA and death in OR and PACU	65–79	68.78	5.29		1.75
	Brazil		≥80	79.33	8.88		8.88
***Rodanant et al.** [5]	2003–2004	23,899	**≥65**	**NR**	**NR**	**39.33**	**NR**
2007	Group of hospitals	Deaths within 24 h					
	Thailand						
***Tamdee et al.** [3]	2003–2007	8,905	**≥65**	**40.42**	**NR**	**31.44**	**NR**
2009	Teaching hospital	CA and death within 24 h	65–75	22.87			
	Thailand	Excluded: cardiac surgery	76–85	67.22			

Table 7. Cont.

Investigators and publication	Time period and data source	Number of patients Time of CA/ death	Age (yr)	CA incidence per 10,000 anesthetics		Mortality incidence per 10,000 anesthetics	
				Perioperative	Anesthesia-related	Perioperative	Anesthesia-related
			>86	148.51			
***Story et al.** [6]	2004, 2007–2008	4,158	**≥70**	**NR**	**NR**	**519.48**	**NR**
2010	Group of hospitals	Deaths within 30 days	70–79			355.4	
	Australia, New Zealand	Excluded: cardiac surgery	80–89			695.6	
			≥90			1219.5	
Goswani et al. [9]	2005 - 2007	223,961	**≥70**	**16.08**	**NR**	**NR**	**NR**
2012	Group of hospitals	CA in OR					
	USA	Excluded: cardiac surgery					
		peripheral nerve block					
		trauma cases					
		transplant cases					
Current study	1996–2010	18,367	**≥60**	**54.44**	**3.26**	**37.02**	**1.63**
	Teaching hospital	CA and death in OR and PACU	60–74	52.41	2.95	35.43	1.47
	Brazil		75–90	61.05	4.36	41.43	2.18
			≥91	42.55	0	42.55	0

*Studies that included only older patients; CA: cardiac arrest; NR: not reported; OR: operating room; ASA = American Society of Anesthesiologists; PACU: postanesthesia care unit.

In contrast to our current study, many prior works have identified advanced age (>75 yr) as a risk factor for perioperative CA [3,6,8,15], and also did not find age itself to be an independent risk factor [10].

Sex was not a risk factor for intraoperative CA in our study. Sex is known to be a significant risk factor for perioperative CA and mortality in young men suffering from trauma [7]. In our study, trauma was the fifth highest cause of intraoperative CA and death in older surgical patients. The elderly are less predisposed to trauma and violence than young persons.

Our study showed that general anesthesia was a predictor of intraoperative CA. However, this may be attributable to the fact that many high-risk surgeries (cardiac, thoracic, vascular, gastroenterological) in older patients were performed under general anesthesia. Another possible confounding factor in this case is that the anesthesiologist often prefers to give general anesthesia to the most fragile patients, independently of the type of surgery.

In our study, respiratory causes of anesthesia-related CA were less frequent (33%) than medication causes (67%). In a recent study in all age groups [22], the authors verified that 64% of anesthesia-related CAs were caused by airway complications. There were three cases of CA after the administration of neuroaxial anesthesia. After neuroaxial anesthesia, a condition in which the loss of sympathetically mediated vasoconstriction may decrease vascular resistance, and the loss of sympathetically mediated cardiac stimulation may diminish both the heart rate and stroke volume. The vasodilatation may permit the peripheral pooling of blood and lower the end-diastolic volume, stroke volume and cardiac output in older patients [23]. In the last five years of our study, we preferentially used isobaric bupivacaine for spinal anesthesia in older patients. This local anesthetic determines lower levels of sympathetic block with lower cardiovascular effects than hyperbaric bupivacaine in older patients [24].

There may have been some methodological weaknesses in our study. First, the data are derived from adverse events reported by faculty and residents. Underreporting is likely in this situation, even though filling out the form for each case was mandatory. To minimize the risk of underreporting CAs and deaths, the information was cross-checked with the operating theater records and hospital administration. Second, this study is representative of the experience in one tertiary referral center. Practices specific to our institution may have influenced our results and may not represent the entire spectrum of elderly patient care practices. A multi-institutional anesthesia database would not only provide useful insights into injury mechanisms, but would also facilitate the development of universally applicable strategies [25].

Conclusions

Our study has identified high incidence of intraoperative CA with high mortality in older patients. The majority of CAs and deaths were caused by factors not related to anesthesia. Anesthesia-related CA and death rates were 3.26 and 1.63 per 10,000 anesthetics, respectively. Improvements achieved in anesthesia safety in the older patients in our institution allowed no anesthesia-related CA and mortality in the last five years of the study and no anesthesia-related CA in ASA I-II physical status older patients. Major predictor of CA and death was a preoperative indicator of health, the ASA physical status, followed by emergency surgery. The fact that all anesthesia-related CAs were associated with medication administration or airway management is important for the development of prevention strategies. The high fatality rate in older surgical patients due to poor physical status suggests that primary prevention might be the key to reducing mortality from intraoperative CA. These findings indicate the need to improve medical perioperative practices for older people with highly complex medical problems in a demonstrably effective manner in under-resourced settings.

Acknowledgments

J. C. Nunes was granted a scholarship from CAPES/DINTER and T. S. Oliveira was granted a scholarship from PIBIC/CNPq. CAPES and CNPq are Brazilian governmental agencies dedicated to promoting scientific research.

Author Contributions

Conceived and designed the experiments: JCN JRCB LGB. Performed the experiments: JCN JRCB LGB. Analyzed the data: JCN JRCB TSO LRDC YMMC LGB. Contributed to the writing of the manuscript: JCN JRCB TSO YMMC LGB.

References

1. World Health Organization website. Available: http://www.who.int/features/factfiles/ageing/en/index.html. Accessed 2013 July 18.
2. Ward SA, Parikh S, Workman B (2011) Health perspectives: international epidemiology of ageing. Best Pract Res Clin Anaesthesiol 25: 305–317.
3. Tamdee D, Charuluxananan S, Punjasawadwong Y Tawichasri C, Kyokong O, et al. (2009) Factors related to 24-hour perioperative cardiac arrest in geriatric patients in a Thai university hospital. J Med Assoc Thai 92: 198–207.
4. Tuchinda L, Sukchareon I, Kusumaphanyo C, Suratsunya T, Hintong T, et al. (2010) The Thai Anesthesia Incident Monitoring Study (Thai AIMS): an analysis of perioperative complication in geriatric patients. J Med Assoc Thai 93: 698–707.
5. Rodanant O, Hintong T, Chua-in W, Tanudsintum S, Sirinanmd C, et al. (2007) The Thai anesthesia incidents study (THAI Study) of perioperative death in geriatric patients. J Med Assoc Thai 90: 1375–1381.
6. Story DA, Leslie K, Myles PS, Fink M, Poustie SJ, et al. (2010) Complications and mortality in older surgical patients in Australia and New Zealand (the REASON study): a multicentre, prospective, observational study. Anaesthesia 65: 1022–1030.
7. Braz LG, Módolo NS, do Nascimento P Jr, Bruschi BA, Castiglia YM, et al. (2006) Perioperative cardiac arrest: a study of 53,718 anesthetics over 9 yr from a Brazilian teaching hospital. Br J Anaesth 96: 569–575.
8. Biboulet P, Aubas P, Dubourdieu J, Rubenovitch J, Capdevila X, et al. (2001) Fatal and non fatal cardiac arrests related to anesthesia. Can J Anaesth 48: 326–332.
9. Goswami S, Brady JE, Jordan DA, Li G (2012) Intraoperative cardiac arrests in adults undergoing noncardiac surgery: incidence, risk factors, and survival outcome. Anesthesiology 117: 1018–1026.
10. Kawashima Y, Seo N, Morita K, Irita K, Iwao Y, et al. (2002) Anesthesia-related mortality and morbidity in Japan (1999). J Anesth 16: 319–331.
11. Braz LG, Braz DG, Cruz DS, Fernandes LA, Módolo NS, et al. (2009) Mortality in anesthesia: a systematic review. Clinics 64: 999–1006.
12. Bainbridge D, Martin J, Arango M, Cheng D (2012) Perioperative and anaesthetic-related mortality in developed and developing countries: a systematic review and meta-analysis. Lancet 380: 1075–1081.
13. Olsson GL, Hallen B (1988) Cardiac arrest during anaesthesia: A computer-aided study in 250,543 anaesthetics. Acta Anaesthesiol Scand 32: 653–664.
14. Marx GF, Mateo CV, Orkin LR (1973) Computer analysis of postanesthetic deaths. Anesthesiology 39: 54–58.
15. Aubas S, Biboulet P, Daures JP, du Cailar J (1991) Incidence and etiology of cardiac arrest occurring during the peroperative period and in the recovery room. A propos of 102,468 anesthesia cases. Ann Fr Anesth Reanim 10: 436–442.
16. Kubota Y, Toyoda Y, Kubota H, Ueda Y, Asad A, et al. (1994) Frequency of anesthetic cardiac arrest and death in the operating room at a single general hospital over a 30-year period. J Clin Anesth 6: 227–238.
17. Deshpande JK (2011) Cause and effect or conjecture? A call for consensus on defining "anesthesia-related mortality." Anesth Analg 112: 1259–1261.
18. Silva E, Cavalcanti AB, Bugano DD, Janes JM, Vallet B, et al. (2012) Do established prognostic factors explain the different mortality rates in ICU septic patients around the world? Minerva Anestesiol 78: 1215–1225.
19. Bishop MJ, Souders JE, Peterson CM, Henderson WG, Domino KB (2008) Factors associated with unanticipated day of surgery deaths in Department of Veterans Affairs hospitals. Anesth Analg 107: 1924–1935.

20. Pearse RM, Holt PJ, Grocott MP (2011) Managing perioperative risk in patients undergoing elective non-cardiac surgery. BMJ 343:d5759
21. Kehlet H, Wilmore DW (2008) Evidence-based surgical care and the evolution of fast-track surgery. Ann Surg 248: 189–198.
22. Ellis SJ, Newland MC, Simonson JA, Peters KR, Romberger DJ, et al. (2014) Anesthesia-related cardiac arrest. Anesthesiology 120: 829–838.
23. Rooke GA (2003) Cardiovascular aging and anesthetic implications. J Cardiothorac Vasc Anesth 17: 512–523.
24. Møller IW, Fernandes A, Edström HH (1984) Subarachnoid anaesthesia with 0.5% bupivacaine: effects of density. Br J Anaesth 56: 1191–1195.
25. Morray JP (2011) Cardiac arrest in anesthetized children: recent advances and challenges for the future. Pediatr Anesth 21: 722–729.

Comparative Persistence of the TNF Antagonists in Rheumatoid Arthritis – A Population-Based Cohort Study

Anat Fisher[1,2]*, Ken Bassett[1,2,3], James M. Wright[1,2,4], M. Alan Brookhart[5], Hugh Freeman[4], Colin R. Dormuth[1,2]

1 Therapeutics Initiative, University of British Columbia, Vancouver, Canada, **2** Department of Anesthesiology, Pharmacology & Therapeutics, University of British Columbia, Vancouver, Canada, **3** Department of Family Practice, University of British Columbia, Vancouver, Canada, **4** Department of Medicine, University of British Columbia, Vancouver, Canada, **5** Department of Epidemiology, Gillings School of Global Public Health, University of North Carolina, Chapel Hill, North Carolina, United States of America

Abstract

Objective: To compare persistence with tumor necrosis factor alpha (TNF) antagonists among rheumatoid arthritis patients in British Columbia. Treatment persistence has been suggested as a proxy for real-world therapeutic benefit and harm of treatments for chronic non-curable diseases, including rheumatoid arthritis. We hypothesized that the different pharmacological characteristics of infliximab, adalimumab and etanercept cause statistically and clinically significant differences in persistence.

Methods: We conducted a population-based cohort study using administrative health data from the Canadian province of British Columbia. The study cohort included rheumatoid arthritis patients who initiated the first course of a TNF antagonist between 2001 and 2008. Persistence was measured as the time between first dispensing to discontinuation. Drug discontinuation was defined as a drug-free interval of 180 days or switching to another TNF antagonist, anakinra, rituximab or abatacept. Persistence was estimated and compared using survival analysis.

Results: The study cohort included 2,923 patients, 63% treated with etanercept. Median persistence in years (95% confidence interval) with infliximab was 3.7 (2.9–4.9), with adalimumab 3.3 (2.6–4.1) and with etanercept 3.8 (3.3–4.3). Similar risk of discontinuation was observed for the three drugs: the hazard ratio (95% confidence interval) was 0.98 (0.85–1.13) comparing infliximab with etanercept, 0.95 (0.78–1.15) comparing infliximab with adalimumab and 1.04 (0.88–1.22) comparing adalimumab with etanercept.

Conclusions: Similar persistence was observed with infliximab, adalimumab and etanercept in rheumatoid arthritis patients during the first 9 years of use. If treatment persistence is a good proxy for the therapeutic benefit and harm of these drugs, then this finding suggests that the three drugs share an overall similar benefit-harm profile in rheumatoid arthritis patients.

Editor: Paul Proost, University of Leuven, Rega Institute, Belgium

Funding: The study was supported by the University of British Columbia Graduate Fellowship and a grant to the University of British Columbia from the British Columbia Ministry of Health. The funders had no role in study design, data collection and analysis, decision to publish, or preparation of the manuscript.

Competing Interests: The authors have declared that no competing interests exist.

* Email: anat.fisher@ti.ubc.ca

Introduction

The tumor necrosis factor alpha (TNF) antagonists are a relatively new class of drugs used to treat multiple inflammatory diseases, including rheumatoid arthritis (RA). These drugs bind and inactivate TNF, a cytokine that primarily acts as a proinflammation mediator and is thought to be important in the pathogenesis of RA [1].

Treatment with a TNF antagonist is not a cure [2] but rather reduces the symptoms of inflammation, possibly inducing remission and preventing long-term complications.

Randomized clinical trials (RCTs) are limited in their ability to provide evidence on the relative benefit and harm of TNF antagonists in real-world setting for several reasons. First, there are no head-to-head RCTs comparing two (or more) individual TNF antagonists. Multiple indirect comparisons have reported inconsistent estimates of relative efficacy and safety [3–9]. Second, the duration of RCTs is considerably shorter than the lifetime of the disease. Since RA is characterized by a variation in disease activity and deterioration over time, effects observed in a short-term trial may not be significant in the long-term and a drug which had no short-term effects may prevent complications or progression of the disease over the long-term [10,11]. Last, RA patients who participate in RCTs designed to assess therapeutic benefit and harm of TNF antagonists are not representative of actual RA populations treated with TNF antagonists in routine clinical settings [12–15]. Furthermore, patients eligible to participate in RCTs had an improved response compared to ineligible patients

[12–14], and therefore an overestimation of therapeutic benefit is likely.

Real-life drug persistence was suggested as a simple indirect approach for assessing long-term therapeutic benefit and harm [10]. This suggestion is based on the assumption that when using a drug that reduces symptoms and prevents complications (but does not cure the disease), patients persist with the treatment as long as they experience or perceive a benefit and they do not experience (or perceive) an unacceptable amount of harm. This theoretical perspective on persistence seems to hold for TNF antagonist drugs – the main reasons for discontinuing or switching these drugs in RA were decreased benefit (36–67% of the discontinuations) or perceived harm (30–58%) [16–21].

Estimates of comparative persistence with TNF antagonists in RA patients remain controversial and estimates could not be pooled due to differences in measures of persistence (e.g. median, mean, percentage of persistent patients after 1-year) [22,23]. Hence, high quality research is warrant to provide evidence on comparative persistence of these drugs.

Each TNF antagonist has different pharmacological properties [24–26] and therefore substantive differences in therapeutic benefit and harm are expected. Since most discontinuations of these drugs are due to decreased benefit or increased harm, we hypothesized that differences in therapeutic effects would lead to differences in persistence between the TNF anatgonists in RA patients. The main objective of the current study was to compare persistence with infliximab, adalimumab and etanercept in RA in the Canadian province of British Columbia.

Patients and Methods

Patients were identified using four British Columbia Ministry of Health administrative databases: PharmaNet (pharmacy dispensing data), Medical Service Plan (MSP) registration information (demographic data), MSP payment information (fee-for-service payments to physicians and alternative providers), and the Discharge Abstract Database (hospital separations). The databases were linked using a unique anonymized identifier. Follow-up data were available until December 31, 2009. The study protocol was approved by the Clinical Research Ethics Board of the University of British Columbia. Patient records and physician information were anonymized and de-identified prior to analysis.

The study cohort was identified based on (1) exposure to infliximab, adalimumab or etanercept and (2) diagnosis of RA. Exposure to TNF antagonist was defined as at least one recorded dispensing claim of infliximab, adalimumab or etanercept between March 2001 and December 31, 2008. The index date was the date of the first dispensing event. We defined a pre-study period of three years preceding the index date during which patients were required to have continuous provincial MSP coverage. A gap shorter than 30 days was not considered to be an interruption in MSP coverage. The pre-study period ensured a standard run-in period of at least three years without TNF antagonist exposure and a standard period during which diagnosis of RA was required.

RA patients were selected into the study cohort if they had two outpatient visits in physician clinics with a diagnosis code of RA (ICD-9 714.XX) at least 60 days apart, or at least one hospitalization with a recorded discharge diagnosis of RA in the pre-study period. This method was similar, though not identical, to criteria previously used in British Columbia data [27]. Patients entering the cohort were assigned to mutually exclusive exposure categories based on the first TNF antagonist they received (i.e., infliximab, adalimumab or etanercept). None of the patients was dispensed two or more different TNF antagonists at the index date. Patients were excluded if they were previously treated with anakinra, rituximab or abatacept, or if either sex or date of birth was not available. In addition, patients were excluded if they had a concurrent diagnosis of Crohn's disease (based on at least one outpatient or inpatient diagnosis code in the pre-study period) or if they were younger than 18 years at the index date (to remove patients with juvenile RA).

During the study period, clinical guidelines and the provincial drug coverage policy considered the drugs comparable [28,29]; nevertheless, the choice of a specific TNF antagonist could be associated with factors that influence drug persistence, such as age or disease severity. Demographic and clinical status variables were included in the multivariate regression model to minimize the effect of such possible confounders. Patient demographic variables included sex, age and a proxy variable for socio-economic status (the annual deductible for prescription cost, which was based on family annual income [30]). We used four mutually exclusive age categories: 18–30, 30–70 (reference), 70–80 and >80 years old, based on a preliminary analysis that demonstrated homogeneous persistence within each age category. Clinical status variables included the number of inpatient and outpatient encounters in the year prior to index, the duration of disease (defined as time from the first recording of diagnostic code of RA in the data to the index) and the presence and severity of comorbidities. We used Quan's algorithm for administrative databases [31] to determine the Charlson comorbidity score [32] during the year preceding the index, but excluding rheumatic diseases. The regression model also contained three variables for other antirheumatic (synthetic) drugs. Two binary variables were: (1) concomitant methotrexate in the 200 days prior to index, where the dispensing period of 200 days reflected average plus two standard deviations of between-dispensing intervals of methotrexate in the study cohort; and (2) dispensing of any nonsteroidal anti-inflammatory drug (NSAID) in the year preceding the index. The third drug variable was the number of previous antirheumatic drugs in the pre-study period. Dispensing records for nine drugs were sought: methotrexate, hydroxychloroquine, sulfasalazine, azathioprine, cyclosporine, minocycline, penicillamine, sodium aurothiomalate, prednisone and intra-articular triamcinolone/methylprednisolone acetate. We included a categorical variable for the calendar year of the index date, which allowed adjustment for possible secular trends in clinical practice [33,34] and late availability of adalimumab (3 years after infliximab and etanercept).

Finally, we included a series of 12 binary variables for high-volume prescribers who initiated more than 70 courses in the study cohort. This series allowed adjustment for differences (an increase or a decrease) in the risk of discontinuing any TNF antagonist in patients treated by a particular physician. We used the prescriber recorded on the first dispensing claim for TNF antagonist as a proxy of the care-providing physician. The prescribers were determined using an anonymized identifier.

Our outcome was persistence (continuous variable), measured in years from index until drug discontinuation. Drug discontinuation was defined as either switching to another 'biologic' antirheumatic drug (TNF antagonists including certolizumab and golimumab, anakinra, rituximab and abatacept) or elapsing of a drug-free interval of 180 days. A drug-free interval was defined as a period without additional dispensing of the same pharmaceutical component after the days-supply of the latest dispensing claim was exhausted. Adding-on a synthetic antirheumatic drug was not considered discontinuation. We selected a long drug free interval that was previously used in similar studies [35] to ensure that we capture events of discontinuation and not only temporary decrease in adherence (patients who had short gaps in treatment and then

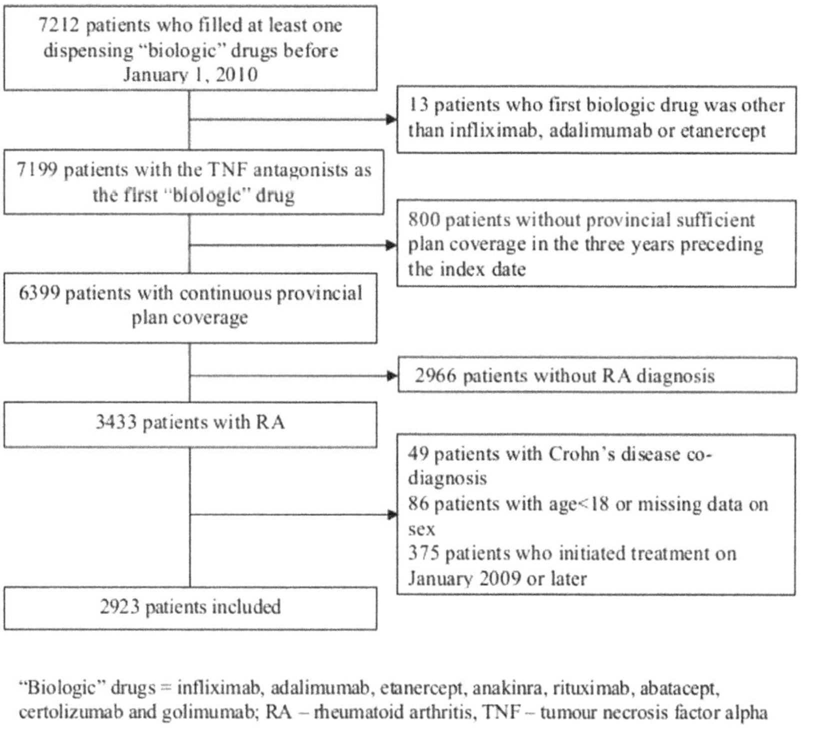

Figure 1. Patients' Flow.

resume the same drug). Discontinuation date was set to the end of days-supply of the latest dispensing event or the date of the first dispensing claim of a different 'biologic' antirheumatic drug, whichever was earliest. Patients were considered censored if they were continuously treated with the first TNF antagonist on December 31, 2009 (end of follow-up period) or during an interruption of more than six days in the provincial MSP coverage. The most common causes of prolonged or infinite interruptions were emigration from the province and death.

Original data on the number of days-supply recorded in PharmaNet were unreliable and frequently did not match the quantity dispensed. Therefore we also calculated days-supply based on dispensed quantity, which, if required, was imputed using the recorded total cost. We considered the prescription cost to be the most accurate and reliable quantity field; given the high cost of these medications, the number of vials or milligrams dispensed could be easily defined. We used the longest duration of days-supply, recorded or calculated, to determine both the length of a drug-free interval and the date of drug discontinuation.

Statistical Methods

Baseline characteristics were presented and compared across the three drug groups. We assumed normality of continuous variables and the significance of differences between groups was assessed with one-way analysis of variance (ANOVA) F-test for continuous variables and the Pearson's Chi-square test for categorical variables. The crude and adjusted hazard ratios for drug discontinuation were estimated using Cox proportional hazards regression. Three pairwise comparisons were presented: infliximab versus adalimumab, infliximab versus etanercept and adalimumab versus etanercept. Drug-sex and drug-age interactions were examined but were included in the final models only if the overall significance was <0.1. We also presented the adjusted hazard ratios for all variables included in the model. We tested linearity of continuous variables and categorized non-linear variables. We also tested model assumptions including the proportional hazards and absence of interactions and found them to be valid. All calculations were performed using the SAS software package Version 9.1 (SAS Institute Inc., Cary, NC).

Results

The study cohort included 2,923 RA patients who initiated TNF antagonists by December 31, 2008 and met all selection criteria (Figure 1). The cohort was predominantly women (72%) and patients treated with etanercept (63%) (Table 1). Ages ranged from 18–92 years (median 56). Patients treated with infliximab had the highest prevalence of concomitant methotrexate therapy and patients with etanercept the lowest. This reflects differences in the indications mentioned in the product monographs; while infliximab is indicated for use in combination with methotrexate [36], the monograph of etanercept mentioned that it "can be initiated in combination with methotrexate ... or used alone" [37]. Similarly, while the provincial special authority policy requires that infliximab is used in combination with methotrexate (or other drug), such requirement does not exist for treatment with etanercept or adalimumab [29].

The three TNF antagonist drugs had similar persistence (median roughly 3.5 years, Figure 2). In the multivariable analysis, the estimated adjusted hazards were comparable for the three TNF antagonists (Table 2). Drug-sex and drug-age interactions were insignificant and were not included in the final model.

The following patients' subgroups had a decreased discontinuation hazard (improved persistence): males, age 30–70, patients without admission to hospital in the year preceding treatment initiation, patients on concomitant MTX or NSAIDs treatment

Table 1. Baseline Characteristics of Patients.

Factor	Infliximab (n = 620, 21%)	Adalimumab (N = 474, 16%)	Etanercept (n = 1829, 63%)
Females, n (%)	438 (71)	344 (73)	1322 (72)
Age	56 (18–87)	58 (22–91)	56 (18–92)
Low deductible ($1–500), n (%)	34 (5)	56 (12)	162 (9)
Medium deductible ($501–2250) n (%)	96 (15)	118 (25)	356 (19)
High deductible (>$2250) n (%)	40 (6)	46 (10)	169 (9)
No deductible n (%)	49 (8)	83 (18)	213 (12)
Number of outpatient visits	33 (3–158)	31 (2–112)	32 (3–136)
Number of admissions	0 (0–6)	0 (0–5)	0 (0–8)
Number of comorbidity	0 (0–6)	0 (0–8)	0 (0–7)
RA duration in years	9.1 (0.1–17.9)	7.7 (0.3–17.9)	8.2 (0–17.8)
MTX users n (%)	417 (67)	277 (59)	902 (49)
NSAID users n (%)	332 (54)	224 (47)	983 (54)
Number of previous drugs	4 (0–8)	4 (0–8)	4 (0–9)
Calendar year	2003 (2001–2008)	2007 (2004–2008)	2005 (2001–2008)

Values are median (range) unless otherwise specified. Please refer to text (Patients and methods) for further details on the variables.
%- percent; MTX- methotrexate; NSAID- nonsteroidal anti-inflammatory drug; RA – rheumatoid arthritis; $ Canadian dollars.

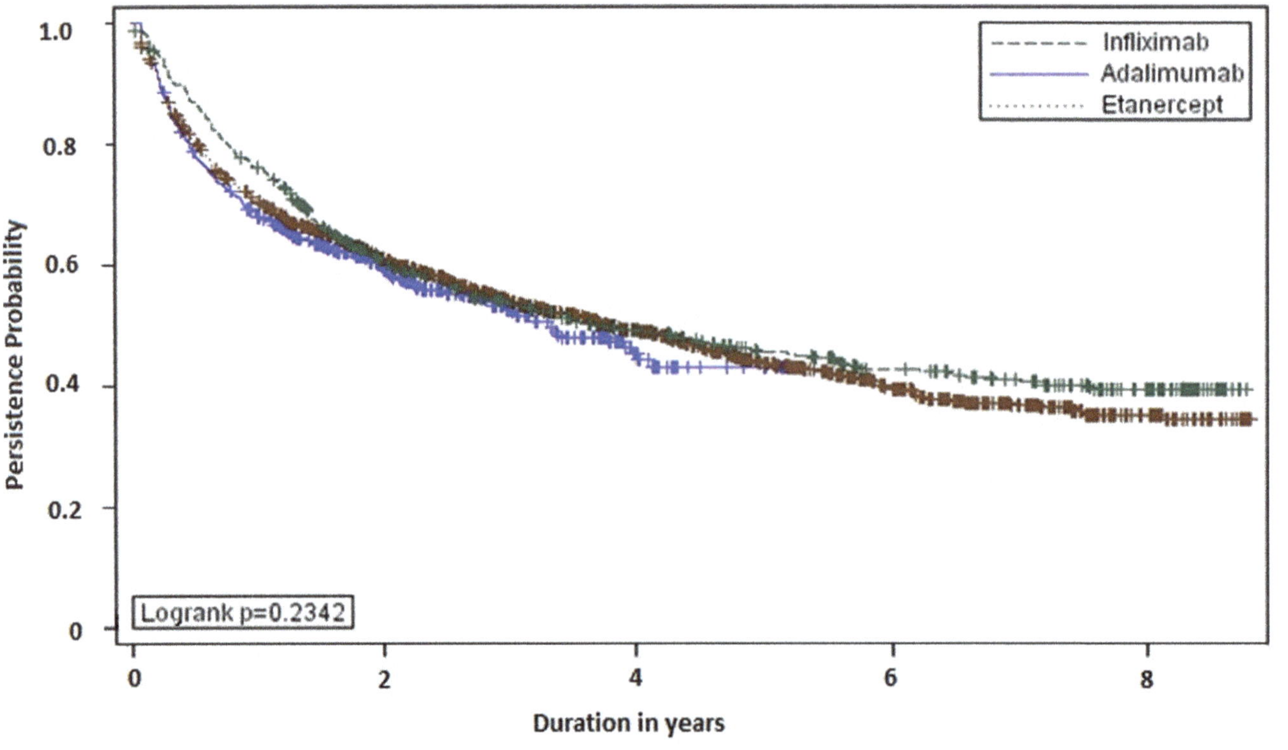

	Number of patients	Events	Censored	Median survival (95% confidence interval)
Infliximab	620	53% (328)	47% (292)	3.68 (2.88-4.95)
Adalimumab	474	46% (219)	54% (255)	3.33 (2.63-4.10)
Etanercept	1829	52% (960)	48% (869)	3.78 (3.31-4.32)

Figure 2. Drug Persistence Curves.

Table 2. Hazard Ratios for Discontinuation of Tumor Necrosis Factor Alpha Antagonists.

Comparison	Crude hazard ratio (95% CI)	Adjusted hazard ratio (95% CI)
Infliximab versus etanercept	0.92 (0.81–1.04)	0.98 (0.85–1.13)
Infliximab versus adalimumab	0.87 (0.73–1.03)	0.95 (0.78–1.15)
Adalimumab versus etanercept	1.06 (0.92–1.23)	1.04 (0.88 1.22)

CI – confidence interval.

and patients previously treated with less than 7 antirheumatic drugs (Table 3).

We demonstrated variation in prescribing practice between the physicians, expressed as differences in the risk for discontinuing any TNF antagonist in patients treated by different physicians (Table 3). Physician-specific risk was estimated through a series of binary variables for each of 12 heavy-volume prescribers who initiated more than 70 courses in the study cohort. Each binary variable represented deviation in 'baseline risk of discontinuing' for patients treated by a particular prescriber. We found that patients treated by two 'heavy-volume' prescribers had an increased risk of discontinuation (hazard ratios significantly higher than 1) and patients treated by another two had a significantly lower risk (hazard ratios significantly lower than 1) (Table 3) compared to patients treated with low to medium-volume prescribers. This physician-specific baseline risk of discontinuation was a significant predictor of persistence (p-value of log likelihood test <0.0001). None of the remaining covariates were associated with persistence.

Discussion

This study found no significant difference in persistence between infliximab, adalimumab and etanercept prescribed for RA patients in British Columbia despite known differences in their pharmacological properties. The theory that treatment persistence can serve as a measurable proxy for real-world therapeutic benefit and harm implies similar long-term benefit and harm of the three drugs in RA patients. In the absence of any safety concerns that are specific to a particular TNF antagonist, it would be reasonable to base the TNF antagonist drug formulary, at least in part, on non-therapeutic factors such as cost, convenience and availability. Even if persistence is not a suitable proxy for harm-benefit in these patients, we showed that differences in convenience of administration - intravenous infusion of infliximab compared with subcutaneous injection of etanercept and adalimumab - were not associated with differences in persistence and therefore should not be considered when selecting a treatment.

Three alternative explanations are suggested for the finding of similar persistence with the three drugs. First, similar persistence could reflect similarities in the benefits and harms of the three drugs despite their different pharmacological properties. This explanation is based on the assumption that not all pharmacological properties strongly influence therapeutic effects, and the differences in these properties between the drugs would therefore not influence the clinical outcome of these drugs.

Second, similar persistence amongst the three TNF antagonists may result from benefit and harm differences in different directions. For example, some properties of infliximab might cause increased benefits compared to etanercept (e.g. apoptosis of

Table 3. Predictors of Discontinuation of Tumor Necrosis Factor Alpha Antagonists.

Factor (reference)	P value (log likelihood test)	Adjusted hazard ratio (95% CI)
Sex (female)	<0.0001	0.76 (0.68–0.86)
Age (30–69 years)	<0.0001	18–29 years 1.53 (1.20–1.96); 70–79 years 1.32 (1.14–1.54); ≥80 years 1.83 (1.39–2.41
Deductible	0.8	
Outpatient visits	0.051	
Admissions (no admission)	0.006	1 admission 1.26 (1.09–1.47); 2 admissions 1.10 (0.86–1.42); >2 admissions 1.51 (1.09–2.10)
Comorbidity	0.23	
RA duration	0.07	
MTX use	<0.0001	0.79 (0.71–0.88)
NSAIDs use	0.03	0.89 (0.80–0.99)
Previous drugs (3–6 RA drugs)	0.03	No drug 1.38 (0.99–1.92); 1–2 drugs 1.04 (0.90–1.20); 7–9 drugs 1.40 (1.09–1.81)
Index year (categories)	0.08	
Prescriber-specific risk (a group of prescribers with <70 courses)	<0.0001	Physician 0.57 (0.42–0.76); physician 0.67 (0.47–0.98); physician 1.38 (1.03–1.84); physician 1.57 (1.26–1.96)

Hazard ratios are presented only for factors that are significant predictors of persistence (p-value of log likelihood test ≤0.05) and for 4 prescribers with hazard ratios that are significantly different than the reference.
CI – confidence interval, MTX – methotrexate; NSAID – nonsteroidal anti-inflammatory drug, RA – rheumatoid arthritis.

activated T cells and circulating monocytes [38] or lack of binding of lymphotoxin alpha. [39,40]). Potentially cancelling the increased benefit is the higher immunogenicity of infliximab which could lead to harm such as an infusion reaction [41] or the wide fluctuations in serum concentration of infliximab [39] which could increase the risk of exceeding the maximum tolerated concentration (leading to harm), or reaching suboptimal concentrations (leading to lack of therapeutic benefit).

Alternatively, persistence may be influenced by factors unrelated to therapeutic benefit or harm and the influence of these factors might be different between the drugs. For example, infliximab requires intravenous administration by health care professionals while both adalimumab and etanercept are self-injectable (subcutaneous administration). Patients treated with infliximab may discontinue treatment due to patient or physician preference for subcutaneous administered drugs [42]. This negative influence on persistence due to intravenous administration may be counter balanced by regular physician follow-up that has been shown to improve adherence and persistence to drug therapy in a variety of diseases [43,44].

Similar persistence with the infliximab, adalimumab and etanercept has previously been demonstrated in some studies [45–48], while differences in persistence was observed in others [18,19,49–55]. Controversial results of previous studies may be due to different population or methodology (e.g. crude versus adjusted estimates). An in-depth systematic exploration of the reasons for the differences between the studies is beyond the scope of current study and requires further research.

The two main strengths of our study are: the characteristics of the data used and accounting for differences in practice between physicians. The universal nature of the Canadian health care system minimized selection bias and thus increased the external validity of our results. Patients were included regardless of age, employment status, socioeconomic status and heath facility use, all factors that could potentially caused biases in previous research that used administrative data, clinical chart review, or registries. Furthermore, the British Columbia Ministry of Health uses a largely systematic and standardized approach to data collection, which ensures the better representativeness of real life treatment patterns and drug-taking behavior. Access to complete information on all dispensed prescription drugs and multiple sources of data (physician encounters, hospital separation and pharmacies) contributed to the usefulness of the data. The data also granted a large sample (N = 2923), which provided ample power, as well as relatively long durations of follow up; roughly nine years.

We accounted for differences in prescribing practice between physicians by adjusting for the baseline risk of discontinuing any TNF antagonist in patients treated by different physicians. Differences in prescribing habits could be caused by differences in knowledge or adherence to different guidelines. Alternatively, patients treated by the same physician may be more similar than patients treated by different physicians in parameters such as geography, socioeconomic status, ethnic background, or age [56], and that could cause differences in the baseline risk of discontinuation. Confirming our finding, Zhang et al 2011 [57] demonstrated differences in physician response to decreased benefit with TNF antagonist therapy.

Several limitations are apparent in in analysis of administrative health data and are caused by absence of clinical information. We were unable to identify reasons for drug discontinuation in our cohort. However, based on previous studies, we assumed that the most common reasons were decreased benefit or increased harm. We also did not have access to possible clinical confounders, and therefore used proxies. This may result in residual confounding that has the potential to bias the results.

Diagnostic accuracy might be compromised or biased because disease diagnoses are coded and recorded in the databases for payment purpose. In addition, differences in accuracy of codes between the care-providers (e.g., different physicians) and variation in coding precision in different diseases are to be expected. To minimize the effect of these sources of inaccuracy, and in the absence of validated algorithm appropriate for our data, we designed a disease algorithm requiring at least two outpatient encounters with RA diagnosis.

We identified errors in recording days-supply in our data, which may be the result of refill policy of the provincial drug-coverage plan, different interpretations of days-supply, or dose titration. To overcome these inaccuracies we used a conservative estimate of days-supply (the longest among several possible approaches to estimation) that might have led to underestimation of the actual length of drug-free intervals, false late ascertainment of drug discontinuation and overestimation of drug persistence. Dispensing data for the three drugs were treated similarly to ensure that the relative hazard ratios were not systematically biased in this regard.

Inaccuracies in recording days-supply also limited our ability to identify patients with dose adjustment. Two analyses of administrative databases [48,55] previously evaluated the frequency of dose escalation in RA patients treated with TNF antagonists showed that dose escalating was more common in patients treated with infliximab. The limited ability to identify dose adjustment in our study may have resulted in overestimation of the days-supply for patients who experienced dose escalation, mainly patients treated with infliximab, and biased estimated comparative persistence of infliximab versus adalimumab or etanercept.

We used a long drug-free interval to ascertain discontinuation rather than direct recording of discontinuation (e.g., medical records or patient reporting). This long drug-free interval algorithm minimized the number of patients considered discontinuers for a temporary interruption. We claim that temporary interruptions should be considered noncompliance, not discontinuation. By using short drug-free intervals, previous studies captured a complex measure of both persistence and compliance and therefore the end point in these studies should not be considered discontinuation. However, by using a long drug-free interval, our analysis was more vulnerable to immortal person-time bias. Patients were required to be alive at the end of drug-free interval to be considered discontinuers; otherwise, their data was censored. Patients who died due to drug effects (harm) were not considered discontinuers but their follow-up time was accounted for. This bias might have affected our comparative estimates if death related to drug effects was significantly more frequent with one of the drug, a condition we did not expected to exist.

The study results indicate that persistence with infliximab, adalimumab and etanercept is similar in RA patients – a finding that does not disapproves the hypothesis that the drugs' benefit and harm could be considered equivalent. Accordingly, clinical and policy decisions for treatment with TNF antagonist could be based on convenience and cost. Even if persistence is not a suitable proxy for harm-benefit profile, our results show that persistence should not be a consideration when selecting a TNF antagonist in RA patients.

Author Contributions

Conceived and designed the experiments: AF KB JMW MAB HF CRD. Performed the experiments: AF. Analyzed the data: AF. Contributed reagents/materials/analysis tools: AF MAB CRD. Contributed to the writing of the manuscript: AF KB JMW MAB HF CRD.

References

1. Brennan FM, Maini RN, Feldmann M (1992) TNF alpha–A pivotal role in rheumatoid arthritis? Br J Rheumatol 31: 293–298.
2. Feldmann M, Maini RN (2001) Anti-TNF alpha therapy of rheumatoid arthritis: What have we learned? Annu Rev Immunol 19: 163–196.
3. Hochberg MC, Tracy JK, Hawkins-Holt M, Flores RH (2003) Comparison of the efficacy of the tumour necrosis factor alpha blocking agents adalimumab, etanercept, and infliximab when added to methotrexate in patients with active rheumatoid arthritis. Ann Rheum Dis 62: ii13–ii16.
4. Gartlehner G, Hansen RA, Jonas BL, Thieda P, Lohr KN (2006) The comparative efficacy and safety of biologics for the treatment of rheumatoid arthritis: A systematic review and metaanalysis. J Rheumatol 33: 2398–2408.
5. Nixon RM, Bansback NJ, Brennan A (2007) Using mixed treatment comparisons and meta-regression to perform indirect comparison to estimate the efficacy of biologic treatments in rheumatoid arthritis. Stat Med 26: 1237–1254.
6. Singh JA, Christensen R, Wells GA, Suarez-Almazor ME, Buchbinder R, et al. (2009) Biologics for rheumatoid arthritis: An overview of Cochrane reviews. Cochrane Database Syst Rev 4: CD007848.
7. Ingham M, Carter C (2010) Meta-analysis and biologics comparing apples to apples: An example using radiographic outcomes in rheumatoid arthritis Arthritis Rheum 62: 76.
8. Wiens A, Venson R, Correr CJ, Otuki MF, Pontarolo R (2010) Meta-analysis of the efficacy and safety of adalimumab, etanercept, and infliximab for the treatment of rheumatoid arthritis. Pharmacotherapy 30: 339–353.
9. Devine EB, Alfonso-Cristancho R, Sullivan SD (2011) Effectiveness of biologic therapies for rheumatoid arthritis: An indirect comparisons approach. Pharmacotherapy 31: 39–51.
10. Wolfe F (1995) The epidemiology of drug treatment failure in rheumatoid arthritis. Baillieres Clin Rheumatol 9: 619–632.
11. Pincus T, Sokka T (2004) Clinical trials in rheumatic diseases: Designs and limitations. Rheum Dis Clin North Am 30: 701–724.
12. Kievit W, Fransen J, Oerlemans AJ, Kuper HH, van der Laar MA, et al. (2007) The efficacy of anti-TNF in rheumatoid arthritis, a comparison between randomised controlled trials and clinical practice. Ann Rheum Dis 66: 1473–1478.
13. Zink A, Strangfeld A, Schneider M, Herzer P, Hierse F, et al. (2006) Effectiveness of tumor necrosis factor inhibitors in rheumatoid arthritis in an observational cohort study: Comparison of patients according to their eligibility for major randomized clinical trials. Arthritis Rheum 54: 3399–3407.
14. Berthelot JM, Benoist-Gerard S, le Goff B, Muller-Chevalet F, Maugars Y (2010) Outcome and safety of TNFalpha antagonist therapy in 475 consecutive outpatients (with rheumatoid arthritis or spondyloarthropathies) treated by a single physician according to their eligibility for clinical trials. Joint Bone Spine 77: 564–569.
15. Sokka T, Pincus T (2003) Eligibility of patients in routine care for major clinical trials of anti-tumor necrosis factor alpha agents in rheumatoid arthritis. Arthritis Rheum 48: 313–318.
16. Hyrich KL, Lunt M, Watson KD, Symmons DPM, Silman AJ (2007) Outcomes after switching from one anti-tumor necrosis factor alpha agent to a second anti-tumor necrosis factor alpha agent in patients with rheumatoid arthritis: Results from a large UK national cohort study. Arthritis Rheum 56: 13–20.
17. Carmona L, Gomez-Reino JJ, on behalf of the BIOBADASER Group (2006) Survival of TNF antagonists in spondylarthritis is better than in rheumatoid arthritis. Data from the Spanish registry BIOBADASER. Arthritis Res Ther 8: R72.
18. Hetland ML, Christensen IJ, Tarp U, Dreyer L, Hansen A, et al. (2010) Direct comparison of treatment responses, remission rates, and drug adherence in patients with rheumatoid arthritis treated with adalimumab, etanercept, or infliximab: Results from eight years of surveillance of clinical practice in the nationwide danish DANBIO registry. Arthritis Rheum 62: 22–32.
19. Fernandez-Nebro A, Irigoyen MV, Urena I, Belmonte-Lopez MA, Coret V, et al. (2007) Effectiveness, predictive response factors, and safety of anti-tumor necrosis factor (TNF) therapies in anti-TNF-naive rheumatoid arthritis. J Rheumatol 34: 2334–2342.
20. Kievit W, Fransen J, Adang EMM, den Broeder AA, Bernelot Moens HJ, et al. (2011) Long-term effectiveness and safety of TNF-blocking agents in daily clinical practice: Results from the Dutch rheumatoid arthritis monitoring register. Rheumatology (Oxford) 50: 196–203.
21. Filippini M, Bazzani C, Favalli EG, Marchesoni A, Atzeni F, et al. (2010) Efficacy and safety of anti-tumour necrosis factor in elderly patients with rheumatoid arthritis: An observational study. Clin Rev Allergy Immunol 38: 90–96.
22. Blum MA, Koo D, Doshi JA (2011) Measurement and rates of persistence with and adherence to biologics for rheumatoid arthritis: A systematic review. Clin Ther 33: 901–913.
23. Koncz T, Pentek M, Brodszky V, Ersek K, Orlewska E, et al. (2010) Adherence to biologic DMARD therapies in rheumatoid arthritis. Expert Opin Biol Ther 10: 1367–1378.
24. Anderson PJ (2005) Tumor necrosis factor inhibitors: Clinical implications of their different immunogenicity profiles. Semin Arthritis Rheum 34: 19–22.
25. Nestorov I (2005) Clinical pharmacokinetics of TNF antagonists: How do they differ? Semin Arthritis Rheum 34: 12–18.
26. Rigby WF (2007) Drug insight: Different mechanisms of action of tumor necrosis factor antagonists-passive-aggressive behavior? Nat Clin Pract Rheumatol 3: 227–233.
27. Lacaille D, Anis AH, Guh DP, Esdaile JM (2005) Gaps in care for rheumatoid arthritis: A population study. Arthritis Rheum 53: 241–248.
28. Furst DE, Keystone EC, Braun J, Breedveld FC, Burmester GR, et al. (2011) Updated consensus statement on biological agents for the treatment of rheumatic diseases, 2010. Ann Rheum Dis 70: i2–i36. 10.1136/ard.2010.146852.
29. British Columbia Ministry of Health (2011) Special authority request; abatacept/ adalimumab/ certolizumab/ etanercept/ golimumab/ infliximab rheumatoid arthritis (initial or switch). British Columbia Ministry of Health website. Available: https://www.health.gov.bc.ca/exforms/pharmacare/5345fil.pdf. Accessed 2012 May 14.
30. British Columbia Ministry of Health (2011) Your level of fair PharmaCare coverage in fair PharmaCare. British Columbia Ministry of Health website. Available: http://www.health.gov.bc.ca/pharmacare/plani/planiindex.html#7. Accessed 2011 Mar 29.
31. Quan H, Sundararajan V, Halfon P, Fong A, Burnand B, et al. (2005) Coding algorithms for defining comorbidities in ICD-9-CM and ICD-10 administrative data. Med Care 43: 1130–1139.
32. Charlson ME, Pompei P, Ales KL, MacKenzie CR (1987) A new method of classifying prognostic comorbidity in longitudinal studies: Development and validation. J Chronic Dis 40: 373–383.
33. Bensen B, Atkins C, Sheriff M, Kelsall J, Khalil H (2011) Profile of patients with rheumatoid arthritis treated with infliximab in Canada-trends toward less DMARD use prior to a biologic, earlier use of infliximab and differences in baseline disease [abstract]. J Rheumatol 38: 1155.
34. Hyrich KL, Watson KD, Lunt M, Symmons DP, on behalf of the British Society for Rheumatology Biologics Register (BSRBR) (2011) Changes in disease characteristics and response rates among patients in the United Kingdom starting anti-tumour necrosis factor therapy for rheumatoid arthritis between 2001 and 2008. Rheumatology (Oxford) 50: 117–123.
35. Ogale S, Hitraya E, Henk HJ (2011) Patterns of biologic agent utilization among patients with rheumatoid arthritis: A retrospective cohort study. BMC Musculoskelet Disord 12: 204.
36. eCPS (online Compendium of Pharmaceuticals and Specialties) (2008) Remicade® (infliximab). 2008. 2009 Jun.
37. eCPS (online Compendium of Pharmaceuticals and Specialties) (2009) Enbrel® (etanercept). 2009. 2009 Jun.
38. Furst DE, Wallis R, Broder M, Beenhouwer DO (2006) Tumor necrosis factor antagonists: Different kinetics and/or mechanisms of action may explain differences in the risk for developing granulomatous infection. Semin Arthritis Rheum 36: 159–167.
39. Tracey D, Klareskog L, Sasso EH, Salfeld JG, Tak PP (2008) Tumor necrosis factor antagonist mechanisms of action: A comprehensive review. Pharmacol Ther 117: 244–279.
40. Ware CF (2005) Network communications: Lymphotoxins, LIGHT, and TNF. Annu Rev Immunol 23: 787–819.
41. Emi Aikawa N, de Carvalho JF, Artur Almeida Silva C, Bonfa E (2010) Immunogenicity of anti-TNF-alpha agents in autoimmune diseases. Clin Rev Allergy Immunol 38: 82–89.
42. Vander Cruyssen B, Van Looy S, Wyns B, Westhovens R, Durez P, et al. (2006) Four-year follow-up of infliximab therapy in rheumatoid arthritis patients with long-standing refractory disease: Attrition and long-term evolution of disease activity. Arthritis Res Ther 8: R112.
43. Amuah JE, Hogan DB, Eliasziw M, Supina A, Beck P, et al. (2010) Persistence with cholinesterase inhibitor therapy in a population-based cohort of patients with alzheimer's disease. Pharmacoepidemiol Drug Saf 19: 670–679.
44. Brookhart MA, Patrick AR, Schneeweiss S, Avorn J, Dormuth C, et al. (2007) Physician follow-up and provider continuity are associated with long-term medication adherence: A study of the dynamics of statin use. Arch Intern Med 167: 847–852. 10.1001/archinte.167.8.847.
45. Finckh A, Simard JF, Gabay C, Guerne PA, SCQM physicians (2006) Evidence for differential acquired drug resistance to anti-tumour necrosis factor agents in rheumatoid arthritis. Ann Rheum Dis 65: 746–752.
46. Flendrie M, Creemers MCW, Welsing PMJ, Den Broeder AA, Van Riel PLCM (2003) Survival during treatment with tumour necrosis factor blocking agents in rheumatoid arthritis. Ann Rheum Dis 62: i30–i33.
47. Pocock JM, Albreshni S, Slack R, Polydoropoulou V, O'Reilly D, et al. (2009) A comparison of drug survival times for infliximab, adalimumab and etanercept [abstract]. Rheumatology (Oxford) 48: 69.
48. Wu E, Chen L, Birnbaum H, Yang E, Cifaldi M (2008) Retrospective claims data analysis of dosage adjustment patterns of TNF antagonists among patients with rheumatoid arthritis. Curr Med Res Opin 24: 2229–2240.
49. Du Pan SM, Dehler S, Ciurea A, Ziswiler HR, Gabay C, et al. (2009) Comparison of drug retention rates and causes of drug discontinuation between anti-tumor necrosis factor agents in rheumatoid arthritis. Arthritis Rheum 61: 560–568.

50. Kristensen LE, Saxne T, Nilsson JA, Geborek P (2006) Impact of concomitant DMARD therapy on adherence to treatment with etanercept and infliximab in rheumatoid arthritis. results from a six-year observational study in southern Sweden. Arthritis Res Ther 8: R174.
51. Marchesoni A, Zaccara E, Gorla R, Bazzani C, Sarzi-Puttini P, et al. (2009) TNF-alpha antagonist survival rate in a cohort of rheumatoid arthritis patients observed under conditions of standard clinical practice. Ann N Y Acad Sci 1173: 837–846.
52. Brocq O, Roux CH, Albert C, Breuil V, Aknouche N, et al. (2007) TNFalpha antagonist continuation rates in 442 patients with inflammatory joint disease. Joint Bone Spine 74: 148–154.
53. Kristensen LE, Saxne T, Geborek P (2006) The LUNDEX, a new index of drug efficacy in clinical practice: Results of a five-year observational study of treatment with infliximab and etanercept among rheumatoid arthritis patients in southern Sweden. Arthritis Rheum 54: 600–606.
54. Ostergaard M, Unkerskov J, Linde L, Krogh NS, Ravn T, et al. (2007) Low remission rates but long drug survival in rheumatoid arthritis patients treated with infliximab or etanercept: Results from the nationwide Danish DANBIO database. Scand J Rheumatol 36: 151–154.
55. Yazici Y, Krasnokutsky S, Barnes JP, Hines PL, Wang J, et al. (2009) Changing patterns of tumor necrosis factor inhibitor use in 9074 patients with rheumatoid arthritis. J Rheumatol 36: 907–913.
56. Donner A, Klar N (2000) Design and analysis of cluster randomization trials in health research. London: Arnold. 178 p.
57. Zhang J, Shan Y, Reed G, Kremer J, Greenberg JD, et al. (2011) Thresholds in disease activity for switching biologics in rheumatoid arthritis patients: Experience from a large US cohort. Arthritis Care Res 63: 1672–1679. 10.1002/acr.20643; 10.1002/acr.20643.

6

Treatment Efficacy for Non-Cardiovascular Chest Pain

Jakob M. Burgstaller[1]*, Boris F. Jenni[1], Johann Steurer[1], Ulrike Held[1], Maria M. Wertli[1,2]

1 Horten Center for Patient Oriented Research and Knowledge Transfer, Department of Internal Medicine, University of Zurich, Zurich, Switzerland, **2** Cantonal Hospital Winterthur, Winterthur, Switzerland

Abstract

Background: Non-cardiovascular chest pain (NCCP) leads to impaired quality of life and is associated with a high disease burden. Upon ruling out cardiovascular disease, only vague recommendations exist for further treatment.

Objectives: To summarize treatment efficacy for patients presenting with NCCP.

Methods: Systematic review and meta-analysis. In July 2013, Medline, Web of Knowledge, Embase, EBSCOhost, Cochrane Reviews and Trials, and Scopus were searched. Hand and bibliography searches were also conducted. Randomized controlled trials (RCTs) evaluating non-surgical treatments in patients with NCCP were included. Exclusion criteria were poor study quality and small sample size (<10 patients per group).

Results: Thirty eligible RCT's were included. Most studies assessed PPI efficacy for gastroesophageal reflux disorders (GERD, n = 10). Two RCTs included musculoskeletal chest pain, seven psychotropic drugs, and eleven various psychological interventions. Study quality was high in five RCTs and acceptable in 25. PPI treatment in patients with GERD (5 RCTs, 192 patients) was more effective than placebo [pooled OR 11.7 (95% CI 5.5 to 25.0, heterogeneity $I^2 = 6.1\%$)]. The pooled OR in GERD negative patients (4 RCTs, 156 patients) was 0.8 (95% CI 0.2 to 2.8, heterogeneity $I^2 = 50.4\%$). In musculoskeletal NCCP (2 RCTs, 229 patients) manual therapy was more effective than usual care but not than home exercise [pooled mean difference 0.5 (95% CI −0.3 to 1.3, heterogeneity $I^2 = 46.2\%$)]. The findings for cognitive behavioral treatment, serotonin reuptake inhibitors, tricyclic antidepressants were mixed. Most evidence was available for cognitive behavioral treatment interventions.

Limitations: Only a small number of studies were available.

Conclusions: Timely diagnostic evaluation and treatment of the disease underlying NCCP is important. For patients with suspected GERD, high-dose treatment with PPI is effective. Only limited evidence was available for most prevalent diseases manifesting with chest pain. In patients with idiopathic NCCP, treatments based on cognitive behavioral principles might be considered.

Editor: Sam Eldabe, The James Cook University Hospital, United Kingdom

Funding: The authors have no support or funding to report.

Competing Interests: The authors have declared that no competing interests exist.

* Email: jakob.burgstaller@usz.ch

Background

In the United States, 6 million patients present to emergency departments with chest pain each year, at an annual cost of $8 billion [1,2]. Sixty to ninety percent of the patients that present to emergency departments with chest pain have no underlying cardiovascular disease [3–6]. The proportion of patients with cardiovascular disease is higher in specialized units (cardiology emergency departments, CCU, ICU) [7] and lower in the primary care setting [6,8–10]. After serious illnesses have been ruled out, physicians often assume that patients with non-cardiovascular chest pain (NCCP) have an excellent prognosis [11,12]. However, patients with NCCP have a high disease burden; many patients that seek care for NCCP complain of persisting symptoms in a 4-year follow-up [13]. Furthermore, patients with non-cardiac chest pain experience an impaired quality of life and greater number of medical visits compared with patients with cardiac pain [14].

In patients with chest pain, the diagnostic work-up focuses primarily on cardiovascular disease and is often performed by cardiologists. Upon ruling out cardiovascular disease, only vague recommendations exist for further treatment, delaying appropriate treatment and causing uncertainty for patients [15]. A recent systematic synthesis of diagnostic tests [16] showed that patients with gastroesophageal reflux disorder (GERD) can be identified by their response to proton pump inhibitor (PPI) treatment, and certain clinical findings can guide clinicians to the most appropriate treatments (e.g., pain increase with movement or decrease on medication were associated with musculoskeletal chest pain). However, limited data are available regarding the efficacy of treatments for patients with NCCP.

The present systematic review aimed to summarize the current evidence about the efficacy of different treatments based on randomized controlled trials (RCTs) for patients that seek care for NCCP.

Methods

Literature search and study selection

This search, conducted in July 2013, followed the PRISMA statement [17]. We searched six databases: Medline (OvidSP), including In-Process & Other Non-Indexed Citations, Daily and OLDMEDLINE; Web of Knowledge, including Biosis and Web of Science; Embase (OvidSP); EBSCOhost, including CINAHL and PsycINFO; Cochrane Reviews and Trials; and Scopus. We used the following search terms as medical subject headings (MeSH terms) and other subject headings: 'thoracic pain', 'chest pain', 'non-cardiac chest pain', 'atypical chest pain', 'musculoskeletal chest pain', 'esophageal chest pain', and 'thoracic spine pain'. The findings were limited to studies published in the last 20 years. We applied no limits regarding study setting or language. **Table S1** depicts two detailed search strategies.

To ensure search completeness, one reviewer (BJ) conducted a thorough search of the bibliographies of all included studies. Potential eligible references were also included in the full text review.

Eligibility criteria

Eligible studies were randomized controlled trials (RCTs) published in the last 20 years. Inclusion criteria were studies reporting on patients aged ≥18 years seeking care for NCCP. NCCP was defined as chest pain after cardiac or other vascular disease (e.g., cardiovascular disease, aortic dissection, pulmonary embolism) had been ruled out. Studies with less than 10 patients per group were excluded.

Study selection, data extraction, and synthesis

Two reviewers (MW and BJ) independently screened 5372 references by title and abstract. Both reviewers independently reviewed the full text of 62 studies that met the eligibility criteria. Disagreements were discussed and resolved by consensus or third party arbitration (JS). Researchers with specific language proficiencies reviewed non-English language references. When the same study was included in several publications without change in treatment, outcome, or follow-up, the most recent publication was chosen and missing information was added from previous publications.

All information regarding the treatment and control groups, treatment duration, follow-up duration, and patient population was extracted and grouped according to the disease investigated.

Quality assessment

Study quality was assessed using the Scottish Intercollegiate Guidelines Network (SIGN) methodology checklist for RCTs [18]. Overall bias risk and study quality were rated according to the SIGN recommendations. The ratings included high quality (++; the majority of criteria met; little or no risk of bias; results unlikely to be changed by further research.), acceptable quality (+; most criteria met; some flaws in the study with an associated risk of bias; conclusions may change in the light of further studies), and low quality (0; either most criteria not met, or significant flaws relating to key aspects of study design; conclusions likely to change in the light of further studies).

It was not possible to include all studies in the meta-analysis because data was missing for some outcomes. It may have happened that the studies originally considered several different outcome measures, but only reported the measures that provided significant results. Copas et al. [19] refer to this as outcome reporting bias, which is defined as outcome reporting driven by the significance and/or direction of the effect size. All studies that were not included in the meta-analyses were assessed for a potential outcome reporting bias using the 9-item outcome reporting in trails (ORBIT) tool [20]. Risk of bias was rated from low (outcome of interest was not measured) to high [trial report states that outcome was analyzed, but only reports that the result was not significant (typically stating $p>0.05$)].

Outcome

The outcome of primary interest was chest pain, including chest pain frequency and intensity.

We also assessed psychological outcome measures. In particular, we aimed to assess the efficacy of treatment interventions on anxiety, depression, and panic disorders. All measures were extracted, and validity of the outcome measure used was assessed.

Statistical analysis

Descriptive statistics were used to summarize findings across all groups of diagnostic studies. These included number of patients, mean patient age, and gender distribution.

In order to summarize findings across studies, different pain score scales were re-scaled to a 0- to 10-point scale where necessary. In addition, the frequency scores were homogenized to present results on a monthly basis. To present counted pain events in the treatment and control arms as odds ratios, we used number of events and number of patients in both groups, with a cut-off of >50% improvement. To present changes from baseline to follow-up in the treatment and control arms as mean differences, we used mean change, standard deviation of change, and number of patients in both groups. If the necessary information was not directly available from the original publication, we derived these quantities following instructions described in the Cochrane Handbook [21]. We assumed a random effects model to obtain a pooled estimate of the effect if more than one trial was available in a subgroup. A restricted maximum-likelihood estimator was used to quantify the amount of heterogeneity.

Risk of bias was assessed using a funnel plot. Funnel plot asymmetry was assessed with the regression test proposed by Egger [22].

Analyses were performed using R statistical software and the "metafor" package [23,24].

Results

Study selection

Figure 1 summarizes the search and inclusion process. Out of 5372 records, 62 were reviewed in full text, resulting in the exclusion of 5310 studies. In total, the analysis included 32 publications based on 30 RCTs. Reasons for the exclusion of 30 publications are provided in Figure 1.

Study characteristics

Table 1 presents the study characteristics and included patients. Ten RCTs (33%) included patients with underlying gastrointestinal cause. Most RCTs ($n=8$, 1037 patients) evaluated the treatment efficacy of a PPI in patients with NCCP [25–32]. Other

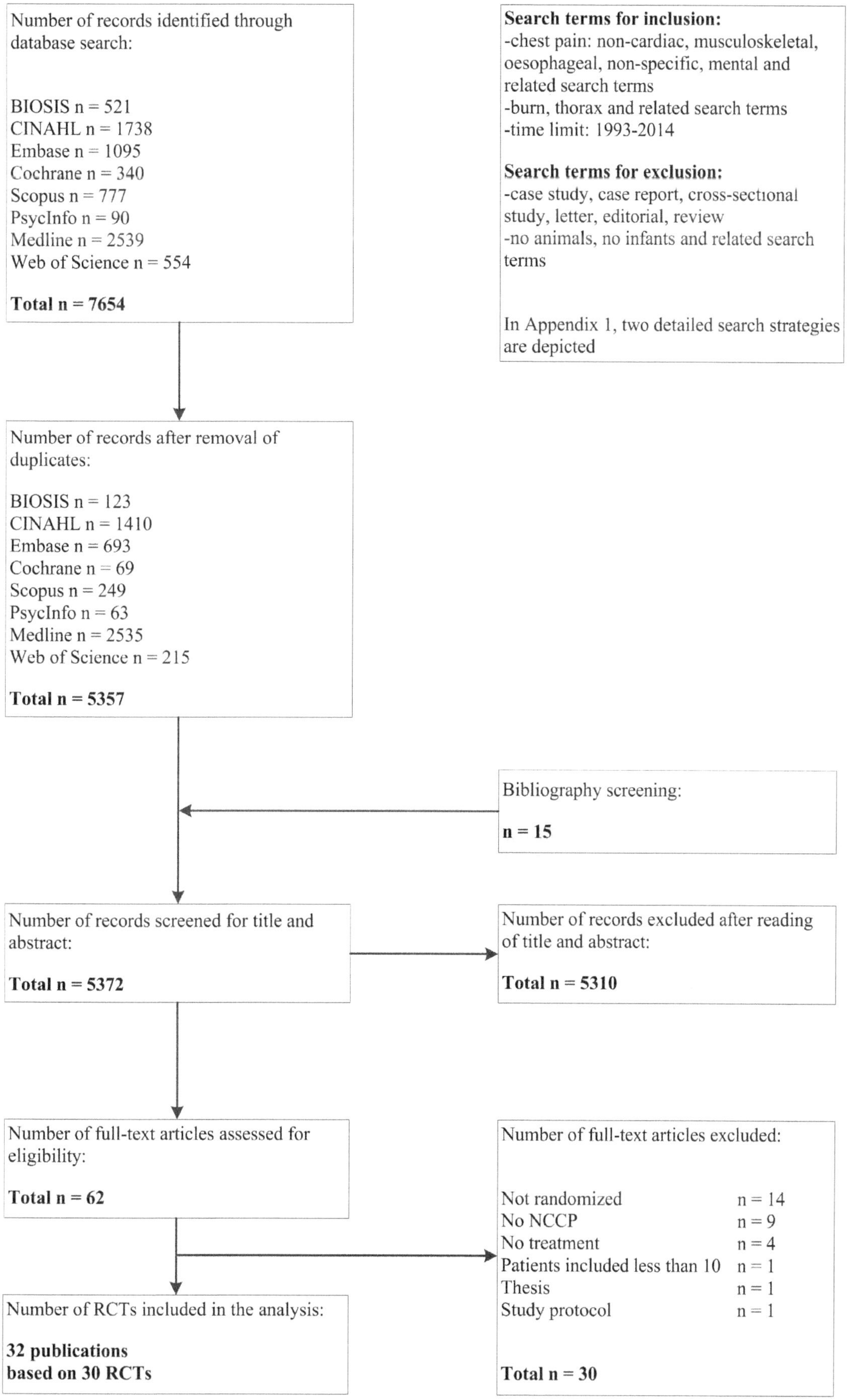

Figure 1. Study flow.

Table 1. Basis characteristics.

Author, year	Setting	Inclusion criteria	Exclusion criteria	Intervention	Number of patients (women)	Age: years (SD or Range)	Duration of disease: days (SD)
GI-symptoms							
Achem, 1997 [25]	Randomized, double-blind trial of 36 patients referred to the University of Florida/Jacksonville for evaluation of the main complaint of NCCP during the period of January 1992 to September 1992, USA	Chest pain retrosternal and suggestive of coronary artery disease (squeezing or oppressive and related to effort and/or emotion) with a duration of at least six months prior to entry and a frequency of at least three episodes per week. Patients may have had other esophageal symptoms, such as pyrosis or dysphagia, but the dominant complaint that brought the patient to medical attention was NCCP. GERD was documented by 24-hr ambulatory pH testing. All patients were deemed not to have cardiac disease by a cardiologist (coronary angiography or stress thallium test), all patients had a normal echocardiogram.	Other sources of chest pain : cardiac disease, epicardial coronary artery disease and valvular heart disease, musculoskeletal causes of chest pain, reproduction of chest pain on palpation of the chest wall or during arm/neck motion	Omeprazole 20 mg orally twice daily vs. placebo for 8 weeks	36 (23)	52 (N.R.)	<1
Bautista, 2004 [26]	Randomized, double-blind, placebo-controlled, crossover trial of 40 patients who were referred by a cardiologist after a comprehensive evaluation, with at least three episodes per week of unexplained chest pain as the predominant symptom, USA	At least three episodes per week of unexplained chest pain (angina like pain behind the breast bone) for a minimum of 3 months, normal or insignificant findings on coronary angiogram, or had insufficient evidence for ischemic heart disease using exercise treadmill, stress thallium, technetium 99 m tetrofosmin or technetium 99 m methoxy isobutyl isonitrile testing	Cardiac abnormality, severe liver, lung, renal, hematological or any other underlying disorder, previous empirical anti-reflux regimen, history of peptic ulcer disease or gastrointestinal surgery, unwilling or incapable of providing informed consent, and inability to fully complete all phases of the study, duodenal or gastric ulcer as well as other significant lesions on upper endoscopy	Lansoprazole 60 mg AM and 30 mg PM vs. placebo for 7 days	40 (9)	54 (3)	N.R.

Table 1. Cont.

Author, year	Setting	Inclusion criteria	Exclusion criteria	Intervention	Number of patients (women)	Age: years (SD or Range)	Duration of disease: days (SD)
Cossentin, 2012 [33]	Randomized, controlled, double-blinded trial with 43 GERD patients with abnormal 24-h pH tests seen in the Gastroenterology Service at the Walter Reed Army Medical Center, 2011, USA	18 years of age or older, have at least one symptom consistent with GERD (to include, but not limited to heartburn, acid taste in the mouth, regurgitation, burning epigastric pain and/or dyspepsia) and evidence of upright (percentage time >6.3) or supine (percentage time >1.2) reflux on 24-h pH testing	Prior gastric or esophageal surgery for the treatment of GERD, severe co-morbid illnesses, history of allergy to baclofen and pregnancy	Baclofen vs. placebo for 14 days	43 (16)	49 (14)	N.R.
Dickman, 2005 [27]	Randomized, double-blind, placebo-controlled, crossover trial of 35 patients with non-cardiac chest pain referred by a cardiologist after a comprehensive cardiac work-up, USA	At least three episodes per week of unexplained chest pain (angina alike pain behind the breast bone) for a minimum of 3 months, normal or insignificant findings on coronary angiogram, or had insufficient evidence for ischemic heart disease using exercise treadmill, stress thallium technetium 99 m tetrofosmin or technetium 99 m methoxy isobutyl isonitrile testing	Severe liver, lung, renal, hematological or any other severe co-morbidity, previous empirical anti-reflux regiment, history of peptic ulcer disease or gastrointestinal surgery, unwilling or incapable of providing informed consent, and inability to fully complete all phases of the study	Rabeprazole 20 mg AM before breakfast and 20 mg PM before dinner vs. placebo for 7 days	35 (12)	56 (10)	N.R.
Dore, 2007 [28]	Randomized controlled study of 266 consecutive patients with heartburn and/or regurgitation, dysphagia and/or odynophagia, with or without esophagitis attending the University Hospital of Sassari, Italy	Heartburn and/or regurgitation, dysphagia and/or odynophagia, with or without esophagitis	Previous endoscopy and or a defined diagnosis of ERD or NERD, upper gastrointestinal (GI) surgery and malignancy, anti-secretory drugs or PPIs during the 4 months before enrollment	Rabeprazole 20 mg vs pantoprazole 20 mg vs esomeprazole 20 mg vs lansoprazole 20 mg for 12 weeks	266 (190)	48 (18–82)	N.R.
Fass, 1998 [29]	Randomized, double-blind, placebo-controlled, crossover trial of 39 patients who were referred by a cardiologist after a comprehensive evaluation, with at least three episodes per week of unexplained chest pain as the predominant symptom, between January and December 1996, USA	At least three episodes per week of unexplained chest pain, insignificant disease or normal anatomy on cardiac angiogram, or lack of evidence of ischemic heart disease on exercise treadmill, stress thallium, technetium 99 m tetrofosmin or technetium 99 m methoxy isobutyl isonitrile testing	Medical contraindication for omeprazole therapy, had already been empirically treated with an anti-reflux regimen, reported a history of peptic ulcer disease or gastrointestinal surgery, or were unwilling or unable to provide informed consent, patients who were unable to fully complete all stages of the study	Omeprazole 40 mg AM and 20 mg PM vs. placebo for 7 days	39 (1)	50 (2)	N.R.

Table 1. Cont.

Author, year	Setting	Inclusion criteria	Exclusion criteria	Intervention	Number of patients (women)	Age: years (SD or Range)	Duration of disease: days (SD)
Jones, 2006 [34]	Randomized controlled, single blinded, trial of 28 patients attending the regional cardiothoracic center with angina-like chest pain in whom a coronary angiography was normal, UK	Angina like chest pain in whom coronary angiography was normal, to be able to attend the department over a period of at least 17 weeks, have no coexistent disease, and experience chest pain at least once a week	Esophageal reflux, proton pump inhibitor (it was necessary for them not to have responded to this medication)	4 week baseline period Hypnotherapy: by a therapist, initial tutorial (about condition and factors that may be involved), hypnosis induced by eye closure, followed by progressive muscular relaxation and standard deepening techniques vs. Supportive therapy plus placebo: by a research assistant, counseling and support, placebo medication total 12 sessions over a 17 week period	28 (18)	57	N.R.
Lind, 1997 [30]	Randomized, double-blind study of patients with heartburn, without endoscopic signs of esophagitis, treatment with omeprazole, 20 or 10 mg once daily, or placebo, for 4 weeks (n = 509) at 25 centers in Denmark and Sweden	Both sexes, 18 years or older, with a history of heartburn as the predominant symptom during the past 12 months, with episodes of heartburn occurring on at least 2 days weekly, and without any endoscopic signs of esophagitis	Presence or history of gastric or duodenal peptic ulcer disease or erosive/ulcerative esophagitis, presence of Barrett's esophagus or an esophageal stricture, previous esophagogastric surgery, treatment with any investigational compound or with anti-secretory agents such as histamine H2-receptor antagonists or PPI in ulcer-healing doses within the month before endoscopy, concurrent cardiovascular, renal, or hepatic disease likely to complicate the evaluation of the study, suspected or confirmed malignancy, clinically significant abnormal findings in the pre-study laboratory screen, or pregnancy or lactation	Omeprazole 20 mg daily vs. 10 mg daily vs. placebo for 4 weeks	509 (303)	50 (N.R.)	N.R.
Pandak, 2002 [31]	Prospective, double-blind, placebo-controlled, parallel, crossover trial of 42 patients who presented with unexplained recurrent chest pain and subsequently had negative results on MIBI testing, ruling out a cardiac etiology, between May 1997 and August 1999, USA.	At least three episodes of chest pain per week of 6 months' duration or longer	Gastric or duodenal ulcer, were already using anti-reflux medications, had omeprazole contraindications, had prior gastric surgery, or could not comply with the study protocol. Patients with physical exam or chest x-ray abnormalities that would explain their chest pain.	Omeprazole 40 mg orally twice daily vs. placebo for 2 weeks	42 (24)	45 (N.R.)	N.R.

Table 1. Cont.

Author, year	Setting	Inclusion criteria	Exclusion criteria	Intervention	Number of patients (women)	Age: years (SD or Range)	Duration of disease: days (SD)
Xia, 2003 [32]	Prospective, single-blind, placebo-controlled trial of 68 patients with chest pain for at least 12 weeks in the preceding 12 months, who were referred to the Cardiology Division of Queen Mary Hospital for evaluation by cardiac catheterization between November 1998 and February 2000, China	Patients who had a normal coronary angiograph, and whose chest pain was considered by a cardiologist to be non-cardiac in origin	Patients with apparent heartburn, acid reflux, dysphagia and dyspepsia	Lansoprazole 30 mg daily vs. placebo for 4 weeks	70 (42)	58 (10)	N.R.
musculoskeletal							
Lehtola, 2010 [35]	Randomized, assessor-blinded, placebo-controlled trial of 114 female patients (referred by their GPs) aged 20–60 years with pain in the thoracic spine area during the period of September 1998 to May 2001, Finland	Female subjects, problems in the thoracic area, duration of the symptoms had to be less than 3 months prior to the study	The primary subjective problem was some pain other than thoracic pain (headache, neck pain etc.), a contra-indication to manipulation or acupuncture, and not having experienced pain in the thoracic area within the last 7 days	Facet-traction manipulation: as many segments between the area T3-T8 as necessary, lasted 10–15 min. vs. Acupuncture: points GB21, GV14, GV9–12, BL13–18 la, BL60 la, points GV9–12, lasted 30 min. vs. Placebo: interference-electrotherapy with suction cups without electricity, sucking between 0 and 0.2 bar, lasted 20 min	114 (114)	43 (N.R.)	N.R.
Stochkendahl, 2012 [36,37]	A non-blinded, randomized controlled trial undertaken at an emergency cardiology department and 4 outpatient chiropractic clinics, 115 consecutive patients with acute chest pain of musculoskeletal origin, between August 2006 and March 2008, Denmark	Aged 18 to 75 years, have had a primary complaint of acute chest pain for less than 7 days duration, should be a resident of the local county, and should be able to read and understand Danish. Participants should have undergone diagnostic procedures to rule out ACS and should not have shown significant comorbidity or contraindications for spinal manipulative therapy.	Previous ACS, prior percutaneous coronary intervention or coronary artery bypass grafting, inflammatory joint disease, insulin-dependent diabetes, fibromyalgia, malignant disease, major osseous anomaly, osteoporosis, apoplexy or dementia, inability to cooperate, and pregnancy	Chiropractic: individual treatment strategy, 1 of 8 experienced chiropractors, high-velocity, low-amplitude manipulation directed toward the thoracic and/or cervical spine, a maximum of 10 treatment sessions of approximately 20 minutes' duration each, 1 to 3 times per week for 4 weeks vs 15-minute consultation that chest pain generally had a benign, self-limiting course and, based on the clinical evaluation, gave individual instructions regarding posture and 2 to 3 home exercises aimed at increasing spinal movement or muscle stretch	115 (48)	51 (11)	N.R.

Table 1. Cont.

Author, year	Setting	Inclusion criteria	Exclusion criteria	Intervention	Number of patients (women)	Age: years (SD or Range)	Duration of disease: days (SD)
psychiatric drugs							
Cannon, 1994 [49]	60 consecutive patients with chest pain underwent cardiac, esophageal, psychiatric, and pain-sensitivity testing and then participated in a randomized, double-blind, placebo controlled three week trial of clonidine, imipramine with a morning placebo, or placebo twice daily. This treatment phase was compared with an identical period of twice-daily placebo for all patients (placebo phase), USA	Normal coronary angiograms and no epicardial coronary-artery spasm after the intravenous administration of ergonovine (0.15 mg), normal left ventricular function at rest, no evidence of left ventricular hypertrophy or valvular heart disease (including mitral-valve prolapse) or echocardiography, blood pressure no higher than 160/100 mmHg when they were receiving no medication, and no musculoskeletal sensitivity that accounted for their characteristic chest pain	N.R.	Clonidine 0.05 mg at 9 AM and 9 PM for 1 week, then 0.1 mg for both doses thereafter vs. imipramine 25 mg at 9 PM for 1 week, then 50 mg nightly, always with a matching placebo at 9 AM vs. placebo at 9 AM and 9 PM	60 (40)	50 (29–72)	1590
Cox, 1998 [50]	Randomized, double-blind, cross-over trial of imipramine 50 mg daily vs placebo in 18 women with chest pain and normal coronary angiograms who were suffering at least two anginal episodes per week despite conventional anti-anginal medication, UK	Completely normal coronary angiogram; at least two episodes of anginal pain per week despite anti-anginal medication	Non-cardiac causes of chest pain and patients receiving anti-depressant therapy for previously diagnosed psychiatric disorders	Imipramine 50 mg daily vs. placebo for 5 weeks	18 (18)	53 (35–72)	1500
Doraiswamy, 2006 [51]	Single-site, double-blind, placebo-controlled study of the efficacy and safety of paroxetine in the treatment of chest pain in 50 patients with normal coronary angiograms or stress tests, USA	Males and females between the ages of 18 and 85 experiencing chest pain at minimum 1 to 2 times per week and with a documented normal coronary angiogram or stress test	Treatment with another antidepressant within the 2 weeks (5 weeks for fluoxetine) of beginning double-blind therapy. Medications: narcotics, reserpine, methyldopa, guanethidine, clonidine, local or general anesthetics, and any other psychotropic medication with the exception of hypnotics or benzodiazepines on a minimal, case-by-case basis	Paroxetine 10 mg for 1 week, then increased to 20 mg daily or adjusted to a maximum of 50 mg daily based on clinical response vs. placebo for 8 weeks	50 (21)	53 (N.R.)	1158

Table 1. Cont.

Author, year	Setting	Inclusion criteria	Exclusion criteria	Intervention	Number of patients (women)	Age: years (SD or Range)	Duration of disease: days (SD)
Keefe, 2011 [52]	Randomized clinical trial examined the separate and combined effects of CST and antidepressant medication (sertraline) in participants with non-cardiac chest pain. 115 patients diagnosed with NCCP were randomly assigned to one of four treatments: CST plus sertraline, CST plus placebo, sertraline alone, or placebo alone. Participants were recruited from Duke University Medical Center, satellite clinics, and the community from February 2002 to October 2005, USA	Complaints of chest pain in the previous 6 months, received a negative stress test within the past 2 years, normal coronary angiogram within the past 2 years, or had a survival probability >98% at 2 years, a low likelihood of significant coronary artery disease (<25%) on the National Cholesterol Education Program's (NCEP) modification of the Framingham Risk Calculator (FRC), able to swallow oral medication, and age 18–85 years	Other cardiac problems associated with chest pain, current use of antidepressant medications or medications significantly affecting pain, a history of drug or alcohol abuse within the past 6 months, pregnancy, severe psychopathology (i.e., suicidal patients, severe depression, or psychosis), or treatment with another antidepressant within a period of less than five times the half-life of the drug concerned (e.g. fluoxetine within 5 weeks of beginning double-blind therapy)	Sertraline alone: started at 50 mg daily, adjusted to a maximum of 200 mg within the initial 10 weeks, then dose level stabilized for the remaining 24 weeks vs. CST: 6 sessions, lasted 60 min., bi-weekly for 10 weeks, then 6 follow-up sessions monthly for 6 months with placebo vs. CST with sertraline vs. placebo alone	115 (77)	48 (12)	N.R.
Rao, 2007 [53]	Randomized, controlled, double-blind study with 24 patients with unexplained noncardiac chest pain who were referred to a tertiary care center, USA	At least 12 weeks, which need not be consecutive, in the preceding 12 months of: (a) midline chest pain or discomfort that is not of burning quality and (b) absence of pathologic gastroesophageal reflux, achalasia, or other motility disorder with a recognized pathologic basis. Also, they were required to have a negative cardiac stress test (treadmill exercise stress test, stress thallium test, or stress technetium 99 m-methoxy isobutyl isonitrile [MIBI]) or negative coronary angiography, normal chest X-ray, normal upper GI endoscopy, normal esophageal manometry, and either a normal 24-h pH study (% fraction time of pH <4.0 was <5) or no improvement in chest pain after 2 months of b.i.d. proton pump inhibitor (PPI) therapy	Referred by cardiologists or after a cardiac source for chest pain, muscular-skeletal sources of chest pain, patients who were hospitalized, or those who had significant comorbid illnesses such as cardiac, pulmonary, renal, or hepatic disease or those with diabetes, neuropathy, history of peptic ulcer disease, seizures, or bronchial asthma and those with known allergy or adverse reaction to theophylline, history of psychiatric disorders or who were under treatment with psychotropic drugs	Theophylline oral capsules of 200 mg daily vs. placebo for 4 weeks after meals (crossover: 1 week washout period, then alternate treatment)	24 (16)	44 (22–70)	>84

Table 1. Cont.

Author, year	Setting	Inclusion criteria	Exclusion criteria	Intervention	Number of patients (women)	Age: years (SD or Range)	Duration of disease: days (SD)
Varia, 2000 [54]	Single-site, double-blind, placebo-controlled study of the efficacy, tolerability, and safety of sertraline in the treatment of chest pain in 30 outpatients who otherwise had normal coronary angiograms or stress tests, USA	Men and women 18 to 85 years of age who were able to swallow oral medication and who had noncardiac chest pain, negative stress test or normal coronary angiogram. Patients who agreed to abstain from alcohol and to adhere to protocol requirements.	DSM-IV criteria for major depression, panic disorder, or drug or alcohol abuse or dependence. Patients with any active or clinically significant condition, including sensitivity to sertraline, which could possibly affect absorption, distribution, or metabolism of the study drug, Treatment with a depot neuroleptic drug, another antidepressant, fluoxetine, monoamine oxidase inhibitors, reserpine, methyldopa, guanethidine, or clonidine, local or general anesthetic agents, drugs known to interact with sertraline, antidepressants, other psychotropic medications, or medications significantly affecting pain	Sertraline started at 50 mg daily, adjusted to a maximum of 200 mg vs. placebo for 8 weeks	30 (N.R.)	N.R.	N.R.
Wulsin, 2002 [55]	Randomized, controlled, non-blind, trial of a protocol intervention to initiate panic disorder treatment of 156 enrolled participants, all at low to moderate risk for acute coronary syndrome, admitted to the University Hospital Chest Pain Center in the ED during a 14- month period (March 1998 to May 1999), USA	All adult (≥18 years)	Cognitive impairment, active severe substance abuse, and bipolar disorder	Intervention: patient education by the research assistant about panic disorder according to study protocol, initiation of treatment with a 1-month supply of paroxetine 20 mg/d vs. Usual care: consisted of reassurance that the patient has no cardiac disease, care as needed through primary care physician, telephone follow-up at 3 months	50 (35)	43 (N.R.)	N.R.
psychological interventions							
Arnold, 2009 [38]	Single center, non-blinded, randomized controlled trial of 700 consecutive patients with acute chest pain and no clear diagnosis at initial presentation referred to the chest pain unit of an emergency department between May 2006 and September 2007, UK	Chest pain of possible cardiac origin, were aged over 25, had no changes for acute coronary syndrome on a diagnostic electrocardiogram	Suspected life threatening non-cardiac disease, known coronary heart disease presenting with recurrent or prolonged episodes of cardiac-type chest pain	Standard verbal advice or verbal advice followed by an information sheet	700 (269)	49 (12)	N.R.

Table 1. Cont.

Author, year	Setting	Inclusion criteria	Exclusion criteria	Intervention	Number of patients (women)	Age: years (SD or Range)	Duration of disease: days (SD)
Esler, 2003 [39]	Randomized controlled, non-blinded, trial with 59 patients who presented to a large, university-affiliated Level One Trauma Center ED with chief complaints of chest pain and were determined to have NCCR, USA	No known history or suspected history of coronary artery disease, other significant medical illness (e.g. congestive heart failure, pulmonary embolism, or lung disease), and no obvious proximal cause of their chest pain (e.g. pneumonia, bronchitis, or chest trauma)	Current psychosis, suicidal or homicidal ideation, and those who were intoxicated from alcohol or other drugs at the time of admission to the ED	CBT (cognitive behavioral treatment) intervention (involving psycho education, diaphragmatic breathing exercises, and cognitive restructuring about physical symptoms), 60 min, 1 psychologist vs. treatment-as-usual	59 (27)	41 (12)	<30: 45.8%, 30–180: 15.3%, 180–720: 5.1%, >720: 33.9%
Gasiorowska, 2008 [56]	A randomized, controlled pilot study of 39 patients with at least three episodes per week of unexplained chest pain for 3 consecutive months, Gastroenterology Service, University of Arizona Health Sciences Center, USA	at least three episodes per week of unexplained chest pain for 3 consecutive months, either insignificant coronary artery disease, normal coronary arteries on cardiac angiogram or lack of evidence of ischaemic heart disease on an exercise treadmill, stress thallium, technetium 99 m tetrofosmin or technetium 99 m sestamibi testing, normal upper endoscopy, pH testing and esophageal manometry	severe underlying comorbidities, upper airway symptoms such as hoarseness, wheezing and laryngospasm, diabetes mellitus, scleroderma, gastroparesis, peptic ulcer disease, history of gastrointestinal surgery, depression, autonomic or peripheral neuropathy or neuromuscular disorder, patients using narcotics, benzodiazepines, tricyclic antidepressants or selective serotonin reuptake inhibitors, patients unable to complete the upper endoscopy, 24-hour esophageal pH monitoring or esophageal manometry, patients demonstrating erosive esophagitis, Barrett's esophagus or other GERD-related complications during upper endoscopy, abnormal pH test or manometry results	Johrei treatment (process of transmission of healing energy) delivered by an experienced and certified Johrei practitioner in a hospital clinic with minimal interaction with the patient. Each Johrei treatment session usually lasts 20 min. vs. waiting list	39 (13)	54.5 (11.9)	N.R.
Hess, 2012 [40]	Randomized controlled, single blinded, trial of 204 patients attending the ED of Saint Mary's Hospital at the Mayo Clinic with symptoms suggestive of ACS, USA	Aged >17 years who presented to the ED with primary symptoms of non-traumatic chest pain and who were being considered for admission to the ED observation unit for monitoring and cardiac stress testing within 24 hours	Elevated initial cardiac troponin T levels above the 99th percentile reference limit (99th percentile, <0.01 ng/mL; lower limit of detection, 0.01 ng/mL; 10% coefficient of variation, 0.035 ng/mL), known coronary artery disease (defined as 1 50% stenosis on cardiac catheterization; prior electrocardio-graphic changes indicative of ischemia, e.g. ST-segment depression, T-wave inversion, or left bundle branch block, perfusion defects or wall motion abnormalities on previous exercise, pharmacological, or rest imaging studies; previous documentation of acute myocardial infarction, or if no records were available, patient self-report of coronary artery disease), cocaine use within the previous 72 hours by clinician history, or pregnancy	Decision aid (information paper): included a 100-person pictograph depicting the pretest probability of acute coronary syndrome and available management options (observation unit admission and stress testing or 24–72 hours outpatient follow-up) after initial evaluation (ECG, interpretation, results of initial cardiac troponin testing, plan for serial cardiac markers) vs. usual care	204 (120)	54.7 (11.9)	0.5 (2)

Table 1. Cont.

Author, year	Setting	Inclusion criteria	Exclusion criteria	Intervention	Number of patients (women)	Age: years (SD or Range)	Duration of disease: days (SD)
Jonsbu, 2011 [41]	A randomized controlled, non-blinded, trial of 40 patients with persistent complaints six months after a negative evaluation at a cardiological outpatient clinic between May 2006 and May 2007 at Molde Hospital, Norway	Aged between 18 and 65 years, persistent symptoms or limitations in activity six months after the cardiac evaluation: at least weekly symptoms of chest pain or palpitations, at least "some impact" on family life, social life, or work from the symptoms, at least "rare but sometimes" avoidance of physical activity because of worry about the heart	Cardiac disease in need of treatment	Intervention: cognitive behavioral treatment (CBT), 3 sessions, lasted 60–90 min., at the Psychiatric Outpatient Clinic at Molde Hospital vs. Control group: usual care from their general practitioner, free to use the health care system when needed	40 (26)	52 (22–65)	360
Lahmann, 2008 [42]	A randomized, controlled, clinical investigation of 22 patients presenting with non-specific chest pain at the University Hospital of Regensburg, Germany	Over the age of 18 years who presented with NSCP	Any underlying somatic disorders; any severe and disabling psychiatric disorder, such as schizophrenia or dementia; as well as patients undergoing psychotherapy and those current enrolled for retirement payment	Functional relaxation: started with a 60-minute psychosomatic-education session, then 10 group-therapy sessions (each 90 min) during 6 weeks vs. enhanced medical care: treatment-as-usual plus 2 case-management counseling interviews (personal-care skills, shared decision-making)	22 (12)	44.35	1773 (2218.5)
Mayou, 1997 [44]	Randomized controlled, non-blinded, trial of 37 patients presenting with chest pain and reassured by a cardiologist they do not have heart disease, UK	Aged 18–65, presence of persisting non-cardiac chest pain occurring at least once a week in the month before the assessment	Cardiac diagnosis, current major depression, living outside the country and being unable to speak English	Cognitive behavioral treatment: consisted of up to 12 sessions of individual therapy with a research counseling psychologist (D.S.) trained and supervised by a clinical psychologist (I.K.) vs. usual care	37 (22)	49 (N.R.)	<180: 11, 180–720: 12, >720: 11
Mayou, 2002 [43]	A randomized controlled, single-blind, trial within a cardiology clinic (referred from primary care practice) at a district general hospital, 80 consecutive patients diagnosed as having benign palpitation ± either palpitation due to awareness of extrasystoles or sinus rhythm ± with associated distress or disability, UK	Aged 17 or over referred to a district cardiac clinic for the assessment of palpitation, suffering from benign palpitation and who described distress or disability	Subjects with very short histories or who did not describe distress or disability	Intervention group: usual care plus nurse-delivered intervention based on cognitive-behavioral principles coordinated with cardiological care, derived from experience with the early treatment of NCCP vs. Control group: usual cardiological care, with no contact with a cardiac nurse either in out-patients or by telephone	80 (57)	44 (N.R.)	N.R.

Table 1. Cont.

Author, year	Setting	Inclusion criteria	Exclusion criteria	Intervention	Number of patients (women)	Age: years (SD or Range)	Duration of disease: days (SD)
Potts, 1999 [45]	Randomized, non-blinded, trial of 60 patients who had continuing chest pain despite cardiological reassurance following haemodynamically normal angiography in the Departments of Cardiology of the Royal Infirmary and Western General Hospitals in Edinburgh, Scotland	Aged 18–70, recent (within the last year) coronary angiography for the investigation of chest pain revealed coronary arteries which were either normal or <50% stenosed, chest pain continuing at least twice weekly after angiography, despite reassurance by the cardiology team, and residence within easy travelling distance of Edinburgh	Past history of myocardial infarction, or serious concurrent physical or psychiatric illness	Intervention (CBT): small groups with a maximum of six subjects. Groups met weekly for 4 weeks, then every two weeks for a further 4 weeks. Each session lasted 2 h	60 (36)	54 (N.R.)	
Sanders, 1997 [46]	Randomized controlled, single-blind, study of 57 consecutive patients with chest pain and normal angiograms over a 12-month period, UK	Normal coronary arteries, not need further medical investigations	All those who were either admitted to a Day Case Unit, and went home once they had received the results of the angiogram, or else stayed overnight on the cardiac ward	1-hour intervention: individualized information and discussion session by a specially trained cardiac nurse, together with a handout and cassette providing information and advice and telephone follow-up to discuss progress, answer questions and reiterate advice vs. usual care	57 (36)	N.R.	<180: 16, <720: 21, >720: 19
Van Peski, 1999 [48]	Randomized controlled, non-blinded, trial of 72 patients presenting with chest pain referred by their general practitioners to the cardiology clinic of the Leiden University Hospital or the Diaconessenhuis Hospital between 1992 and the first months of 1996 and who had received a discharge diagnosis of NCCP, Netherlands	18 to 75 years old with chest pain as the main complaint, who had a normal cardiovascular system according to a cardiologist	Proven coronary artery disease or myocardial ischemia, as demonstrated by coronary angiography, exercise testing, laboratory examination, electrocardiogram, or chest x-ray, a history of typical angina pectoris; insufficient fluency in Dutch, current psychiatric treatment for NCCP, current diagnosis of an organic mental syndrome, psychotic disorder; major depression, bipolar disorder, or use of psychoactive substances (excluding nicotine) within 3 months before study entry	Cognitive behavioral treatment: 4 to 12 weekly sessions of 45 to 60 minutes, depending on the severity of the patient's problem, the maximum duration of therapy was 6 months. Treatment was modeled after cognitive-behavioral therapy for panic, hypochondriasis, and unexplained physical symptoms, each patient received written information about the therapy model and treatment procedures. The therapists were a physician with basic training in cognitive-behavioral therapy and a senior psychologist trained in cognitive-behavioral therapy vs. Usual care: free to use health resources as they saw fit. They were seen in the cardiology clinic for the follow-up assessments 6 months and 12 months after the baseline interview	72 (36)	49 (11)	1500 (1770)

ACS, acute coronary syndrome; CBT, cognitive behavioral therapy; CST, coping skills training; ECG, electrocardiogram; GERD, gastroesophageal reflux disease; GI, gastro-intestinal; mg, milligram; MIBI, methoxy-isobutyl-isonitril; min, minutes; n.r., not reported; NCCP, non-cardiac chest pain; NSAID, nonsteroidal antiinflammatory drugs; PPI, proton-pump inhibitor; vs., versus.

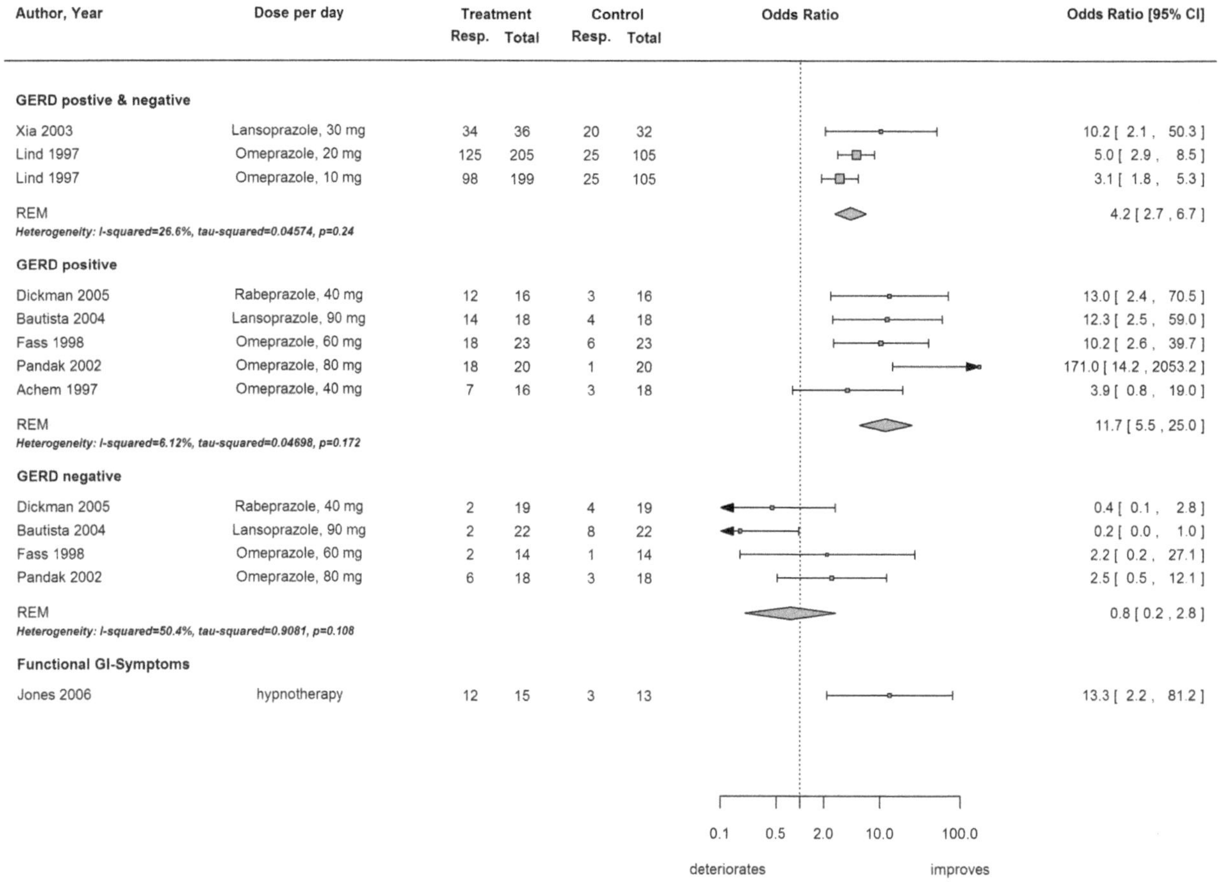

Figure 2. Efficacy of Proton Pump Inhibitor (PPI) treatment in patients with NCCP.

treatments included baclofen [33] and hypnotherapy [34]. Two RCTs included patients with musculoskeletal chest pain (7%, 229 patients): one compared the efficacy of manual therapy to acupuncture and sham intervention [35], while the other compared chiropractic treatment to self-management [36,37]. The efficacy of treatments based on cognitive behavioral principles was assessed in eleven RCTs (37%, 1370 patients) [38–48]. The use of psychotropic drugs compared with placebo was evaluated in seven RCTs (23%, 347 patients) [49–55]. Study quality was high in 5 RCTs (17%) and acceptable in 25 (83%; **Table S2**). No studies had to be excluded because of poor study quality. All studies included in the systematic review but not in the meta-analysis were rated to have low (n = 6) to no (n = 3) risk of outcome reporting bias.

Treatment efficacy for NCCP due to gastroesophageal reflux disease (GERD)

Only similar RCTs (n = 7, 771 patients) were included in the meta-analysis (Figure 2). A PPI was administered in most RCTs twice daily for 1 to 8 weeks. In two RCTs, GERD-positive and GERD-negative patients were not distinguished [30,32]; in both of these studies, the efficacy of treatment was more effective than placebo. The pooled odds ratio for a reduction in chest pain of ≥ 50% was 4.2 (95% CI 2.7 to 6.7, heterogeneity $I^2 = 26.6\%$).

When patients with GERD [n = 5, 192 patients, GERD-positive: confirmed by upper endoscopy and/or 24-h pH manometry [25–27,29,31]] were compared with patients without GERD [n = 4, 156 patients, GERD-negative [26,27,29,31]] the treatment efficacy of the PPI treatment increased. The pooled OR for GERD-positive patients with NCCP was 11.7 (95% CI 5.5 to 25.0, heterogeneity $I^2 = 6.1\%$); in comparison, the pooled OR for patients without GERD was 0.8 (95% CI 0.2 to 2.8, heterogeneity $I^2 = 50.4\%$).

While the heterogeneity among GERD-positive patients was low and three of five RCTs emanated from the same center [26,27,29], there was some heterogeneity among the GERD-negative patients. Regarding GERD-negative patients, two RCTs found a trend toward more chest pain in the treatment group [26,27] while two RCTs found a trend toward less chest pain in the PPI group [29,31]. Funnel plots for the three groups (GERD-positive and GERD-negative mixed, GERD-positive alone, and GERD-negative alone) are depicted in **Figure S1**. There was no evidence for funnel plot asymmetry in the mixed group (GERD-positive and GERD-negative, p = 0.27) or in the GERD-negative group (p = 0.68); however, some evidence of funnel plot asymmetry was observed in the GERD-positive group (p = 0.04), as assessed using Egger's regression test [22]. We refrained from statistical adjustment for outcome reporting bias as proposed by Copas et al. [19] because only one PPI treatment study was not included in our meta-analysis [28]. Dore et al. did not analyze the outcome of interest in our study and therefore the study was associated with a low risk of outcome reporting bias (**Table S3**). Jones et al. investigated the efficacy of hypnotherapy in patients with functional gastrointestinal symptoms (Figure 2) [34]. Baclofen treatment was associated with more chest pain (Figure 3) at the 2-

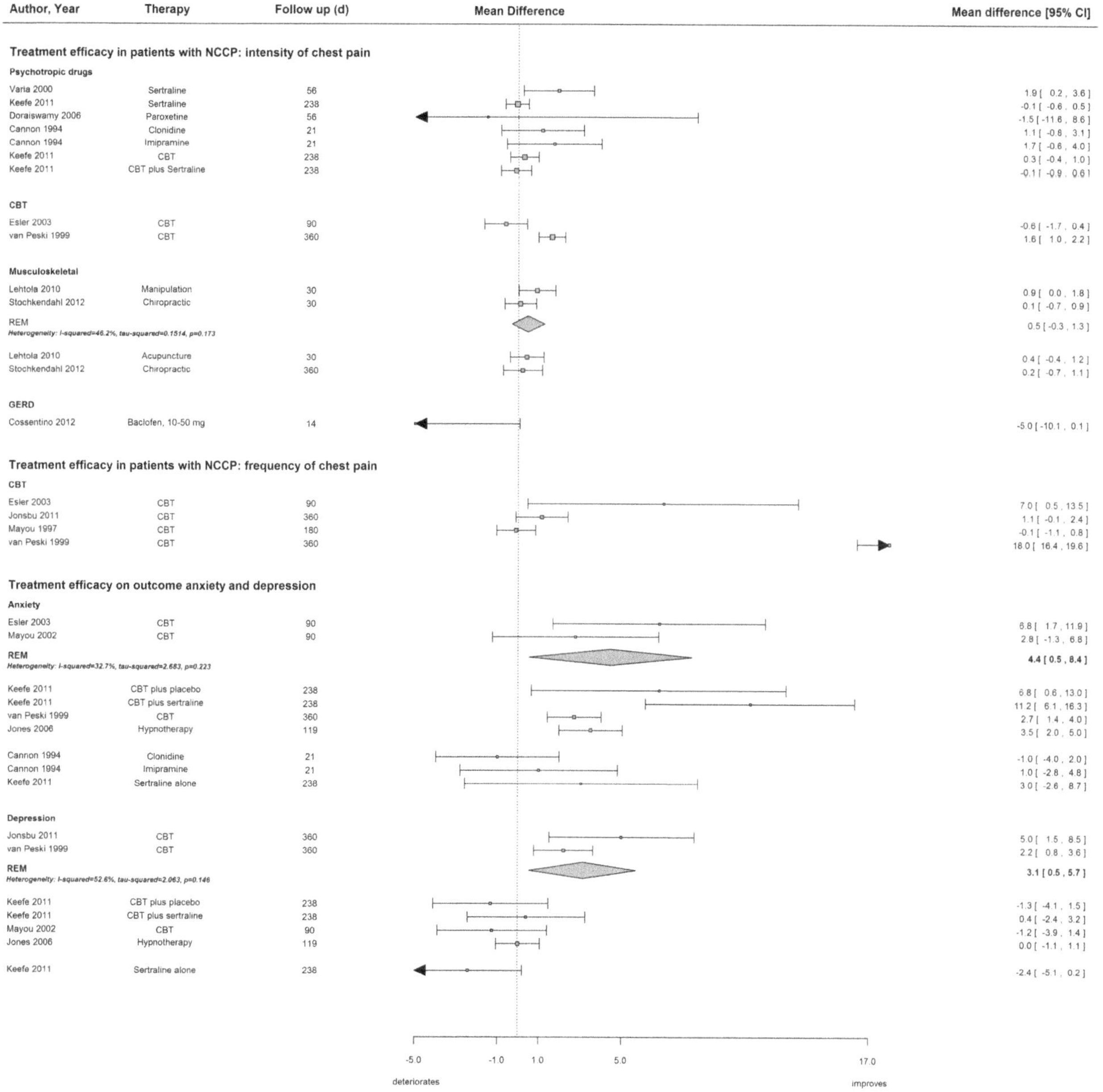

Figure 3. Treatment efficacy in patients with NCCP: intensity and frequency of chest pain.

week follow-up [33]. Detailed results for all studies are summarized in **Table S4**.

Treatment efficacy regarding the intensity and frequency of non-cardiac chest pain

Treating patients with NCCP without a specific diagnosis of psychiatric disease with the selective serotonin reuptake inhibitor sertraline was more effective after 2 months [54], but not after 8 months of follow-up for chest pain intensity (Figure 3) [52]. Although use of the tricyclic antidepressant imipramine exhibited a trend towards less chest pain intensity, the effect was not statistically significant [49]. Findings were mixed regarding treatments based on the principles of cognitive behavioral therapy (CBT). One study showed that CBT (4 to 12 60-min sessions) more effectively reduced chest pain intensity at 1 year than usual care at the cardiology department [48]. Another study found that cognitive skill training (5 bi-weekly and 6 30-min monthly sessions), alone or supplemented with sertraline, was no more effective than placebo or sertraline alone in reducing chest pain intensity at 8 months of follow-up [52]. A brief CBT intervention was not more effective in reducing chest pain intensity (Figure 3), but more effectively reduced chest pain frequency (Figure 3) at 3 months of follow-up [39]. Two smaller RCTs found no [44] or only a trend towards [41] less frequent chest pain after CBT interventions (Figure 3). In a small pilot study Johrei, a process of transmission of healing energy, was compared to a waiting list [56]. While the treatment group experienced a significant improvement in symptom intensity these findings need further validation. The heterogeneity of the study settings and treatments used prevented us from conducting a meta-analysis.

One study of patients with musculoskeletal NCCP found that manipulation reduced pain more effectively than acupuncture and usual care (Figure 3) [35]. Another study found that chiropractic treatment and home exercise were similarly effective [36]. The pooled mean difference for the manipulation therapy was 0.5 (95% CI −0.3 to 1.3, heterogeneity $I^2 = 46.2\%$).

Efficacy of treatment regarding anxiety and depression

Only similar studies were included in meta-analyses. CBT more effectively reduced anxiety scores in all studies (Figure 3). The pooled mean difference for CBT in two similar studies [39,43] was 4.4 (95% CI 0.5 to 8.4, heterogeneity $I^2 = 32.7\%$).

CBT treatment reduced depression scores more effectively than usual general practitioner (GP) care after 1 year [41,47]. The pooled mean difference for CBT was 3.1 (95% CI 0.5 to 5.7, heterogeneity $I^2 = 52.6\%$). A study with four arms compared CBT or no treatment and sertraline or placebo [52]. While CBT with and without sertraline was more effective at reducing anxiety scores, they were no more effective at reducing depression scores than placebo. At baseline, depression scores were lower than anxiety scores in this study population (depression 8.9–10.2, range 0–63; anxiety 34–41, range 20–80).

Discussion

Main findings

The systematic analysis of 30 RCTs involving patients with NCCP demonstrated that PPI treatment was effective in patients with GERD. In NCCP patients without GERD, PPI treatment was no more effective than placebo. Treatment based on cognitive behavioral principles reduced chest pain frequency compared with 'general practitioner treatment' in three RCTs, while one study found no effect. Most studies that compared the efficacy of serotonin antagonists or tricyclic agents with placebo demonstrated no difference or only a trend towards less pain intensity in the treatment arms. Manipulative treatment interventions produced conflicting results for patients with musculoskeletal chest pain, and acupuncture was no more effective than usual care. For most prevalent diseases that manifested with chest pain, only a few studies were available.

Results in light of the existing literature

To our knowledge, this is the first comprehensive systematic review and meta-analysis to summarize the current evidence on treatment efficacy based on RCTs for various diseases presenting in patients with NCCP. Recently new therapies for NCCP of gastrointestinal origin were discussed [57]. Treatment interventions including nitrates, Phosphodiesterase-5 inhibitors, anticholinergics, calcium channel blockers, and endoscopic injection of botulinum toxin may be effective in a subset of patients with gastrointestinal diseases. Most of these interventions have been studied in non-randomized trials or case series [58]. This systematic review and meta-analysis confirms that limited RCTs are available for many interventions and highlights the need for further studies. Non-randomized trials tend to overestimate treatment effects [59]. Further, this comprehensive overview addresses the need for interdisciplinary evaluation and care in patients with NCCP and summarizes the evidence for treatment interventions in underlying diseases oftentimes not considered. A recent systematic review found evidence that NCCP patients have similar levels of psychological morbidity than patients with cardiac chest pain and higher levels than healthy controls [60]. While gastroesophageal diseases are common these findings indicate that other diseases might not be diagnosed.

Only limited evidence was available for most prevalent diseases that manifest with chest pain. Only two RCTs investigated treatment efficacy of manual therapy in patients with musculoskeletal chest pain [35,36]. The efficacy of psychotropic drugs on chest pain intensity, anxiety and depression scores were in line with a recently published meta-analysis that analyzed the efficacy of CBT compared with pharmacotherapy in adults with major depressive disorder (21 RCTs, 2027 patients) or anxiety disorder (21 RCTs, 1266 patients) [61]. The authors found CBT to be equally effective as pharmacotherapy in patients with depression whereas CBT was somewhat more effective than pharmacotherapy in anxiety disorders [61]. It has been shown that patients discharged from the emergency department with the diagnosis of NCCP had elevated anxiety levels compared to healthy individuals [62]. Anxiety disorder might be an underlying disease for subjects with chest symptoms to seek evaluation in emergency departments. Interestingly, CBT was more effective in patients with panic disorders [61]. This information may be relevant for further management of patients with unexplained chest pain. No study was identified that investigated panic disorders in patients with NCCP. However, in patients that present with NCCP to the emergency department, panic disorders are often not diagnosed [63,64].

A recent meta-analysis using a hierarchical Bayesian model demonstrated the diagnostic value of the response to high-dose PPI treatment in patients with GERD [posterior mean sensitivity 0.89 and specificity of 0.88 [16]]. Together with the current findings in patients with NCCP, in which GERD is suspected, PPI treatment should be initiated early and PPI treatment response should be evaluated after 2 weeks [16]. While the findings are in line with previous published meta-analyses on PPI treatment studies [65,66], this is the first meta-analysis to assess study quality and the risk for outcome reporting bias. In comparison to Kahrilas et al. [65,66] and Cremonini et al. [65,66], one additional study was included [30]. Further, Cremonini et al. [65,66] included open-label studies and did not distinguish between GERD-positive and GERD-negative patients. We also used odds ratios as the effect measure for pooling because of its favorable mathematical properties over the relative risk. This includes that the odds ratio is unbounded regardless of the underlying event rate [67]. Our study expands on a relevant aspect in the clinical setting where the PPI response is often used for the diagnosis of GERD. We showed that the effect in a mixed patient sample is smaller compared to patients where GERD was diagnosed by a reference test (e.g. 24-hour pH monitoring). Therefore, a lack of response to PPI treatment after 2 weeks should lead to discontinuation of PPI treatment, while a response indicates underlying GERD for which PPI treatment is effective.

Strengths and limitations

This review comprehensively evaluates the currently available studies. The search was inclusive; no language restrictions were applied, a thorough bibliographic search was conducted to identify all relevant studies, and rigorous methodology was applied. The extraction process was performed in accordance with current guidelines and supported by an experienced statistician. Potential factors influencing treatment efficacy were identified by a multidisciplinary team (an internist, general practitioner, statistician, and methodologist).

The main limitation of this systematic review and meta-analysis was the limited number of RCTs. Many interventions used in clinical practice in patients with NCCP were not assessed in RCTs. Of the included studies, many were only of moderate methodological quality. Furthermore, NCCP is a collective term with potentially different underlying diseases and therefore might present differently. Treatment efficacy in one population in which the prevalence for one disease is high might be entirely different for another population [68]. In addition, the heterogeneity of the outcome measures used and follow-up durations reported prevented us from including most studies in our meta-analysis. The results of these studies should be interpreted on an individual study level within the context of the study population. We have tried to balance this by providing a thorough description of the studies inclusion and exclusion criteria and the study settings. This information will allow readers to judge to whom various study results apply.

Research implications

Additional research should compare diagnostic indicators (e.g., pain increase with movement or decrease on medication were associated with musculoskeletal chest pain) [16] plus a corresponding treatment intervention to usual care alone in defined patient populations (e.g., emergency departments, primary care). Future research should also aim to contribute to our knowledge about diagnostic processes and treatment decisions for patients with NCCP. Although most patients with chest pain consult primary care physicians [69], few studies are performed in this setting. Additional research is needed to strengthen the evidence in a primary care setting. Screening questionnaires for panic and anxiety disorders could be used to identify patients that need further specialized assessment and would respond well to treatments based on cognitive behavioral principles. No such study was found in the current analysis.

Implication for practice

Patients with NCCP incur high healthcare costs owing to extensive and often invasive diagnostic testing, as well as the effect of NCCP on quality of life. Early identification of underlying diseases is essential to avoid delayed treatment and chronicity of complaints. Symptoms and clinical findings may provide important information to guide treatment of an underlying illness [16]. In patients with typical GERD symptoms, twice-daily high-dose PPI treatment is the most efficient diagnostic and therapeutic approach. GERD is very likely if a positive treatment response occurs after 1 week, and is unlikely if there is no response after 4 weeks of PPI treatment [16]. In patients that do not respond to PPI, PPI treatment should be stopped if an endoscopy reveals no pathological findings.

Panic and anxiety disorders are often missed in clinical practice [70]. For patients with anxiety, treatments based on cognitive behavioral principles might be more effective than pharmacologic treatment. To date, evidence for the efficacy of serotonin antagonists or tricyclic agents in patients with NCCP is weak.

Conclusion

Timely diagnostic evaluation and treatment of the underlying disease is important for patients with NCCP. The current systematic review and meta-analysis showed a lack of RCTs for many diseases presenting with NCCP or treatment interventions proposed in the literature. Only limited evidence was available for prevalent diseases that manifest with chest pain. In addition, many treatment interventions that have been shown to be effective in non-randomized trials have not been studied in RCTs and might overestimate treatment efficacy. In patients suspected to have GERD high-dose treatment with a PPI is effective. In otherwise unexplained NCCP treatments based on cognitive behavioral principles might be considered. There is a need for further high quality studies addressing the gaps highlighted in this review.

Supporting Information

Figure S1 Risk of bias assessment by using Funnel Plot.
(TIF)

Table S1 Search Strategy July Week 28, 2013.
(DOCX)

Table S2 Summary of the SIGN quality assessment.
(DOCX)

Table S3 Risk for Outcome Reporting Bias in Trials (ORBIT) in studies excluded from Meta-analyses.
(DOCX)

Table S4 Detailed summary of results.
(DOCX)

Checklist S1 PRISMA checklist.
(DOC)

Author Contributions

Conceived and designed the experiments: JB BJ UH MW JS. Performed the experiments: JB BJ MW. Analyzed the data: JB BJ UH MW JS. Contributed reagents/materials/analysis tools: JB BJ UH MW JS. Contributed to the writing of the manuscript: JB BJ UH MW JS.

References

1. Eslick GD, Coulshed DS, Talley NJ (2002) Review article: The burden of illness of non-cardiac chest pain. Alimentary Pharmacology and Therapeutics 16: 1217–1223.
2. Kahn SE (2000) The challenge of evaluating the patient with chest pain. Arch Pathol Lab Med 124: 1418–1419.
3. Cayley WE Jr (2005) Diagnosing the cause of chest pain. Am Fam Physician 72: 2012–2021.
4. Blatchford O, Capewell S, Murray S, Blatchford M (1999) Emergency medical admissions in Glasgow: General practices vary despite adjustment for age, sex, and deprivation. British Journal of General Practice 49: 551–554.
5. Rosengren A, Wilhelmsen L (1998) Respiratory symptoms and long-term risk of death from cardiovascular disease, cancer and other causes in Swedish men. Int J Epidemiol 27: 962–969.
6. Buntinx F, Knockaert D, Bruyninckx R, De Blaey N, Aerts M, et al. (2001) Chest pain in general practice or in the hospital emergency department: Is it the same? Fam Pract 18: 586–589.
7. Rosengren A, Wilhelmsen L, Hagman M, Wedel H (1998) Natural history of myocardial infarction and angina pectoris in a general population sample of middle-aged men: a 16-year follow-up of the Primary Prevention Study, Goteborg, Sweden. J Intern Med 244: 495–505.
8. Nilsson S, Scheike M, Engblom D, Karlsson LG, Molstad S, et al. (2003) Chest pain and ischaemic heart disease in primary care. British Journal of General Practice 53: 378–382.
9. Verdon F, Burnand B, Herzig L, Junod M, Pecoud A, et al. (2007) Chest wall syndrome among primary care patients: a cohort study. BMC Fam Pract 8: 51.
10. Svavarsdottir AE, Jonasson MR, Gudmundsson GH, Fjeldsted K (1996) Chest pain in family practice. Diagnosis and long-term outcome in a community setting. Can Fam Physician 42: 1122–1128.
11. Wilcox RG, Roland JM, Hampton JR (1981) Prognosis of patients with "chest pain ?cause". Br Med J (Clin Res Ed) 282: 431–433.
12. Robertson N, Javed N, Samani NJ, Khunti K (2008) Psychological morbidity and illness appraisals of patients with cardiac and non-cardiac chest pain attending a rapid access chest pain clinic: a longitudinal cohort study. Heart 94: e12.
13. Eslick GD, Talley NJ (2008) Natural history and predictors of outcome for non-cardiac chest pain: a prospective 4-year cohort study. Neurogastroenterol Motil 20: 989–997.
14. Eslick GD, Talley NJ (2004) Non-cardiac chest pain: predictors of health care seeking, the types of health care professional consulted, work absenteeism and interruption of daily activities. Aliment Pharmacol Ther 20: 909–915.
15. Stochkendahl MJ, Christensen HW (2010) Chest pain in focal musculoskeletal disorders. Med Clin North Am 94: 259–273.

16. Wertli MM, Ruchti KB, Steurer J, Held U (2013) Diagnostic indicators of non-cardiovascular chest pain: a systematic review and meta-analysis. BMC Med 11: 239.
17. Moher D, Liberati A, Tetzlaff J, Altman DG (2009) Preferred reporting items for systematic reviews and meta-analyses: the PRISMA statement. PLoS Med 6: e1000097.
18. Eslick GD, Talley NJ (2000) Non-cardiac chest pain: squeezing the life out of the Australian healthcare system? Med J Aust 173: 233–234.
19. Copas J, Dwan K, Kirkham J, Williamson P (2013) A model-based correction for outcome reporting bias in meta-analysis. Biostatistics.
20. Kirkham JJ, Dwan KM, Altman DG, Gamble C, Dodd S, et al. (2010) The impact of outcome reporting bias in randomised controlled trials on a cohort of systematic reviews. BMJ 340: c365.
21. Higgins JPT, Green S (2011) Cochrane Handbook for Systematic Reviews of Interventions. The Cochrane Collaboration.
22. Egger M, Davey Smith G, Schneider M, Minder C (1997) Bias in meta-analysis detected by a simple, graphical test. BMJ 315: 629–634.
23. R Development Core Team (2011) R: A language and environment for statistical computing. In: R Foundation for Statistical Computing V, Austria, editor. Vienna, Austria: R Foundation for Statistical Computing.
24. Viechtbauer W (2010) Conducting Meta-Analyses in R with the metafor Package. Journal of Statistical Software 36: 1–48.
25. Achem SR, Kolts BE, MacMath T, Richter J, Mohr D, et al. (1997) Effects of omeprazole versus placebo in treatment of noncardiac chest pain and gastroesophageal reflux. Dig Dis Sci 42: 2138–2145.
26. Bautista J, Fullerton H, Briseno M, Cui H, Fass R (2004) The effect of an empirical trial of high-dose lansoprazole on symptom response of patients with non-cardiac chest pain - A randomized, double-blind, placebo-controlled, crossover trial. Alimentary Pharmacology and Therapeutics 19: 1123–1130.
27. Dickman R, Emmons S, Cui H, Sewell J, Hernandez D, et al. (2005) The effect of a therapeutic trial of high-dose rabeprazole on symptom response of patients with non-cardiac chest pain: A randomized, double-blind, placebo-controlled, crossover trial. Alimentary Pharmacology and Therapeutics 22: 547–555.
28. Dore MP, Pedroni A, Pes GM, Maragkoudakis E, Tadeu V, et al. (2007) Effect of antisecretory therapy on atypical symptoms in gastroesophageal reflux disease. Digestive Diseases & Sciences 52: 463–468.
29. Fass R, Fennerty MB, Ofman JJ, Gralnek IM, Johnson C, et al. (1998) The clinical and economic value of a short course of omeprazole in patients with noncardiac chest pain. Gastroenterology 115: 42–49.
30. Lind T, Havelund T, Carlsson R, Anker-Hansen O, Glise H, et al. (1997) Heartburn without oesophagitis: efficacy of omeprazole therapy and features determining therapeutic response. Scand J Gastroenterol 32: 974–979.
31. Pandak WM, Arezo S, Everett S, Jesse R, DeCosta G, et al. (2002) Short course of omeprazole: a better first diagnostic approach to noncardiac chest pain than endoscopy, manometry, or 24-hour esophageal pH monitoring. J Clin Gastroenterol 35: 307–314.
32. Xia HHX, Lai KC, Lam SK, Hu WHC, Wong NYH, et al. (2003) Symptomatic response to lansoprazole predicts abnormal acid reflux in endoscopy-negative patients with non-cardiac chest pain. Alimentary Pharmacology and Therapeutics 17: 369–377.
33. Cossentino MJ, Mann K, Armbruster SP, Lake JM, Maydonovitch C, et al. (2012) Randomised clinical trial: the effect of baclofen in patients with gastro-oesophageal reflux - a randomised prospective study. Aliment Pharmacol Ther 35: 1036–1044.
34. Jones H, Cooper P, Miller V, Brooks N, Whorwell PJ (2006) Treatment of non-cardiac chest pain: a controlled trial of hypnotherapy. Gut 55: 1403–1408.
35. Lehtola V, Korhonen I, Airaksinen O (2010) A randomised, placebo-controlled, clinical trial for the short-term effectiveness of manipulative therapy and acupuncture on pain caused by mechanical thoracic spine dysfunction. International Musculoskeletal Medicine 32: 25–32.
36. Stochkendahl MJ, Christensen HW, Vach W, Hoilund-Carlsen PF, Haghfelt T, et al. (2012) Chiropractic treatment vs self-management in patients with acute chest pain: a randomized controlled trial of patients without acute coronary syndrome. J Manipulative Physiol Ther 35: 7–17.
37. Stochkendahl MJ, Christensen HW, Vach W, Hoilund-Carlsen PF, Haghfelt T, et al. (2012) A randomized clinical trial of chiropractic treatment and self-management in patients with acute musculoskeletal chest pain: 1-year follow-up. J Manipulative Physiol Ther 35: 254–262.
38. Arnold J, Goodacre S, Bath P, Price J (2009) Information sheets for patients with acute chest pain: randomised controlled trial. BMJ: British Medical Journal (Overseas & Retired Doctors Edition) 338: 700–702.
39. Esler JL, Barlow DH, Woolard RH, Nicholson RA, Nash JM, et al. (2003) A brief-cognitive behavioral intervention for patients with noncardiac chest pain. Behavior Therapy 34: 129–148.
40. Hess EP, Knoedler MA, Shah ND, Kline JA, Breslin M, et al. (2012) The chest pain choice decision aid: a randomized trial. Circulation Cardiovascular Quality & Outcomes 5: 251–259.
41. Jonsbu E, Dammen T, Morken G, Moum T, Martinsen EW (2011) Short-term cognitive behavioral therapy for non-cardiac chest pain and benign palpitations: a randomized controlled trial. J Psychosom Res 70: 117–123.
42. Lahmann C, Loew TH, Tritt K, Nickel M (2008) Efficacy of functional relaxation and patient education in the treatment of somatoform heart disorders: a randomized, controlled clinical investigation. Psychosomatics 49: 378–385.
43. Mayou R, Sprigings D, Birkhead J, Price J (2002) A randomized controlled trial of a brief educational and psychological intervention for patients presenting to a cardiac clinic with palpitation. Psychol Med 32: 699–706.
44. Mayou RA, Bryant BM, Sanders D, Bass C, Klimes I, et al. (1997) A controlled trial of cognitive behavioural therapy for non-cardiac chest pain. Psychol Med 27: 1021–1031.
45. Potts SG, Lewin R, Fox KA, Johnstone EC (1999) Group psychological treatment for chest pain with normal coronary arteries. QJM 92: 81–86.
46. Sanders D, Bass C, Mayou RA, Goodwin S, Bryant BM, et al. (1997) Non-cardiac chest pain: why was a brief intervention apparently ineffective? Psychol Med 27: 1033–1040.
47. Van Peski-Oosterbaan AS, Spinhoven P, Van der Does AJ, Bruschke AV, Rooijmans HG (1999) Cognitive change following cognitive behavioural therapy for non-cardiac chest pain. Psychotherapy & Psychosomatics 68: 214–220.
48. Van Peski-Oosterbaan AS, Spinhoven P, Van Rood Y, Van der Does JW, Bruschke AV, et al. (1999) Cognitive-behavioral therapy for noncardiac chest pain: A randomized trial. American Journal of Medicine 106: 424–429.
49. Cannon RO, Quyyumi AA, Mincemoyer R, Stine AM, Gracely RH, et al. (1994) Imipramine in Patients with Chest Pain Despite Normal Coronary Angiograms. New England Journal of Medicine 330: 1411–1417.
50. Cox ID, Hann CM, Kaski JC (1998) Low dose imipramine improves chest pain but not quality of life in patients with angina and normal coronary angiograms. Eur Heart J 19: 250–254.
51. Doraiswamy PM, Varia I, Hellegers C, Wagner HR, Clary GL, et al. (2006) A randomized controlled trial of paroxetine for noncardiac chest pain. Psychopharmacol Bull 39: 15–24.
52. Keefe FJ, Shelby RA, Somers TJ, Varia I, Blazing M, et al. (2011) Effects of coping skills training and sertraline in patients with non-cardiac chest pain: a randomized controlled study. Pain 152: 730–741.
53. Rao SS, Mudipalli RS, Remes-Troche JM, Utech CL, Zimmerman B (2007) Theophylline improves esophageal chest pain–a randomized, placebo-controlled study. American Journal of Gastroenterology 102: 930–938.
54. Varia I, Logue E, O'Connor C, Newby K, Wagner HR, et al. (2000) Randomized trial of sertraline in patients with unexplained chest pain of noncardiac origin. Am Heart J 140: 367–372.
55. Wulsin L, Liu T, Storrow A, Evans S, Dewan N, et al. (2002) A randomized, controlled trial of panic disorder treatment initiation in an emergency department chest pain center. Ann Emerg Med 39: 139–143.
56. Gasiorowska A, Navarro-Rodriguez T, Dickman R, Wendel C, Moty B, et al. (2009) Clinical trial: the effect of Johrei on symptoms of patients with functional chest pain. Aliment Pharmacol Ther 29: 126–134.
57. Maradey-Romero C, Fass R (2014) New therapies for non-cardiac chest pain. Curr Gastroenterol Rep 16: 390.
58. Hershcovici T, Achem SR, Jha LK, Fass R (2012) Systematic review: the treatment of noncardiac chest pain. Aliment Pharmacol Ther 35: 5–14.
59. Kunz R, Vist G, Oxman AD (2007) Randomisation to protect against selection bias in healthcare trials. Cochrane Database Syst Rev: MR000012.
60. Webster R, Norman P, Goodacre S, Thompson A (2012) The prevalence and correlates of psychological outcomes in patients with acute non-cardiac chest pain: a systematic review. Emergency Medicine Journal 29: 267–273.
61. Roshanaei-Moghaddam B, Pauly MC, Atkins DC, Baldwin SA, Stein MB, et al. (2011) Relative effects of CBT and pharmacotherapy in depression versus anxiety: is medication somewhat better for depression, and CBT somewhat better for anxiety? Depress Anxiety 28: 560–567.
62. Smeijers L, van de Pas H, Nyklicek I, Notten PJ, Pedersen SS, et al. (2014) The independent association of anxiety with non-cardiac chest pain. Psychol Health 29: 253–263.
63. White KS, Raffa SD, Jakle KR, Stoddard JA, Barlow DH, et al. (2008) Morbidity of DSM-IV Axis I disorders in patients with noncardiac chest pain: Psychiatric morbidity linked with increased pain and health care utilization. Journal of consulting and clinical psychology 76: 422.
64. Fleet RP, Dupuis G, Marchand A, Burelle D, Arsenault A, et al. (1996) Panic disorder in emergency department chest pain patients: prevalence, comorbidity, suicidal ideation, and physician recognition. The American journal of medicine 101: 371–380.
65. Cremonini F, Wise J, Moayyedi P, Talley NJ (2005) Diagnostic and therapeutic use of proton pump inhibitors in non-cardiac chest pain: A metaanalysis. American Journal of Gastroenterology 100: 1226–1232.
66. Kahrilas PJ, Hughes N, Howden CW (2011) Response of unexplained chest pain to proton pump inhibitor treatment in patients with and without objective evidence of gastro-oesophageal reflux disease. Gut 60: 1473–1478.
67. Egger M, Smith GD, Altman D (2008) Systematic reviews in health care: meta-analysis in context. Wiley. com.
68. Wilhelmsen L, Rosengren A, Hagman M, Lappas G (1998) "Nonspecific" chest pain associated with high long-term mortality: results from the primary prevention study in Goteborg, Sweden. Clin Cardiol 21: 477–482.
69. Bosner S, Becker A, Hani MA, Keller H, Sonnichsen AC, et al. (2010) Chest wall syndrome in primary care patients with chest pain: presentation, associated features and diagnosis. Fam Pract 27: 363–369.
70. Katerndahl DA, Trammell C (1997) Prevalence and recognition of panic states in STARNET patients presenting with chest pain. J Fam Pract 45: 54–63.

7

Blocking TRPV1 in Nucleus Accumbens Inhibits Persistent Morphine Conditioned Place Preference Expression in Rats

Li-Jun Heng[1,2⑨], Bo Huang[1⑨], Heng Guo[3⑨], Lian-Ting Ma[2], Wei-Xin Yuan[1], Jian Song[2], Peng Wang[1,2], Guo-Zheng Xu[2]*, Guo-Dong Gao[1]*

1 Department of Neurosurgery, Tangdu Hospital of Fourth Military Medical University, Xi'an, Shaanxi, China, **2** Department of Neurosurgery, Wuhan General Hospital of Guangzhou Military Command, Wuhan, Hubei, China, **3** Department of Neurosurgery, PLA Chengdu General Hospital, Chengdu, Sichuan, China

Abstract

The function of TRPV1 (transient receptor potential vanilloid subfamily, member 1) in the central nervous system is gradually elucidated. It has been recently proved to be expressed in nucleus accumbens (NAc), a region playing an essential role in mediating opioid craving and taking behaviors. Based on the general role of TRPV1 antagonist in blocking neural over-excitability by both pre- and post-synaptic mechanisms, TRPV1 antagonist capsazepine (CPZ) was tested for its ability to prohibit persistent opioid craving in rats. In the present study, we assessed the expression of TRPV1 in nucleus accumbens and investigated the effect of CPZ in bilateral nucleus accumbens on persistent morphine conditioned place preference (mCPP) in rats. We also evaluated the side-effect of CPZ on activity by comparing cross-beam times between groups. We found that morphine conditioned place preference increased the TRPV1 expression and CPZ attenuated morphine conditioned place preference in a dose-dependent and target-specific manner after both short- and long-term spontaneous withdrawal, reflected by the reduction of the increased time in morphine-paired side. CPZ (10 nM) could induce prolonged and stable inhibition of morphine conditioned place preference expression. More importantly, CPZ did not cause dysfunction of activity in the subjects tested, which indicates the inhibitory effect was not obtained at the sacrifice of regular movement. Collectively, these results indicated that injection of TRPV1 antagonist in nucleus accumbens is capable of attenuating persistent morphine conditioned place preference without affecting normal activity. Thus, TRPV1 antagonist is one of the promising therapeutic drugs for the treatment of opioid addiction.

Editor: Yael Abreu-Villaça, Universidade do Estado do Rio de Janeiro, Brazil

Funding: This work is supported by National Natural Science Foundation of China (31070940 to GDG, 31100778 to LJH), Military 12th Five-year Program of China (BWS11J006 to GZX), Scientific Research Foundation for the Returned Overseas Chinese Scholars, State Education Ministry (SRFROCS1711 to LJH), Tangdu Outstanding Talents Surporting Project (Tangdu5084 to LJH) and China Postdoctoral Science Foundation. The funders had no role in study design, data collection and analysis, decision to publish, or preparation of the manuscript.

Competing Interests: The authors have declared that no competing interests exist.

* Email: gaogd@outlook.com (GDG); xu-gz@163.com (GZX)

⑨ These authors contributed equally to this work.

Introduction

Opioid addiction is a type of complex brain disorder, which is characterized by uncontrollable opioid craving and compulsive opioid seeking and taking behavior regardless of consequences. High incidence of drug craving and relapse to drug seeking and taking behaviors is the main obstacle for treatment [1]. As traditional therapy fail to work well in preventing relapse in opioid addicts, more effective and target-specific pharmacotherapies with little side effect are in demand.

TRPV1 (transient receptor potential vanilloid subfamily, member 1) is a nonselective cation channel that could be activated by heat, proton, capsaicin and endogenous ligands endovanilloids [2–4]. TRPV1 distributed in a variety of areas in the central nervous system [5–8]. It has been gradually established that TRPV1 had important role in a series of physiological and pathological status, such as neural development, anxiety and depression. There is still limited information about the function of central TRPV1 in drug addiction, especially in opioid addiction. Previous research suggested that repeated systematic blockade of TRPV1 by capsazepine (CPZ), a TRPV1 antagonist, significantly reduced naloxone-induced withdrawal symptoms [9]. However, there was no further tests of the effect of CPZ on morphine craving or relapse, which is the core process of addiction [1]. Recently, it has been reported that TRPV1 antagonist decreased cocaine-induced cocaine-seeking behavior [10]. Both findings suggest the engagement of TRPV1 in drug addiction behaviors. However, considering the limitation of the animal model used, the difference between opioid and psychostimulant dependence [11] and the peripheral effects accompanying systematic delivery of TRPV1 blocker, further studies are needed to clarify the central action site and behavioral role for TRPV1 in opioid relapse.

Nucleus accumbens (NAc) was known as a critical region in mediating opioid relapse, and has been found to express TRPV1 [5,6]. Anatomical and electrophysiological studies suggest the possible subcellular localization of NAc TRPV1 is mainly in the presynaptic terminals and the cell bodies [5,6,12,13]. Presynaptic TRPV1 has been proved to facilitate glutamate release and accordingly potentiate glutamatergic transmission in widespread brain areas [13–21]. Importantly, the enhancement of glutamatergic synaptic strength via increased presynaptic release in NAc is an essential neuroadaptation during withdrawal associated with opioid dependence [22]. Blockade or attenuation of NAc glutamatergic transmission to reduce the excitatory drive may prevent relapse to opioid use [23–25]. In another aspect, TRPV1 present in the cell bodies are proposed to modulate neuronal activity [20]. TRPV1 agonist could increase the spike frequency of neurons in ventral tegmental area [26]. These observations strongly suggested that NAc TRPV1 antagonism might perform anti-relapse effect by limiting neuronal activity and diminishing the efficacy of excitatory inputs from presynaptic terminals, which could reduce morphine conditioned place preference (mCPP) expression [27].

Taken together, the TRPV1 receptor in nucleus accumbens could be a potential target for preventing opioid relapse. In the present study, we test the effect of blocking TRPV1 in NAc on persistent mCPP expression in rats and assess the influence of TRPV1 antagonist on motor activity in the same subjects.

Materials and Methods

Subjects and surgery

Male Sprague–Dawley rats (initial weight 200–250 g; Centre of Experimental Animals, Fourth Military Medical University, Xi'an, Shaanxi, China) were individually housed in a temperature- and humidity-controlled vivarium on a 12-hour light/dark cycle. All rats were allowed ad libitum access to food and water. Rats were acclimated to handling daily and allowed to adapt for at least 3 days before the experiment. This study was carried out in strict accordance with the Chinese Animal Welfare Act. The protocol was approved by the Committee on the Ethics of Animal Experiments of Tangdu Hospital of Fourth Military Medical University (Permit Number: TD-5084). All surgery was performed under chloral hydrate anesthesia, and all efforts were made to minimize suffering.

Rats were anesthetized with chloral hydrate (400 mg/kg, i.p.) and implanted with cannulas (0.67 mm of external diameter; Rewardsales, Shenzhen, Guangdong, China) positioned 1.5 mm above each target. The coordinates (Paxinos and Watson, 2005) were as follows respectively: NAc core: anteroposterior (AP), + 1.5 mm and mediolateral (ML), ±1.6 mm from bregma; dorsoventral (DV), −6.0 mm from the skull surface; Dorsal striatum (DS): AP, +0.9 mm; ML, ±3.4 mm; DV, −3.8 mm. The cannulas were anchored to the skull with stainless steel screws and dental cement. A stainless steel probe with a plastic cap was inserted into each cannula to keep them unblocked and prevent infection. Rats were allowed to recover from surgery for at least 5d before morphine conditioned preference training. Food intake and body weights were assessed before and after the surgery.

Morphine conditioned place preference

All experiments were performed in a dimly lit room. The CPP apparatus is composed of two equally sized wooden chambers(25.3×20.1×20.3 cm) separated by a guillotine door. The two chambers differ in their color and floor texture to provide distinct contexts that were paired with morphine or saline injections. One chamber consisted of white walls and a smooth PVC-covered floor with hollow tranverse lines. The other chamber had black walls and a coarse PVC-covered floor with hollow longitudinal lines. The procedure consisted of three different phases: preconditioning test (day 1), conditioning (day 2-day 6), and postconditioning tests, as indicated in Results. In the preconditioning test, each rat was placed in the white compartment with the door open to allow the animal to freely explore the apparatus for 15 min. Animals showing a strong unconditioned preference (>540 s in any chamber), which were 7 of the 135 rats totally used, were discarded. In the subsequent 5 days, conditioning was conducted using a counterbalanced protocol, such that one-half of the animals in each experimental group were conditioned to the spontaneously preferred side and the other half to the spontaneously nonpreferred side. In each conditioning day, the animals received an injection of either morphine (1 mg/kg, 3 mg/kg, 10 mg/kg, s.c.) or saline (1 ml/kg, s.c.) at 9:00–9:30 and were confined for 45 min in the assigned chamber before returning to their home cages. Six hours later, the animals received an injection of vehicle solution (saline, 1 ml/kg, s.c.) and were confined to the alternative chamber for 45 min. In the postconditioning phase, the expression of CPP was tested in withdrawal day 1, 7 (1 w, short-term withdrawal), 14 (2 w) and 21 (3 w, long-term withdrawal) after the last training session. The postconditioning test consisted of placing the animal into the white chamber and allowing it to freely access both chambers for 15 min. Videos of all 15 min tests were captured online and analyzed offline. The amount of time that the animals spend in the conditioned chamber was recorded as CPP score (in seconds).

Intra-NAc application of CPZ

All rats firstly received mCPP training with 10 mg/kg morphine as described earlier. CPZ was dissolved in DMSO and stored at the concentration of 100 μM, which was diluted to different concentrations for intracranial injection with at most 0.1% DMSO in final solution. Vehicle solutions were prepared accordingly. CPZ (0.1 nM, 1 nM, 10 nM) or vehicle was injected bilateral intra-NAc daily from 3 days before the mCPP expression test during short-term (1 w) or long-term (3 w) withdrawal. CPZ (1 μl) was delivered over 3 min for each side of target. The CPP test was

Table 1. The food intake and body weight of animals after surgery (Means±SEM).

Measured parameters	Control	Surgery
Food intake (g/d)	23.01±4.93	22.76±4.09
Initial body weight (g)	208.96±10.07	211.10±11.28
Body weight after recover (g)	219.92±7.16*	221.20±9.51*

*$p<0.05$, compared to the initial body weight.

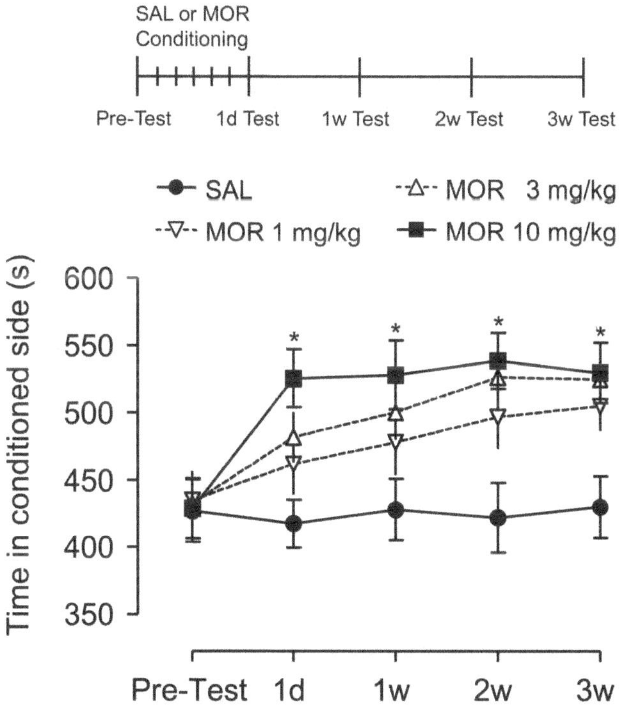

Figure 1. Repeated morphine conditioning induced persistent conditioned place preference (CPP) during withdrawal. Morphine conditioned place preference scores (time spent in drug-paired chamber) increased during morphine withdrawal. Sustained increase of mCPP score during morphine withdrawal occurred in high-dose morphine group (10 mg/kg) but not in low- (1 mg/kg) or moderate-dose (3 mg/kg) groups (n = 3). *$p<0.01$, *vs* SAL group. SAL, saline; MOR, morphine.

performed 30 min after the last CPZ injection. Furthermore, to examine the target specific effect of CPZ on mCPP, CPZ (10 nM) was injected unilateral NAc or bilateral DS before mCPP test during short-term (1 w) withdrawal.

Motor activity assessment

To assess the effects of CPZ on motor activity, crossline times were counted manually from the video of mCPP test after CPZ injection. Crossline times was defined as sum of the counts of the subject moving cross the two putative transverse lines trisecting each chamber and the counts of the subject crossing the guillotine door.

Immunoelectron microscopy

After the behavior test, rats were anesthetized with chloral hydrate (400 mg/kg, i.p.) and perfused intracardially with 100 ml of physiological saline (0.9% NaCl), followed by perfusion with a fixative containing 0.05% glutaraldehyde, 4% paraformaldehyde and 15% picric acid. The brain was removed from the skull and post-fixed in the above fixative without glutaraldehyde at room temperature for 2 hours. Vibratome sections 50 μm in thickness were cut from the blocks. Following washing in 0.01 M PBS, the sections were cryoprotected in 30% sucrose until they sunk. The sections were washed in 0.01 M PBS and incubated in blocking solution (5% NGS+5% BSA) at room temperature for 3 hours. After washing in 0.01 M PBS, the sections were incubated in rabbit anti-TRPV1 antibodies (1:150, Santa Cruz Biotechnology) and containing 1% BSA for 48 hours at 4°C. Following incubation with the primary antiserum, the sections were processed for immunogold labeling of rabbit TRPV1 antiserum. The tissue was rinsed in PBS and incubated overnight at 4°C in a 1:50 dilution of colloidal gold conjugated to goat anti-rabbit IgG (Nanoprobes) in 1% BSA. The sections were rinsed in PBS and post-fixed in 2% glutaraldehyde for 45 minutes. They were then rinsed in deionized water 10 times, and the gold particles were silver intensified by a 9-minute incubation in an HQ Silver silver enhancer (Nanoprobes). After rinsing in deionized water and 0.1 M PB 6 times, the sections were osmicated (0.5% OsO_4, 1 hour, room temperature), dehydrated and embedded in Durcupan. After examination by light microscopy, the areas of interest were re-embedded and ultrathin-sectioned for electron microscopy. Ultrathin serial sections were collected on formvar-coated single slot grids, stained with lead citrate and washed in distilled water. Sections were observed under an electron microscope (JEM-1230).

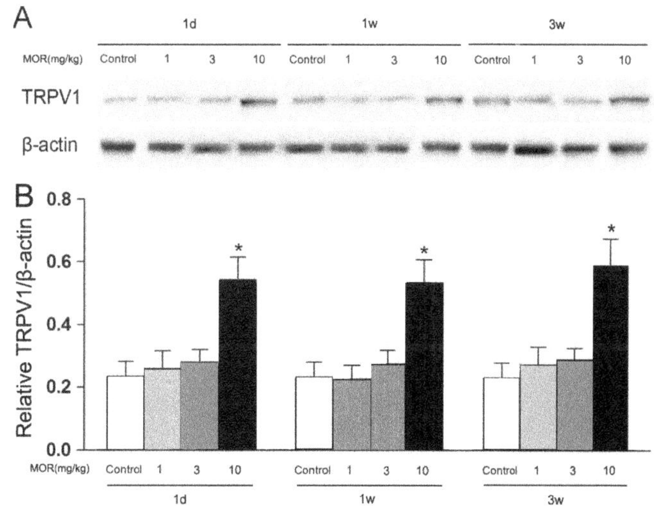

Figure 2. Analysis of western blot results of TRPV1 expression in the nucleus accumbens (NAc). (A) Representative blots of TRPV1. β-actin showed similar protein loading in each group. (B) Densitometric analyses of TRPV1 expression in NAc. The changes were expressed as the ratio to β-actin. Data represent Mean±SEM (n = 3), *$p<0.01$, *vs* control group.

The quantity of the symmetric and asymmetric synapses established by TRPV1-positive axon terminals was examined in the NAc. Serial ultrathin sections were made from a depth of ~3 μm from the surface of the vibratome sections. Every 8th section the TRPV1-stained terminals were analyzed in order, following the rules of systematic random sampling, to avoid sampling the same axon terminals. The number of TRPV1 terminals forming symmetric and asymmetric synapses was calculated for each group and normalized to 3000 μm^2 to quantify the exact changes in the number of stained terminals in each group. To assess any changes occurring in the density of TRPV1 per terminal, the number of gold particles located in the membrane of the axon terminals was counted and normalized to 1 μm of the terminal's perimeter. Image-Pro Plus 6.0 was used to make the above measurements.

Western blot

After sacrifice, the brain was dissected, chilled on a glass plate on ice and then cut into slices. The trace of the entry needle was checked to confirm the injection site. According to Atlas of The Rat Brain by George Paxinos & Charles Watson, the area of Bregma ±1.6 mm was removed from the slices and cut limited tissue of NAc, and homogenized in ice-cold homogenizing buffer (50 mM Tris-Cl, pH 7.4, 150 mM NaCl, 5 mM EDTA, 0.1% SDS, 1% NP-40, 1% deoxycholate, 1% Triton X-100, 10 mM PMSF, 50 mM sodium vanadate and 0.1% protease inhibitors cock-tail (Roche, Switzerland)). After centrifugation at 12,000×g for 15 min at 4 °C, the supernatant was collected and the protein content was subsequently assayed by using a BCA Protein Assay Kit (Pierce, Rockford, IL, USA). Equal quantities of total protein (75 μg per lane) were separated by sodium dodecyl sulfate-polyacrylamide gel electrophoresis (SDS-PAGE), followed by transfer to nitrocellulose membranes. The membranes were incubated in 5% milk at room temperature for 2 h. Blots were then incubated with rabbit polyclonal antibody against TRPV1 (1:1000, Santa Cruz Biotechnology), or β-actin (1:2000). After washing with buffer, the blots were incubated in anti-rabbit (Zhong Shan, Beijing, China, 1:1000) secondary antibody conjugated with horseradish peroxide in TBS-T with 5% milk at 4 °C overnight. The blots were visualized using a West Pico Chemiluminescent Kit (Pierce, Rockford, IL, USA), and the density of protein bands quantified by transmittance densitometry using volume integration with LumiAnalyst Image Analysis software.

Histology

At the end of the behavioral experiments, rats were anesthetized with chloral hydrate (400 mg/kg, i.p.) and perfused intracardially with 10% PBS-buffered formalin. The brains were removed, post-fixed overnight in a 30% sucrose/formalin solution, and then cryoprotected in 30% sucrose/saline. To verify the location of the cannula tips, 40 μm coronal sections were cut through the targeted area (NAc or DS), and stained with cresyl violet, and examined under a light microscope. Rats with off-target cannula placements in only one side of Nac were involved in the Uni-off Nac group for analyses. Rats with incorrect cannula placements were excluded from the study. Overall, six rats were excluded for this reason.

Data analysis

Data were expressed as Mean ±SEM. Statistical analyses were performed using repeated measures analysis of variance (ANOVA) followed by Duncan *post hoc* tests for multiple comparisons. The accepted level of statistical significance is $p<0.05$.

Results

Food intake and body weight after surgery

As shown in Table.1, the daily food intake of surgery animals was similar with control group after the surgery under anesthetized with chloral hydrate. All animals showed increasing body weight after 5-day raise. There were not significant differences of both initial and recovering body weight between control and surgery groups.

Morphine conditioned place preference

Higher mCPP scores were observed in morphine conditioned groups (Fig.1). In 1 mg/kg and 3 mg/kg morphine groups, the mCPP expression was numerically increased, but this difference was not significant ($F=0.375$, $p=0.960$). However, comparing to control group, significantly higher mCPP scores in all the 4

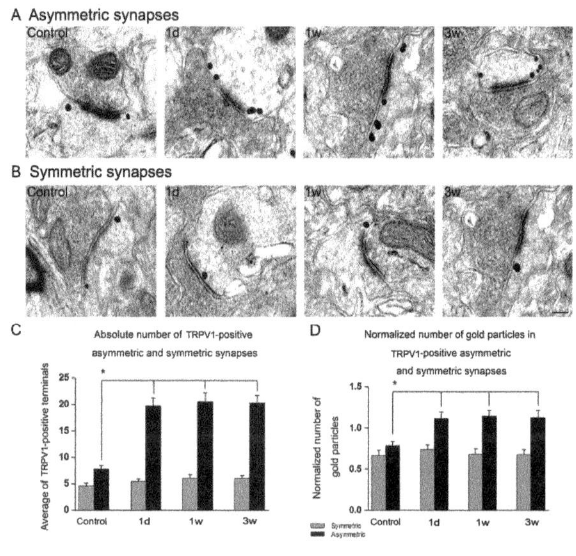

Figure 3. Quantitative changes in TRPV1 expression at the ultrastructural level in morphine withdrawal groups. High-power electron micrographs from the NAc of different groups showing TRPV1 immunogold labeling in the axon terminals forming asymmetric, excitatory-type synapses (A) and symmetric, inhibitory-type synapses (B). In the morphine withdrawal groups the number of gold particles on terminals forming asymmetric synapses increased (A). Graph (C) shows changes in the average number of TRPV1-positive asymmetric and symmetric synapses in each group. The number of TRPV1-positive asymmetric synapses in the morphine withdrawal groups was significantly higher than the control group. However, no difference was found in the normalized number of TRPV1-positive symmetric synapses among all groups. The number of TRPV1-positive symmetric synapses of control were 4.72±0.77, 4.72±0.47 and 4.74±1.00 for 1 d, 1 w and 3 w group respectively. The number of TRPV1-positive asymmetric synapses of control were 7.74±1.38, 7.75±0.77 and 7.74±1.28 for 1 d, 1 w and 3 w group respectively. Graph (D) shows the normalized number of gold particles in TRPV1-positive asymmetric and symmetric synapses. No difference appeared in the normalized number of gold particles in TRPV1-positive symmetric synapses. In contrast, a significant increase occurred in the normalized number of gold particles in TRPV1-positive asymmetric synapses of morphine withdrawal groups versus control group. The normalized number of gold particles in TRPV1-positive symmetric synapses of control were 0.68±0.17, 0.68±0.03 and 0.69±0.04 for 1 d, 1 w and 3 w group respectively. The normalized number of gold particles in TRPV1-positive asymmetric synapses of control were 0.78±0.07, 0.79±0.13 and 0.79±0.03 for 1 d, 1 w and 3 w group respectively. Scale: 200 nm. Data represent Mean±SEM (n = 3), *$p<0.05$, *vs* control group.

postconditioning tests performed at 1 d, 1 w, 2 w, 3 w after last training session were observed in high-dose (10 mg/kg) morphine conditioned group ($F = 8.144$, $p = 0.006$). There was no significant difference for mCPP score among four time point of postconditioning tests in 10 mg/kg morphine group ($p>0.05$), which indicated that morphine with 10 mg/kg induced a persistent and relatively stable mCPP expression. We chose 10 mg/kg morphine for conditioning training in the CPZ-intervening experiments.

Morphine increased TRPV1 expression in NAc meurons

Levels of TRPV1 in the nucleus accumbens were detected by Western blot and quantitatively analyzed (Fig. 2). Control group revealed the moderate expression of TRPV1 in the nucleus accumbens. There were not significant changes of TRPV1 expression in 1 mg/kg and 3 mg/kg morphine treated groups. However, TRPV1 immunoreactivity was increased markedly in 10 mg/kg morphine withdrawal animals compared with the control group ($F = 79.288$, $p<0.01$). There were not significant differences of TRPV1 immunoreactivity between 1 week and 3 week morphine withdrawal groups ($p>0.05$).

Increased TRPV1 located in asymmetric synapses

Transmission electron microscopy was used to examine the expression of TRPV1 in synapse. The immunogold-positive axon terminals were found in both asymmetric synapses (excitatory-type) and symmetric synapses (inhibitory-type) (Fig. 3,Peters et al., 1991).

Two vibratome sections from each of three rats in each group were calculated for the absolute number of TRPV1 positive asymmetric and symmetric synapses, and each vibratome section was normalized to 3000 μm^2. Compared to the control group, a significant increase was found in the number of TRPV1 positive asymmetric synapses in the morphine withdrawal groups (Fig.3C, $F = 75.321$, $p<0.05$), but no significant change was found in the number of TRPV1 positive symmetric synapses in morphine withdrawal groups (Fig.3C, $p = 0.622$).

To quantify the changes in the number of immunogold particles in certain terminals of the NAc of rats, the number of gold particles in the membranes of TRPV1 stained axon terminals forming symmetric or asymmetric synapses was counted and normalized to the unit perimeter (1 μm) of the axon terminal membrane. Significant increase was observed in the number of immunogold particles in axon terminals forming asymmetric synapses between the control group and morphine withdrawal groups (Fig.3D, $F = 36.547$, $p<0.05$). In contrast, the number of immunogold particles showed no difference in axon terminals forming symmetric synapses between the control group and morphine withdrawal groups (Fig.3D, $p = 0.056$).

Intra-NAc CPZ decreased persistent mCPP expression in a target specific manner

To determine whether NAc endovanilloid receptor TRPV1 is involved in the expression of mCPP, rats were given bilaterally repeated intra-NAc injections of different doses of TRPV1 antagonist CPZ during morphine withdrawal. When CPZ was applied during short-term morphine withdrawal, as shown in

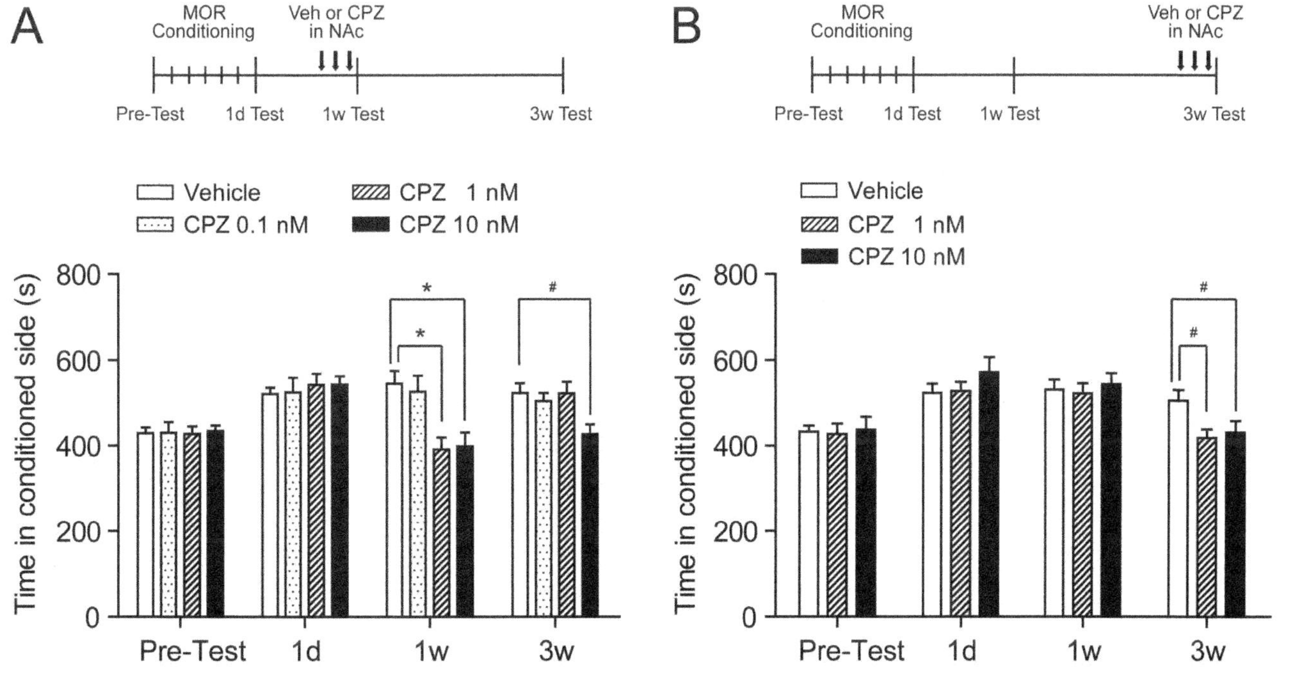

Figure 4. TRPV1 antagonist CPZ administered in bilateral NAc core decreased persistent morphine CPP after both short-(1 w) and long-term(3 w) withdrawal. (A) Dose-dependent effect of CPZ on persistent mCPP expression. Repeated high-dose CPZ (10 nM) injection during short-term morphine withdrawal could induce a complete and prolonged inhibition on mCPP expression. The moderate-dose CPZ (1 nM) has similar but temporary prohibiting effect on mCPP expression, as it could only be observed at 1 w but not 3 w of morphine withdrawal. The low-dose CPZ (0.1 nM) has no influence on mCPP. The upper schedule panel shows the rats were trained conditioned to morphine and received repeated CPZ injections in NAc core after short-term(1 w) withdrawal ($n = 11$ of Vehicle and CPZ 0.1 nM group, $n = 10$ of CPZ 1 nM group, and $n = 9$ of CPZ 10 nM group). (B) CPZ (1 nM and 10 nM) administration eliminated mCPP ($n = 7$). The upper schedule panel shows the rats were conditioned to morphine and received CPZ injections in NAc core after long-term(3 w) withdrawal. *$p<0.01$, *vs* control group; #$p<0.05$, *vs* control group. MOR, morphine; Veh, vehicle; CPZ, capsazepine; NAc, nucleus accumbens.

Fig. 4A, both 1 nM and 10 nM of CPZ significantly decreased mCPP expression at 1 w test (CPZ 1 nM, 370.9±20.2 s; CPZ 10 nM, 371.9±32.5 s; vehicle, 562.0±28.9 s; $F = 12.28$, $p<0.01$) (Fig. 4A). but the inhibitory effect of 1 nM CPZ was completely eliminated when tested at 3 w with the mCPP score reverted similar to control level (CPZ 1 nM, 522.6±26.4 s; vehicle, 523.3±22.5 s; $p>0.05$) (Fig. 4A). However, the inhibition of 10 nM CPZ could last to 3 w after morphine withdrawal (CPZ 10 nM, 426.8±23.2 s; vehicle, 523.3±22.5 s; $p<0.05$) (Fig. 4A). No active effect of low dose of CPZ (0.1 nM) was observed when tested at 1 w ($p>0.05$) (Fig. 4A). We used higher dose (1 nM or 10 nM) of CPZ for experiments during long-term (3 w) withdrawal. After three times injection, significant inhibition of mCPP expression was observed in both dose of CPZ (CPZ 1 nM, 418.4±19.9 s; CPZ 10 nM, 430.9±26.9 s; vehicle, 505.1±24.6 s; $F = 14.86$, $p<0.05$) (Fig. 4B). Thus, blocking TRPV1 in NAc disrupts the mCPP expression in both short- and long-term withdrawal. Figure 5 showed the Distribution of infusion sites in nucleus accumbens core.

To investigate whether CPZ inhibition on mCPP is a target-specific effect, we applied CPZ (10 nM) randomly in unilateral NAc, or bilateral DS during short-term (1 w) morphine withdrawal. Data from rats initially prepared for the bilateral CPZ administration study but with off-NAc cannula placements in only one side confirmed with staining was also analyzed here. As depicted in Figure 6A, in Uni-NAc group, no alteration of mCPP was detected after CPZ injection (CPZ, 549.1±29.7 s; vehicle, 539.0±15.9 s; $F = 0.245$, $p = 0.959$). Similarly, CPZ injection did not decrease mCPP in the Uni-off NAc group (Fig. 6A). Furthermore, when we examined the CPZ effect on mCPP in

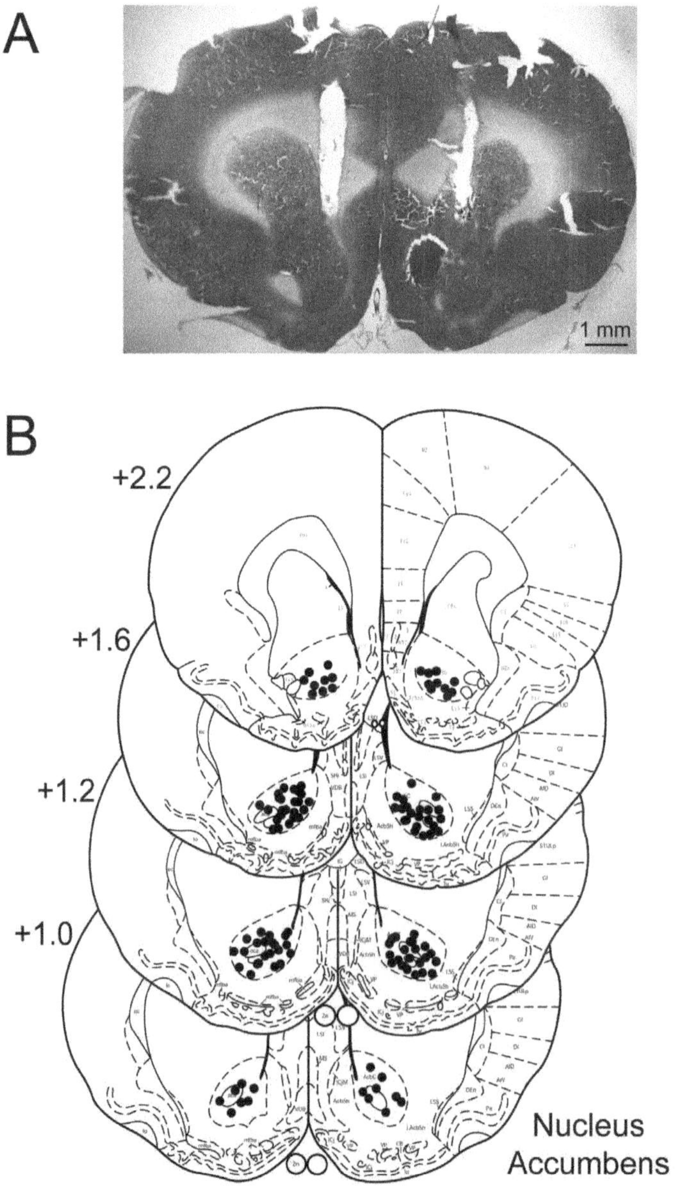

Figure 5. Distribution of infusion sites in nucleus accumbens core. (A) Photograph of representative cannula placements. The cannulas are implanted 1.5 mm above the target. (B) Schematic representations of vehicle or capsazepine injection sites in nucleus accumbens core at the labeled coronal planes. The numbers are the coordinates anterior (+) to bregma in millimeters according to Paxinos and Watson (2005).

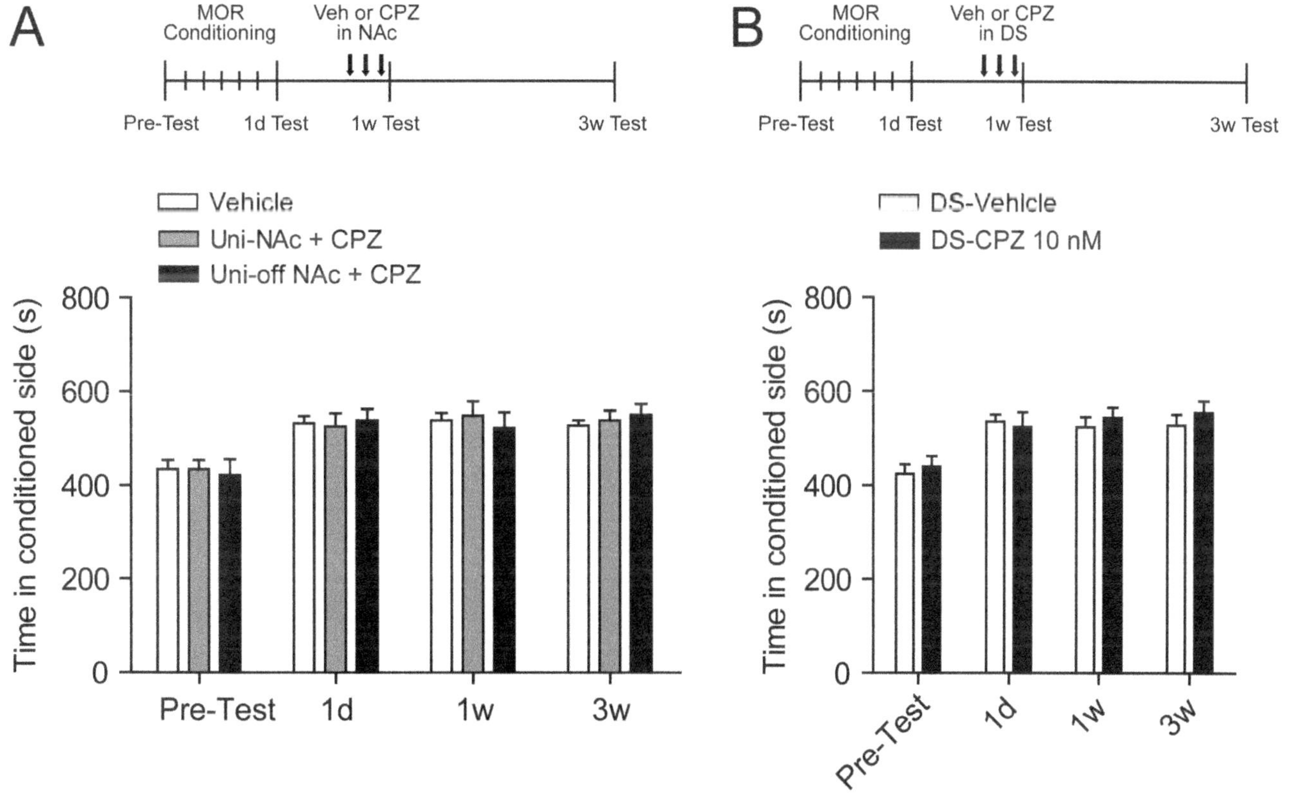

Figure 6. Injection of TRPV1 antagonist CPZ in unilateral of NAc or DS did not change persistent mCPP expression after short-term(1 w) withdrawal. (A) Unilateral NAc CPZ injection (10 nM) or one side off-target during bilateral NAc CPZ infusion (1 nM or 10 nM) failed to affect the sustained mCPP. The upper panel shows the scheme for morphine conditioning, CPZ treatment and mCPP test. Values are Mean ±SEM (n = 7 of Vehicle and Uni-NAc+CPZ group and n = 3 of Uni-off NAc+CPZ group). (B) CPZ (10 nM) injection in DS failed to influence persistent morphine CPP. The upper panel shows rats were conditioned to morphine and received CPZ injections in bilateral DS after short-term withdrawal. Values are mean ±SEM (n = 6 of DS-Vehicle group and n = 7 of DS-CPZ 10 nM group). MOR, morphine; Veh, vehicle; CPZ, capsazepine; NAc, nucleus accumbens; Uni, unilateral; DS, dorsal striatum.

the target outside NAc, we found the effective dose of CPZ (10 nM) in DS failed to influence the persistent mCPP expession ($F = 0.261$, $p = 0.853$) (Fig. 6B).

To assess the possible effect of intra-NAc CPZ on motor activity, which could indirectly influence mCPP expression, crossline times of the rats during mCPP tests were analyzed. As shown in Fig.7, there was no statistical difference ($F = 1.13$, $p > 0.05$) in crossline times among all groups after CPZ injection in both short-term (1 w) and long-term (3 w) withdrawal. The results confirmed that the alteration of all parameters in the mCPP expression test did not result from changes in motor abilities of rats.

Discussion

It is suggested that the NAc glutamatergic system is a key candidate for mediating morphine withdrawal-related addictive behaviors [28,29]. Alcantara et al. reported that morphine treatment increase the number of synapses of NAc, which was due primarily to an increase in the number of asymmetric synapses, and Asymmetric synapses in the accumbens are characteristic of glutamatergic synapses formed by inputs from other area such as prefrontal cortex, hippocampus and so on [30]. In the present study, we demonstrated that TRPV1 was increased in the nucleus accumbens of rats after morphine conditioned. Significant increase was observed in the number of immunogold particles in axon terminals forming asymmetric synapses between the control group and morphine withdrawal groups. In contrast, it showed no difference in axon terminals forming symmetric synapses, which suggested that the TRPV1 expression at asymmetric synapses might involve in morphine induced CPP. Antagonism of TRPV1 by the selective TRPV1 antagonist CPZ suppressed persistent mCPP expression in rats either during short-term or long-term morphine withdrawal. This inhibitory effect is target-specific, unique for NAc. Conversely, effective doses of CPZ in NAc did not cause significant side-effect on motor activity of the subjects, suggesting the decrease of mCPP expression is not due to motor inhibitory properties of TRPV1 antagonist. Collectively, these results not only extend our understanding on the role of central TRPV1 in drug addiction, but also indicate that TRPV1 antagonist may be a promising type of medication for inhibiting morphine conditioned behaviour.

Morphine withdrawal increased TRPV1 expression in NAc meurons

TRPV1 is a calcium-permeable cation channel [31,32]. In the central nervous system, TRPV1 is widely expressed in brain regions including postsynaptic dendrite spines, cell somata [33], and in various layers of the cortex [6,34]. Previous studies suggested that activation of postsynaptic TRPV1 channels triggered long-term depression in the NAc [12]. Activation of TRPV1 receptors is coupled to glutamate release, which in turn

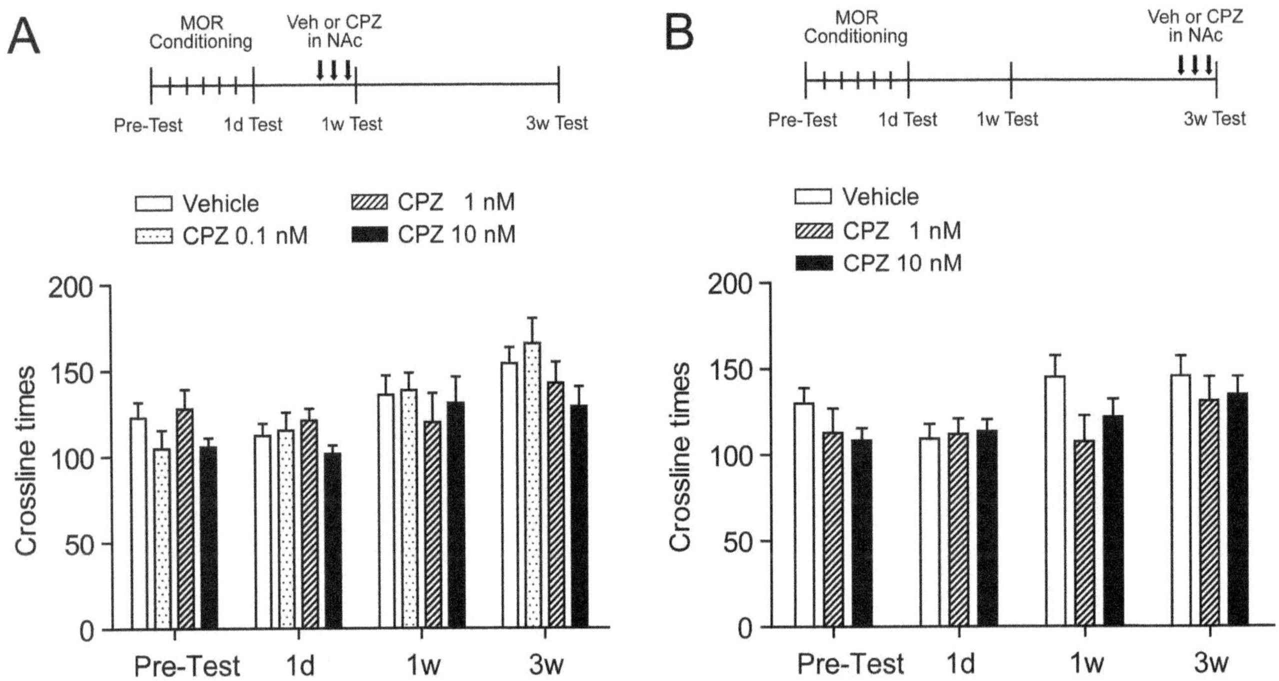

Figure 7. TRPV1 antagonist CPZ administered in bilateral NAc fail to affect normal activity after both short-(1 w) and long-term(3 w) withdrawal. (A) All doses of CPZ tested failed to influence the activity of animal measured by photobeam breaks during the 15-min mCPP test (n = 11 of Vehicle and CPZ 0.1 nM group, n = 10 of CPZ 1 nM group, and n = 9 of CPZ 10 nM group). The upper schedule panel shows the rats were trained conditioned to morphine and received repeated CPZ injections in NAc core after short-term (1 w) withdrawal. (B) Both effective doses of CPZ (1 nM and 10 nM) in eliminating sustained mCPP expression fail to affect activity (n = 7). The upper schedule panel shows the rats were conditioned to morphine and received CPZ injections in NAc core after long-term (3 w) withdrawal.Values are mean ±SEM. MOR, morphine; Veh, vehicle; CPZ, capsazepine; NAc, nucleus accumbens.

affects the release of GABA, dopamine, and other catecholamines [35,36]. Activation of TRPV1 in the ventral tegmental area caused excitation of dopaminergic neurons and increased dopamine release in NAc after a painful stimulus [26]. AMPA receptors and GABAA receptors activation are associated with facilitation of motivated behaviors [37].

In the present study, we found that morphine with 10 mg/kg induced persistent and relatively stable mCPP expression lasting from short-term (1 w) to long-term (3 w) withdrawal, which dose has been continuously confirmed to induce sustained mCPP expression in rodents [38,39]. Accordingly, the expression of TRPV1 in the NAcc was elevated in morphine conditioned animals and maintained in high levels after 1 w and 3 w withdrawal compared to the control group. The increased TRPV1 distributed on the presynaptic membrane of asymmetric synapses. The results indicated that increasing expression of TRPV1 on the presynaptic membrane of asymmetric synapses in NAcc might play an important role in morphine conditioned place preference.

Intra-NAc CPZ reduced mCPP expression

To confirm the role of TRPV1 in morphine induced conditioned place preference, we injected TRPV1 antagonist CPZ intra-NAc and found that blocking TRPV1 in NAc disrupts the mCPP expression in both short- and long-term withdrawal. Previous study has shown that repeated systematic administration of CPZ could reduce naloxone-induced acute withdrawal symptoms in mice [9]. These findings together reveal the important role of TRPV1 in both psychological and physical aspects of opioid-related behaviors.

At least two possible mechanisms may underlie the inhibitory behavioral effect of TRPV1 antagonist in NAc on mCPP. Firstly, blockade of TRPV1 in NAc may prevent it from overdrive by excitatory inputs essential for CPP. Previous studies have shown that potentiation of glutamatergic inputs on NAc medium spiny neurons is a critical type of neuroadaptation happened during prolonged opioid withdrawal and is associated with relapse [22,24,40]. Furthermore, fully or partially blockade of glutamatergic inputs has been proved to disrupt reinstatement to opioid seeking and taking behaviors [23–25,40]. It has been proved that TRPV1 activation facilitate presynaptic neurotransmitter release in variety of brain regions [3,13–17,19–21] and the existence of TRPV1 mRNA in main glutamatergic areas innervating NAc [7]. In the present study, significant increase of the number of TRPV1 positive asymmetric synapses was observed and more immunogold particles in axon terminals in the morphine conditioned rats, which suggested that the inhibitory effect of TRPV1 antagonist on synaptic efficacy should be taken into account when evaluating its inhibitory effect on CPP. Supporting this idea, our finding that the time window for the effectiveness of NAc TRPV1 antagonist on mCPP persisting from short- to long-term drug withdrawal overlapped with the period for NAc glutamate inputs potentiation reported before [22,41]. Secondly, reduction of NAc neuronal activity by TRPV1 antagonist may also contribute to its effect on mCPP expression. Wu et al [22] reported the increase of intrinsic excitability in NAc neurons during opioid withdrawal, which suggested an enhanced response capability of these neurons. In agreement with these data, increased NAc immediate early gene expression during opioid withdrawal and reinstatement supports the upregulation of NAc neural reactivity during withdrawal

[42,43]. Conversely, blocking NAc activity could reduce mCPP expression and prevent opioid relapse [27]. As is shown previously, membrane depolarization and increase of spiking are essential manifestations after central TRPV1 activation [20,26], which is mediated by its modulatory on K^+ and Ca^{2+} conductance or direct Ca^{2+} and Na^+ influx via the channel itself. Accordingly, blockade of NAc TRPV1, may contribute to limit neural activity in this region, which was confirmed to have relapse preventing effect [27]. Further studies are necessary to elucidate the above and other mechanisms involved in the action of central, especially NAc, TRPV1 antagonism on drug addiction.

Intra-NAc CPZ administration did not affect on motor activity

Our data showed that the effective dose of NAc CPZ in preventing mCPP expression failed to influence the locomotor activity. Consistent with previous studies [44,45], we showed together that this dose range of CPZ is not sufficient to produce behavioral effect on general activity in rats when given alone. However, stimulation of TRPV1 by application of its ligand externally has been shown to suppress spontaneous activity in rodents [15,45–47]. Moreover, blockade of TRPV1 by CPZ has been proved to attenuate hypolocomotor effect of anandamide [47,48], a ligand for both cannabinoid receptor and TRPV1, which revealed that anandamide induced activity disruption is caused by a TRPV1-dependent mechanism. Collectively, these findings indicate that targeting central TRPV1 may modulate activity of the subject. Nevertheless, discrepancies between these findings and our result implicated that blocking TRPV1 by endogenous ligands in the brain, at least in NAc, may not be sufficient to affect activity, in another word, tonic TRPV1 activation in NAc isn't involved in regulating basal activity. The finding that TRPV1 gene knockout mice showed normal locomotor activity further supports this viewpoint [12]. Thus, blocking TRPV1 in NAc will result in non-effect on activity and the inhibition of CPZ on prolonged mCPP expression is not due to its influence on moving ability of the rats.

In conclusion, the present study indicated the importance of TRPV1 in the NAc in morphine addiction. The increased expression of TRPV1 in the presynaptic membranes of asymmetric synapses in NAc during morphine withdrawal may be one of the mechanisms of mCPP expression. We further demonstrated the inhibitory effect of NAc TRPV1 antagonism on prolonged mCPP expression, which confirmed the involvement of NAc TRPV1 in persistent opioid addiction. Our results support for further mechanism assessment and developing novel treatment targeting central, especially NAc, TRPV1 for mCPP prevention.

Author Contributions

Conceived and designed the experiments: LJH GZX GDG LTM. Performed the experiments: LJH BH HG. Analyzed the data: LJH WXY JS PW. Contributed to the writing of the manuscript: LJH GDG GZX.

References

1. O'Brien CP (1997) A range of research-based pharmacotherapies for addiction. Science 278: 66–70.
2. Wu LJ, Sweet TB, Clapham DE (2010) International Union of Basic and Clinical Pharmacology. LXXVI. Current progress in the mammalian TRP ion channel family. Pharmacol Rev 62: 381–404.
3. Matta JA, Ahern GP (2011) TRPV1 and synaptic transmission. Curr Pharm Biotechnol 12: 95–101.
4. Ho KW, Ward NJ, Calkins DJ (2012) TRPV1: a stress response protein in the central nervous system. Am J Neurodegener Dis 1: 1–14.
5. Micale V, Cristino L, Tamburella A, Petrosino S, Leggio GM, et al. (2009) Altered responses of dopamine D3 receptor null mice to excitotoxic or anxiogenic stimuli: Possible involvement of the endocannabinoid and endovanilloid systems. Neurobiol Dis 36: 70–80.
6. Roberts JC, Davis JB, Benham CD (2004) [3H]Resiniferatoxin autoradiography in the CNS of wild-type and TRPV1 null mice defines TRPV1 (VR-1) protein distribution. Brain Res 995: 176–183.
7. Tian YH, Lee SY, Kim HC, Jang CG (2010) Repeated methamphetamine treatment increases expression of TRPV1 mRNA in the frontal cortex but not in the striatum or hippocampus of mice. Neurosci Lett 472: 61–64.
8. Cristino L, de Petrocellis L, Pryce G, Baker D, Guglielmotti V, et al. (2006) Immunohistochemical localization of cannabinoid type 1 and vanilloid transient receptor potential vanilloid type 1 receptors in the mouse brain. Neuroscience 139: 1405–1415.
9. Nguyen TL, Nam YS, Lee SY, Kim HC, Jang CG (2010) Effects of capsazepine, a transient receptor potential vanilloid type 1 antagonist, on morphine-induced antinociception, tolerance, and dependence in mice. Br J Anaesth 105: 668–674.
10. Adamczyk P, Miszkiel J, McCreary AC, Filip M, Papp M, et al. (2012) The effects of cannabinoid CB1, CB2 and vanilloid TRPV1 receptor antagonists on cocaine addictive behavior in rats. Brain Res 1444: 45–54.
11. Badiani A, Belin D, Epstein D, Calu D, Shaham Y (2011) Opiate versus psychostimulant addiction: the differences do matter. Nat Rev Neurosci 12: 685–700.
12. Grueter BA, Brasnjo G, Malenka RC (2010) Postsynaptic TRPV1 triggers cell type-specific long-term depression in the nucleus accumbens. Nat Neurosci 13: 1519–1525.
13. Musella A, De Chiara V, Rossi S, Prosperetti C, Bernardi G, et al. (2009) TRPV1 channels facilitate glutamate transmission in the striatum. Mol Cell Neurosci 40: 89–97.
14. Benninger F, Freund TF, Hajos N (2008) Control of excitatory synaptic transmission by capsaicin is unaltered in TRPV1 vanilloid receptor knockout mice. Neurochem Int 52: 89–94.
15. de Lago E, de Miguel R, Lastres-Becker I, Ramos JA, Fernandez-Ruiz J (2004) Involvement of vanilloid-like receptors in the effects of anandamide on motor behavior and nigrostriatal dopaminergic activity: in vivo and in vitro evidence. Brain Res 1007: 152–159.
16. Marinelli S, Di Marzo V, Berretta N, Matias I, Maccarrone M, et al. (2003) Presynaptic facilitation of glutamatergic synapses to dopaminergic neurons of the rat substantia nigra by endogenous stimulation of vanilloid receptors. J Neurosci 23: 3136–3144.
17. Marinelli S, Vaughan CW, Christie MJ, Connor M (2002) Capsaicin activation of glutamatergic synaptic transmission in the rat locus coeruleus in vitro. J Physiol 543: 531–540.
18. Mori F, Ribolsi M, Kusayanagi H, Monteleone F, Mantovani V, et al. (2012) TRPV1 channels regulate cortical excitability in humans. J Neurosci 32: 873–879.
19. Sasamura T, Sasaki M, Tohda C, Kuraishi Y (1998) Existence of capsaicin-sensitive glutamatergic terminals in rat hypothalamus. Neuroreport 9: 2045–2048.
20. Xing J, Li J (2007) TRPV1 receptor mediates glutamatergic synaptic input to dorsolateral periaqueductal gray (dl-PAG) neurons. J Neurophysiol 97: 503–511.
21. Yokoyama T, Saito T, Ohbuchi T, Hashimoto H, Suzuki H, et al. (2010) TRPV1 gene deficiency attenuates miniature EPSC potentiation induced by mannitol and angiotensin II in supraoptic magnocellular neurons. J Neurosci 30: 876–884.
22. Wu X, Shi M, Wei C, Yang M, Liu Y, et al. (2012) Potentiation of synaptic strength and intrinsic excitability in the nucleus accumbens after 10 days of morphine withdrawal. J Neurosci Res 90: 1270–1283.
23. Ma YY, Chu NN, Guo CY, Han JS, Cui CL (2007) NR2B-containing NMDA receptor is required for morphine-but not stress-induced reinstatement. Exp Neurol 203: 309–319.
24. LaLumiere RT, Kalivas PW (2008) Glutamate release in the nucleus accumbens core is necessary for heroin seeking. J Neurosci 28: 3170–3177.
25. Bossert JM, Gray SM, Lu L, Shaham Y (2006) Activation of group II metabotropic glutamate receptors in the nucleus accumbens shell attenuates context-induced relapse to heroin seeking. Neuropsychopharmacology 31: 2197–2209.
26. Marinelli S, Pascucci T, Bernardi G, Puglisi-Allegra S, Mercuri NB (2005) Activation of TRPV1 in the VTA excites dopaminergic neurons and increases chemical- and noxious-induced dopamine release in the nucleus accumbens. Neuropsychopharmacology 30: 864–870.
27. Esmaeili MH, Sahraei H, Ali-Beig H, Ardehari-Ghaleh M, Mohammadian Z, et al. (2012) Transient inactivation of the nucleus accumbens reduces both the expression and acquisition of morphine-induced conditioned place preference in rats. Pharmacol Biochem Behav 102: 249–256.
28. Siggins GR, Martin G, Roberto M, Nie Z, Madamba S, et al. (2003) Glutamatergic transmission in opiate and alcohol dependence. Ann N Y Acad Sci 1003: 196–211.

29. Gass JT, Olive MF (2008) Glutamatergic substrates of drug addiction and alcoholism. Biochem Pharmacol 75: 218–265.
30. Alcantara AA, Lim HY, Floyd CE, Garces J, Mendenhall JM, et al. (2011) Cocaine- and morphine-induced synaptic plasticity in the nucleus accumbens. Synapse 65: 309–320.
31. Caterina MJ, Schumacher MA, Tominaga M, Rosen TA, Levine JD, et al. (1997) The capsaicin receptor: a heat-activated ion channel in the pain pathway. Nature 389: 816–824.
32. Szallasi A, Blumberg PM (1999) Vanilloid (Capsaicin) receptors and mechanisms. Pharmacol Rev 51: 159–212.
33. Toth A, Boczan J, Kedei N, Lizanecz E, Bagi Z, et al. (2005) Expression and distribution of vanilloid receptor 1 (TRPV1) in the adult rat brain. Brain Res Mol Brain Res 135: 162–168.
34. Mezey E, Toth ZE, Cortright DN, Arzubi MK, Krause JE, et al. (2000) Distribution of mRNA for vanilloid receptor subtype 1 (VR1), and VR1-like immunoreactivity, in the central nervous system of the rat and human. Proc Natl Acad Sci U S A 97: 3655–3660.
35. Jin YH, Bailey TW, Li BY, Schild JH, Andresen MC (2004) Purinergic and vanilloid receptor activation releases glutamate from separate cranial afferent terminals in nucleus tractus solitarius. J Neurosci 24: 4709–4717.
36. Li DP, Chen SR, Pan HL (2004) VR1 receptor activation induces glutamate release and postsynaptic firing in the paraventricular nucleus. J Neurophysiol 92: 1807–1816.
37. Yuan WX, Heng LJ, Ma J, Wang XQ, Qu LJ, et al. (2013) Increased expression of cannabinoid receptor 1 in the nucleus accumbens core in a rat model with morphine withdrawal. Brain Res 1531: 102–112.
38. Li YQ, Li FQ, Wang XY, Wu P, Zhao M, et al. (2008) Central amygdala extracellular signal-regulated kinase signaling pathway is critical to incubation of opiate craving. J Neurosci 28: 13248–13257.
39. Milekic MH, Brown SD, Castellini C, Alberini CM (2006) Persistent disruption of an established morphine conditioned place preference. J Neurosci 26: 3010–3020.
40. Shen H, Moussawi K, Zhou W, Toda S, Kalivas PW (2011) Heroin relapse requires long-term potentiation-like plasticity mediated by NMDA2b-containing receptors. Proc Natl Acad Sci U S A 108: 19407–19412.
41. Bajo M, Crawford EF, Roberto M, Madamba SG, Siggins GR (2006) Chronic morphine treatment alters expression of N-methyl-D-aspartate receptor subunits in the extended amygdala. J Neurosci Res 83: 532–537.
42. Koya E, Spijker S, Voorn P, Binnekade R, Schmidt ED, et al. (2006) Enhanced cortical and accumbal molecular reactivity associated with conditioned heroin, but not sucrose-seeking behaviour. J Neurochem 98: 905–915.
43. Kuntz KL, Patel KM, Grigson PS, Freeman WM, Vrana KE (2008) Heroin self-administration: II. CNS gene expression following withdrawal and cue-induced drug-seeking behavior. Pharmacol Biochem Behav 90: 349–356.
44. Aguiar DC, Terzian AL, Guimaraes FS, Moreira FA (2009) Anxiolytic-like effects induced by blockade of transient receptor potential vanilloid type 1 (TRPV1) channels in the medial prefrontal cortex of rats. Psychopharmacology (Berl) 205: 217–225.
45. Lee J, Di Marzo V, Brotchie JM (2006) A role for vanilloid receptor 1 (TRPV1) and endocannabinnoid signalling in the regulation of spontaneous and L-DOPA induced locomotion in normal and reserpine-treated rats. Neuropharmacology 51: 557–565.
46. Di Marzo V, Lastres-Becker I, Bisogno T, De Petrocellis L, Milone A, et al. (2001) Hypolocomotor effects in rats of capsaicin and two long chain capsaicin homologues. Eur J Pharmacol 420: 123–131.
47. Panlilio LV, Mazzola C, Medalie J, Hahn B, Justinova Z, et al. (2009) Anandamide-induced behavioral disruption through a vanilloid-dependent mechanism in rats. Psychopharmacology (Berl) 203: 529–538.
48. Tzavara ET, Li DL, Moutsimilli L, Bisogno T, Di Marzo V, et al. (2006) Endocannabinoids activate transient receptor potential vanilloid 1 receptors to reduce hyperdopaminergia-related hyperactivity: therapeutic implications. Biol Psychiatry 59: 508–515.

8

A Preliminary Pilot Randomized Crossover Study of Uzara (*Xysmalobium undulatum*) versus Ibuprofen in the Treatment of Primary Dysmenorrhea

Karim H. I. Abd-El-Maeboud*, Mohamed A. M. F. Kortam, Mohamed S. Ali, Mostafa I. Ibrahim, Radwa M. M. Z. Mohamed

Department of Obstetrics and Gynecology, Faculty of Medicine, Ain Shams University, Cairo, Egypt

Abstract

Objective: Preliminary evaluation of efficacy and safety of uzara use in treatment of moderate and severe primary dysmenorrhea in comparison to ibuprofen.

Materials and Methods: This randomized, comparative two way cross-over study comprised 60 single female students at Faculty of Medicine, Ain Shams University, Egypt, aged 19–28 years with moderate (n = 46) or severe (n = 14) primary dysmenorrhea. Participants were randomized to take either uzara (80 mg/8 hours for two doses, then 40 mg/8 hours) then ibuprofen (400 mg/6 hours) in two subsequent cycles or vice versa. The pain intensity, using VAS, was recorded immediately before taking the medication (0 hour) and after 4, 12, 24, 48–60, 96–120 hours. Main outcome measures included effectiveness of pain relief defined as drop of VAS to 3 or less, patient's global evaluation of the drug, absence from school, the use of a rescue medication, and, in those who continued the treatment, the pain intensity difference (PID) at different points after start of medication and its sum (SPID).

Results: Uzara was comparably effective to ibuprofen (78.3% vs. 86.7% of cycles; respectively), with comparable rates of effectiveness on global evaluation (being around 50% for either drug), and rates of school absences (11.7% vs. 13.3%; respectively). The need for rescue medication was different (18.3% and 10%; respectively), albeit with no statistical significance. The means of PID at different time points and SPID were comparable, with significantly lower average mean of VAS scores compared to that felt with no medication (1.6 vs. 6.8, $p<0.001$). Side effects were less with uzara than ibuprofen (0% vs. 8.3%, $p<0.05$).

Conclusions: Uzara might be as effective as ibuprofen in management of primary dysmenorrhea but with less side effects. These findings need to be confirmed by a properly designed trial with a larger sample size.

Trial Registration: Current Controlled Trials ISRCTN25618258

Editor: Kristina Gemzell-Danielsson, Karolinska Institutet, Sweden

Funding: This work was fully funded by the authors.

Competing Interests: The authors have declared that no competing interests exist.

* Email: Kabdelmaeboud@yahoo.com

Introduction

Primary dysmenorrhea is a common gynecological problem [1–3]. Nonsteroidal anti-inflammatory drugs (NSAIDs) are well established as first-line therapy. Common side effects are nausea, vomiting, dyspepsia and diarrhea; with less common serious ones [4]. They act by suppressing the production of endometrial prostaglandins [2]. They are significantly more effective in relieving pain when compared to placebo or paracetamol. However, they have an overall treatment failure rate of approximately 25%. Regarding effectiveness and safety, evidence is still lacking to determine the best individual NSAID in treatment of dysmenorrhea [2,5]. The combined oral contraceptives pills (COCPs), which act by decreasing menstrual fluid volume and prostaglandin production have been advocated to treat primary dysmenorrhea, however there is insufficient evidence for pain relief with their use [6]. Other alternative therapeutic modalities include acupuncture [7], transcutaneous electrical nerve stimulation (TENS) [8], laparoscopic presacral neurectomy [9], spinal manipulation [10], behavioral interventions [11], Zingiber officinale R. rhizomes (ginger) [12], and herbal and dietary therapies (including magnesium, vitamin B6, vitamin B1, vitamin E, omega-3 fatty acids, and Japanese herbal combination) [13].

Uzarae radix. is a herbal remedy extracted from the uzara root, which constitutes of the dried underground parts of the 2–3 year-old plants Xysmalobium undulatum, This important medicinal plant has been historically used by the native inhabitants of South Africa to treat digestive complaints. It is approved by Commission E to treat acute nonspecific diarrhea [14]. Although the inhibition of active chloride secretion has been recently suggested to play a

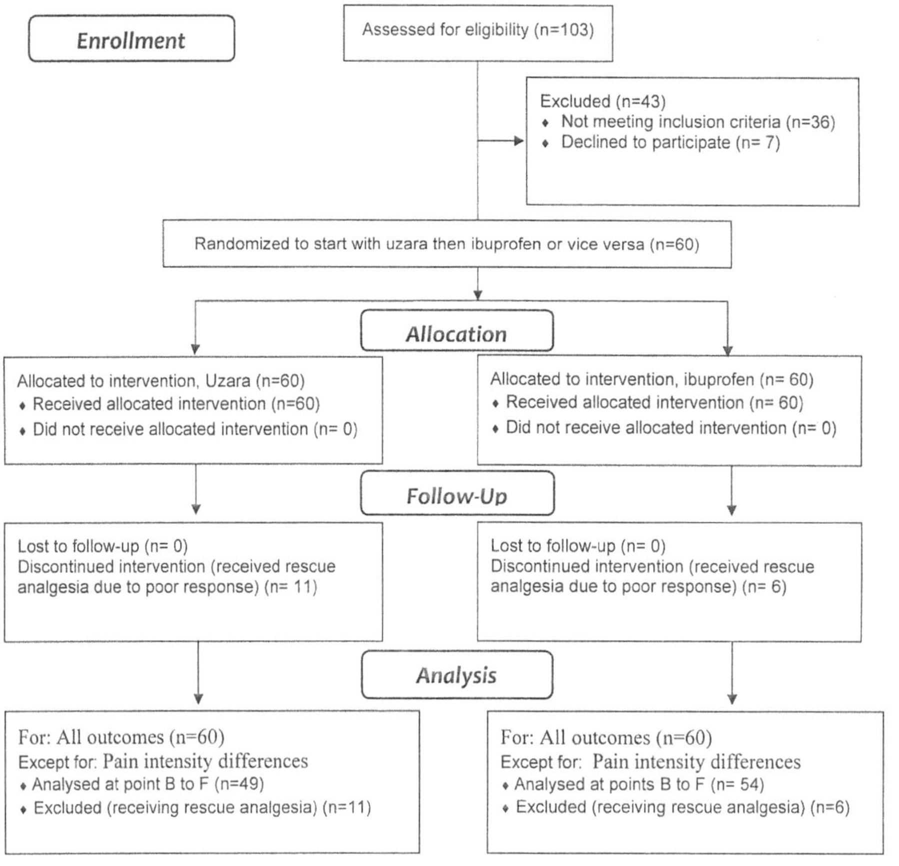

Figure 1. Flow-Chart of study participants.

role [15], the anti-diarrheal action of uzara root extracts is thought to be mainly through inhibiting the motility of visceral smooth muscle. The action is qualitatively similar to that of papaverine [16]. Uzara root extracts inhibit motility in the small intestine and urogenital tract with traditional uses including afterbirth cramps and dysmenorrhea [17]. Strangely enough, there are no published studies evaluating its use as a treatment option for menstrual cramps although its use has been suggested since 1913 [18]. Also, no health hazards or side effects are known [19] and recent studies have failed to find significant cardiovascular pharmacodynamic effects with its oral administration [20]. Uzara contains glycosides with cardenolide structure (uzarin and xysmalorin) which have been reported to cross-react with the conventional digitalis assays [20,21], thus not to be administered concomitantly with other cardioactive glycosides [14,21].

The aim of this study is to evaluate the efficacy, safety and tolerability of uzara in comparison to ibuprofen, a NSAID, in the treatment of primary dysmenorrhea.

Materials and Methods

This was a pilot phase III randomized comparative, two way cross-over assignment, safety and efficacy study, aiming at preliminary evaluation of uzara versus ibuprofen in the treatment of primary dysmenorrhea. The protocol for this trial and supporting CONSORT checklist are available as supporting information; see Protocol S1 and Checklist S1.The study protocol approval was obtained on 29th August 2010 (FMASU 773/2010) from the Ethics and Research Committee of the Faculty of Medicine, Ain Shams University 00006444. The authors confirm that all their ongoing and related trails for uzara in their institute are registered. The participants were 60 women with moderate or severe primary dysmenorrhea, recruited from female students attending clinical classes in medicine (Faculty of Medicine) or nursing (High Institute of Nursing). The inclusion criteria were: age between 18 and 28 years, regular cycles (21–35 days) with duration of 3 to 7 days, a history of at least 6 consecutive months of moderate to severe primary dysmenorrhea as determined by the verbal rating scale (VRS, a 4-point self-rated verbal score: 0, none; 1, mild; 2, moderate; and 3, severe menstrual pain) [22], with the pain lasting for at least 2 days and who required analgesia in each of the last 3 consecutive cycles, preceding participation in the study. The exclusion criteria were planning to get married during the study period; known or suspected secondary dysmenorrhea and other causes of chronic pelvic pain (previous major abdominal or pelvic surgery, endometriosis, pelvic inflammatory disease, ovarian cysts, pathological vaginal secretion, chronic abdominal pain, inflammatory bowel disease, irritable bowel syndrome); hormonal therapy during the last 6 months or planning to take hormonal therapy during the study period; regular intake of pain medications (including NSAIDs) for other reason than dysmenorrhea, digoxin, antidepressants, tranquilizers, hypnotics, sedatives, or sex hormones; any concomitant disease or condition that might require any intake of analgesic medication; history of significant chronic constipation or recurrent colitis; evidence of clinically relevant serious condition whether gynecological, cardiovascular, hematological, hepatic, gastrointestinal, renal, pulmonary endocrinological, autoimmune diseases, neurologic or psychiatric

Table 1. Participants' Characteristics (n = 60).*

Characteristic	Median/No.	IQR/Percent
Age (years)	23	20.5–24
BMI	22.5	21.1–25.6
Age at menarche (years)	12	11–13
Cycle (days)	28	27–28
Flow (days)	6	5–7
Flow: Average	52	86.7
Heavy	8	13.3
Age at Onset of Dysmenorrhea (Years)	13	12–14
Duration of Dysmenorrhea (days):		
One	14	23.3
Two	32	53.3
Three	11	18.3
Four	3	5
Onset of Dysmenorrhea in relation to Onset of Menses:		
−2 days	11	18.3
−1 day	16	26.7
Same day	26	43.3
+1 day	6	10
+2 days	1	1.7
Peak of Dysmenorrhea in relation to Onset of Menses:		
−2 days	3	5
−1 day	9	15
Same day	32	53.3
+1 day	11	18.3
+2 days	5	8.3
Peak of Dysmenorrhea in relation to Flow of Menses:		
Mild flow	21	35
Moderate flow	22	36.7
Heavy flow	17	28.3
Absence from Work during Menses:		
None	17	28.3
Occasional	24	40
Alternate menses	8	13.3
Every menses	11	18.3

* Results are median/number (No) and interquartile range (IQR)/percentage (percent)

disease, based on a clinical assessment and routine laboratory investigations; unwillingness to comply with the protocol, or participation in another clinical trial in the 3 months prior to the start of this study.

Each participant completed a case record form, including demographic details and past medical and surgical history. A transabdominal ultrasonographic scanning (TAS) was performed in all participants to exclude any pelvic pathology. Severity of dysmenorrhea in all participants was initially assessed by two validated pain scales: visual analogue scale (VAS), verbal rating scale (VRS) [23]. VAS is a one-dimensional linear scale of 0–10 cm (0 cm representing no pain; 10 cm, severe pain) with values greater than 5 defined as moderate or severe. Marked limitation of daily activities evidenced by absence from school was recorded.

The objective of the study was explained to eligible participants, who all signed a written informed consent. The randomization sequence was computer generated and kept concealed by the first author (KA) who played no role in patients' recruitment. Other co-authors -indulged in patients' recruitment and consenting to the study- were continuously updated regarding number of participants with assigned sequence. They collaborated together to allocate the next available number to each participant in order of her enrollment in the study. Subsequently, the first author (KA) was contacted and asked to release the sequence (order of drug intake, uzara/ibuprofen or vice versa).

Uzara is a coated tablet, contained purely vegetable active substance 40 mg dry extract of roots of uzara plant, *Xysmalobium undulatum* (4–6:1) [extracting medium: methanol 60% (V/V)] and glucose, lactose, sucrose, and fortifying wheat (Uzara 40 mg,

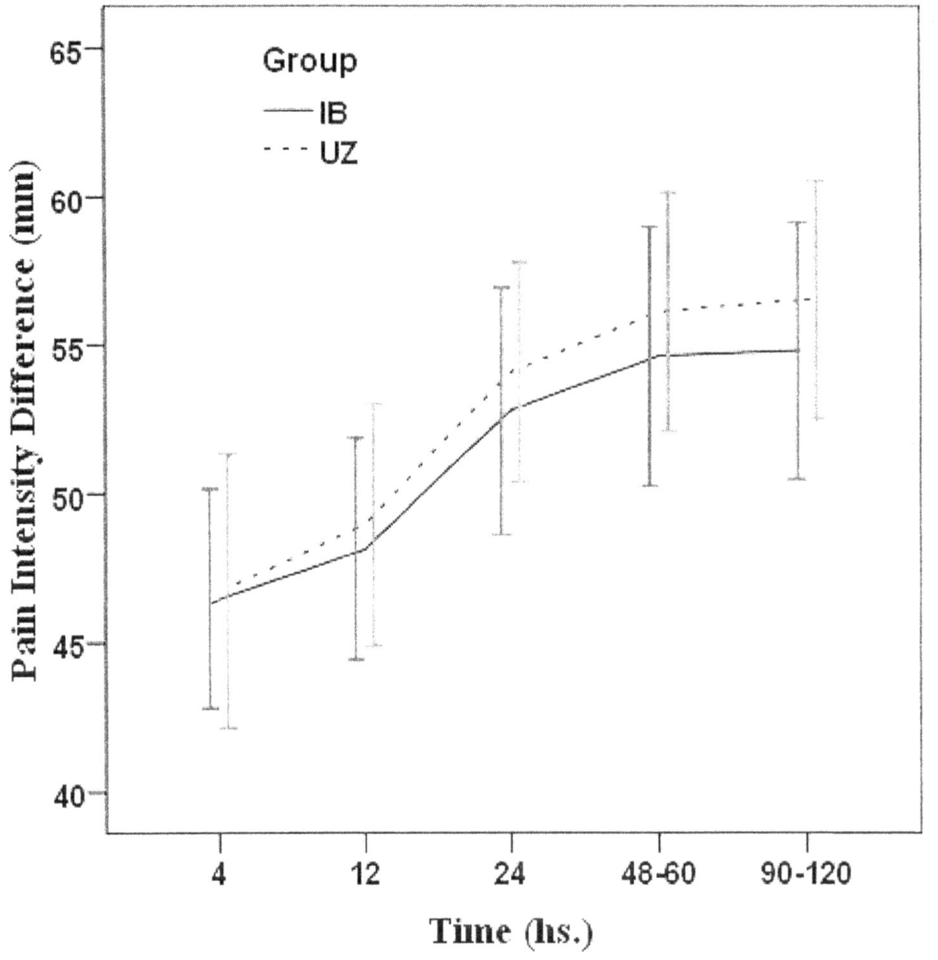

Figure 2. Pain intensity difference (PID) – mean scores of visual analog scale (error bars: 95% C.I., confidence interval) based on drug start at each cycle with Uzara (UZ) or Ibuprofen (IB) (Cycles: UZ, *N*=49; IB, *N*=54), excluding 17 cycles where rescue analgesia was used.

Registration owner: STADA GmbH, Bad Vilbel, Manufacturer: HEMOPHARM GmbH, Germany). The control drug was ibuprofen 400 mg sugar coated tablets (Brufen 400 mg, Kahira Pharm. & Chem. Ind. Co., Cairo, Egypt; under license from Abbott Laboratories). Treatment was commenced with the onset of menstruation or when pain is felt to be impending (up to two days before the expected start of menstruation) and stopped when there was mild or no pain (VAS score 3 or less) 6–8 hours from the last test tablet or after 5 days treatment duration. Both drugs were taken orally; uzara two tablets every 8 hours for 2 doses then one tablet every 8 hours (maximum daily dose 200 mg), Ibuprofen one tablet every 6 hour (maximum daily dose 1600 mg). Each of the two drugs, ibuprofen and uzara, has a short serum half-life, being 1.8–2 hours [24] versus 8.87 $\pm$ 2.20 hours [25]; respectively. It is reported that the duration of washout time should be approximately 10$\times$ the plasma apparent terminal elimination half-life to provide for 99.9% of the administered dose to be eliminated from the body [26]. So, the incorporation of a relatively long washout period (3 weeks between treatment periods, i.e. two successive menses) in the cross over design of the present study was assumed to diminish safely the impact of carryover effects and eliminate the need for testing for carry over effects. In both treatment cycles, participants recorded the pain intensity they experienced, using visual analogue scale (VAS) at 6 time-points: immediately before starting the tested medication (0 hour) and after 4, 12, 24, 48–60 and 96–120 hours. The occurrence of school absence as a result of confirmed marked limitation of physical activity in relation to dysmenorrhea was recorded. The use of other analgesics was allowed for those receiving little or no pain relief i.e., rescues medication. This was permitted 1 hour after the intake of the tested drug. The type, dose, frequency of administration and the response using VAS were recorded after the intake of the rescue drug, if needed. Adverse reactions and tolerability to all medications were recorded. After the end of the each treatment cycle, participants' global evaluation of the study medication was recorded as effective or non-effective.

In the present study, the primary outcomes measures –all related to analgesic effect- were: a drop in VAS score to $\leq$3 at point B (4 hours after receiving the medication), participant's global evaluation of the drug, absence from school, the use of a rescue medication, and in those who continued the treatment, the pain intensity difference (PID) at certain points after start of medication and its sum (SPID). Secondary outcome measures included adverse reactions and drug tolerability recorded at the end of each cycle.

Being a preliminary pilot study to assess the use of uzara in dysmenorrhea compared to the standard therapy (ibuprofen) in knowledgeable medical students, who might be skeptic about its

Table 2. Risk analysis for the main outcome measures (Direction: Uzara minus Ibuprofen).

Outcome	Uzara group (n = 60)				Ibuprofen group (n = 60)				RR	95% CI	ARR	95% CI	NNT	95% CI
	Favorable outcome	Unfavorable outcome	AR	95% CI	Favorable outcome	Unfavorable outcome	AR	95% CI						
VAS	47(78.3%)	13 (21.7%)	0.22	0.11 to 0.32	52 (86.7%)	8 (13.3%)	0.13	0.05 to 0.22	1.63	0.73 to 3.63	−0.08	−0.22 to 0.05	−12.0	−4.58 to 19.30
Global outcome	29 (48.3%)	31(51.7%)	0.52	0.39 to 0.64	31(51.7%)	29 (48.3%)	0.48	0.36 to 0.61	1.07	0.75 to 1.53	−0.03	−0.21 to 0.15	−30.0	−4.71 to 6.87
School absenteeism	53 (88.3%)	7 (11.7%)	0.12	0.04 to 0.20	52 (86.7%)	8(13.3)	0.13	0.05 to 0.22	0.88	0.34 to 2.26	0.02	−0.10 to 0.13	60.0	−9.84 to 7.41
Rescue analgesic use	49 (81.7%)	11 (18.3%)	0.18	0.09 to 0.28	54 (90%)	6 (10%)	0.10	0.02 to 0.18	1.83	0.72 to 4.64	−0.08	−0.21 to 0.04	−12.0	−4.83 to 24.66

AR, absolute risk; ARR, absolute risk reduction; CI, confidence interval; NNT, number needed to treat; RR, relative risk.

effectiveness, we opted to include a sample size (60 subjects) larger than usual to avoid a false negative result which would preclude the opportunity to further examination of uzara in this respect. All analyses were performed with SPSS 17 (SPSS, Inc., Chicago, IL, USA). The Student t tests (for independent and dependent parameters) were used for continuous variables whereas Fisher's exact test was used for categorical variables. For all analyses, a two-tailed p value of less than 0.05 was considered statistically significant. Intention-to-treat (ITT) analysis was performed for all outcomes except for pain intensity difference (PID) over time. The latter was analyzed in those receiving study medications (uzara versus ibuprofen) as "modified intention-to-treat" or "per protocol"; a non-randomized, observational comparison. For those receiving rescue medications, as pre-specified in study protocol, the response using VAS scoring was recorded and analyzed separately to avoid confounding the analgesic effect of study medications. Risk analysis was done to estimate the risk of untoward outcomes in either study group. The relative risk (RR) was then calculated as the risk in the uzara group relative to the ibuprofen group. Absolute risk reduction (ARR) was calculated by subtraction of the risk in the ibuprofen group from that in the uzara group. The number needed to treat (NNT) was then calculated as the reciprocal of the ARR. All risk estimates were presented along with their 95% C.I. (confidence interval).

Results

To save time as the researchers were late in registering the study internationally, the study was announced during lectures so that those students suffering from dysmenorrhea and willing to volunteer in a trial of a new therapeutic line were invited to register themselves in a preliminary list for interview. This lasted till January 31st 2011when the trial was registered (Trial registration number: ISRCTN25618258; Registry website: http://www.controlled-trials.com). Following this, the first 103 subjects, in order, were interviewed with full explanation of the study protocol and assessment for eligibility. Patients' enrollment (60 subjects) followed with signing a well-informed consent, use of medications, and follow up till March 28, 2012 when the trial ended (Figure 1). Initial assessment, using VRS scoring, revealed that dysmenorrhea was moderate in 46 patients and severe in 14 patients, all virgin with absence of prior sexual intercourse. The general characteristics of the participants are shown in Table 1. Medical advice was sought in 16.7% (10/60); with an analgesic being prescribed to the participants by a lay relative in 85% (51/60) of cases. Family history of primary dysmenorrhea - in mother, a sister, or both – was positive in 50% of participants (30/60).

Thirty participants started with uzara, while the other 30 started with ibuprofen. There was no significant difference between uzara and ibuprofen cycles regarding the number of doses taken by the participants (2.12 ± 0.97 vs. 2.28 ± 0.76, p = 0.371; with median being 2 and range 1–4 vs. 1–6; respectively). The effectiveness of uzara and ibuprofen were comparable (Table 2) in terms of the reduction of VAS score to 3 or less (78.3% vs. 86.7%; respectively, p = 0.337) and participant's global evaluation (48.3% vs. 51.7%; respectively, p = 0.855). Satisfactory relief of pain, as indicated by the absent need of rescue drug, was lower with uzara compared to Ibuprofen (81.7% vs. 90%) groups, albeit with no statistical significance (p = 0.295). Of note, 2 (3.3%) participants with severe dysmenorrhea received a rescue drug with both tested medications, i.e. both medications failed to relief their pain. Discordant response with only one drug being effective and reported failure with the other was also noticed; uzara alone was effective in 2 participants, while ibuprofen only was effective in 9 participants.

Table 3. Effectiveness based on pain intensity difference (PID) at different time points after drug start and their sum (SPID) with Uzara (UZ) and Ibuprofen (IB) (Cycles: UZ, *N* = *49*; IB, *N* = *54*), with exclusion of 17cycles where rescue analgesia was used.

Effectiveness measure (Visual analogue sscale)	Uzara (Mean ± S.E.M.)	Ibuprofen (Mean ± S.E.M.)	P	Mean Difference (95% C.I.)
Basal VAS	67.35 ± 2.12	66.30 ± 1.93	0.714	1.051 (−4.622 to 6.723)
Pain Intensity Difference (PID) by hour after drug intake:				
4 hs.	46.73 ± 2.29	46.48 ± 1.83	0.931	0.253 (−5.511 to 6.018)
12 hs.	48.98 ± 2.03	48.15 ± 1.85	0.762	0.831 (−4.602 to 6.265)
24 hs.	54.08 ± 1.84	52.78 ± 2.07	0.642	1.304 (−4.240 to 6.848)
48–60 hs.	56.12 ± 2.02	54.63 ± 2.18	0.618	1.493 (−4.427 to 7.413)
90–120 hs.	56.53 ± 2.01	54.81 ± 2.16	0.565	1.716 (−4.172 to 7.604)
Sum (SPID)	262.45 ± 9.19	256.85 ± 9.6	0.676	5.597 (−20.887 to 32.081)

CI, confidence interval; P, probability; S.E.M., standard error of mean.

School absence rates were comparable; being 11.7% (7/60) for uzara and 13.3% (8/60) for ibuprofen, ($p>0.05$); both being lower than the participants' historical school absence rate (19/60 or 31.7%; $p<0.01$). In those who continued the study medications, the means of pain intensity difference (PID) at different time points after their start and its sum (SPID) were comparable (Figure 2, and Table 3). The mean post-treatment VAS scores in both uzara and ibuprofen cycles were comparable (1.63±0.86 vs. 1.61±0.83; respectively), being both significantly lower than the initial (pre-treatment) VAS (6.77±1.57; $p<0.001$). In those using rescue medications, the average VAS scores after drug use were 2.7±2.7 and 3±0.8; respectively ($p>0.05$).

All participants tolerated uzara well with 0% (0/60) side effects compared to 8.3% (5/60) with ibuprofen ($p<0.05$). These were all gastro-intestinal side effects including nausea (two participants), vomiting (one participant), stomach cramps alone (one participant) or with nausea (one participant).

Discussion

This study has assessed the efficacy, safety and tolerability of uzara in comparison to ibuprofen, a NSAID, in the treatment of primary dysmenorrhea. Our analyses showed that the effectiveness of uzara was comparable to that of ibuprofen, a standard first line therapy. The failure rates of uzara (21.7%) and Ibuprofen (13.3%) were comparable to other reported NSAIDs [2,5]. Two participants failed to respond to both drugs, while discordant response with only one drug being effective was also noticed in 11 participants. All participants tolerated uzara well with no reported side effects compared to 8.3% in Ibuprofen cycles.

A point of strength of our study is the prospective randomized design with crossover assignment of medication to allow each participant to act as her own control. Also, to provide clinically meaningful results, two measurement of severity of dysmenorrhea, visual analogue scale (VAS) and verbal rating scale (VRS), were used [22]. Although, some investigators considered a reduction of 3 points of pain severity in the VAS as an outcome to define successful treatment [23], a reduction of VAS score to 3 or less was chosen to indicate effectiveness in the present study as this would indicate a mild degree of pain likely to be acceptable to the woman. Retrospective participant's global evaluation of each medication showed also comparable efficacy; albeit with lower figures which might be explained by subject's expectation to have complete analgesia. One limitation is failure to double blind this study, due to lack of technical facilities to manufacture ibuprofen tablet identical to that of uzara. Non-blinding of the participants might have being disadvantageous to uzara, being acknowledged by them as a test medication with potential loss of trust and lowered expectations regarding efficacy. This could be a source of bias against uzara with apparently less effectiveness (78.3% vs. 86.7% of cycles of ibuprofen; respectively), and higher need for rescue drug usage (18.3% and 10%; respectively), though being statistically insignificant. Other limitations are the apparently lower number of study participants and belonging to a special cultural sector with medical background. Since all study participants were virgin with absence of prior sexual intercourse, an assumption based on strict religious banning of pre-marital sex in our society, our results can be safely generalized to unmarried or abstinent young females. In fact, one might assume that this would not interfere with overall generalizability due to elimination of other confounding factors, such as IUD or pelvic infection, which can interfere with dysmenorrhea.

We hypothesized that uzara is effective in treating primary dysmenorrhea. Catecholamines can theoretically cause either excitation or inhibition of the uterus depending on whether alpha or beta adrenergic receptors predominate. The adrenergic responsiveness of the myometrium appears to be regulated by steroid hormones [27]. It is suggested that stress-associated enhancement of sympathetic activity leads to exacerbation of uterine contraction and increased menstrual pain. This activity might be decreased via exercise with subsequent symptomatic relief [28]. The mechanism of analgesic effect of uzara is apparently through inhibiting the motility of visceral smooth muscle of the uterus, probably via the local stimulation of sympathetic nerves with an inhibitory effect on smooth muscles; an action similar to that suggested for its anti-diarrheal action [16]. This is further supported by earlier use of beta2-adrenoceptor agonists in the treatment of women with primary dysmenorrhea. Despite the failure of hydroxyphenyl-orciprenalin [29], and isoxsuprine [30], to show any benefit in previous studies, another one reported pain relief with a combination of isoxsuprine, acetaminophen and caffeine [31]. Moreover, two studies reported pain relief in severe primary dysmenorrhea with terbutaline administered via spray inhalations [32] or intravenous injection, along with inhibition of the myometrial activity and increased uterine blood flow [33]. A recent review on the use beta2-adrenoceptor agonists for dysmenorrhea found that adverse effects with all these medications were reported in up to a quarter of the total number of participants and they included nausea, vomiting, dizziness, tremors and palpitations. Although this mechanism for relieving dysmenorrhea fell into disrepute for over 30 years due to high incidence of adverse effects in these few, relatively small-sized and inadequate quality studies [34], this does not preclude the assertion that uterine sympathetic supply plays a role in the pathogenesis of primary dysmenorrhea. The response to uzara in the present study supports this view. Therefore, uzara might benefit women by relieving dysmenorrhea via this mechanism of action, but without significant risk of side effects, which preclude the use of beta2-adrenoceptor agonists as an acceptable clinical treatment option.

This study suggests that uzara might be as effective as ibuprofen in treatment of primary dysmenorrhea. Considering its better tolerability, shorter contraindication list and lower incidence of side effects, uzara might be considered as an alternative agent to NSAIDs in women who have failed response, contraindications or side effects. With suggested different mechanism of action of uzara, one might wonder whether combining it with NSAIDs would have a good additive effect evidenced by a better success rate and the need of lower doses of NSAIDs with lower adverse effects. Therefore, further large-scale studies are warranted to confirm and explore uzara's role in the management of primary dysmenorrhea.

Supporting Information

Checklist S1 CONSORT Checklist.
(DOC)

Protocol S1 Trial Protocol.
(DOC)

Author Contributions

Conceived and designed the experiments: KHIA-E-M MAMFK MSA MII RMMZM. Performed the experiments: MAMFK MSA MII RMMZM. Analyzed the data: KHIA-E-M MAMFK MSA MII RMMZM. Contributed reagents/materials/analysis tools: KHIA-E-M MAMFK MSA MII RMMZM. Wrote the paper: KHIA-E-M MAMFK MSA MII RMMZM.

References

1. Coco AS (1999) Primary Dysmenorrhoea. Am Fam Physician 60(2):489–96.
2. Dawood MY (2006) Primary Dysmenorrhea - Advances in pathogenesis and management. Obstet Gynecol 108(2):428–41.
3. Harlow SD, Park M (1996) A longitudinal study of risk factors for the occurrence, duration and severity of menstrual cramps in a cohort of college women. Br J Obstet Gynaecol 103: 1134–42.
4. Marjoribanks J, Proctor M, Farquhar C, Derks RS (2010) Nonsteroidal anti-inflammatory drugs for dysmenorrhoea. Cochrane Database of Systematic Reviews, Issue 1. Art. No.:CD001751.pub2.
5. Modaress Nejad V, Asadipour M (2006) Comparison the effectiveness of Fennel and Mefenamic acid on pain intensity in dysmenorrhea. East Med Health J 12(3/4):423–7.
6. Wong CL, Farquhar C, Roberts H, Proctor M (2009) Oral contraceptive pill for primary dysmenorrhoea. Cochrane Database of Systematic Reviews, Issue 4. Art. No.:CD002120.pub3.
7. Smith CA, Zhu X, He L, Song J (2011) Acupuncture for dysmenorrhoea. Cochrane Database of Systematic Reviews, Issue 1. Art. No.: CD007854.pub2.
8. Proctor M, Farquhar C, Stones W, He L, Zhu X, et al. (2002) Transcutaneous electrical nerve stimulation for primary dysmenorrhoea. Cochrane Database of Systematic Reviews, Issue 1. Art. No.: CD002123.
9. Proctor M, Latthe P, Farquhar C, Khan K, Johnson N (2005) Surgical interruption of pelvic nerve pathways for primary and secondary dysmenorrhoea. Cochrane Database of Systematic Reviews, Issue 4. Art. No.: CD001896.pub2.
10. Proctor M, Hing W, Johnson TC, Murphy PA, Brown J (2006) Spinal manipulation for dysmenorrhoea. Cochrane Database of Systematic Reviews, Issue 3. Art. No.: CD002119.pub3.
11. Proctor M, Murphy PA, Pattison HM, Suckling JA, Farquhar C (2007) Behavioural interventions for dysmenorrhoea. Cochrane Database of Systematic Reviews, Issue 3. Art. No.: CD002248.pub3.
12. Rahnama P, Montazeri A, Huseini HF, Kianbakht S, Naseri M (2012) Effect of Zingiber officinale R. rhizomes (ginger) on pain relief in primary dysmenorrhea: a placebo randomized trial. BMC Complement Altern Med 12: 92.
13. Proctor M, Murphy PA (2001) Herbal and dietary therapies for primary and secondary dysmenorrhoea. Cochrane Database of Systematic Reviews, Issue 2. Art. No.:CD002124.
14. Kraft K, Hobbs C (2004) Pocket guide to herbal medicine. Stuttgart: Georg Thieme Veralg. p.124.
15. Schulzke JD, Andres S, Amasheh M, Fromm A, Günzel D (2011) Anti-diarrheal mechanism of the traditional remedy Uzara via reduction of active chloride secretion. PLoS One. 6(3):e18107.
16. Schulz V, Hänsel R, Blumenthal M, Tyler VE (2004) Rational Phytotherapy: A Reference Guide for Physicians and Pharmacists. Berlin: Springer-Veralg, Fifth Ed, p.264
17. Schmelzer GH (2011) Xysmalobium undulatum (L.) WT Aiton. In: Schmelzer G.H. & Gurib-Fakim A. (Editors). Prota 11(2): Medicinal plants/Plantes médicinales 2. [CD-Rom]. PROTA, Wageningen, Netherlands. Available: http://database.prota.org/PROTAhtml/Xysmalobium%20undulatum_En.htm. Accessed: 2013 Jun 1.
18. Novak J (1913) in Wien. Klin. Woch., December 11th, 1913. Cited by Anonymous: An Epitome of Current Medical Literature: 139. Atropine In Dysmenorrhoea. The Br Med J March7, 1914, p.39.
19. Blumenthal M, Busse W, Goldberg A, Gruenwald J, Hall T, et al. (1998) The Complete German Commission E monographs: Therapeutic Guide to Herbal Medicines. Austin/Texas: American Botanical Council, First Edn, p.226.
20. Schmiedl S, Ritter A, Szymanski J, Schneider F, Plecko T, et al. (2012) Cardiovascular effects, pharmacokinetics and cross-reactivity in digitalis glycoside immunoassays of an antidiarrheal uzara root extract. Int J Clin Pharmacol Ther 50(10): 729–40.
21. Thürmann PA, Neff A, Fleisch J (2004) Interference of Uzara glycosides in assays of digitalis glycosides. Int J Clin Pharmacol Ther 42(5):281–4.
22. Lara-Muñoz C, Ponce de Leon S, Feinstein AR, Puente A, Wells CK (2004) Comparison of Three Rating Scales for Measuring Subjective Phenomena in Clinical Research: I. Use of Experimentally Controlled Auditory Stimuli. Arch Med Res 35(1):43–8.
23. Lee JS, Hobden E, Stiell IG, Wells GA (2003) Clinically important change in the visual analog scale after adequate pain control. Acad Emerg Med 10: 1128–30.
24. Available: http://www.drugs.com/pro/ibuprofen.html. Accessed: 2014 May 5.
25. Thürmann PA, Neff A, Fleisch J (2004) Interference of uzara glycosides in assays of digitalis glycosides. International Journal of Clinical Pharmacology and Therapeutics 42(5): 281–284.
26. Guidance for Industry: BIOEQUIVALENCE GUIDANCE. Docket No. 94D-0401. U.S. Department of Health and Human Services, Food and Drug Administration. Center for Veterinary Medicine (CVM) November 8, 2006, p.15. Available: http://www.fda.gov/downloads/AnimalVeterinary/GuidanceComplianceEnforcement/GuidanceforIndustry/ucm052363.pdf Accessed: 2014 May 5.
27. Williams LT, Lefkowitz RJ (1977) Regulation of rabbit myometrial alpha adrenergic receptors by estrogen and progesterone. J Clin Invest 60(4):815–8.
28. Ganon L (1986) The potential of exercise in the alleviation of menstrual disorders and menopausal symptom. Women Health 14(2): 105–7.
29. Hansen MK, Secher NJ (1975) Beta-receptor stimulation in essential dysmenorrhea. Am J Obstet Gynecol 121(4):566–7.
30. Nesheim BI, Walloe L (1976) The use of isoxsuprine in essential dysmenorrhea. A controlled clinical study. Acta Obstet Gynecol Scand 55(4):315–6.
31. Gallegos-Torres J, Flores-Mercado F (1975) Isoxsuprine in primary dysmenorrhoea. Its effectiveness in premenstrual tension. J Int Med Res 3 (3):194–201.
32. Kullander S, Svanberg L (1981) Terbutaline inhalation for alleviation of severe pain in essential dysmenorrhea. Acta Obstet Gynecol Scand 60(4):425–7.
33. Akerlund M, Andersson KE, Ingemarsson I (1976) Effects of terbutaline on myometrial activity, uterine blood flow, and lower abdominal pain in women with primary dysmenorrhoea. Br J Obstet Gynaecol 83(9):673–8.
34. Fedorowicz Z, Nasser M, Jagannath VA, Beaman JH, Ejaz K, et al. (2012) Beta2-adrenoceptor agonists for dysmenorrhoea (Review). The Cochrane Collaboration. Published by JohnWiley & Sons, Ltd. The Cochrane Library, Issue 5.

9

Increased Risk of Urinary Tract Cancer in ESRD Patients Associated with Usage of Chinese Herbal Products Suspected of Containing Aristolochic Acid

Shuo-Meng Wang[1,4], Ming-Nan Lai[2], Alan Wei[3], Ya-Yin Chen[1,2], Yeong-Shiau Pu[1], Pau-Chung Chen[4], Jung-Der Wang[5,6]*

1 Department of Urology, National Taiwan University Hospital, Taipei, Taiwan, **2** Department of Statistics, Feng Chia University, Taichung, Taiwan, **3** School of Medicine, Stony Brook University, Stony Brook, New York, United States of America, **4** Institute of Occupational Medicine and Industrial Hygiene, College of Public Health, National Taiwan University, Taipei, Taiwan, **5** Department of Public Health, National Cheng Kung University Medical College, Tainan City, Taiwan, **6** Departments of Internal Medicine and Occupational and Environmental Medicine, National Cheng Kung University Hospital, Tainan City, Taiwan

Abstract

Introduction: Both end-stage renal disease (ESRD) and urothelial cancer (UC) are associated with the consumption of Chinese herbal products containing aristolochic acid (AA) by the general population. The objective of this study was to determine the risk of UC associated with AA-related Chinese herbal products among ESRD patients.

Methods: We conducted a cohort study using the National Health Insurance reimbursement database to enroll all ESRD patients in Taiwan from 1998–2002. Cox regression models were constructed and hazard ratios and confidence intervals were estimated after controlling for potential confounders, including age, sex, residence in region with endemic black foot disease, urinary tract infection, and use of non-steroidal anti-inflammatory drugs and acetaminophen.

Results: A total of 38,995 ESRD patients were included in the final analysis, and 320 patients developed UC after ESRD. Having been prescribed Mu Tong that was adulterated with Guan Mu Tong (*Aristolochia manshuriensis*) before 2004, or an estimated consumption of more than 1–100 mg of aristolochic acid, were both associated with an increased risk of UC in the multivariable analyses. Analgesic consumption of more than 150 pills was also associated with an increased risk of UC, although there was little correlation between the two risk factors.

Conclusion: Consumption of aristolochic acid-related Chinese herbal products was associated with an increased risk of developing UC in ESRD patients. Regular follow-up screening for UC in ESRD patients who have consumed Chinese herbal products is thus necessary.

Editor: Francisco X. Real, Centro Nacional de Investigaciones Oncológicas (CNIO), Spain

Funding: This study was supported by the National Health Research Institutes of Taiwan (intramural project EO-100-EO-PP04), and a grant from the Headquarters of University Advancement at the National Cheng Kung University. The funders had no role in study design, data collection and analysis, decision to publish, or preparation of the manuscript.

Competing Interests: The authors have declared that no competing interests exist.

* Email: jdwang121@gmail.com

Introduction

Aristolochic acid nephropathy—a progressive form of renal interstitial fibrosis—was first reported in a group of young Belgian patients with end-stage renal disease in 1993, and was thought to be caused by the use of Chinese herbal medicines that contained aristolochic acid [1–3]. Aristolochic acid has been shown to be associated with urothelial cancer (UC) in many studies of clinical cases around the world, in animal models, and by the detection of aristolochic acid–DNA adducts in the kidney and ureteral tissues [4][5,6]. Prior studies observed increased risks of developing UC and ESRD in the general population in association with the consumption of Chinese herbal products [7][8], and patients with ESRD have a higher incidence of malignancies than the general population [9–12]. We have noticed an extraordinarily high incidence of UC in uremic or ESRD patients in the past decade in Taiwan [13–16], but the reason for this remains unknown. Some researchers suggest that chronic bladder irritation, a decreased urinary washout effect, atrophic involution of the bladder, compound analgesic abuse [17–19], use of Chinese herbs [4,5,20], groundwater intake (arsenic exposure) [21,22], and uremia per se [15,16] may play roles in the development of UC. A report published by the International Agency in Research on Cancer (IARC) [23] stated that the risk factors associated with UC include analgesics (phenacetin), herbal usage (aristolochic acid), heavy metals (arsenic) and tobacco smoking.

Although the IARC classifies aristolochic acid as a group 1 carcinogen, to the best of our knowledge there have been no cohort studies that examine the association between urinary tract cancer and the use of herbs or herbal products containing aristolochic acid in ESRD patients. In March of 1995, Taiwan established the National Health Insurance (NHI) program, which covers more than 99% of the population [24]. The NHI routinely reimburses enrollees for the cost of prescribed medicines, including Chinese herbal products containing aristolochic acid, which were widely prescribed before being banned in December 2003. We thus used the NHI reimbursement database to conduct an ESRD population-based cohort study to examine the association between having been prescribed Chinese herbal products that contain substantial amounts of aristolochic acid, including Guan Mu Tong and Guang Fangchi, and the risk of urinary tract cancer, as well as the possibility of a dose–response relationship between the two.

Materials and Methods

Study Population

Established in Taiwan in March 1995, the National Health Insurance program (NHI) covers over 99% of the population residents [24]. Standard mixtures of Chinese herbal products (CHP) are included in the regular schedule of reimbursement. The National Health Research Institutes (NHRI) transformed the NHI reimbursement data into files suitable for use by researchers, and which contain detailed information about the usage of conventional drugs and CHP [25]. This study was conducted using ESRD patient data obtained from the database of approximately more than 22 million people enrolled in the NHI. The data collection period began in 1996, but became more comprehensive after January 1997. As noted above, the NHRI anonymized and converted the reimbursement data into research-ready files, called the National Health Insurance Research Database (NHIRD) [25]. The identification numbers of all the individuals in the database were doubly encrypted to ensure their privacy.

The dataset to which we had access provided detailed demographic data (including birth date and sex) and information regarding the health-care services provided for each patient, including all payments for outpatient visits, hospitalizations, and prescriptions, as well as where each patient lived. The data for each hospitalization contained up to five diagnoses that were coded according to the International Classification of Diseases, Ninth Revision (ICD-9) [26], all drugs prescribed and the doses (i.e., conventional medicines, including generic and commercial brands of acetaminophen and non-steroidal anti-inflammatory drugs, as well as Chinese herbal products), and the date of each prescription. During the study period (i.e., from January 1, 1998, to December 31, 2002), all prescribed medications were covered under the NHI of Taiwan, and no drug could be dispensed at a pharmacy without a doctor's prescription.

To select potential case subjects for this study, we first obtained the NHI catastrophic illness registry files for all patients who were diagnosed with end-stage renal disease from January 1, 1998, to December 31, 2002. Because all patients who are registered as having a catastrophic illness are exempt from all copayments, their data is very comprehensive and has been carefully validated. A diagnosis of urinary tract cancer or end-stage renal disease made by doctors and officials of the NHI is usually accurate: urinary tract cancer must be proven by tissue pathology, and is classified as cancer of the upper urinary tract, which includes the renal pelvis and ureter (ICD-9 codes 189.1 and 189.2, respectively) or bladder cancer (ICD-9 code 188). The database contains 38,675 Non-UTC and 839 UTC prevalent cases of end-stage renal disease that were diagnosed from January 1, 1998, to December 31, 2002.Within this population, we identified 320 patients who were newly diagnosed with urinary tract cancer from January 1, 2001, to December 31, 2002, to allow at least four years between January 1, 1997, and the date of diagnosis to give sufficient time for the case subjects to accumulate sufficient doses of herbal products to induce UTC.

Exposure Assessment

The reimbursement database contained all the details of the prescribed conventional medicines, which included acetaminophen and the commercial names of 45 kinds of non-steroidal anti-inflammatory drugs (NSAIDs), shown in the File S1.

As phenacetin has been totally banned by the Department of Health since 1986, it was not included. Doses of each drug were determined according to the number of pills prescribed and cumulative doses were calculated before ESRD. The use of 600–1000 pills of acetaminophen, NSAIDs, or mixed analgesics has been associated with an increased risk of renal damage or renal cancer in previous studies [27,28]. We thus accumulated the total number of analgesics pills for each subject before dialysis during 1998–2002.

According to the standard prescription recommended by the Committee on Chinese Medicine and Pharmacy (CCMP) in Taiwan, the following Chinese herbal products may contain AA: Xi-Xin (Asarum heterotoppoides), Guan-Mu-Tong (Aristolochia manshuriensis), and Guang-Fangchi (A. fangchi). However, Guan-Mu-Tong and Guang-Fangchi were once offered under the names Mu-Tong (Akebia sp.) and Fangchi (Stephania sp.), respectively, in Taiwan before 2003, because of similarities of gross morphology and common practices [29]. In addition, according to an investigation by the Bureau of Food and Drug Analysis in Taiwan, as well as some studies, approximately 89.2–100% of Fangchi preparations were actually Guang-Fangchi [30–32] and 84% of Mu-Tong were actually Guan-Mu-Tong [33]. These three herbs were prescribed as single products or included as components of some mixed CHP. Each pharmaceutical company has published and submitted the detailed composition of every product it produces, and data on this can be retrieved from the website of the Committee on Chinese Medicine and Pharmacy of the Department of Health [29]. With this information, the original amounts of herbs, in grams, could be determined for each mixture of CHP, and the cumulative dose for each herb prescribed to an individual before developing ESRD could thus be calculated. We also calculated the estimated cumulative dose of aristolochic acid for each subject by using the following estimates obtained in previous studies: the estimated average doses of aristolochic acid per 1 g of Guan Mu Tong, Guang Fangchi, and Xi Xin are 2.59 mg, 2.04 mg, and 0.042 mg, respectively [30,32–35].

The reimbursement database also has data on where all the subjects lived. We identified subjects who lived in the four townships in Taiwan that have been reported to be areas endemic for black foot disease—Pu-Tai and Yi-Chu in Chiayi County, and Hsueh-Chia and Pei-Men in Tainan County [36,37]. Black foot disease is a peripheral vascular disease that has been endemic to the coastal region of Taiwan for the past 60 years, and is associated with drinking water from artesian wells containing arsenic, and has been documented to be associated with an increased incidence of bladder cancer [36,37]. We controlled for this factor (townships) as a surrogate for arsenic exposure.

According to the Committee on Chinese Medicine and Pharmacy [29], Mu Tong is usually prescribed for the treatment of hepatitis, urinary tract infection, rhinitis, dysmenorrhea, and eczema. Recurrent or chronic urinary tract infection, associated with Schistosomiasis or prolonged indwelling catheters in patients with spinal cord injury, is associated with an increase risk of bladder cancer [38,39], whereas urinary tract infection from other causes does not show any consistent association with bladder cancer risk [38,40]. We thus defined patients with chronic urinary tract infection (UTI) as those who had such a diagnosis at least 12 times up to one year before the diagnosis of UC, and we controlled for the above potential confounders during the risk-estimate analysis. The patients with diabetes or hypertension were also ascertained based on the related diagnosis numbers in ICD-9 before ESRD diagnosis.

Statistical Analyses

To assess the independent association of various risk factors with new occurrences of UC, univariate and multivariable Cox regression models were used to analyze the population of ESRD patients and those cases that developed UC subsequent to ESRD diagnosis. Potential risk factors, including age, sex, hypertension, diabetes mellitus, chronic UTI, and prescriptions of NSAIDs, acetaminophen or any of the aforementioned Chinese herbs suspected to contain AA, were assessed for independent association with new occurrences of UC. We constructed models for two different types of exposure assessment: prescribed dosages of Chinese herbs (model 1) and different estimated dosages of AA as risk factors (model 2). The dose–response association between cumulative dose of Chinese herbs, analgesics and occurrence of UC was tested by the Mantel–Haenszel extension for the trend. For each potential risk factor, multivariate Cox proportional hazards models were constructed to estimate the relative risk and its 95% confidence interval (CI) for UC incidence. An estimate with the 95% CI that did not contain the number 1 was considered statistically significant. We also ran a correlation analysis between the total numbers of analgesics pills and cumulative doses (in mg) of AA. All the above analyses were conducted using the SAS ver. 9.2 software package (SAS Institute, Cary, NC, USA).

Results

After excluding people with incomplete data or aged over 100 years, a total of 39,514 prevalent cases of end-stage renal disease were included in the data, with 839 of these developing UTC between January 1, 1998 and December 31, 2002. Among these patients, there were 38,675 cases without UTC and 320 UTC cases who were newly diagnosed with urinary tract cancer between January 1, 2001 and December 31, 2002. A total of 38,995 ESRD patients were thus included in the final analysis, with 18,522 (47.5%) men and 20,473 (52.5%) women. There were high prevalence rates of hypertension (88.5%) and diabetes mellitus (55.7%). The average crude incidence rate of UTC for these ESRD patients was 1,368 per million person-years.

Table 1 summarizes the frequency data of the ESRD patient population with respect to different potential risk factors, including sex, age, follow-up time after ESRD diagnosis, residence in township with endemic black foot disease, hypertension, diabetes, chronic UTI, and analgesics (NSAID and acetaminophen) consumption. The patient population was also characterized in terms of Chinese herb consumption for individual herbs (Mu-Tong, Fangchi, and Xi-Xin), as well as total estimated consumption of AA calculated based on total consumption of Chinese herbs containing this substance. The incidence rate of UTC appears to increase with the time after diagnosis of ESRD (Table 1).

Because only one UTC patient and 254 non-UTC controls had lived in area with endemic black foot disease (Table 1), we decided to exclude subjects with this characteristic in the final analysis for both cases and controls.

The number of new UTC cases and adjusted hazard ratios (aHR) calculated from the Cox regression models for multiple risk factors (sex, age, diabetes, hypertension, chronic UTI, analgesics and cumulative doses for different herbs) are summarized in Table 2. The crude and adjusted HR (aHR) for development of UTC increased significantly for older patients, whereas the crude and adjusted HR for development of UTC was not significantly related to either hypertension or diabetes. Crude HR's also increased for prescribed cumulative doses of Mu-Tong greater than 1 g, Fangchi 1–30 g, >100 g, as well as for prescribed Xi-Xin and for estimated AA consumptions of 1–100 mg, 101–200 g, and >300 mg. Prescription of analgesics also increased the crude HR. After control of potential confounding by other risk factors, we found that the aHR for development of UTC increased for ESRD patients prescribed Mu Tong, and that the various estimated consumptions of AA were each associated with an increased risk of UTC in the multivariable analyses (Mu Tong: at 1–30 g, aHR = 1.8, 95% CI = 1.3 to 2.6, and each 30 g increase, aHR = 1.3, 95% CI = 1.2 to 1.5; AA: at 1–100 mg, aHR = 2.1, 95% CI = 1.6 to 2.6, and each 100 mg increase, aHR = 1.6, 95% CI = 1.4 to 1.8). Prescription of analgesics is associated with a greater risk of urothelial cancer, with an increased aHR of 1.3 (95% CI = 1.2 to 1.4) for each increment of 150 pills, as summarized in models 1 and 2 of Table 2. However, there is little association between the prescribed numbers of analgesic pills and cumulative doses of AA, as shown in Figure 1.

Discussion

To the best of our knowledge, this is the first population-based study to document a linear dose–response relationship between prescription of Chinese herbal products containing AA and the risk of UTC in ESRD patients after controlling for confounding by age, sex, living in a township endemic for black foot disease (a surrogate of arsenic contamination in the water supply), analgesic consumption, and history of chronic urinary tract infection. In fact, because the NHI reimbursement database collects all prescription information prospectively, we can rule out the possibility of recall bias for the intake doses of various Chinese herbal products. Since we included all ESRD patients newly diagnosed in Taiwan from 1998 to 2002, and the diagnosis of urinary tract cancer or end-stage renal disease made by doctors and officials of the NHI is usually accurate, we can also rule out the possibility of selection bias. Moreover, we excluded all subjects who had lived in townships endemic for black foot disease (a surrogate of high arsenic exposure) to prevent confounding the results due to the carcinogenic effects of arsenic exposure. Although increased prescription of analgesics was also associated with UTC (Table 2), the effect has been controlled in the multivariable regression model, and Figure 1 also shows no association between the number of analgesics pills and cumulative dose of AA. Finally, this study has documented a dose-dependent association between the cumulative estimated prescribed dose of AA and urinary tract cancer, as well as a dose-dependent association between the cumulative prescribed dose of Mu-Tong and UTC. We thus tentatively conclude that the urothelial cancers developed by ESRD patients are associated with prescription of AA-associated Chinese herbal products.

This study found a consistent dose-response relationship between the estimated intake of AA (or prescribed dose of AA-containing CHP) and urinary tract cancer in ESRD patients, suggesting that AA may be responsible for increased cancer risk of these patients. Fangchi and Xi-Xin both showed increased hazard ratios at higher doses, but these results did not reach statistical significance after adjustment for risk factors, likely due to the small number of case subjects. However, the increased hazard ratios for the occurrence of UC were found to be significantly higher in

Table 1. Frequency distributions of various risk factors for the occurrence of urinary tract cancers (UTC) stratified by different inclusion criteria in 38,995 patients with end-stage renal disease (ESRD).

	All ESRD Patients	
Risk Factors	**UTC Cases (n = 320)**	**Non-UTC Cases (n = 38675)**
Sex		
Men	131 (40.94%)	18391 (47.55%)
Women	189 (59.06%)	20284 (52.45%)
Age (year)		
<50	67 (20.94%)	9804 (25.35%)
50–59	80 (25.00%)	7790 (20.14%)
60–69	99 (30.94%)	10572 (27.34%)
70–99	74 (23.13%)	10509 (27.17%)
Residence in township where black foot disease was endemic		
No	319 (99.69%)	38421 (99.34%)
Yes	1 (0.31%)	254 (0.66%)
Hypertension		
No	68 (21.25%)	4297 (11.11%)
Yes	252 (78.75%)	34378 (88.89%)
Diabetes		
No	219 (68.44%)	17045 (44.07%)
Yes	101 (31.56%)	21630 (55.93%)
Chronic UTI		
No	312 (97.50%)	38511 (99.58%)
Yes	8 (2.50%)	164 (0.42%)
Analgesics *(pills) NSAID & acetaminophen		
0–150	123 (38.44%)	16116 (41.65%)
151–300	74 (23.13%)	8187 (21.16%)
351–450	32 (10.00%)	4405 (11.40%)
451–600	25 (7.81%)	2665 (6.90%)
>600	66 (20.63%)	7306 (18.88%)
Mu-Tong (g) total amount prescribed		
0	286 (89.38%)	35968 (93.00%)
1–30	20 (6.25%)	1845 (4.77%)
30–60	3 (0.94%)	348 (0.90%)
61–100	3 (0.94%)	179 (0.46%)
101–200	4 (1.25%)	164 (0.42%)
>200	4 (1.25%)	171 (0.44%)
Fangchi (g) total amount prescribed		
0	295 (92.19%)	35731 (92.39%)
1–30	19 (5.94%)	2417 (6.25%)
31–60 (31–100)	4 (1.25%)	271 (0.70%)
61–100	0 (0%)	121 (0.31%)
101–200 (>100)	2 (0.63%)	86 (0.22%)
>200	0 (0%)	49 (0.13%)
Xi-Xin (g) total amount prescribed		
0	283 (88.44%)	34679 (89.67%)
1–30	22 (6.88%)	2995 (7.74%)
31–60	5 (1.56%)	465 (1.20%)
61–100	5 (1.56%)	231 (0.60%)
101–200	3 (0.94%)	185 (0.48%)
>200	2 (0.63%)	120 (0.32%)
Aristolochic acid (mg) estimated total consumption		

Table 1. Cont.

	All ESRD Patients	
Risk Factors	UTC Cases (n = 320)	Non-UTC Cases (n = 38675)
0	270 (84.38%)	32550 (84.16%)
1–100	33 (10.31%)	5363 (13.09%)
101–200	4 (1.25%)	464 (1.20%)
201–300	4 (1.25%)	197 (0.51%)
>300	9 (2.81%)	.04%)

Analgesics *, sum of acetaminophen and non-steroidal anti-inflammatory drugs (NSAIDs).

ESRD patients when over 1–30 g of Mu-Tong or over 1–100 mg cumulative AA were prescribed. Because these doses are much smaller than those reported by Belgian scholars [4] and our previous report [7], it suggests that patients with ESRD might be more vulnerable to the carcinogenic effects of AA. Although these subgroups do not correlate with a cumulative dose of higher than 147-mg AA, as reported in the Belgian report [4], the observation of increased hazard ratios at lower cumulative levels of AA-containing Chinese herbal products in ESRD patients who consume these products suggests potential pathogenic effects at lower doses, and this is an issue that deserves further investigation, with more long-term follow-up of these patients.

Forty-five percent of the UTC cases in this study were upper urinary tract cancer, which is similar to the rates seen in the general population, as reported by the National Cancer Registry and in a previous clinical report examining pathology-confirmed urinary tract cancer cases in Taiwan [41]. However, these rates are much higher than those in other countries, in which less than 10% of all UTC cases are upper urinary tract cancer. In this study, prescription of Chinese herbal products was associated with urothelial cancers that occurred in all parts of the urinary tract, similar to what was reported in a recent case study of Belgian women who received kidney transplants for end-stage AA nephropathy, in which 44.7% had upper urinary tract cancer and 39.5% had bladder cancer [42]. We thus hypothesize that AA induces urothelial cancers in the upper urinary tract and bladder with approximately equal tendency.

We also found a dose-dependent association between analgesics and occurrence of UTC among patients with ESRD, corroborating previous reports [17–19]. Unfortunately, we did not have a sufficiently large sample size to further explore this issue. Future studies are thus recommended to collect more UTC cases among patients with ESRD, and determine if the effect is associated with acetaminophen, aspirin, or any other NSAID.

There are some limitations to this study, as follows. First, because patient identities were not obtainable from the NHI reimbursement database, histopathology reports were unavailable to confirm the diagnoses. However, accurate diagnosis of UTC in the NHI database is based on pathology and/or cytology evidence and made after serious consideration with histopathologic proof in 95% of bladder cancers and 91%–92% of upper urinary tract cancers [43]. Second, we were unable to contact patients directly about their use of herbs due to anonymization of the database; therefore, we were unable to rule out the possibility that subjects may have taken additional nephrotoxic herbs or agents that were not prescribed. However, the comprehensive coverage and copayment for prescriptions is universally 50 NT$ (approximately equal to US $1.5), which is generally less than the cost of herbs

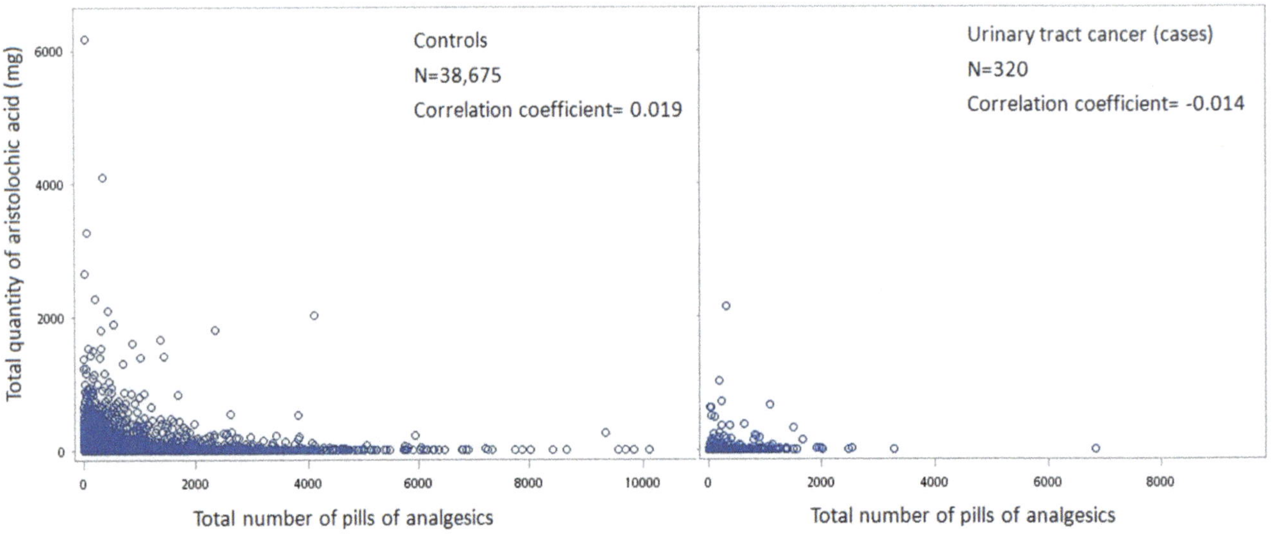

Figure 1. Correlation analysis between prescription of analgesics (number of pills) and cumulative dose of aristolochic acid for both cases and controls.

Table 2. Crude and adjusted hazards ratios (HR), and 95% confidence intervals (CI) estimated from multivariate Cox regression models for urinary tract cancer developed in patients with ESRD.

		Model 1	Model 2
Risk Factors	**Crude HR (95% CI)**	**Adjusted HR (95% CI)†**	**Adjusted HR (95% CI)†**
Sex			
Men	1	1	1
Women	1.02 (0.82 to 1.27)	0.89 (0.71 to 1.12)	0.91 (0.73 to 1.14)
Age (years)			
<50	1	1	1
50–59	1.38 (1.04 to 1.85)*	1.43 (1.06 to 1.93)*	1.44 (1.07 to 1.92)*
60–69	1.77 (1.34 to 2.35)**	1.75 (1.30 to 2.36)**	1.73 (1.29 to 2.32)**
70–99	1.93 (1.39 to 2.66)**	1.90 (1.35 to 2.67)**	1.83 (1.31 to 2.56)**
Diabetes			
No	1	1	1
Yes	1.12 (0.90 to 1.40)	0.95 (0.76 to 1.20)	0.94 (0.75 to 1.19)
Hypertension			
No	1	1	1
Yes	1.00 (0.78 to 1.29)	0.74 (0.57 to 0.97)*	0.78 (0.60 to 1.01)
Chronic UTI			
No	1	1	1
Yes	4.77 (2.46 to 9.26)**	6.85 (3.52 to 13.34)**	6.68 (3.43 to 12.99)**
Analgesics (pills)			
0–150	1	1	1
151–300	2.03 (1.54 to 2.67)**	1.91 (1.44 to 2.53)**	1.93 (1.46 to 2.55)**
301–450	2.26 (1.55 to 3.28)**	1.97 (1.35 to 2.89)**	2.02 (1.39 to 2.95)**
451–600	2.92 (1.93 to 4.43)**	2.70 (1.75 to 4.15)**	2.72 (1.78 to 4.16)**
>600	3.36 (2.51 to 4.49)**	2.98 (2.19 to 4.06)**	2.83 (2.09 to 3.83)**
Each 150 pills increase	1.35 (1.26 to 1.44)**	1.32 (1.23 to 1.41)**	1.31 (1.22 to 1.40)**
Mu-Tong (g) total amount prescribed			
0	1	1	-
1–30	2.38 (1.79 to 3.16)**	1.83 (1.30 to 2.57)**	-
31–60	2.21 (1.29 to 3.82)‡	1.98 (1.07 to 3.69)*	-
61–100	3.08 (1.58 to 6.02)**	2.51 (1.19 to 5.28)*	-
101–200	2.73 (1.61 to 4.63)**	3.16 (1.63 to 6.14)**	-
>200	3.45 (1.88 to 6.36)**	3.46 (1.70 to 7.03)**	-
Each 30 g increase	1.33 (1.23 to 1.44)**	1.31 (1.17 to 1.48)**	-
Fangchi (g) total amount prescribed			
0	1	1	-
1–30	2.24 (1.73 to 2.92)**	1.23 (0.91 to 1.67)	-
31–100	1.41 (0.75 to 2.66)	0.84 (0.43 to 1.62)	-
>100	3.18 (1.31 to 7.70)*	1.89 (0.76 to 4.68)	-
Each 30 g increase	1.56 (1.33 to 1.84)**	1.22 (1.00 to 1.48)	-
Xi-Xin (g) total amount prescribed			
0	1	1	-
1–30	2.02 (1.55 to 2.63)**	1.27 (0.91 to 1.78)	-
31–60	2.40 (1.44 to 3.99)**	1.50 (0.84 to 2.70)	-
61–100	2.90 (1.62 to 5.20)**	1.34 (0.69 to 2.60)	-
101–200	2.47 (1.26 to 4.83)‡	1.17 (0.53 to 2.59)	-
>200	2.25 (1.15 to 4.21)*	0.78 (0.34 to 1.81)	-
Each 30 g increase	1.28 (1.18 to 1.39)**	1.02 (0.89 to 1.16)	-
Aristolochic acid (mg) estimated total consumption			
0	1	-	1

Table 2. Cont.

		Model 1	Model 2
Risk Factors	**Crude HR (95% CI)**	**Adjusted HR (95% CI)†**	**Adjusted HR (95% CI)†**
1–100	1.21 (0.83 to 1.78)	-	2.05 (1.61 to 2.60)**
101–200	2.16 (0.80 to 5.80)	-	2.84 (1.66 to 4.86)**
201–300	4.80 (1.79 to 12.91)‡	-	2.42 (0.89 to 6.55)
>300	6.29 (3.23 to 12.26)**	-	5.18 (2.86 to 9.40)**
Each 100 mg increase	1.56 (1.40 to 1.74)**	-	1.57 (1.40 to 1.75)**

†Logistic regression models for different dosages of Chinese herbs (model 1) and different estimated dosages of aristolochic acid as risk factors (model 2) were adjusted for age, sex, residence in township with endemic black foot disease, and history of chronic UTI.
*$P<0.05$.
‡$P<0.01$.
**$P<0.001$.

sold in Taiwan's markets. It is thus unlikely that the subjects purchased AA-containing herbs or nephrotoxic drugs without a prescription. Third, we also could not validate the actual intake of prescribed herbal product by the patients. Because 95% of the dosing frequenciesfor Chinese herbal products last for only one week [44], a large cumulative dose indicates that patients on long-term prescriptions actually consumed the prescribed medication. However, if the patients did not take all of the prescribed medication, our findings would underestimate the effects of AA-related Chinese herbal consumption. Fourth, because the NHI data did not include smoking history, we could not control for this variable in our models. However, because smoking rates in Taiwan in the last two decades have ranged from 47% to 62% and from 2.3% to 5.3%, for males and females, respectively, male patients with ESRD would be expected to have a higher risk of developing UTC if smoking were a major contributing risk factor [45]. As we did not find any increased risk of UTC in males compared to females, our results do not seem to be confounded by smoking.

Conclusions

This study finds that AA from Chinese herbal products and analgesics is associated with increased risk of developing UTC in ESRD patients, due to these having been prescribed low doses of Mu-Tong. The linear dose-response relationships found in this work may be useful in consideration of a total ban or establishment of limits on the consumption of such herbal products among patients with ESRD and/or chronic kidney disease. More studies are needed to examine the potential carcinogenic effects of analgesics on patients with ESRD and/or chronic renal failure. In addition, regular follow-up screening for UC in ESRD patients who have consumed AA-related Chinese herbal products is also necessary.

Supporting Information

File S1 The commercial names of 45 kinds of non-steroidal anti-inflammatory drugs in the reimbursement database.
(DOCX)

Author Contributions

Conceived and designed the experiments: SMW JD. Performed the experiments: JDW PC. Analyzed the data: SMW. Contributed reagents/materials/analysis tools: PCC. Wrote the paper: SMW. Contributed to the idea and design in this work: MNL AW YYC YSP.

References

1. Vanherweghem JL, Depierreux M, Tielemans C, Abramowicz D, Dratwa M, et al. (1993) Rapidly progressive interstitial renal fibrosis in young women: association with slimming regimen including Chinese herbs. Lancet 341: 387–391.
2. Vanhaelen M, Vanhaelen-Fastre R, But P, Vanherweghem JL (1994) Identification of aristolochic acid in Chinese herbs. Lancet 343: 174.
3. Cosyns JP (2003) Aristolochic acid and 'Chinese herbs nephropathy': a review of the evidence to date. Drug safety : an international journal of medical toxicology and drug experience 26: 33–48.
4. Nortier JL, Martinez MC, Schmeiser HH, Arlt VM, Bieler CA, et al. (2000) Urothelial carcinoma associated with the use of a Chinese herb (Aristolochia fangchi). N Engl J Med 342: 1686–1692.
5. Cosyns JP, Jadoul M, Squifflet JP, Wese FX, van Ypersele de Strihou C (1999) Urothelial lesions in Chinese-herb nephropathy. American journal of kidney diseases : the official journal of the National Kidney Foundation 33: 1011–1017.
6. Arlt VM, Stiborova M, Schmeiser HH (2002) Aristolochic acid as a probable human cancer hazard in herbal remedies: a review. Mutagenesis 17: 265–277.
7. Lai MN, Wang SM, Chen PC, Chen YY, Wang JD (2010) Population-based case-control study of Chinese herbal products containing aristolochic acid and urinary tract cancer risk. J Natl Cancer Inst 102: 179–186.
8. Lai MN, Wang SM, Chen PC, Chen YY, Wang JD (2009) Population-based case-control study of Chinese herbal products containing aristolochic acid and urinary tract cancer risk. J Natl Cancer Inst 102: 179–186.
9. Matas AJ, Simmons RL, Kjellstrand CM, Buselmeier TJ, Najarian JS (1975) Increased incidence of malignancy during chronic renal failure. Lancet 1: 883–886.
10. Port FK, Ragheb NE, Schwartz AG, Hawthorne VM (1989) Neoplasms in dialysis patients: a population-based study. American journal of kidney diseases : the official journal of the National Kidney Foundation 14: 119–123.
11. Kjellstrand CM (1979) Are malignancies increased in uremia? Nephron 23: 159–161.
12. Maisonneuve P, Agodoa L, Gellert R, Stewart JH, Buccianti G, et al. (1999) Cancer in patients on dialysis for end-stage renal disease: an international collaborative study. Lancet 354: 93–99.
13. Chuang CH, Lee CT, Tsai TL, Chen JB, Hsu KT, et al. (2002) Urological malignancy in chronic dialysis patients. Acta Nephrologica 16: 19–24.
14. Chang CH, Yang CM, Yang AH (2007) Renal diagnosis of chronic hemodialysis patients with urinary tract transitional cell carcinoma in Taiwan. Cancer 109: 1487–1492.
15. Ou JH, Pan CC, Lin JS, Tzai TS, Yang WH, et al. (2000) Transitional cell carcinoma in dialysis patients. European urology 37: 90–94.
16. Chen KS, Lai MK, Huang CC, Chu SH, Leu ML (1995) Urologic cancers in uremic patients. American journal of kidney diseases : the official journal of the National Kidney Foundation 25: 694–700.
17. Gonwa TA, Corbett WT, Schey HM, Buckalew VM, Jr. (1980) Analgesic-associated nephropathy and transitional cell carcinoma of the urinary tract. Annals of internal medicine 93: 249–252.

18. Swindle P, Falk M, Rigby R, Petrie J, Hawley C, et al. (1998) Transitional cell carcinoma in renal transplant recipients: the influence of compound analgesics. British journal of urology 81: 229–233.
19. Kliem V, Thon W, Krautzig S, Kolditz M, Behrend M, et al. (1996) High mortality from urothelial carcinoma despite regular tumor screening in patients with analgesic nephropathy after renal transplantation. Transplant international : official journal of the European Society for Organ Transplantation 9: 231–235.
20. Vanherweghem LJ (1998) Misuse of herbal remedies: the case of an outbreak of terminal renal failure in Belgium (Chinese herbs nephropathy). Journal of alternative and complementary medicine 4: 9–13.
21. Chiang HS, Guo HR, Hong CL, Lin SM, Lee EF (1993) The incidence of bladder cancer in the black foot disease endemic area in Taiwan. British journal of urology 71: 274–278.
22. Chiou HY, Chiou ST, Hsu YH, Chou YL, Tseng CH, et al. (2001) Incidence of transitional cell carcinoma and arsenic in drinking water: a follow-up study of 8,102 residents in an arseniasis-endemic area in northeastern Taiwan. American journal of epidemiology 153: 411–418.
23. Wiessler M (1994) DNA adducts of pyrrolizidine alkaloids, nitroimidazoles and aristolochic acid. IARC Sci Publ: 165–177.
24. TaiwanYearbook2009 Public Health: Health Insurance.
25. NHRI-Taiwan (2003) National Health Research Database.
26. Centers_for_Disease_Control_and_Prevention (2009) International Classification of Diseases, Ninth Revision (ICD-9). Atlanta, Georgia.
27. Perneger TV, Whelton PK, Klag MJ (1994) Risk of kidney failure associated with the use of acetaminophen, aspirin, and nonsteroidal antiinflammatory drugs. N Engl J Med 331: 1675–1679.
28. Gago-Dominguez M, Yuan JM, Castelao JE, Ross RK, Yu MC (1999) Regular use of analgesics is a risk factor for renal cell carcinoma. Br J Cancer 81: 542–548.
29. Committee Chinese Medicine and Pharmacy DOH-T (2002) Unified Formulas.
30. Hsu Y, Tseng H, Wen K (1997) Determination of aristolochic acid in Fangchi radix. Ann Rept NLFD Taiwan ROC: 136–142 (In Chinese).
31. Tung C, Ho Y, Tsai H, Chong Y (1999) Studies on the commonly musused and adulterated Chinese crude drug species in Taiwan. Chin Med Coll J: 35–46.
32. Deng J (2002) Quality evaluation of Fang-Ji and analysis of marker constituents [dissertation]. Taiwan: Institute of Chiense Pharmaceutical Sciences, China Medical University: 75–77.
33. Chuang M, Hsu Y, Chang H, Lin J, Liao C (2002) Studies on adulteration and misusage of marketed Akebiae caulisn. Ann Rept NLFD Taiwan ROC: 104–119 (In Chinese).
34. Jong TT, Lee MR, Hsiao SS, Hsai JL, Wu TS, et al. (2003) Analysis of aristolochic acid in nine sources of Xixin, a traditional Chinese medicine, by liquid chromatography/atmospheric pressure chemical ionization/tandem mass spectrometry. J Pharm Biomed Anal 33: 831–837.
35. Hsu Y, Lo C, Chang H, Lin J (2003) Studies on adulteration and misusage of Asari radi in the market. Ann Rept NLFD Taiwan ROC: 153–167 (In Chinese).
36. Chen CJ, Chuang YC, Lin TM, Wu HY (1985) Malignant neoplasms among residents of a blackfoot disease-endemic area in Taiwan: high-arsenic artesian well water and cancers. Cancer research 45: 5895–5899.
37. Chen CJ, Chuang YC, You SL, Lin TM, Wu HY (1986) A retrospective study on malignant neoplasms of bladder, lung and liver in blackfoot disease endemic area in Taiwan. British journal of cancer 53: 399–405.
38. Johansson SL, Cohen SM (1997) Epidemiology and etiology of bladder cancer. Seminars in surgical oncology 13: 291–298.
39. Groah SL, Weitzenkamp DA, Lammertse DP, Whiteneck GG, Lezotte DC, et al. (2002) Excess risk of bladder cancer in spinal cord injury: Evidence for an association between indwelling catheter use and bladder cancer. Archives of Physical Medicine and Rehabilitation 83: 346–351.
40. Jiang X, Castelao JE, Groshen S, Cortessis VK, Shibata D, et al. (2009) Urinary tract infections and reduced risk of bladder cancer in Los Angeles. British journal of cancer 100: 834–839.
41. (2008) Cancer Incidence Rate in Taiwan, 1998–2002 & 2003–2007 http://tcr.cph.ntu.edu.tw/main.php?Page = N2: Taiwan cancer registry.
42. Achenbach H, Fischer A (1997) 6-O-beta-D-glucoside of aristolochic acid IIIa and other components from the roots of Aristolochia baetica. Planta Med 63: 579.
43. TaiwanCancerRegistry (2009) Cancer incidence rate in Taiwan, 1998–2002.
44. Hsieh SC, Lai JN, Lee CF, Hu FC, Tseng WL, et al. (2008) The prescribing of Chinese herbal products in Taiwan: a cross-sectional analysis of the national health insurance reimbursement database. Pharmacoepidemiology and drug safety 17: 609–619.
45. (2013) Adult Smoking Behavior Surveillance System,ASBS. Taipei, Taiwan.

10

Habituation to Experimentally Induced Electrical Pain during Voluntary-Breathing Controlled Electrical Stimulation (BreEStim)

Shengai Li[1,2], Tracy Hu[1,2], Maria A. Beran[1,2], Sheng Li[1,2]*

1 Department of Physical Medicine and Rehabilitation, University of Texas Health Science Center at Houston, Houston, Texas, United States of America, 2 Neurorehabilitation Research Laboratory TIRR Memorial Hermann Research Center, Houston, Texas, United States of America

Abstract

Objective: Painful peripheral electrical stimulation to acupuncture points was found to cause sensitization if delivered randomly (EStim), but induced habituation if triggered by voluntary breathing (BreEStim). The objective was to systematically compare the effectiveness of BreEStim and EStim and to investigate the possible mechanisms mediating the habituation effect of BreEStim.

Methods: Eleven pain-free, healthy subjects (6 males, 5 females) participated in the study. Each subject received the BreEStim and EStim treatments in a random order at least three days apart. Both treatments consisted of 120 painful but tolerable stimuli to the ulnar nerve at the elbow on the dominant arm. BreEStim was triggered by voluntary breathing while EStim was delivered randomly. Electrical sensation threshold (EST) and electrical pain threshold (EPT) were measured from the thenar and hypothenar eminences on both hands at pre-intervention and 10-minutes post-intervention.

Results: There was no difference in the pre-intervention baseline measurement of EST and EPT between BreEStim and EStim. BreEStim increased EPT in all tested sites on both hands, while EStim increased EPT in the dominant hypothenar eminence distal to the stimulating site and had no effect on EPT in other sites. There was no difference in the intensity of electrical stimulation between EStim and BreEStim.

Conclusion: Our findings support the important role human voluntary breathing plays in the systemic habituation effect of BreEStim to peripheral painful electrical stimulation.

Editor: Mikhail A. Lebedev, Duke University, United States of America

Funding: This study was supported in part by an NIH grant (NIH/NINDS R01NS060774) and a research grant (013-109) from Mission Connect, a program of TIRR Foundation. The funders had no role in study design, data collection and analysis, decision to publish, or preparation of the manuscript.

Competing Interests: Sheng Li holds U.S. Patent No. 8,229,566 "Method and Apparatus of Breathing-Controlled Electrical Stimulation for Skeletal Muscles", issued on 7/24/2012 and U.S. Patent No. 8,588,919 "Method and Apparatus of Breathing-Controlled Electrical Stimulation for Skeletal Muscles" Divisional of Application No. 12/146,176 (issued as U.S. Patent 8,229,566). This does not alter the authors' adherence to PLOS ONE policies on sharing data and materials.

* Email: sheng.li@uth.tmc.edu

Introduction

Pain is multi-dimensional and includes distinct sensory and affective (i.e., unpleasantness) components [1]. Memory mechanisms play a significant role in the persistent awareness of chronic neuropathic pain as well as in the reinforcement of the associated distress. Neuropathic pain is very common, difficult to manage, and has increasingly been recognized as a major contributor to suffering, poor rehabilitation outcomes and reduced quality of life of the persons who are suffering from chronic neuropathic pain [2–4]. Various neurostimulation techniques [5], such as transcutaneous electrical nerve stimulation (TENS) [6], electroacupuncture [7], spinal cord stimulation [8], deep brain stimulation [9], and transcranial direct current stimulation [10–13] have been used for management of neuropathic pain.

We recently proposed an innovative treatment – breathing-controlled electrical stimulation (BreEStim) for neuropathic pain management [14,15]. This technique was developed from our discovery of the systemic effect of human voluntary breathing on motor function and pain perception [14–20]. In the BreEStim treatment (see details in [14]), human voluntary breathing signal triggers an external electrical stimulator. A single-pulse electrical stimulation is then delivered to peripheral acupuncture points. After receiving a week of daily BreEStim treatment to the acupuncture points on the ipsilateral forearm, a patient with constant shooting phantom pain secondary to an above-the-knee amputation reported no more shooting phantom pain, although he was still able to feel the occasional non-painful shooting sensation in the phantom limb [15]. A similar analgesic effect was also reported in a patient with spinal cord injury [14]. To account for this analgesic effect, we hypothesized that BreEStim integrates multiple internal pain coping mechanisms during voluntary breathing [15], such as electroacupuncture effect, habituation to aversive stimuli, analgesia effect from voluntary breathing, anterograde amnesia of aversive stimuli and activation of the reward system. As a result, the BreEStim treatment has a measurable clinical analgesic effect by increasing pain tolerance, i.e., increased pain threshold.

In a recent study [21], we compared the effects of BreEStim and EStim on sensory thresholds in healthy subjects. Electrical pain threshold (EPT) increased after BreEStim, but decreased after EStim. Neither intervention affected other sensory thresholds (mechanical sensation threshold, thermal thresholds). In this study [21], the same protocol (100 painful electrical stimuli at similar intensities delivered to acupuncture points, Neiguan and Weiguan, on the forearm) led to the opposite findings of habituation after BreEStim and sensitization after EStim. This protocol, however, had - a few confounding factors. The location of the acupuncture point (Neiguan) is very close to the path of the median nerve. Thus, electrical stimulation to the acupuncture points would stimulate the median nerve as well. Both repeated aversive electrical stimulation and electro-acupuncture are reported to have analgesic effects [7,22,23], but the sensitization effect was only observed after EStim. Following unilateral electrical median nerve stimulation, there was bilateral activation of primary somatosensory cortex [22] and increased pain threshold of the contralateral index finger [23]. In contrast, the sensitization effect was seen in both stimulated and contralateral symmetrical area after EStim in the previous study [21]. In the present study, we aimed to compare BreEStim and EStim by examining these factors (nerve stimulation vs. acupuncture, unilateral vs. contralateral or systemic effects).

Methods

Subjects

Eleven young and healthy subjects (6 male, 5 female, averaged 29.7 years of age, ranging from 25–44) volunteered in this experiment. According to daily use in writing and eating, one subject was left-handed, and the rest were right-headed. All subjects had no known history of neuromuscular diseases and were pain free. All subjects gave written informed consent prior to participation. This study was approved by the Committee for the Protection of Human Subjects at the University of Texas Health Science Center at Houston and TIRR Memorial Hermann Hospital.

Experimental procedures and BreEStim/EStim interventions

In the present study, we adopted our recently published protocol [21]. Each subject received two intervention sessions – EStim and BreEStim. Each intervention was given at least 3 days apart and the order of the sessions was randomized and balanced across subjects to minimize the order effect. Each intervention session consisted of 120 stimuli and took about 30–40 min. Details of each intervention are available on the open access methodology video article at: http://www.jove.com/video/50077/.

During each intervention session, subjects were seated comfortably with both arms and hands on the experiment table in approximately symmetrical positions with the elbow joint of the dominant arm flexed at about 90 degrees (Figure 1). A pair of surface electrodes was placed on the medial aspect on the elbow joint. One electrode was at the joint line level and the other was approximately 3 cm above proximally along the path of ulnar nerve. Surface electrodes were trimmed to a size of one inch by one inch prior to placement.

Delivery of electrical stimulation was the key difference between EStim and BreEStim. During EStim, single-pulse electrical stimuli were randomly delivered every 4 to 8 seconds using a computer program. During BreEStim, subjects wore a face mask connected indirectly to the experimental computer via a pneumotach system (Hans Rodulph Inc). A single-pulse electrical stimulus was triggered if a preset threshold was met by voluntary inhalation signals, usually every 4 to 8 seconds. During voluntary inhalation, subjects were instructed to take a deep breath, similar to routine deep breaths, but faster and stronger. To ensure this, subjects were explicitly instructed to expand their chest walls during voluntary, effortful inhalation. Experimentally, the airflow rate was monitored on the computer. When the airflow rate reached 40% of its peak, an electrical pulse was triggered. When wearing a face mask, subjects usually tolerated such breathing well. As in our previous studies [14,15,18], no hyperventilation was reported. For both EStim and BreEStim, rest was allowed upon request. Length of rest and number of rest breaks were also upon request.

The intensity of the electrical stimulation started from the pain threshold and increased to the highest level as tolerated. At that level, subjects may find the electrical stimulation annoying, noxious or painful, but still tolerable even if received repetitively. The experimenter(s) verbally encouraged subjects to increase the level of electrical stimulation gradually as tolerated and pointed out that aversion to electrical stimulation was part of the intervention. Subjects were advised that the expected pain level was equivalent to 6~7 on the 0–10 VAS scale. However, it is important to point out that the intensity of electrical stimulation was adjusted by the subjects themselves according to their subjective feeling of aversiveness. The intensity of electrical stimulation was recorded at the 20th, 40th, 60th, 80th, 100th and 120th trial of each intervention.

Electrical sensation and pain thresholds

Electrical sensation (EST) and pain (EPT) thresholds were the primary quantitative sensory testing measures. To standardize the tests, EST and EPT testing was performed before and 10 minutes after each intervention (EStim and BreEStim) as in our recent publication [21]. Both EST and EPT were assessed on the thenar and hypothenar eminences of both dominant (treatment) and non-dominant (non-treatment) hands to compare the outcomes of the interventions. The order of EST and EPT assessments on the sites (hypothenar and thenar eminences) was randomized and balanced between two hands.

The same trimmed electrodes were used to assess EST and EPT using the same stimulator (electrical stimulator 7SA, Digitimer). A pair of electrodes was spaced next to each other centered on the thenar or hypothenar eminence. The border of each electrode was marked to ensure consistent placement before and after the intervention. For EST, subjects were instructed to close their eyes and to say "yes" when they explicitly felt electrical stimulation. The intensity of electrical stimulation started from zero and gradually increased in increments of 0.1 mA. For EPT, the intensity of electrical stimulation started from the sensation threshold level and increased in increments of 1 mA. The level of electrical stimulation was recorded as EPT when subjects first reported the electrical stimulation as painful. To improve consistency among subjects, they were advised that the pain threshold level was equivalent to 1 on the 0–10 VAS scale. For both EST and EPT assessments, thresholds from three trials were recorded and averaged.

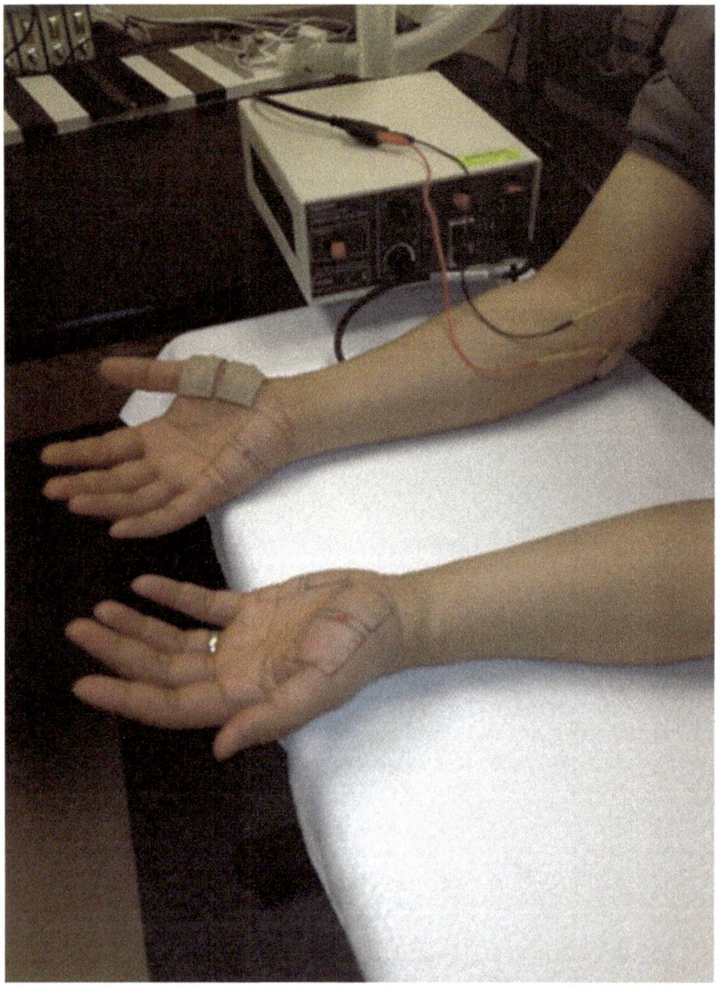

Figure 1. Experimental Set-up.

Data analysis and statistical analysis

EST and EPT were measured at the thenar and hypothenar eminences on both treated (dominant) and non-treated (non-dominant) hands before and after each intervention. Paired t-tests were used to compare the baseline thresholds prior to BreEStim and EStim treatment on different days. The thresholds were similar across each hand and data were collapsed for the baseline analysis. The pre-treatment baseline value was obtained by averaging across testing sites (thenar and hypothenar) and hands (dominant and non-dominant) for EST and EPT. To assess the effect of each intervention, a repeated measures three-way ANOVA with factors of TREATMENT (2 levels, pre- and post-intervention) and HAND (2 levels, dominant and non-dominant) and SITE (2 levels, thenar and hypothenar) was performed. The effect of each intervention was first calculated using the following equation: percent change = (post-intervention – pre-invention)/ pre-interventionx100%. To further compare the effects of intervention on EST and EPT between BreEStim and EStim, a repeated-measures three-way ANOVA with factors of INTERVENTION (2 levels, BreEStim and EStim), SITE and HAND was performed. A repeated measures two-way ANOVA was performed with factors INTERVENTION and TRIAL (7 levels, 0, 20, 40, 60, 80, 100, 120) to compare possible differences in the intensity between the two interventions. Post hoc Tukey's HSD tests were performed when there was a significant effect in ANOVA tests. The alpha level required for all statistical significance was set at .05. Data were reported as means in the text and as means ± standard errors in the figures and in the table.

Results

The pre-intervention baseline EST and EPT values were averaged across sites and hands to compare baseline assessment on different days. EST and EPT are summarized in Table 1. There were no statistically significant differences in these pre-intervention thresholds on different days (paired t-tests, p value: 0.66 for EST and 0.98 for EPT).

BreEStim systematically increased EPT across sites and hands (Fig 2, upper panel), without changing EST. For EPT, a repeated measures 3-way ANOVA showed main effects of TREATMENT ($F_{[1,\ 10]} = 10.18$, $p = .009$) and SITE ($F_{[1,\ 10]} = 6.98$, $p = .025$). No main effects of HAND or significant interactions were found. EPT averaged across sites and hands significantly increased after BreEStim (Pre vs. Post: 25.7 mA vs. 29.2 mA). EPT was significantly greater in the hypothenar eminence (29.4 mA) than in the thenar eminence (25.5 mA) both before and after BreEStim. A similar ANOVA for EST only showed a main effect of SITE ($F_{[1,\ 10]} = 11.55$, $p = .007$). EST was 4.17 mA in the thenar

Table 1. Electrical sensation threshold and electrical pain threshold from the thenar and hypothenar eminences of the treatment (dominant) and non-treatment (non-dominant) hands before and after BreEStim and EStim.

	Electrical sensation threshold (EST)				Electrical pain threshold (EPT)			
	Treatment		Non-treatment		Treatment		Non-treatment	
	Thenar	Hypothenar	Thenar	Hypothenar	Thenar	Hypothenar	Thenar	Hypothenar
Pre-BreEStim(mean)	4.12	5.25	4.22	5.20	24.28	27.21	23.99	27.46
Pre-BreEStim(SE)	*0.3*	*0.6*	*0.3*	*0.5*	*2.7*	*2.8*	*2.3*	*2.8*
Post-BreEStim(mean)	4.25	5.40	4.09	5.14	**26.72**	**31.70**	**27.20**	**31.30**
Post-BreEStim(SE)	*0.3*	*0.6*	*0.3*	*0.4*	*2.5*	*3.1*	*2.6*	*3.1*
Pre-EStim(mean)	4.00	5.32	4.24	5.24	24.16	25.35	23.90	27.43
Pre-EStim(SE)	*0.1*	*0.4*	*0.2*	*0.4*	*2.3*	*2.4*	*2.1*	*2.3*
Post-EStim(mean)	3.83	5.40	4.25	4.98	23.65	**28.37**	23.32	26.39
Post-EStim(SE)	0.2	0.5	0.3	0.4	2.9	3.2	2.1	2.9

Bold numbers indicate significant difference from pre-treatment measurements.

eminence and 5.25 mA in the hypothenar eminence. No main effects of TREATMENT and HAND, or significant interactions were found.

EStim treatment showed a different effect on EPT, (Figure 2). A 3-way ANOVA did not show main effects of TREATMENT and HAND. But there was a main effect of SITE ($F_{[1,\ 10]} = 6.18$, $p = .032$), significant interactions of TREATMENT x HAND ($F_{[1,\ 10]} = 6.42$, $p = .030$) and TREATMENTxHANDxSITE ($F_{[1,\ 10]} = 8.94$, $p = .014$). Post-hoc Tukey HSD tests revealed that EStim significantly increased EPT on the dominant hypothenar eminence distal to the stimulating site (Pre vs. Post: 25.35 mA vs. 28.37 mA in the dominant hypothenar eminence). EStim did not affect EPT on the contralateral site (Pre vs. Post: 27.43 mA vs. 26.39 mA on the thenar eminence of the non-dominant hand) (see Table 1 for details). Like BreEStim, EStim did not significantly affect EST. A similar 3-way ANOVA only revealed a main effect of SITE ($F_{[1,\ 10]} = 12.27$, $p = .006$) (thenar vs. hypothenar: 4.08 mA vs. 5.23 mA). No other main effects or significant interactions were found.

Differences in these pre- and post-intervention thresholds reflected the effect of intervention, since the pre-intervention baseline EST and EPT values on different days were not significantly different. EPT change after BreEStim (15.1%) was significantly different from EPT change after EStim (−1.2%) (Figure 3). A 3-way ANOVA showed a main effect of INTERVENTION ($F_{[1,\ 10]} = 9.11$, $p = .013$). No other main effects or significant interactions were found.

The intensity of electrical stimulation increased progressively during both EStim and BreEStim (Figure 4). According to an INTERVENTION×TRIAL two-way ANOVA, there was a main effect of TRIAL ($F_{[6,\ 60]} = 48.28$, $p < .00001$), indicating progressive increase in the intensity during the course of treatment. Tukey HSD Post-hoc tests revealed that the intensity increased significantly at the end of 20 trials and 40 trials compared to the starting intensity at the pain threshold ($p < 0.001$). There was no statistical significance in the intensity after 40 trials. However, there was no difference in the intensity between two interventions. The ANOVA showed no main effect of INTERVENTION or significant interaction.

Discussion

In the present study, pain-free healthy subjects received the same amount of painful, yet tolerable electrical stimuli (120 stimuli) to the ulnar nerve at the elbow level on the dominant side during EStim and BreEStim interventions at least three days apart. Electrical sensation threshold (EST) and electrical pain threshold (EPT) were measured from both thenar and hypothenar eminences of both hands to compare topographic vs. central effects. The main findings were increased EPT in all sites after BreEStim, i.e., habituation, but no effect on EPT after EStim except for the hypothenar eminence on the stimulated side. There was no significant difference in the intensity of electrical stimulation between EStim and BreEStim. Both interventions had no effect on EST.

Overall, the present findings are consistent with the previous study [21]: BreEStim has systemic analgesic effects to painful stimulation after the intervention, i.e., habituation, while there is no such effect after EStim. In the previous study, painful electrical stimuli were delivered to acupuncture points (Neiguan and Weiguan) of the dominant forearm where the acupuncture point – Neiguan is very close to the path of the median nerve Painful electrical stimuli that was delivered to the ulnar nerve at the elbow level (far from the acupuncture points) resulted in the same pattern

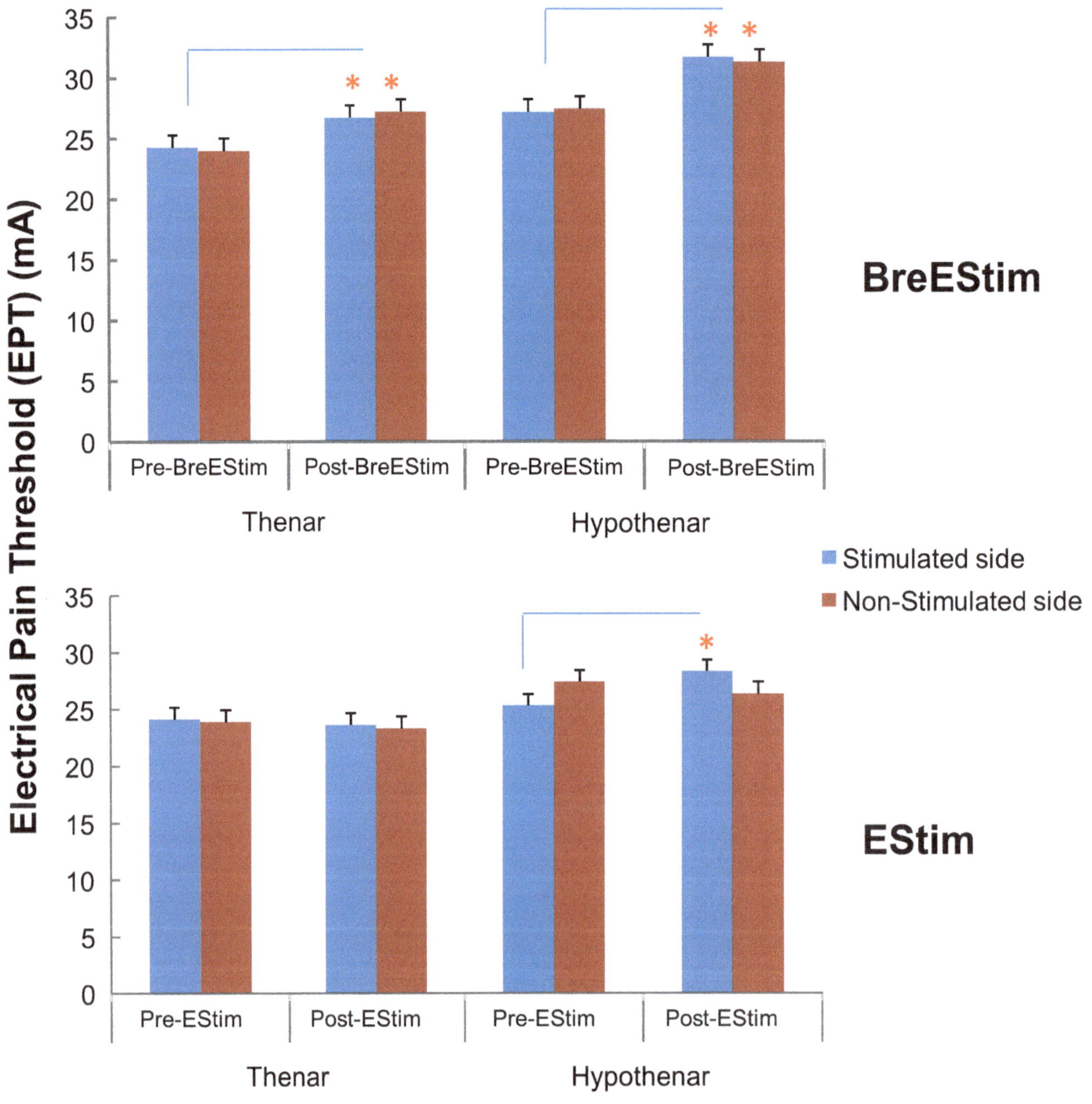

Figure 2. Electrical pain thresholds pre- and post-BreEStim (upper panel) and pre- and post-EStim (lower panel) in all four tested sites on both stimulated and non-stimulated side. Average values and standard errors are shown.

of analgesic effect across subjects. Variations in individual responses could account for the degrees of difference between two studies. Increase in EPT was about 27% after BreEStim in the previous study. It was 15% in this study. If acupuncture-induced analgesia contributed to the difference, we would have seen further decrease in EPT after EStim in this study as compared to 10% decrease in EPT in the previous study. However, there was no change in EPT in the contralateral non-stimulated hand after EStim.

Central sensitization after short-term painful electrical stimulation

Central sensitization after a brief course of painful stimulation is a common phenomenon [24–26]. In a recent study [24], about 105 stimuli at the intensity of 5 on the visual analogue scale ("10" – worst pain, "0" – no pain) applied to the volar area of the middle forearm caused increased activation in the classic pain processing areas, including the anterior cingulate cortex (ACC), insular cortex, as compared to the rest state. The ACC and the insula have been reported to selectively process the aversive quality of noxious stimulation [27,28]. Using advanced fMRI (7 T), Hahn et al. [25] was able to demonstrate additional activation of periaqueductal gray (PAG) which was often not observed using

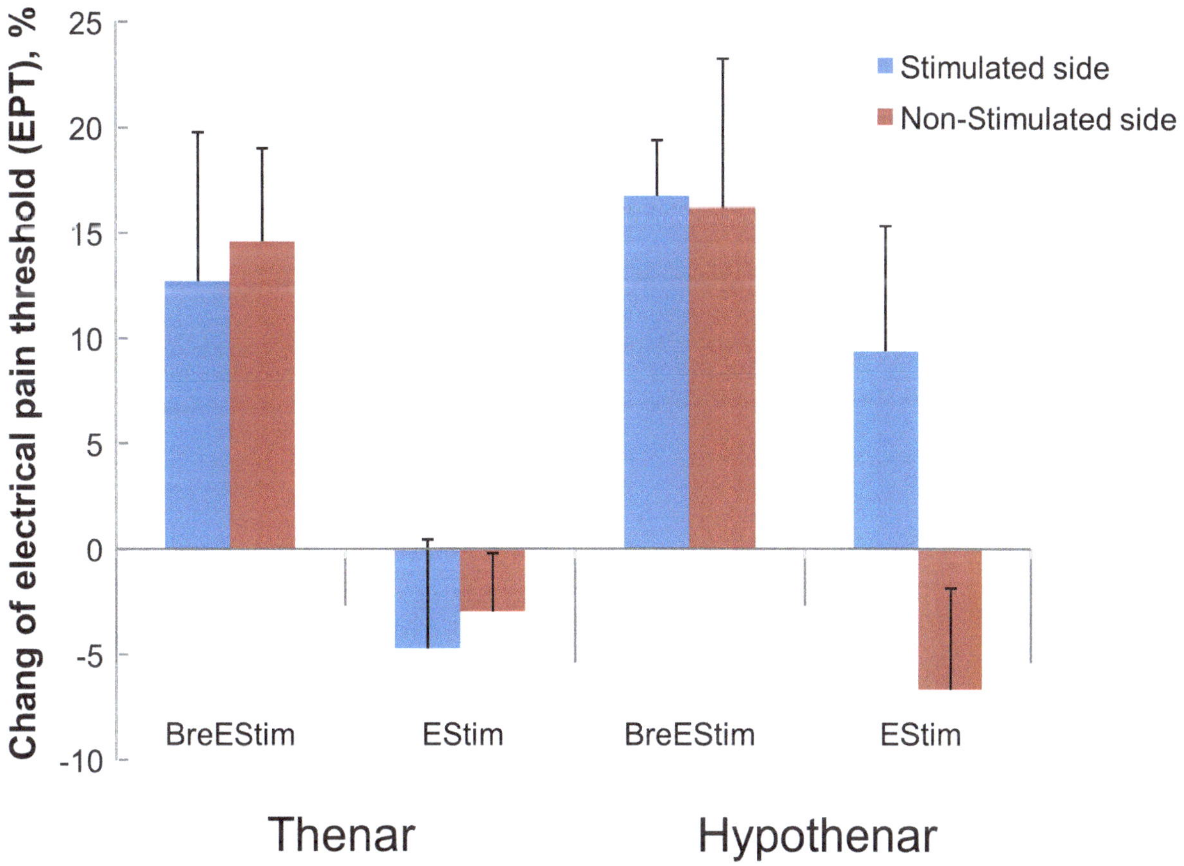

Figure 3. Change of electrical pain threshold as percentage of pre-intervention values after BreEStim and EStim. Average values and standard errors are presented.

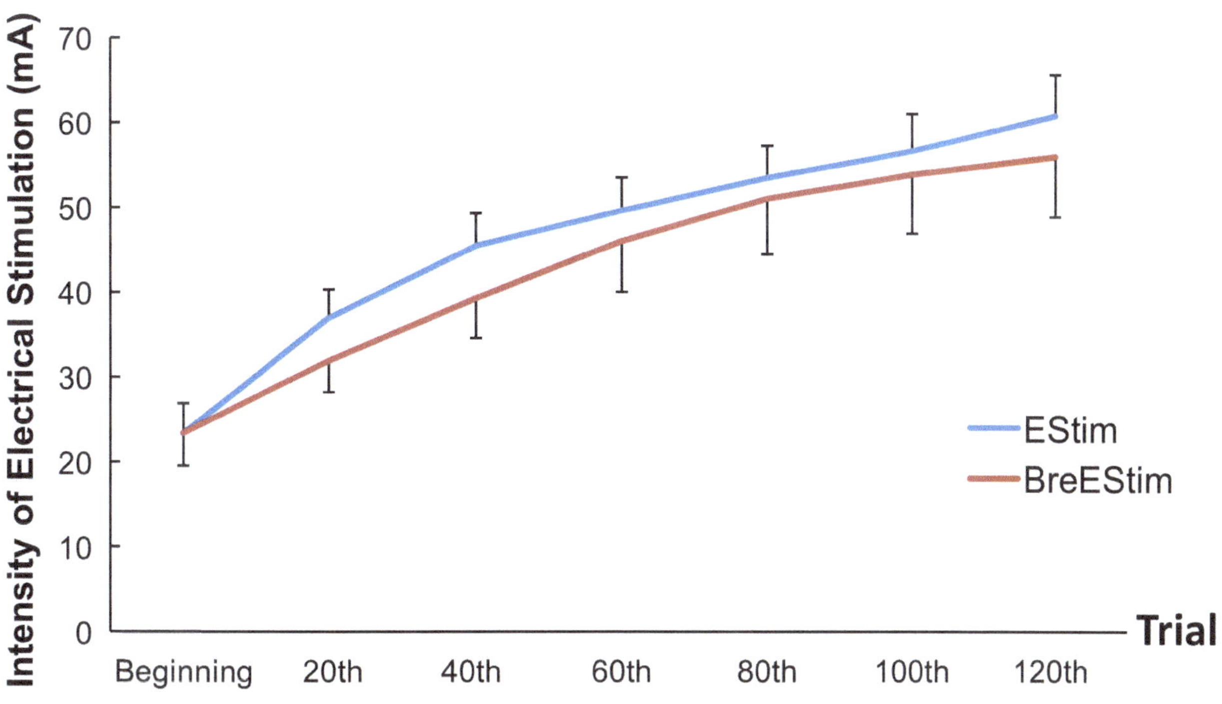

Figure 4. The intensity of electrical stimulation from beginning (trial 0) to the end (trial 120) during BreEStim and EStim. Average values and standard errors are presented.

3T fMRI techniques. PAG is known as a pivot region of the descending pain control system [29–31]. These studies suggest that painful peripheral electrical stimulation triggers central responses to aversiveness of painful stimuli and internal descending pain coping mechanisms at the same time, i.e., central sensitization.

Our previous findings are consistent with this central sensitization effect of painful EStim [21]. We observed decreased EPT in the thenar eminence in both hands after 100 painful electrical stimuli to the forearm (Neiguan and Weiguan) on the dominant side. However, in the current study we observed increased EPT in the hypothenar eminence distal to the ulnar nerve on the dominant side, but no change in EPT in the thenar eminence of the dominant hand and in both thenar and hypothenar eminences of the non-dominant hand. No change in EPT in the areas that are not innervated by the ulnar nerve may be attributed to the possible habituation effect, since we used the same protocol but a higher number of painful electrical stimuli (120 electrical stimuli) in the present study. However, the result of increased EPT only in the hypothenar eminence distal to the ulnar nerve at the stimulating site may be caused by a different factor. Direct nerve stimulation to the ulnar nerve at the elbow may interfere with orthodromic impulse propagation of electrical stimulation from the distal hypothenar area — the "busy line" effect [32]. Further study is needed to investigate this dose effect and its relation to central sensitization.

The habituation effect of BreEStim

The habituation effect of BreEStim in the present study was consistent with our previous study in which electrical stimulation was delivered to acupuncture points [21]. There was no difference in the intensity of electrical stimulation between EStim and BreEStim in the present and previous [21] studies. Therefore, the habituation effect of BreEStim is likely attributable to the effect associated with voluntary breathing. Distinctly different from autonomic breathing, voluntary breathing requires extensive cortical and subcortical activation and suppression of brainstem respiratory center for autonomic breathing [33,34]. According to brain imaging studies, these respiratory-related areas include the primary motor cortex, the premotor cortex, the supplementary motor area, the primary and secondary somatosensory cortices, the insula, the ACC and amygdala, and the dorsolateral prefrontal cortex [35–46].

The habituation effect of BreEStim may be explained by multiple internal pain coping mechanisms. Firstly, voluntary breathing-specific cortical activation is likely to make painful stimulation less unpleasant. There are respiratory specific connections between the insula and the ACC and the activity of pulmonary stretch receptors [47,48]. Secondary to activation of pulmonary stretch receptors from chest wall expansion during voluntary inhalation, the ACC and the insula are thus specifically activated during voluntary inhalation. The ACC and the insula have been reported to selectively process the aversive quality of noxious stimulation [27,28], but does not influence sensation of the stimulation [49]. The breathing-associated activation in the ACC and the insula has been related to reduction in pain ratings in certain conditions, such as meditation [50]. Secondly, memory of peripheral electrical stimulation is not consolidated. It has been reported that during activation of the insular cortex by localized micro-stimulation, peripheral aversive stimulation leads to item-specific impairment of aversive memory reconsolidation, i.e., anterograde amnesia [51]. In other words, peripheral painful electrical stimulation is likely to be remembered to a lesser degree during BreEStim. In contrast, memory of aversive electrical stimulation is likely to be consolidated during EStim in which electrical stimulation is delivered during normal breathing. Lastly, the descending pain control mechanism is further enhanced by BreEStim. A recent human study supports the important role of the PAG in regulation of both respiration and pain [27]. Activation of PAG is likely further enhanced during voluntary breathing [52], in addition to painful stimulation-induced reflexive activation to peripheral painful electrical stimulation. Thus, the descending pain control role of PAG is further strengthened. Further neuroimaging studies are needed, however, to substantiate the above mechanisms.

Our findings support the important role voluntary breathing plays in habituation to painful peripheral electrical stimulation during BreEStim. The multi-faceted effects on affective and sensation dimensions of pain could explain the effectiveness of BreEStim on pain reduction in amputation and spinal cord injury patients [14,15]. This is essentially consistent with previous reports of the effect of regulated breathing on reduction in pain perception [50,53,54]. After repetitive exposure to thermal pain pulses, pain intensity and unpleasantness were reduced during slow breathing (half of normal rate) as compared to normal breathing in both healthy subjects and subjects with fibromyalgia syndrome. It is worth mentioning that slow breathing also requires voluntary control of breathing. Future imaging studies may be able to detect different activation patterns between effortful and fast vs. slow voluntary breathing.

Conclusion

In summary, BreEStim increased EPT in all tested sites in both hands, while EStim increased EPT in the hypothenar eminence distal to the stimulating nerve and has no effect on EPT in other sites not innervated by stimulating nerve in pain-free healthy human subjects.

Acknowledgments

This study was supported in part by an NIH grant (NIH/NINDS R01NS060774) and a research grant (013-109) from Mission Connect, a program of TIRR Foundation. The funders had no role in study design, data collection and analysis, decision to publish, or preparation of the manuscript.

Author Contributions

Conceived and designed the experiments: SL TH MB SL. Performed the experiments: SL TH MB SL. Analyzed the data: SL SL. Contributed reagents/materials/analysis tools: SL SL. Contributed to the writing of the manuscript: SL SL. Discussed and interpreted the data: SL TH MB SL.

References

1. Price DD (2000) Psychological and neural mechanisms of the affective dimension of pain. Science 288: 1769–1772.
2. Norrbrink Budh C, Hultling C, Lundeberg T (2005) Quality of sleep in individuals with spinal cord injury: a comparison between patients with and without pain. Spinal Cord 43: 85–95.
3. Stormer S, Gerner HJ, Gruninger W, Metzmacher K, Follinger S, et al. (1997) Chronic pain/dysaesthesiae in spinal cord injury patients: results of a multicentre study. Spinal Cord 35: 446–455.
4. Jensen MP, Chodroff MJ, Dworkin RH (2007) The impact of neuropathic pain on health-related quality of life: review and implications. Neurology 68: 1178–1182.
5. Kotze A, Simpson KH (2008) Stimulation-produced analgesia: acupuncture, TENS and related techniques. Anaesthesia and Intensive Care Medicine 9: 29.
6. Norrbrink Budh C, Lundeberg T (2004) Non-pharmacological pain-relieving therapies in individuals with spinal cord injury: a patient perspective. Complement Ther Med 12: 189–197.

7. Ulett GA, Han S, Han JS (1998) Electroacupuncture: Mechanisms and clinical application. Biol Psychi 44: 129.
8. Finnerup NB, Yezierski RP, Sang CN, Burchiel KJ, Jensen TS (2001) Treatment of spinal cord injury pain. Pain Clin Updates 9: 1–6.
9. Murphy D, Reid DB (2001) Pain treatment satisfaction in spinal cord injury. Spinal Cord 39: 44–46.
10. Fregni F, Boggio PS, Lima MC, Ferreira MJ, Wagner T, et al. (2006) A sham-controlled, phase II trial of transcranial direct current stimulation for the treatment of central pain in traumatic spinal cord injury. Pain 122: 197–209.
11. Boggio PS, Zaghi S, Fregni F (2009) Modulation of emotions associated with images of human pain using anodal transcranial direct current stimulation (tDCS). Neuropsychologia 47: 212–217.
12. Boggio PS, Zaghi S, Lopes M, Fregni F (2008) Modulatory effects of anodal transcranial direct current stimulation on perception and pain thresholds in healthy volunteers. Eur J Neurol 15: 1124–1130.
13. Plow EB, Pascual-Leone A, MacHado A (2012) Brain stimulation in the treatment of chronic neuropathic and non-cancerous pain. J Pain 13: 411–424.
14. Li S (2013) Breathing-controlled Electrical Stimulation (BreEStim) for management of neuropathic pain and spasticity. J Vis Exp: e50077.
15. Li S, Melton DH, Berliner JC (2012) Breathing-controlled electrical stimulation (BreEStim) could modify the affective component of neuropathic pain after amputation: a case report. J Pain Res 5: 71–75.
16. Li S, Laskin JJ (2006) Influences of ventilation on maximal isometric force of the finger flexors. Muscle Nerve 34: 651–655.
17. Li S, Park WH, Borg A (2012) Phase-dependent respiratory-motor interactions in reaction time tasks during rhythmic voluntary breathing. Motor Control 16: 493–505.
18. Li S, Rymer WZ (2011) Voluntary breathing influences corticospinal excitability of nonrespiratory finger muscles. J Neurophysiol 105: 512–521.
19. Li S, Yasuda N (2007) Forced ventilation increases variability of isometric finger forces. Neurosci Lett 412: 243–247.
20. Ikeda ER, Borg A, Brown D, Malouf J, Showers KM, et al. (2009) The valsalva maneuver revisited: the influence of voluntary breathing on isometric muscle strength. J Strength Cond Res 23: 127–132.
21. Li S, Berliner JC, Melton DH, Li S (2013) Modification of electrical pain threshold by voluntary breathing-controlled electrical stimulation (BreEStim) in healthy subjects. PLoS One 8: e70282.
22. Nihashi T, Naganawa S, Sato C, Kawai H, Nakamura T, et al. (2005) Contralateral and ipsilateral responses in primary somatosensory cortex following electrical median nerve stimulation–an fMRI study. Clin Neurophysiol 116: 842.
23. Kastrup A, Baudewig J, Schnaudigel S, Huonker R, Becker L, et al. (2008) Behavioral correlates of negative BOLD signal changes in the primary somatosensory cortex. NeuroImage 41: 1364–1371.
24. Nickel FT, Ott S, Möhringer S, Saake M, Dörfler A, et al. (2014) Brain correlates of short-term habituation to repetitive electrical noxious stimulation. Eur J Pain 18: 56–66.
25. Hahn A, Kranz GS, Seidel EM, Sladky R, Kraus C, et al. (2013) Comparing neural response to painful electrical stimulation with functional MRI at 3 and 7T. NeuroImage 82: 336–343.
26. Seifert F, Bschorer K, De Col R, Filitz J, Peltz E, et al. (2009) Medial prefrontal cortex activity is predictive for hyperalgesia and pharmacological antihyperalgesia. J Neurosci 29: 6167–6175.
27. Von Leupoldt A, Sommer T, Kegat S, Eippert F, Baumann HJ, et al. (2009) Down-regulation of insular cortex responses to dyspnea and pain in asthma. Am J Respir Critl Care Med 180: 232.
28. LaGraize SC, Borzan J, Peng YB, Fuchs PN (2006) Selective regulation of pain affect following activation of the opioid anterior cingulate cortex system. Exp Neurol 197: 22.
29. Freund W, Wunderlich AP, Stuber G, Mayer F, Steffen P, et al. (2011) The role of periaqueductal gray and cingulate cortex during suppression of pain in complex regional pain syndrome. Clin J Pain 27: 796–804.
30. Valet M, Sprenger T, Boecker H, Willoch F, Rummeny E, et al. (2004) Distraction modulates connectivity of the cingulo-frontal cortex and the midbrain during pain–an fMRI analysis. Pain 109: 399–408.
31. Linnman C, Moulton EA, Barmettler G, Becerra L, Borsook D (2012) Neuroimaging of the periaqueductal gray: state of the field. Neuroimage 60: 505–522.
32. Sluka KA, Walsh D (2003) Transcutaneous electrical nerve stimulation: Basic science mechanisms and clinical effectiveness. J Pain 4: 109.
33. Haouzi P, Chenuel B, Barroche G (2006) Interactions between volitional and automatic breathing during respiratory apraxia. Resp Physiol Neurobiol 152: 169–175.
34. Guz A (1997) Brain, breathing and breathlessness. Respir Physiol 109: 197–204.
35. Colebatch JG, Adams L, Murphy K, Martin AJ, Lammertsma AA, et al. (1991) Regional cerebral blood flow during volitional breathing in man. J Physiol 443: 91–103.
36. Maskill D, Murphy K, Mier A, Owen M, Guz A (1991) Motor cortical representation of the diaphragm in man. J Physiol 443: 105–121.
37. Ramsay SC, Adams L, Murphy K, Corfield DR, Grootoonk S, et al. (1993) Regional cerebral blood flow during volitional expiration in man: a comparison with volitional inspiration. J Physiol 461: 85–101.
38. Fink GR, Adams L, Watson JD, Innes JA, Wuyam B, et al. (1995) Hyperpnoea during and immediately after exercise in man: evidence of motor cortical involvement. J Physiol 489 (Pt 3): 663–675.
39. Macey KE, Macey PM, Woo MA, Harper RK, Alger JR, et al. (2004) fMRI signal changes in response to forced expiratory loading in congenital central hypoventilation syndrome. J Appl Physiol 97: 1897–1907.
40. Macey PM, Macey KE, Henderson LA, Alger JR, Frysinger RC, et al. (2003) Functional magnetic resonance imaging responses to expiratory loading in obstructive sleep apnea. Respir Physiol Neurobiol 138: 275–290.
41. Evans KC, Shea SA, Saykin AJ (1999) Functional MRI localisation of central nervous system regions associated with volitional inspiration in humans. J Physiol 520 Pt 2: 383–392.
42. Smejkal V, Druga R, Tintera J (1999) Control of breathing and brain activation in human subjects seen by functional magnetic resonance imaging. Physiol Res 48: 21–25.
43. Smejkal V, Druga R, Tintera J (2000) Brain activation during volitional control of breathing. Physiol Res 49: 659–663.
44. Mazzone SB, McLennan L, McGovern AE, Egan GF, Farrell MJ (2007) Representation of Capsaicin-evoked Urge-to-Cough in the Human Brain Using Functional Magnetic Resonance Imaging. Am J Respir Crit Care Med 176: 327–332.
45. Evans KC (2010) Cortico-limbic circuitry and the airways: Insights from functional neuroimaging of respiratory afferents and efferents. Biological Psychology 84: 13.
46. Evans KC, Dougherty DD, Schmid AM, Scannell E, McCallister A, et al. (2009) Modulation of spontaneous breathing via limbic/paralimbic-bulbar circuitry: An event-related fMRI study. NeuroImage 47: 961.
47. Hanamori T, Kunitake T, Kato K, Kannan H (1998) Neurons in the posterior insular cortex are responsive to gustatory stimulation of the pharyngolarynx, baroreceptor and chemoreceptor stimulation, and tail pinch in rats. Brain Res 785: 97–106.
48. Gaytan SP, Pasaro R (1998) Connections of the rostral ventral respiratory neuronal cell group: an anterograde and retrograde tracing study in the rat. Brain Res Bull 47: 625–642.
49. LaBuda CJ, Fuchs PN (2005) Attenuation of negative pain affect produced by unilateral spinal nerve injury in the rat following anterior cingulate cortex activation. Neurosci 136: 311.
50. Zeidan F, Martucci KT, Kraft RA, Gordon NS, McHaffie JG, et al. (2011) Brain mechanisms supporting the modulation of pain by mindfulness meditation. J Neurosci 31: 5540–5548.
51. Stehberg J, Levy D, Zangen A (2009) Impairment of aversive memory reconsolidation by localized intracranial electrical stimulation. Eur J Neurosci 29: 964–969.
52. Green AL, Wang S, Purvis S, Owen SLF, Bain PG, et al. (2007) Identifying cardiorespiratory neurocircuitry involved in central command during exercise in humans. J Physiol 578: 605.
53. Zautra AJ, Fasman R, Davis MC, Craig AD (2010) The effects of slow breathing on affective responses to pain stimuli: an experimental study. Pain 149: 12–18.
54. Chalaye P, Goffaux P, Lafrenaye S, Marchand S (2009) Respiratory effects on experimental heat pain and cardiac activity. Pain Med 10: 1334–1340.

11

Systematic Evaluation of "Compliance" to Prescribed Treatment Medications and "Abstinence" from Psychoactive Drug Abuse in Chemical Dependence Programs: Data from the Comprehensive Analysis of Reported Drugs

Kenneth Blum[1,2,6,7*], David Han[3], John Femino[4], David E. Smith[5], Scott Saunders[6], Thomas Simpatico[7], Stephen J. Schoenthaler[8], Marlene Oscar-Berman[9], Mark S. Gold[1]

1 Department of Psychiatry and McKnight Brain Institute, University of Florida, College of Medicine, Gainesville, Florida, United States of America, **2** Department of Clinical Neurology, PATH Foundation NY, New York, New York, United States of America, **3** Department of Management Science and Statistics, University of Texas at San Antonio, San Antonio, Texas, United States of America, **4** Meadows Edge Recovery Center, North Kingstown, Rhode Island, United States of America, **5** David Smith and Associates and Institute of Health and Aging, University of California San Francisco School of Medicine, San Francisco, California, United States of America, **6** Dominion Diagnostics, LLC, North Kingstown, Rhode Island, United States of America, **7** Human Integrated Services Unit University of Vermont Center for Clinical and Translational Science, and Department of Psychiatry, UVM College of Medicine, Burlington, Vermont, United States of America, **8** Department of Sociology, California State University, Turlock, California, United States of America, **9** Departments of Psychiatry, Neurology, and Anatomy and Neurobiology, Boston University School of Medicine, and Department of Veterans Affairs Healthcare System, Boston, Massachusetts, United States of America

Abstract

This is the first quantitative analysis of data from urine drug tests for compliance to treatment medications and abstinence from drug abuse across "levels of care" in six eastern states of America. Comprehensive Analysis of Reported Drugs (CARD) data was used in this *post-hoc* retrospective observational study from 10,570 patients, filtered to include a total of 2,919 patients prescribed at least one treatment medication during 2010 and 2011. The first and last urine samples (5,838 specimens) were analyzed; compliance to treatment medications and abstinence from drugs of abuse supported treatment effectiveness for many. Compared to non-compliant patients, compliant patients were marginally less likely to abuse opioids, cannabinoids, and ethanol during treatment although more likely to abuse benzodiazepines. Almost 17% of the non-abstinent patients used benzodiazepines, 15% used opiates, and 10% used cocaine during treatment. Compliance was significantly higher in residential than in the non-residential treatment facilities. Independent of level of care, 67.2% of the patients ($n = 1963$; $P < .001$) had every treatment medication found in both first and last urine specimens (compliance). In addition, 39.2% of the patients ($n = 1143$; $P < .001$) had no substance of abuse detected in either the first or last urine samples (abstinence). Moreover, in 2010, 16.9% of the patients ($n = 57$) were abstinent at first but not at last urine (deteriorating abstinence), the percentage dropped to 13.3% ($n = 174$) in 2011; this improvement over years was statistically significant. A longitudinal analysis for abstinence and compliance was studied in a randomized subset from 2011, ($n = 511$) representing 17.5% of the total cohort. A statistically significant upward trend ($p = 2.353 \times 10^{-8}$) of abstinence rates as well as a similar but stronger trend for compliance (($p = 2.200 \times 10^{-16}$) was found. Being cognizant of the trend toward drug urine testing being linked to medical necessity eliminating abusive screening, the interpretation of these valuable results require further intensive investigation.

Editor: Kent E. Vrana, Penn State College of Medicine, United States of America

Funding: The preparation and review of the manuscript were supported in part by funds from the National Institutes of Health, National Institute on Alcohol Abuse and Alcoholism (R01-AA07112 and K05-AA00219) and the Medical Research Service of the US Department of Veterans Affairs (MOB). TS is the recipient of the following grants: United States Department of Human Services, Public Health Service, Substance Abuse and Mental Service Administration (SAMHSA) [SM058809]; Attorney General's Office, Chittenden County, Vermont, Pilot Study; Medical Services, US Veterans Administration, Chittenden County, Vermont. Dominion Diagnostics, LLC, provided consultant money to KB, JF, DES, and DH. These cited funders had no role in study design, data analysis, decision to publish, or preparation of the manuscript.

Competing Interests: SS of Dominion Diagnostics, LLC, de-identified the post hoc collected data. There is a conflict of interest involving KB, DH, JF, DES, and TS, who are members of the Scientific Advisory Board of Dominion Diagnostics, LLC. SS is a full-time paid employee of Dominion Diagnostics, LLC. KB is the recipient of a grant from Life Extension Foundation, Ft. Lauderdale, Florida.

* Email: drd2gene@gmail.com

These authors contributed equally to this work.

Introduction

The issue

Substance use disorders (SUDs) present a formidable challenge to treatment providers. Multi-faceted factors influence the course of the disorder, treatment outcomes and relapse. Evaluation and quantification of these factors is essential to reduce morbidity and maximize positive outcomes. Most clinicians would agree that compliance to prescribed treatment medications, as well as, patients being abstinent from drugs of abuse during treatment, are important outcome challenges in chemical dependence programs. Surprisingly, a 1-17-14 PUBMED search resulted in only one article that matched the following terminology: "urine analysis and compliance to prescribed treatment medications during *in-patient* and or *out- patient* treatment." A shorter word search did not find any additional articles. One article was found about non-cancer pain patients and the authors concluded: "Regular urine drug testing should be a part of acute and chronic pain management whether or not the patient has any signs or symptoms of drug misuse" (abuse) [1]. Likewise, a 1-17-14 PUBMED search found only four articles that match the following terminology: "urine analysis and abstinence to drugs of abuse during *in-patient* or *out-patient* treatment." While it is believed by some that compliance of treatment medications in patients undergoing treatment has been studied for over 20 years the present article is the only one to evaluate this topic systematically for both compliance to treatment medications and abstinence of licit and illicit drugs during treatment in one sample analysis.

These articles [2–18] were specific to type of intervention and drug of choice but not generalized to the level of care per se or to an entire American state [1,19–21]. While the Institute of Medicine have reviewed information linked to both compliance and abstinence related to drug abuse there is no definitive reported outcome published in the literature to date [6-17-13]. There is one report by Starrels *et al.* [22] that reviewed the literature relating opioid abuse and urine testing and concluded: "Relatively weak evidence supports the effectiveness of opioid treatment agreements and urine drug testing in reducing opioid misuse (abuse) by patients with chronic pain."

Moreover, a review of the overall literature on "addiction" per se revealed that there are 42,162 PUBMED listed articles [7-23-14]. An exhaustive word search and direct analysis of all the papers including an arduous review of a subset of 50 free articles resulted in only one paper concerning Long-acting Methadone (LAAM) utilizing urine analysis that evaluated both compliance and abstinence simultaneously [23]. Additionally, careful review of the largest cohort of approximately 10,000 patients derived from the national Drug Abuse Treatment Outcome Studies (DATOS), found no evidence of coupling both abstinence and compliance during treatment dependent upon level of care. One study by Simpson *et al.* [24] evaluating cocaine abusing patients based on urine analysis found higher severity of patient problems at program intake and shorter stays in treatment (<90 days) were related to higher cocaine relapse rates.

None of the above studies, however, including Simpson *et al.* [24] evaluated the following important question. When each urine sample measures both prescription medication and illicit drug use of patients being treated for drug addiction, are those who comply with prescribed treatment (as measured in baseline urine) more likely to be in remission at the end of treatment (as measured in urine) than patients who did not comply with prescription treatment (as measured in baseline urine)? The treating physician wants to know for each client as treatment commences if ordering urine tests on both prescription medication and illicit drugs is important, for diagnosis and management and are these tests based upon medical necessity criteria.

Based on the paucity of real quantitative data revealed by our systematic review of the literature, we embarked on this comprehensive study. In terms of clinical importance we are cognizant that clinicians want to see the main findings broken down for, each type of drug use, and each type of prescription treatment, each type of setting (residential, outpatient, etc) and by age and gender. Our data herein provides some of these answers although more analysis and research is required.

Importance of Urine Drug Testing

Our clinical experience suggests that randomized urine testing is a crucial part of any successful treatment program and as such deserves consideration. According to DuPont and Gold [25] the dominant characteristic of SUDs, is relapse. One of the lessons learned by DuPont and Skipper [26] was that long-term frequent random urine drug and alcohol testing dramatically reduced relapse in physicians mandated to participate in the physician health program (PHPs). Although partly a reflection of the cohesive nature of the program, only 22% of physicians tested positive at any time during the program and at the five-year point 71% were still licensed and employed [25,27]. The Federal Center for Substance Abuse Treatment also strongly advocates drug urine testing [28]. In fact, Tenore [29] and others [26] emphasized urine toxicology screening as an important standard of care in addiction and pain-treatment settings.

We are cognizant of the trend toward drug urine testing being linked to medical necessity eliminating abusive screening and do not endorse this seemingly *post hoc* abusive screening.

Comprehensive drug monitoring tools have recently been developed to assist clinicians demonstrate precision, at intake, during treatment and for individual and program outcomes [30]. One such clinical tool is the "Comprehensive Analysis of Reported Drugs" (CARD™) a reporting system that uses laboratory results from validated urine drug testing profiles of commonly abused illicit and prescription drugs, their metabolites, biological markers and commercial adulterant screening (that includes: creatinine, specific gravity, pH, and oxidants) and compares them to prescribed and self -reported drug use.

The two key clinical issues during in-patient or out-patient recovery programs are patients' compliance to prescribed treatment medications and patients' abstinence from all non-prescribed licit or illicit psychoactive drugs.

Monitoring compliance

When combined with counseling and other behavioral therapies, medications are an essential treatment element for many patients with SUD.

Adherence has been defined as, the extent to which a person's behavior conforms to medical or health advice [31]. While there is no data available on compliance to typical Food and Drug Administration (FDA) approved drugs for SUD, Chong *et al.* [32] following an extensive review of the literature, suggested that non-adherence or non-compliance with anti-depressant treatment is very common. Four meta-analyses [33–36] have demonstrated that for tricyclic antidepressants and selective serotonin reuptake inhibitors, drop-out rates are in the range of 21–33%. Many psychiatrists and addiction treatment professionals agree that patients attending programs for SUD may likewise not comply with prescribed treatment medications. A literature search revealed a paucity of information regarding this pivotal clinical issue. None of the papers we identified on the subject, used data from biological markers to determine compliance to treatment medications.

Monitoring abstinence

A further review (1-17-14) of the literature [MEDLINE, PsycINFO, EMBASE, Cochrane Central Register of Controlled Clinical Trials] utilizing the term "monitoring drug abuse abstinence by urine analysis" resulted in fifteen citations regarding abstinence. While most of the studies evaluated drugs like alcohol, opioids and psychostimulants individually, none systematically analyzed abstinence data according to state by state outcomes, by treatment modality, as a function of level of care, or trends over time.

It is noteworthy that without data to measure and control for patient characteristics, including severity of drug use and medical and social problems, such comparisons while important must be interpreted with caution and require more intense investigation.

Hypotheses: Two null hypotheses form the basis of this retrospective *post hoc* study. Patients in chemical dependency programs in America: 1) adhere to prescribed treatment medications and 2) abstain from illicit drug use during treatment.

Methods

Comprehensive Analysis of Reported Drugs (CARD)

This is a statistical analysis of unidentifiable data from CARD, privately held at Dominion Diagnostics LLC North Kingston RI, used to evaluate treatment adherence in a large clinical cohort from across a number of eastern states in America. Prior to being accessed for this statistical analysis the data was de-identified by Scott Saunders, MS. The ethics committee from Path Foundation NY on November 29th 2012 waived the approval of an IRB for this post hoc retrospective study of unidentifiable data, as well as the need for individual consent by patients to use the database for research. The non-public anonymized data can be provided to researchers, with prior written approval, by Dominion Diagnostics LLC. A detailed explanation of CARD methodology can be found in the "CARD Rule Sets" in Supporting information S1. This innovative monitoring tool can aggregate data from each client within a clinical practice to establish percentages of clients who are compliant with medications prescribed during treatment. The analysis also detects unexpected illicit drug use (non- abstinence) in patients tested, relative to expected reported drug use and aggregates that data.

Expected or not expected patient behaviors guide treatment plans and measure outcomes. Treatment decisions cannot be determined based on the simplistic nature of a positive or negative drug test. The basis of the CARD methodology is that drugs present in the body, whether prescribed, or self-reported, have been scientifically proven to exhibit specific conditional results on drug tests. Because drugs can metabolize into other reportable substances, the possibility exists that test results can be open to misinterpretation. CARD engages the patient's prescriptions and/ or self-reported drug abuse, their drug test results, and the correlation of thousands of scientifically valid test result conditions to link the ingestion of drugs and subsequent results into classifications of 'Expected', 'Not Expected', or 'Alerts' for physicians. (**See Supporting information S1**). Although we are focused on FDA approved anti-addiction drugs because of duel diagnosis the following drug classes tested included: anabolic steroids, antidepressants, hallucinogens, inhalants, muscle relaxants, opioids, psychostimulants, psychotropic's, sedatives/hypnotics/depressants.

Statistical Analyses

Statistical analyses were conducted using the discrete contingency analyses, the two-level binomial logistic regression model, and the Generalized Linear Mixed Model (GLMM) in the R package version 2.15.0. The Fisher's exact test was used to evaluate differences in adherence to treatment medications and abstinence rates according to the type of treatment (in-patient *vs.* out-patient), level of care and differences in compliance and abstinence rates in 2010 compared to 2011. We also analyzed a subset of 511 patients representing 17.5% of the entire data set for trend relating to longitudinal urine screens up to 52 times for both compliance and abstinence. It is noteworthy that each and every statistical analysis herein comes with a controlled Type-I error rate.

Distribution of Subjects and Specimens Tested. In this analysis data was derived from 10,570 patients at treatment centers across six eastern states of America [Maryland (MD), Maine (ME), North Carolina (NC), Rhode Island (RI), South Carolina (SC) and Vermont (VT)]. The sample size is largely skewed to NC and VT, while SC represents less than 1% of the whole sample (Table 1).

Although initially there was data from a total 84,206 specimens, to ensure uniformity only first and last specimens tested were used in the analysis. As detailed below in a number of cases the first specimen was obtained in year 2010 while the last specimen was collected in 2011. Of 21,140 urine specimens analyzed across two years (2010 to 2011) the dataset was further filtered to include a total of 2,919 patients who were on at least one prescription medication ($n = 2{,}919$; total 5838 specimens). The data was stratified over five different levels of care each with the minimum number of calendar days between the first and last urine specimens analyzed (Table 2). The distribution of the number of calendar days between the first and last urine samples is heavily right skewed ranging from 15 days to 717 days. The median is 176 days with the inter-quartile range of 281 days. The sample mean and sample standard deviation are 226.2 days and 171.0 days, respectively.

The patient distribution across two modalities and five levels of care is presented in Table 3. The sample consisted of the out-patients (OP) 96%, of which one-third was in the opiate treatment program (OTP). It was found that 11.6% of the patients ($n = 338$) had both the first and last urine specimens collected in 2010 while 44.9% ($n = 1311$) first and last collected in 2011. The rest of 43.5% ($n = 1270$) had the first urine specimen collected in 2010 and the last specimen collected in 2011. All the patients were taking at least one prescription medication and 18.0% of the patients ($n = 525$) were found to be on more than one prescription drug. Definitions of the terms used include; *compliance* being when each and every reported prescription drug was detected, *both* refers to the *first* and *last* urine samples together and *abstinence* means that no analytes that could not be attributed to a reported prescription were detected in urine samples tested. The PATH Foundation IRB reviewed the protocol and waived further approval due to post hoc analysis.

Results

Compliance

From both first and last urine specimens, 67.2% of the patients ($n = 1963$; $P < .001$) had every treatment medication found in both urine samples, hence were "compliance both". Every treatment medication was found in the first urine sample, 77.9% of the patients ($n = 2274$; $P < .001$) hence "compliance first", while, 78.4% of the patients ($n = 2289$; $P < .001$) had every treatment

Table 1. Distribution of participants by state.

State	Sample Size
Maryland (MD)	218 (7.5)
Maine (ME)	359 (12.3)
North Carolina (NC)	833 (28.5)
Rhode Island (RI)	542 (18.6)
South Carolina (SC)	28 (1.0)
Vermont (VT)	939 (32.1)
Total	2919

medication found in the last urine sample, hence "compliance last". Over the course of the first and last urine specimen collections, it was found that 10.9% of the patients (n = 319) were not complying at all. Improvement in compliance was shown in 11.2% of the patients (n = 326) who did not comply at first but complied at last. However, 10.7% of the patients (n = 311) showed a deteriorating compliance behavior by complying at first but not complying at last urinalysis.

Abstinence

For the measurement of abstinence, 39.2% of the patients (n = 1143; $P<.001$) had no substance of abuse detected in either of the urine samples, hence "abstinence both". Moreover, 54.0% of the patients (n = 1577; $P<.001$) had no substance of abuse found in the first urine sample, hence "abstinence first", while 57.3% of the patients (n = 1672; $P<.001$) had no substance of abuse found in the last urine sample, hence "abstinence last". Over the course of the first and last urine specimen collections, it was found that 27.9% of the patients (n = 813) were not abstinent at all. Improvement in abstinence was shown in 18.1% of the patients (n = 529) who were not abstinent at first but abstinent at last. The abstinence of 14.9% of the patients (n = 434) deteriorated as they were abstinent at first but not abstinent at last urine drug test.

Contingency Analyses

The rates of compliance and abstinence across the six eastern states are presented in Table 4. Overall, statistically significant differences were found in the compliance rates as well as the abstinence rates among the six states. That is, ME and NC exhibited the highest compliance rates of over 80%, while SC gave the lowest rate of below 50%. SC and MD, however, showed the highest abstinence rates while ME and RI had the lowest. Illicit drug use during treatment for each state differed whereby: MD = 50.9%; ME = 65.5%; NC = 58.6%; RI = 63.8%; SC = 50.0% and VT = 62.0%.

The rates of compliance and abstinence over the patients' modality are presented in Table 5. From Fisher's exact tests, there is statistically significant evidence to conclude that the out-patients adhered to treatment medications better than the in-patients ($P_{both}<.001$; $P_{first}=.005$; $P_{last}<.001$). On the other hand, the abstinence rates were similar between the out-patients and the in-patients except for the case of "abstinence last" where the out-patients showed higher tendency of abusing drugs compared to the in-patients ($P_{last}=.01$).

The rates of compliance and abstinence over the patients' level of care are presented in Table 6. Overall a statistically significant difference in the compliance rates as well as the abstinence rates were found among the five levels of care in this study. The patients in the opiate treatment program (OTP) exhibited the highest compliance rates of over 85%, while those in the residential facility (RES) gave the lowest rate of below 65%. The patients in the residential facility (RES), as well as the intensive out-patients (IOP), however, showed the highest abstinence rates while the out-patients (OP) gave consistently low rates.

Comparison 2010 and 2011

In order to make an annual comparison and examine any trend of the compliance rates and the abstinence rates over time, the dataset was grouped by the year of the collected urine samples. This is important to determine since we hypothesized that familiarity by the staff in using CARD between 2010 when it was first initiated and 2011 one year of experience might help to enhance both compliance and abstinence in respective patients. As already mentioned, 11.6% of the patients (n = 338) had both the first and last urine specimens collected in 2010 while 44.9% (n = 1311) had them collected in 2011. Although no statistically significant difference (each $P>.30$) was found in the compliance rates between 2010 and 2011, Fisher's exact tests revealed that there was statistically significant improvement in the abstinence rates in 2011 compared to 2010 ($P_{both}=.04$; $P_{last}<.001$).

Table 2. Patient level of care and minimum days between samples.

Level of Care	Minimum Days between Samples
In-Patient (IP)	21
Residential facility (RES)	30
Intensive Out-Patient (IOP)	15
Out-Patient (OP)	30
Opiate Treatment Program (OTP)	30

Table 3. Distribution of participants over modality and level of care.

Modality	Sample Size	Level of Care	Sample Size
In-Patient	116 (4.0)	IP	41 (1.4)
		RES	75 (2.6)
Out-Patient	2803 (96.0)	IOP	340 (11.6)
		OP	1558 (53.4)
		OTP	905 (31.0)
Total	2919	**Total**	2919

IP-In-patients; RES = Residential facility; IOP = Intensive outpatients, OP = Outpatient; OPT = Opiate treatment programs.

Regression analyses revealed that over the course of two urine specimen collections, 15.1% of the patients (n = 51) were not complying at all in 2010, while 14.0% of the patients (n = 183) were not complying at all in 2011. In 2010, 60.1% of the patients (n = 203) were continuously complying, and in 2011, 61.5% of the patients (n = 806) were continuously complying. Improvement in compliance was shown in 11.8% of the patients (n = 40) who did not comply at first but complied at last in 2010. This percentage increased to 13.2% (n = 173) in 2011. In 2010, 13.0% of the patients (n = 44) complied at first but did not comply at last, showing a deteriorating compliance behavior. However, this percentage dropped to 11.4% (n = 149) in 2011. Nevertheless, these changes over time were not found to be statistically significant ($P = .72$).

In addition, over the course of two urine specimen collections, it was found that 35.2% of the patients ($n = 119$) were not abstinent at all in 2010, and the percentage dropped to 28.3% ($n = 371$) in 2011. In 2010, 32.8% of the patients ($n = 111$) were continuously abstinent, and in 2011, the percentage increased to 38.0% ($n = 498$). Improvement in abstinence was shown in 15.1% of the patients ($n = 51$) who were not abstinent at first but were abstinent at last in 2010. The percentage increased to 20.4% ($n = 268$) in 2011. In 2010, 16.9% of the patients ($n = 57$) were abstinent at first but were not abstinent at last, a sign of deteriorating abstinence behavior. This percentage dropped to 13.3% ($n = 174$) in 2011. These changes over years were found to be statistically significant ($P = .005$).

Furthermore we evaluated the association between the compliance and the abstinence measured in this study through odds ratios (OR) and the corresponding 95% confidence intervals. There is statistically significant evidence to show that a compliant patient is more likely to be abstinent during treatment compared to a non-compliant patient. In particular, "abstinence both" is more likely for a patient in "compliance both" than not (OR = 1.34; $P<.001$). Also, "abstinence first" is more likely for a patient in "compliance both" than not (OR = 1.19; $P<.001$), and "abstinence both" is more likely for a patient in "compliance first" than not (OR = 1.17; $P = .05$). Lastly, "abstinence first" is more likely for a patient in "compliance first" than not (OR = 1.29; $P = .002$). It seems that "abstinence last" (or "compliance last") does not have a statistically significant association with "compliance both/first/last" (or "abstinence both/first/last") (each $P>.30$).

Longitudinal Analysis

Following our comparison of data collected in 2010 versus 2011 to further elucidate these interesting findings we looked at urine samples at every time point in a randomly selected subset of patients from 2011.

Figure 1 below describes the longitudinal trend of the abstinence of a subset of the patients ($n = 511$; 17.5%) after removing 56 patients who had only one urine specimen from a pool of patients. Their urine samples were collected in several occasions (up to 52 times) in 2011 and analyzed using CARD. In general, a statistically significant upward trend was observed overall ($p = 2.353\times10^{-8}$), which implies improved abstinence rates over time.

The selected subset of the patients also showed 100% compliance to at least one reported prescription drug. Hence, Figure 2 below describes the longitudinal trend of the improved

Table 4. Compliance and abstinence rates of participants across the six U.S. eastern states.

Eastern States	Comp B n(%)	Comp F n(%)	Comp L n(%)	Abs B n(%)	Abs F n(%)	Abs L n(%)
MD	103(47.3)	127(58.3)	138(63.3)	107(49.1)	145(66.5)	142(65.1)
ME	290(80.8)	315(87.7)	326(90.8)	124(34.5)	184(51.3)	184(51.3)
NC	690(82.8)	719(86.3)	788(94.6)	345(41.4)	462(55.5)	503(60.4)
RI	247(45.6)	349(64.4)	310(57.2)	196(36.2)	262(48.3)	293(54.1)
SC	9(32.1)	13(46.4)	13(46.4)	14(50.0)	18(64.3)	20(71.4)
VT	624(66.5)	751(80.0)	714(76.0)	357(38.0)	506(53.9)	530(56.4)
χ^2	292.87	179.26	355.14	17.94	23.74	18.97
***p*-value**	<.001	<.001	<.001	.003	.002	.002

MD = Maryland; ME = Maine; NC = North Carolina; RI = Rhode Island: SC = South Carolina; VT = Vermont. Comp = Compliance; Abs = Abstinence. B = Both; F = First; L = Last.

Table 5. Compliance and abstinence rates by participants according to treatment modality.

Modality	Comp B n(%)	Comp F n(%)	Comp L n(%)	Abs B n(%)	Abs F n(%)	Abs L n(%)
In-Patient (IP)	56 (48.3)	78 (67.2)	73 (62.9)	51 (44.0)	60 (51.7)	80 (69.0)
Out-Patient (OP)	1907 (68.0)	2196 (78.3)	2216 (79.1)	1092 (39.0)	1517 (54.1)	1592 (56.8)
χ^2	19.74	7.98	17.12	1.17	0.26	6.74
p-value	<.001	.005	<.001	.28	.61	.01

Comp = Compliance; Abs = Abstinence. B = Both; F = First; L = Last.

compliance of the same subset of the patients ($n = 511$; 17.5%) after removing 56 patients who had only one urine specimen from a pool of patients. Their urine samples were collected on several occasions (up to 52 times) in 2011 and analyzed using CARD. Again, in general, a statistically significant upward trend was observed overall ($p = 2.200 \times 10^{-16}$), which implies improved compliance rates over time. This upward trend was found to be even stronger than the trend of abstinence.

Drugs of abuse used by non-abstinent patients

The primary drugs abused by the patients ($n = 1776$) who were not abstinent during treatment are given in Table 7. Almost 23% of the non-abstinent patients used psychostimulants, 25% used benzodiazepines, 32% used cannabinoids, and 38% used opioids during treatment. Use of nicotine was not considered in this analysis. The odds ratios (OR) with the corresponding 95% confidence intervals in Table 5 estimated any association between the abused drug and the compliance to the prescription medications by non-abstinent patients. As large *p*-values indicate, there were no statistically significant associations between the drugs abused and the compliance status in most cases. Compared to a non-compliant patient, it was found that a compliant patient was marginally less likely to abuse opioids ($P = .07$), cannabinoids ($P = .04$), and ethanol ($P = .07$) during the treatment. On the other hand, it was also revealed that a compliant patient was more likely to abuse benzodiazepines compared to a non-compliant patient during the treatment ($P = .004$).

Unexpected drug use during treatment in this very large cohort was significant ($p<0.0001$), differed across six eastern states and was significantly greater in non-residential treatment than in residential treatment ($\chi^2 = 6.74$; $p = 0.0094$; OR = 1.69). From Fisher's exact tests, there is statistically significant evidence to conclude that the out-patients adhered to treatment medications better than the in-patients ($P_{both}<.001$; $P_{first} = .005$; $P_{last}<.001$). On the other hand, the abstinence rates were similar between the out-patients and the in-patients except for the case of "abstinence last" where the out-patients showed higher tendency of abusing drugs compared to the in-patients ($P_{last} = .01$). The importance of the last urine tested is underscored by revealing the significant difference between in-patients and out-patients, eliminating guessing and providing real quantification of this issue.

Discussion

Although most clinicians would not be surprised that this analysis of CARD data was not consistent with the null hypothesizes, this is the first report in the chemical dependency literature that quantifies non-adherence to prescribed medication during treatment and the first that found objective evidence of significant drug abuse in recovery (especially during treatment periods). This finding is not surprising especially when we consider the genetic antecedents of addiction and their role in relapse. Recently, Dahlgren [37] found that, 89% (16/18) carriers of the DRD2 A1 allele, reported relapse in contrast to 53% (17/32) in the non-carriers ($p = 0.01$; odds ratio = 7.1). There is also growing recognition nationally that self-report of drug use is often unreliable. Comings *et al.* [38] associated the dopamine D2 receptor gene A1 allele, with immature defense style (lying) responses to a defense-style questionnaire in patients attending addiction treatment. Certainly, genetic factors coupled with potential fear of punitive measures leads to unreliable self- report of drug use in agreement with the present analysis.

According to Katz and Fanciullo, [39] although there is a lack of accepted diagnostic criteria for medication misuse in patients with chronic pain, awareness of a patient's inappropriate use of illicit drugs or medications, is important in good patient

Table 6. Compliance and abstinence rates by participants according to level of care.

Level of Care	Comp B n(%)	Comp F n(%)	Comp L n(%)	Abs B n(%)	Abs F n(%)	Abs L n(%)
IP	22 (53.7)	30 (73.2)	26 (63.4)	14 (34.2)	16 (39.0)	26 (63.4)
RES	34 (45.3)	48 (64.0)	47 (62.7)	37 (49.3)	44 (58.7)	54 (72.0)
IOP	245 (72.1)	281 (82.7)	276 (81.2)	166 (48.8)	228 (67.1)	218 (64.1)
OP	893 (57.3)	1117 (71.7)	1072 (68.8)	553 (35.5)	784 (50.3)	838 (53.8)
OTP	769 (85.0)	798 (88.2)	868 (95.9)	373 (41.2)	505 (55.8)	536 (59.2)
χ^2	222.22	103.78	266.66	27.41	37.38	22.94
p-value	<.001	<.001	<.001	<.001	<.001	<.001

IP = In-Patient; RES = Residential facility; IOP = Intensive Out-Patient; OP = Outpatient; OTP = Opiate Treatment Program. Comp = Compliance; Abs = Abstinence. B = Both; F = First; L = Last.

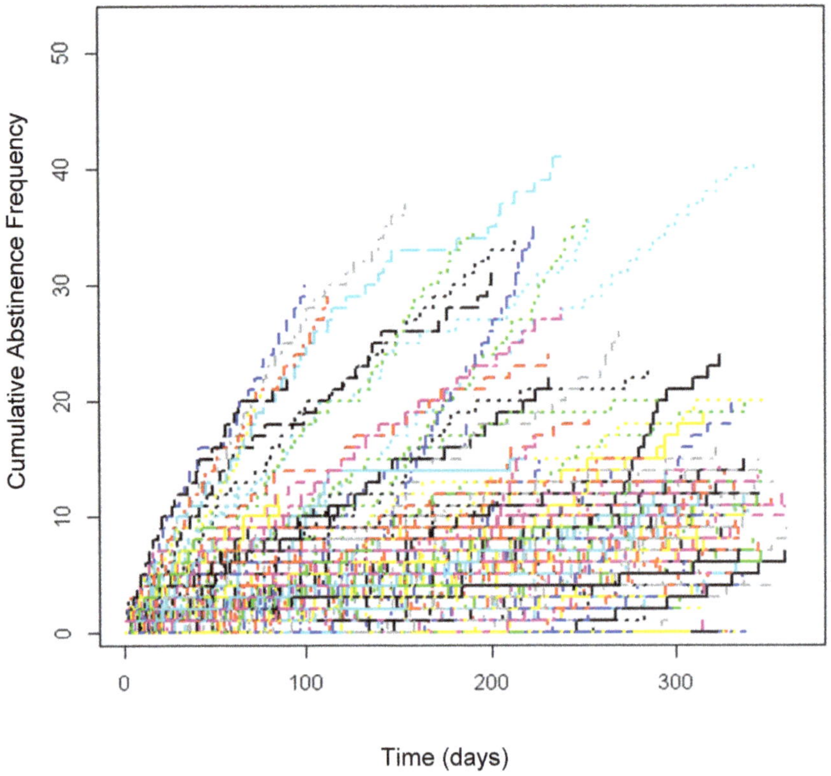

Figure 1. Cumulative Abstinence Frequency over Time.

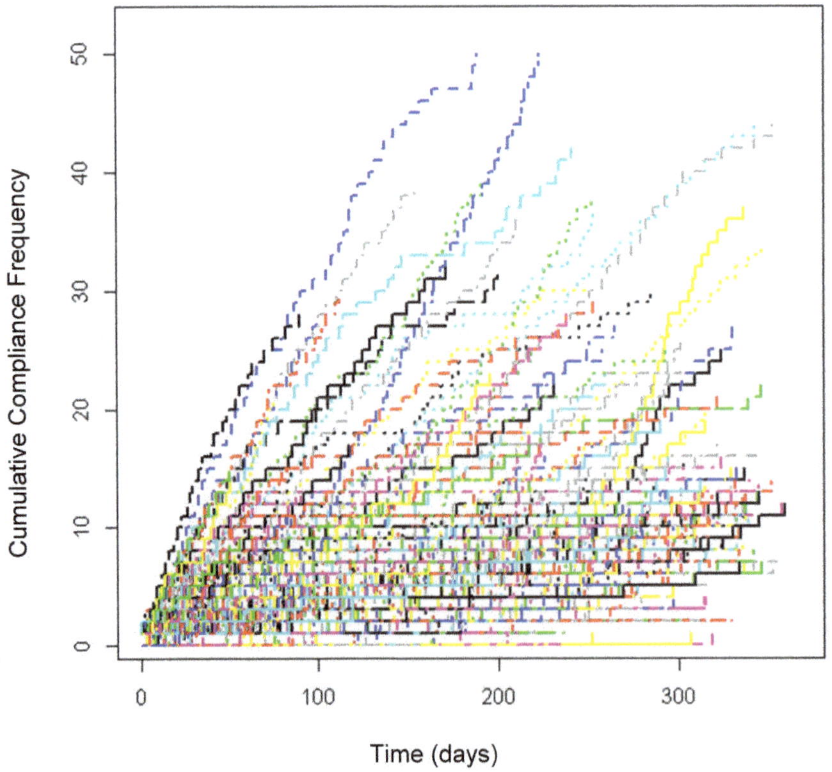

Figure 2. Cumulative Compliance Frequency over Time.

Table 7. Primary drugs abused by non-abstinent patients and association to compliance ($n = 1776$).

Drug Class	N (%)	OR	95% C.I.	*p*-value
Psychostimulants	403 (22.7)	0.93	(0.74, 1.18)	.56
Hallucinogens (PCP, LSD, etc.)	4 (0.2)	0.54	(0.08, 3.87)	.54
Inhalants (hydrocarbons)	0 (0.0)	–	–	–
Opioids (analgesics, antitussives, cough suppressants, opiate antagonists)	676 (38.1)	0.83	(0.68, 1.02)	.07
Benzodiazepines (anti-anxiety)	442 (24.9)	1.40	(1.11, 1.77)	.004
Amphetamines	135 (7.6)	0.83	(0.58, 1.19)	.31
Cannabinoids	563 (31.7)	0.81	(0.66, 0.99)	.04
Ethanol	299 (16.8)	0.79	(0.61, 1.02)	.07
Barbiturates	41 (2.3)	0.69	(0.37, 1.29)	.24

management. It has also been suggested that as the use of opioids for chronic pain increases so does the risk for drug non-adherence, associated drug abuse, potential addiction, and other abnormal drug-related behaviors. McCarberg [30] states that cost-benefit studies suggest that liquid chromatography tests (LUTs) could reduce the costs associated with non-adherence in chronic pain therapy, up to 14.8-fold. Opioids in this present study were indeed the drugs that demonstrated best compliance and were most abused by non-abstinent patients.

Urine drug testing is necessary to determine treatment outcomes and compliance. Input from prescription monitoring programs such as CARD, together with interviews with spouses and medical record reviews may be used to improve patient management and clinical interactions. The finding that abstinence rates improved between 2010 and 2011 and longitudinally during 2011 may be explained by increased honesty in clinical interactions as clinicians gained experience in the use of CARD.

McLellan *et al.* [40] pointed out that relapse rates for addictions are similar to other chronic illnesses, and like diabetes and hypertension, are dependent in-part on adherence to treatment medication. The study finding that compliant patients are more likely to be abstinent during treatment also supports the value of determining non-adherence to medications, which can associate with relapse.

That in-spite of compliance to treatment medications there is a significant unexpected drug use in this large cohort emphasizes the need to find effective anti-relapse treatment modalities to attenuate the known brain-reward circuitry impairment that underpins addiction as defined by ASAM, 2011. In fact, Nora Volkow, irrefutably argues for the development a dopamine D2 agonist that over the long-term up-regulate rather than down regulates these receptors and could provide anti -drug craving and relapse-prevention [41].

The Center for Substance Abuse Treatment already strongly advocates for the use of drug urine testing by treatment program's [28]. Given this context, it would be useful to conduct outcome analyses to further understand why and how some patients and treatment programs are able to get good outcomes and to promote the wide-spread use of practices that successful programs and clinicians employ like, for example, brain reward circuitry balancing especially dopamine up-regulation as observed in epigenetics [42]. Most recently, using genome-wide DNA methylation and gene expression mapping, Zhang observed that in the pre-frontal cortices of deceased alcoholics, compared to matched controls, powerful epigenetics effects impact 126 genes on dopaminergic pathways [43].

Conclusion

As the very first observational study done in this area, we have identified multiple issues and caveats in our analysis. A limitation of this analysis of pre and post treatment changes is the absence of covariates and lack of systematic collection of urine samples between the first and last sample for each patient. Features of the clinical course of treatment should be considered in the design of future analyses, for example, the first urine collected on admission may be expected to be positive for abused drugs in many programs, while, the last urine might be a trigger for termination of treatment.

Further investigation of this novel CARD database may answer more questions in addition future research to expand the longitudinal aspect of the dataset is needed. This will help to identify any trend or pattern of compliance and abstinence rates over a longer period of time under a systematic and controlled design. This study provides strong objective evidence of non-compliance to treatment medications by a cohort of SUD patients. Additionally, significant drug abuse during treatment was observed across the six states. As expected a large number of patients continue to partially meet treatment expectations with over 60% continuing their struggle with drug abuse.

We found evidence for the effectiveness of substance abuse treatment and based on our longitudinal analysis improvement in outcome for many patients when monitoring both compliance and abstinence are routinely incorporated into treatment. However, albeit there are certain limitations, in that our findings related to a subset of (n = 511) 17.5% of the entire data set; they certainly show a very significant trend for improvement in both compliance and abstinence during treatment.

The analysis of first and last urines found that compared to non-compliant patients, compliant patients were less likely to abuse opioids, cannabinoids, and ethanol during treatment. However, compliant patients were significantly more likely to abuse benzodiazepines. Compliance was significantly higher in residential than in non-residential treatment facilities. Moreover, in 2010, 16.9% of the patients ($n = 57$) were abstinent at first but were not abstinent at last, a sign of deteriorating abstinence behavior. This percentage dropped to 13.3% ($n = 174$) in 2011. This improvement over years was statistically significant however requires confirmation and further exploration by our laboratory and other researchers.

Information from this study does provide some quantitative data both about compliance to FDA approved treatment medications and abstinence from psychoactive licit and illicit drugs of abuse. Additional research is required to further test the clinical utility of this novel tool. These important quantitative findings should impact the clinical issues related to both compliance and abstinence in chemical dependency programs based on medicine assisted therapeutics. Notably, both compliance to prescription medication and abstinence from drugs of abuse was found in many patients supporting the effectiveness of treatment. These findings are in agreement with Reisfield *et al.* who proclaimed that drug urine testing is an invaluable resource for primary care [44]. In fact our longitudinal analysis of a subset of patients albeit, independent of level of care revealed significant improvements in both abstinence and compliance whereby compliance was robust. Future studies are being planned to include level of care in longitudinal analyses in a larger cohort.

While encouraging especially when one considers the positive results in our subset longitudinal analyses, addiction is a chronic disease and overall these results indicate the need for novel therapeutic targets and a paradigm shift in both in-patient and out-patient treatment tactics based on additional research and outcome studies.

Supporting Information

Supporting information S1 CARD Rule Sets. (DOCX)

Acknowledgments

The authors are appreciative of Margaret A. Madigan, B.Sc., Dr. Kenneth Blum's Editorial Assistant, who edited the entire manuscript prior to submission; Chris Campanella, B.Sc. Director of Information Services, involving computer programming and data entry and collection for Dominion Diagnostics LLC., who along with others at Dominion Diagnostics LLC., developed the working engines responsible for CARD; Mary Hauser, MA, Vice President of Addiction Services and New Market Development of Dominion Diagnostics LLC for important input on the clinical basis of CARD; Lisa Marzilli, Pharm. D., Pharmacy Services, Dominion Diagnostics, LLC., for clinical input related to patient and chart histories.

Author Contributions

Conceived and designed the experiments: KB SS. Performed the experiments: KB SS. Analyzed the data: DH SS. Contributed reagents/materials/analysis tools: SS. Wrote the paper: KB DH JF DES SS TS SJS MOB MSG. Provided in-depth analysis of DATOS and input into the paper: SJS. Provided important urine testing references: MSG. Provided clinical concepts and framework: DES JF. Conducted and directed all aspects of the data collection, statistical analyses, and writing: KB DH.

References

1. Gilbert JW, Wheeler GR, Mick GE, Storey BB, Herder SL, et al. (2010) Importance of urine drug testing in the treatment of chronic noncancer pain: implications of recent medicare policy changes in Kentucky. Pain Physician 13:167–186.
2. Jacobs W, DuPont R, Gold MS (2000) Drug testing and the DSM V. Psychiat Ann 30: 583–588.
3. Goldberger BA, Frost-Pineda K, Gold MS (2003) Methodone related deaths exceed heroin in the state of Florida. J Addict Dis 22:139.
4. Jacobs WS, Repetto M, Vinson S, Pomm R, Gold MS (2004) Random urine testing as an intervention for drug addiction. Psychiatr Ann 34: 781–785.
5. McCusker RR, Fuehrlein B, Goldberger BA, Gold MS, Cone EJ (2006) Technical brief: caffeine content of decaffeinated coffee. J Anal Toxicol 30: 611–613.
6. Gold MS, Frost-Pineda K (2006) Problem doctors: Is there a system-level solution? Letter to the Editor. Ann Intern Med 144: 861–862.
7. Gold MS, Frost-Pineda K, Goldberger BA, DuPont RL (2006) Physicians and Drug Screening. Letter to the Editor. J Adolesc Health 39: 154–155.
8. Merlo LJ, Gold MS (2008) Increased assessment and monitoring needed for methadone patients. Author reply. Am J Med 121: e25.
9. Merlo L, Gold M (2008) Prescription Opioid Abuse and Dependence Among Physicians: Hypotheses and Treatment. Harv Rev Psychiatry 16: 181–194.
10. Graham NA, Merlo LJ, Goldberger BA, Gold MS (2008) Methadone and heroin-related deaths in Florida. Am J Drug Alcohol Abuse 24: 347–353.
11. DuPont RL, McLellan AT, White WL, Merlo LJ, Gold MS (2009) Setting the standard for recovery: Physicians' Health Programs J Subst Abuse Treat 36: 159–171.
12. Bailey JA, Hurley RW, Gold MS (2010) Crossroads of Pain and Addiction. Pain Med 11: 1803–1818.
13. Reisfield GM, Graham NA, Gold MS (2011) RE: "Estimates of nondisclosure of cigarette smoking among pregnant and nonpregnant women of reproductive age in the United States". Letter to the Editor. Am J Epidemiol 173: 1095–1096.
14. DuPont RL, Goldberger BA, Gold MS (2011) Clinical and legal considerations in drug testing. In: Chris Cavacuiti editor. Principals of Addiction Medicine – The Essentials. Baltimore, MD: Lippincott Williams & Wilkins.
15. Reisfield GM, Goldberger, Gold MS, DuPont RL (2012) The Mirage of Impairing Drug Concentration Thresholds: A Rationale for Zero Tolerance *Per Se* Driving under the Influence of Drugs Laws. J Anal Toxicol 36: 353–356.
16. Goldberger BA, Martin DM, Gold MS (2013) Afghanistan Treatment Center Study: Children's Hair, Oral Fluid, and Urine Random Drug Testing. In: Afghanistan National Urban Drug Use Survey, 2012. Washington, DC: U. S. Department of State, Bureau of International Narcotics and Law Enforcement Affairs. pp. A104–A126.
17. Fuehrlein BS, Gold MS (2013) Medication Assisted Recovery in Alcohol and Opioid Dependence. Dir Psychiatry 33: 15–27.
18. Greene W, Gold MS (2015) Section 16: Drug Abuse. In: Bope ET, Kellerman RD, (Eds.) Conn's Current Therapy 2015. Philadelphia: Saunders, Inc. pp. 946–951.
19. Gerra G, Borella F, Zaimovic A, Moi G, Bussandri M, et al. (2004) Buprenorphine versus methadone for opioid dependence: predictor variables for treatment outcome. Drug Alcohol Depend 75: 37–45.
20. Campbell J, Nickel EJ, Penick EC, Wallace D, Gabrielli WF, et al. (2003) Comparison of desipramine or carbamazepine to placebo for crack cocaine-dependent patients. Am J Addict 12: 122–136.
21. Shaner A, Roberts LJ, Eckman TA, Tucker DE, Tsuang JW, et al. (1997) Monetary reinforcement of abstinence from cocaine among mentally ill patients with cocaine dependence. Psychiatr Serv 48: 807–810.
22. Starrels JL, Becker WC, Alford DP, Kapoor A, Williams AR, et al. (2010) Systematic review: treatment agreements and urine drug testing to reduce opioid misuse in patients with chronic pain. Ann Intern Med 152: 712–720.
23. Longshore D, Annon J, Anglin MD, Rawson RA (2005) Levo-alpha-acetylmethadol (LAAM) versus methadone: treatment retention and opiate use. Addiction 100: 1131–1139.
24. Simpson DD, Joe GW, Fletcher BW, Hubbard RL, Anglin MD (1999) A national evaluation of treatment outcomes for cocaine dependence. Arch Gen Psychiatry 56:507–514.
25. DuPont RL, Gold MS (1995) Withdrawal and reward: Implications for detoxification and relapse prevention. Psychiatr Ann 25: 663–668.
26. DuPont RL, Skipper GE (2012) Six lessons from state physician health programs to promote long-term recovery. J Psychoactive Drugs 44: 72–78.
27. DuPont RL, McLellan AT, Carr G, Gendel M, Skipper GE (2009) How are addicted physicians treated? A national survey of Physician Health Programs. J Subst Abuse Treat 37: 1–7.
28. Standridge JB, Adams SM, Zotos AP (2010) Urine drug screening: a valuable office procedure. Am Fam Physician 81: 635–640.
29. Tenore PL (2010) Advanced urine toxicology testing. J Addict Dis 29: 436–448.
30. McCarberg BH (2011) A critical assessment of opioid treatment adherence using urine drug testing in chronic pain management. Postgrad Med 123: 124–31. doi: 10.3810/pgm.2011.11.2502.
31. Bruer JT (1982) Methodological rigor and citation frequency in patient compliance literature. Am J Public Health 72: 1119–1123.
32. Chong WW, Aslani P, Chen TF (2011) Effectiveness of interventions to improve antidepressant medication adherence: a systematic review. Int J Clin Pract 65:954–975.
33. Anderson IM, Tomenson BM (1995) Treatment discontinuation with selective serotonin reuptake inhibitors compared with tricyclic antidepressants: a meta-analysis. BMJ 310: 1433–1438.
34. Steffens DC, Krishnan KR, Helms MJ (1997) Are SSRIs better than TCAs? Comparison of SSRIs and TCAs: a meta-analysis. Depress Anxiety 6: 10–18.
35. Montgomery SA, Kasper S (1995) Comparison of compliance between serotonin reuptake inhibitors and tricyclic antidepressants: a meta-analysis. Int Clin Psychopharmacol 9: 33–40.
36. Anderson IM (1998) SSRIS versus tricyclic antidepressants in depressed inpatients: a meta-analysis of efficacy and tolerability. Depress Anxiety 7: 11–17.

37. Dahlgren A, Wargelius HL, Berglund KJ, Fahlke C, Blennow K, et al. (2011) Do alcohol-dependent individuals with DRD2 A1 allele have an increased risk of relapse? A pilot study. Alcohol Alcohol 46: 509–513.
38. Comings DE, MacMurray J, Johnson P, Dietz G, Muhleman D (1995) Dopamine D2 receptor gene (DRD2) haplotypes and the defense style questionnaire in substance abuse, Tourette syndrome, and controls. Biol Psychiatry 37: 798–805.
39. Katz N, Fanciullo GJ (2002) Role of urine toxicology testing in the management of chronic opioid therapy. Clin J Pain 18: 76–82.
40. McLellan AT, Lewis DC, O'Brien CP, Kleber HD (2000) Drug dependence, a chronic medical illness: implications for treatment, insurance and outcomes evaluation. JAMA 284: 1689–1695.
41. Volkow ND, Tomasi D, Wang GJ, Telang F, Fowler JS, et al. (2013) Predominance of D2 Receptors in Mediating Dopamine's Effects in Brain Metabolism: Effects of Alcoholism. J Neurosci. 2013: 33: 4527–35.
42. Archer T, Oscar-Berman M, Blum K, Gold M (2013) Epigenetic Modulation of Mood Disorders. J Genet Syndr Gene Ther 4(120): pii: 1000120.
43. Zhang H (2013) Profiling epigenomic and trasciptomic alteration in postmortem prefrontal cortex of human alcoholcs. J Addic. Res. and Therp. 4: 57 (abstract) 2013. Proceedings of 2nd International conference on Addiction Research & Therapy, Las Vegas, NV 22–24, USA.
44. Reisfield GM, Graham NA, Gold MS (2010) Urine drug testing is still an invaluable resource for primary care. Ann Intern Med 153:420; author reply 420–421.

12

A Preclinical Physiological Assay to Test Modulation of Knee Joint Pain in the Spinal Cord: Effects of Oxycodone and Naproxen

Jason A. Miranda[1]*, Phil Stanley[2], Katrina Gore[2], Jamie Turner[1], Rebecca Dias[1], Huw Rees[1]

1 Neusentis Research Unit, Pfizer, Cambridge, United Kingdom, **2** Research Statistics, Clinical Research, Pfizer, Cambridge, United Kingdom

Abstract

Sensory processing in the spinal cord during disease states can reveal mechanisms for novel treatments, yet very little is known about pain processing at this level in the most commonly used animal models of articular pain. Here we report a test of the prediction that two clinically effective compounds, naproxen (an NSAID) and oxycodone (an opiate), are efficacious in reducing the response of spinal dorsal horn neurons to noxious knee joint rotation in the monosodium iodoacetate (MIA) sensitized rat. The overall objective for these experiments was to develop a high quality *in vivo* electrophysiology assay to confidently test novel compounds for efficacy against pain. Given the recent calls for improved preclinical experimental quality we also developed and implemented an Assay Capability Tool to determine the quality of our assay and ensure the quality of our results. Spinal dorsal horn neurons receiving input from the hind limb knee joint were recorded in anesthetized rats 14 days after they were sensitized with 1 mg of MIA. Intravenous administered oxycodone and naproxen were each tested separately for their effects on phasic, tonic, ongoing and afterdischarge action potential counts in response to innocuous and noxious knee joint rotation. Oxycodone reduced tonic spike counts more than the other measures, doing so by up to 85%. Tonic counts were therefore designated the primary endpoint when testing naproxen which reduced counts by up to 81%. Both reductions occurred at doses consistent with clinically effective doses for osteoarthritis. These results demonstrate that clinically effective doses of standard treatments for osteoarthritis reduce pain processing measured at the level of the spinal cord for two different mechanisms. The Assay Capability Tool helped to guide experimental design leading to a high quality and robust preclinical assay to use in discovering novel treatments for pain.

Editor: Theodore John Price, University of Texas at Dallas, United States of America

Funding: All work was funded by Pfizer LTD. Pfizer LTD. provided support in the form of salaries for all authors, but did not have any additional role in the study design, data collection and analysis, decision to publish, or preparation of the manuscript. The specific roles of these authors are articulated in the 'author contributions' section.

Competing Interests: All work was funded by Pfizer LTD., the employer of all authors. There are no patents, products in development or marketed products to declare. This does not alter the authors' adherence to all the PLOS ONE policies on sharing data and materials, as detailed online in the guide for authors.

* Email: jason.miranda2@pfizer.com

Introduction

Knee joint pain processing

Highly characterized animal models of pain sensitization are employed to study pain mechanisms and aid the discovery of novel clinical treatments. Although the relevance of studying mechanisms of human disease in rodents is in question [1,2], many of the fundamental mechanisms underlying pain processing are consistent across vertebrates [3,4]. This is particularly true for sensitized articular tissue and several models attempt to recapitulate symptoms of osteoarthritis including pain [5–7]. In particular, 30–40% of knee joint afferents in the rat and cat contain important modulators of pain and hyperalgesia, such as calcitonin gene-related peptide and substance P [8–10]. Joint afferents also have a higher proportion of high threshold and 'silent' C-fiber afferents [11], which can develop increased mechanical sensitivity when sensitized. Moreover, sensitization is required for many analgesics to be effective against noxious stimulation [12–14] suggesting that these abundant afferents are important in pain processing. Together, this suggests that models of articular sensitization may inform not only drug discovery for joint pain but also general pain mechanisms.

The rat monosodium iodoacetate (MIA) model of knee joint sensitization is one of the most extensively characterized in terms of pain behavior and peripheral physiology. MIA intra-articular injection results in large reductions in weight bearing on the sensitized limb and spontaneous mobility that persist beyond 14 days [15–17]. Consistent with these behavioral changes, C-fiber primary afferents show increased sustained action potential firing in response to noxious joint rotation and compression as well as increased spontaneous firing [12,18]. These patterns of response are common to other knee joint sensitization methods [19,20] as is sustained spiking activity after noxious stimulation has ended [21–23] which is hypothesized to be due to sustained C-fiber activity. MIA sensitized neural responses are also susceptible to pharmacological modulation [12–14].

Despite the characterization of knee joint pain processing in the periphery of sensitized rats, very little is known about the state of processing in the spinal dorsal horn. Cellular and molecular changes do occur in the spinal cord such as increases in COX-1/-2 [24], proinflammatory cytokines [25], pain related neuropeptides [26,27], activation of mitogen activated protein kinases [28] and microglial activation [29–31], suggesting that pain processing in the spinal cord is important to the behavioral effects in this model. Wide dynamic range neurons receiving direct input from the MIA sensitized knee joint have shown increased spontaneous spiking activity [13] but the majority of spinal cord physiology studies focus on secondary sensitization arising in the ipsilateral paw [32,33]. Here we report a test of the prediction that two clinically effective compounds, naproxen (an NSAID) and oxycodone (an opiate), are efficacious in reducing the response of spinal dorsal horn neurons to noxious knee joint rotation in the MIA sensitized rat. The objective for these experiments was to develop a high quality *in vivo* electrophysiology assay to confidently test novel compounds for efficacy against pain.

Assessing experimental quality and assay capability

Recent publications have established there is a high risk of experimental bias and irreproducibility in the majority of preclinical research areas, including pain [34–39]. Recommendations for experimental design and reporting have been proposed by the Collaborative Approach to Meta-analysis and Review of Animal Data in Experimental Studies (CAMARADES) [40], the US National Institute for Neurological Disorders and Stroke [41] and the ARRIVE guidelines from the National Centre for the Replacement, Refinement & Reduction of Animals in Research [42]. Adopting these recommendations may also reduce both animal use and the cost of research projects while at the same time increasing confidence in results [43]. This highlights a clear need for a comprehensive tool to guide experimental design and reporting and, ultimately, standardization across preclinical research. We have designed and implemented a broadly applicable tool, the "Assay Capability Tool" (ACT), to guide the development and assess the quality of our drug discovery assays and exploratory experiments in pain physiology. The ACT complements the ARRIVE reporting guidelines by addressing issues of data quality and reproducibility.

Two issues must be addressed to ensure rigorous and repeatable experiments and/or assays: 1) unbiased experimental design and conduct and 2) adequate reporting. Here we report the results from two separate experiments aimed at addressing these issues. Recent meta-analyses in several research disciplines have highlighted a common failure to use key experimental design components that help guard against biased results [34–38,44,45] including allocation concealment, random experimental treatment allocation, sample size calculation, blinded outcome assessment and replication. In addition, commonly used methods for statistical interpretation of treatment effects are at high risk of introducing bias [46,47]. Second, several groups have called for improved reporting standards to improve reproducibility, rigorous assessment of results and efficient use of animals [41,42,48,49]. A broadly applicable tool would need to incorporate both of these aspects. Using the ACT led to the foundation of a robust assay in which to test novel compounds for preclinical efficacy and its broader implementation may help guide the standardization of experimental quality across preclinical research.

Methods

Experimental animals

Adult male Sprague Dawley rats were ordered from Charles River (Margate, UK), housed in groups of four and given five days to acclimate to the housing facility. Environmental conditions were a temperature of 21°C ±2°, humidity of 55% ±10%, lighting of 350 lux (at bench level) and a 12:12 light:dark cycle with lights on at 0700 and off at 1900. Animals were housed in 595×380×200 mm cages (Techniplast UK, 1354G Eurostandard Type IV) and given access to rat maintenance food (#801002 RMI [E] Diet, Special Diet Services, Witham, UK) and water *ad libitum*. Environmental enrichment included bedding (LBS, Litaspen Premium B6 grade), one red tinted guinea pig hut (Bio-Serv, cat# K3261), one 10 mm×10 mm ×50 mm aspen chew block (LBS, cat# 011590) and one handful of paper wool nesting material (LBS, cat# 033801). During housing, animals were monitored twice daily for health status. No adverse events were observed. At the start of the experiments animals weighed (mean±SD) 202±14 grams. Both the oxycodone and naproxen studies were each conducted using 23 animals with one cell recorded per animal (n = 12 saline versus n = 11 oxycodone and n = 11 saline versus n = 12 naproxen). One animal from each experiment was excluded due to poor electrophysiological isolation of the focal neuron during the recording. The experimenters were blinded to the pharmacological treatment while processing data and making exclusion decisions. All procedures were carried out under an approved Home Office project license (number PPL 80/2578) and in accordance with the Animals (Scientific Procedures) Act, 1986 (UK) (amended 2013). All sections of this report adhere to the ARRIVE Guidelines for reporting animal research [42]. A completed ARRIVE guidelines checklist is included in Checklist S1.

Animal preparation

Rats were anesthetized with a 3% isoflurane O_2 mixture and given a single intra-articular injection of monosodium iodoacetate (MIA, Batch # 021M5300V, Sigma-Aldrich Company Ltd., Dorset, UK) through the infrapatellar ligament of the left knee. The MIA was dissolved in 0.9% sterile saline at 0.04 mg/µl, made up immediately before injection and administered in a volume of 25 µl (1 mg per knee). Animals were returned to the home cage until the day of electrophysiological recording, which was 14–17 days post MIA injection (Figure 1A). Previously this protocol has been shown to sensitize knee joint afferents and induce pain behavior [16,17,50,51].

After 14–17 days rats were anesthetized with isoflurane (induction 5% in O_2 at 4 L/min; reduced to 2.5–3% in O_2 for surgery at a flow rate of 1 L/min). Cannulae (Portex fine bore polyethylene tubing, 0.5 mm ID, 1 mm OD), were inserted into the right jugular vein and carotid artery. The jugular vein cannula was used for administration of compounds and the carotid cannula allowed both recording of blood pressure and blood sampling for PK analysis. The carotid cannula was pre filled with heparinized

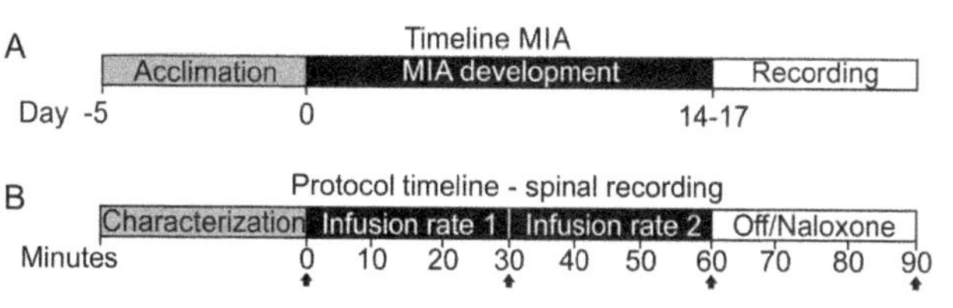

Figure 1. Experimental timelines. (A) MIA Sensitization timeline with recording on a single day between 14–17 days post injection (B) Protocol on the day of recording. Black arrows denote time points at which dried blood spot samples were taken for drug exposure measurement.

saline (250 units/ml) to prevent clotting. Body temperature was maintained throughout the surgery and recording session at 37°C using a homeothermic blanket system (#507221F, Harvard Apparatus Ltd., Kent, UK).

To expose the dorsal spinal cord, an incision was made in the skin on the back of the animal midway between the shoulders and pelvis and the muscle attachments to the dorsal and lateral spinal process cut. The bone was then firmly clamped with lateral bars placed between the dorsolateral and ventrolateral spinal processes at the level of the lumbar enlargement to stabilize the cord for recording. The L3-L5 lumbar cord was exposed by laminectomy, the skin was raised and secured and the cavity filled with warm (37°C) mineral oil (#330779, Sigma-Aldrich Co. Ltd, Dorset, UK) to prevent the exposed tissue from drying out, after which the dura mater was removed.

To stabilize the knee joint for rotation, an incision was made in the skin over the femur of the MIA injected knee and the muscle separated from the femur by blunt dissection. The femur was then clamped to isolate movement to the knee joint during rotation. Once the femur was secured, the isoflurane anesthesia was reduced and maintained at 1.5–2% in O_2 at a flow rate of 1 L/min during the recording session.

Electrophysiology recording

Single-unit activity of dorsal horn neurons responding to outward rotation of the knee joint was recorded using fine tungsten microelectrodes (2–5 MΩ, #573200 and #575300, A-M Systems, Sequim, WA). Signals were amplified (head stage NL100, A.C. Preamp NL104, Digitimer Ltd, Welwyn Garden City, UK), low pass filtered at 5 kHz (Neurolog NL125/126, Digitimer), passed through a 50/60 Hz noise eliminator (Humbug, Quest Scientific Instruments Inc., Vancouver, BC), digitized at 20 kHz sampling frequency (CED1401, Cambridge Electronic Designs, Cambridge, UK) and stored on a computer for offline analysis. All of the cells that responded to joint rotation could be activated by firm pressure applied to the joint with a pair of forceps, and this was used as a search stimulus to identify appropriate cells and check that activity was generated primarily from the knee and not the ankle joint. Once an acceptable cell was identified, the left foot was secured in a custom-made protractor device with tissue glue and Micropore Medical tape. Responses were characterized to clockwise rotation of the protractor (outward rotation), which requires more torque per degree, allowing for noxious stimulation at lower angles when compared to inward rotation [52].

All cells that showed some degree of tonic firing on knee rotation and where the knee could be rotated up to 40° beyond the tonic firing threshold were included in the experiment. In any one electrophysiological recording the first cell that responded in this manner was chosen for study irrespective of any other considerations, i.e. presence or absence of baseline activity or any afterdischarge following rotation. After starting the recording, cells were left for two minutes to settle, the foot and knee were then rotated at 20° increasing increments for eight seconds each to establish the tonic spiking activity threshold and therefore defined the range of the rotation stimulus set that extended up to 40° beyond the threshold. Tonic spiking threshold was determined as the lowest rotation angle that elicited at least five spikes occurring during the first six seconds of the rotation after subtracting phasic spiking occurring during the first one second. Ten minutes later, a rotation set was completed in 20° increments up to 40° beyond the tonic spiking threshold to establish the baseline (0 minute time point). Drug or vehicle infusion was then started and rotation sets completed at 10 minute intervals for a further 90 minutes.

Study conduct

The assay development and study conduct were guided by a novel Assay Capability Tool (ACT). The tool consists of 13 questions and a summary assessment of the experimental capability. Table 1 provides the questions along with explanations of the necessity for each component. The questions are grouped into three sets aimed to address: 1) the alignment of assay capability to the research objectives, 2) managing variation and 3) ensuring objectivity in the conduct of the study. The ACT was used to influence the methodological development of the assay and Table 2 provides the assessment of the experiments in this manuscript.

Randomization and blinding are essential components of good study conduct. A randomized drug and vehicle administration schedule was created using the standard = RAND() function in Microsoft Excel. In an effort to reduce animal use in the long term, randomization was done in two separate blocks, with half the drug and control animals randomly allocated to the first block and half to the second. At the end of block one, data were processed and unblinded to determine whether the whole experiment was likely to be futile. This is akin to futility assessment in clinical trials except that, instead of predetermining strict futility criteria, we simply looked for a complete lack of evidence of an effect. Since we did not see this in either of these experiments we continued with the second randomized and blinded blocks. Coded vials containing the treatment were prepared by a third person not involved in the experiment to maintain blinding.

Drug administration protocols

Figure 1B illustrates the timeline for pharmacological treatments. Rats were i.v. infused with 0.3 mg/ml oxycodone hydrochloride (Sigma-Aldrich Co. LTD, cat# O1378-500MG) dissolved in 0.9% saline, at 0.67 ml/kg/hr for 30 minutes followed by 2 ml/kg/hr for 30 minutes. This infusion protocol was chosen to deliver the highest dose that did not cause severe respiratory depression and fell within the range of clinical plasma concentrations [53]. Vehicle control animals received the same infusion rates with 0.9% saline. During the final 30 minutes, animals randomized to the oxycodone group were infused with 10 mg/ml naloxone hydrochloride (Sigma, cat#N7758-250MG) dissolved in 0.9% saline, at 2 ml/kg/hr for 30 minutes. Animals randomized to the vehicle group were administered saline during the final 30 minutes. The experimenter was blinded to both phases of the treatment. This dose was chosen to ensure a level known to antagonize the antinociceptive effects of oxycodone while avoiding the known antinociceptive effects of Naloxone at low doses [54,55]. Vehicle control animals received the same infusion rates with 0.9% saline.

Naproxen sodium (Sigma, cat# M1275-5G) was administered at 1.5 mg/ml i.v. dissolved in 0.9% saline, at 1 ml/kg/hr for 30 minutes followed by 2 ml/kg/hr for 30 minutes followed by no infusion for 30 minutes. This dose was chosen to produce an unbound plasma concentration consistent with clinical exposures [56]. Vehicle control animals received the same infusion rates with 0.9% saline.

PK analysis

In both experiments, 30 μl blood spots were taken at 0, 30, 60 and 90 minutes for blood concentration analysis by Unilabs York Bioanalytical Solutions (Sandwich, UK) using mass spectrometry. Working solutions were prepared in 25% acetonitrile and used to spike sufficient calibration samples and QC samples in blank fresh rat blood. Calibration samples were prepared to generate a calibration line from 1–1000 ng/ml and QC samples were

Table 1. Assay Capability Tool.

Question to consider:	Why it is important:		
Aligning Assay Capability with Project Objectives			
Q1: Are the scientific objectives for running the assay recorded in a protocol/SOP?	The scientific questions to be answered, the measurements to be obtained and analyzed along with their required precision (as defined by, for example, a standard error or confidence limits) must be stated in the protocol/SOP to prevent data dredging and misinterpretation of the results.		
Q2: What will a successful assay outcome look like in order to guide decision making?	Pre-specifying decision criteria leads to clear decisions and ensures unbiased interpretation of results. A target value should be stated for the primary endpoint. Since all assay results include inherent uncertainty, pre-defining what a successful outcome will look like requires a pre-specified level of uncertainty that can be tolerated for acceptable decision making.		
Q3: Is the experimental design, as described in the protocol/SOP, aligned closely with the objectives?	Is the experimental design and conduct capable of achieving results that meet the objectives? The design and conduct should be revisited in light of current/changing objectives. Once the objectives and definitions of success are defined, consultation with a statistician is essential to ensure the assay is appropriate.		
Enabling Assay Capability by Managing Variation			
Q4: Are the assay's development and validation fully documented?	What work has been done in order to verify that an assay is fit for purpose? The answer should identify key lessons/issues/concerns arising from experiments done while the assay was being developed. Assay developers should document validation runs using positive and negative controls and tool compounds to provide benchmarks and reassurance to the users of the resulting data.		
Q5: Have the sources of variability present in the assay been explored?	All assays exhibit variability and it is important to know what the sources of variability are and their relative sizes. The major sources of variation and the statistical methods that will be used for their control should be summarized in the assay protocol. Understanding and controlling sources of variability in an assay are critical to achieving required precision as captured in the standard errors and confidence intervals for key endpoints.		
Q6: Is the proposed sample size/level of replication fit for purpose?	An assay that enables a clear decision requires sufficient, but not excessive, precision. Sample size should always be based on what is known about the assay's variability in the laboratory where it will be run and the quantitative definition of what a successful assay outcome will look like. Relying on historical precedent or published values should not be the default strategy.		
Q7: Is there a comprehensive protocol/SOP detailing study objectives, key endpoints, experimental design, methods of analysis and a timetable of activities?	A comprehensive assay protocol supports efficient decisions by specifying the methods to be used to control variation (e.g. randomization, blocking, use of covariates and blinding). It helps to ensure uniformity in assay execution resulting in assay results that are reproducible and comparable from one run to another. It promotes transparency by documenting the actual conditions of the assay. This helps decision makers interpret the results.		
Q8: How is assay performance monitored over time? What is the plan for reacting to signs of instability?	Repeated assay use should be tracked to detect changing conditions that may affect the interpretation of results and to understand the natural variability of the assay. Quality control (QC) charts are available to monitor the assay consistency of controls, standard or tool compounds over time. Ongoing monitoring is necessary to understand any changes and their implications for interpreting the results and to trigger remediation when necessary.		
Objectivity in Assay Conduct			
Q9: Are inclusion/exclusion criteria for the assay specified in the protocol/SOP?	Criteria for the inclusion/exclusion of animals, cells, etc. in an assay should be pre-defined and clearly stated in the protocol/SOP. This ensures all the appropriate data are collected and eliminates selection bias.		
Q10: Is the management of subjectivity in data collection and reporting defined in the protocol/SOP?	There is a need to ensure, through the use of randomization and blinding, that the scientist remains unaware of the treatment that the animal has received. Even when the assay measurement is obtained automatically without human intervention there is possibility for bias, and randomization is essential and blinding is highly recommended. Studies of a long duration should be done in blocks to ensure that no bias is introduced by changing conditions over time.		
Q11: If the raw data are processed (e.g. by summarization or normalization) prior to analysis, is the method for doing this specified in the study protocol/SOP?	Methods of processing raw data prior to statistical analysis should be clearly stated in the assay protocol/SOP. For example, is it the raw response data, change from baseline or log transformed data that are to be analyzed; or are the raw data summarized into an area under the curve or average? This ensures that assay methods and results can be reproduced and validated.		
Q12: Are rules for treating data as outliers in the analysis specified in the protocol/SOP?	Rules for treating data as outliers should be clearly stated in the assay protocol/SOP. Rules should be in place for the removal of individual data points, whole animals and dose groups as required. This ensures all the appropriate data are analyzed and eliminates selection bias.		
Q13: Is the analysis specified in the study protocol/SOP? Is it fit for purpose?	The statistical analysis must reflect the study design and assay objectives. Inappropriate analyses can result in misleading conclusions and a false sense of precision. The analysis must incorporate the structure of the data and consultation with a statistician is essential to model the experimental structure appropriately.		
Summary			
	Aligning Assay Capability with Project Objectives	**Enabling Assay Capability by Managing Variation**	**Objectivity in Assay Conduct**
Confidence for decision making	Low/Medium/High	Low/Medium/High	Low/Medium/High
Assay Capability Tool Summary	Summarize the evidence for an overall confidence rating in this assay for a given experiment		
Technical specification			
Target value	Required effect size for decision making		
Required precision	Depends on the identified acceptable level of risk for a given project		
Required replication	Based on a sample size calculation using data from previous experiments or a pilot study		

prepared at 5, 50 and 500 ng/ml. A 5000 ng/ml QC was additionally run diluted 7.2 fold within the assay batch. Mass spectrometry was performed on an API5000, with oxycodone monitored using m/z 316.2–241.2 DP 90 CE 39 and naproxen monitored using m/z 231.1–185.1 DP 100 CE 22. Samples were injected (20 μl) into an HPLC-MS/MS system with oxycodone resolved on a Zorbax XDB-C18 50×3 mm 1.8U column and naproxen resolved on an Accucore Polar Premium 50×3 mm 2.6 U column.

Data processing and analysis

As part of the assay development, four endpoints were measured in the oxycodone experiment: the phasic spike count during the first one second of joint rotation, the tonic spike count during the subsequent six seconds of joint rotation, the ongoing spike count occurring during the 120 seconds preceding the first rotation of a stimulus set, and the afterdischarge spike count 120 seconds following the offset of the last rotation in a stimulus set. Since these responses are counts, they are not normally distributed and the natural log (ln(x+1) to overcome counts of zero) was used to stabilize the variances and reduce the asymmetry of the distributions. All analyses were performed on the log transformed counts, fitting a one-way analysis of covariance using the 0 minute rotation set as the covariate. The results are presented as geometric means, ratios of geometric means and 95% confidence interval estimates of the ratios.

Inferences were made from individual analyses of covariance performed at the 30, 60, and 90 minute rotation sets separately using the 0 minute trial as the covariate. These rotation set time points were identified *a priori* as they represent the end of the separate drug infusions and therefore the time of maximum drug exposure. All analyses were carried out using GenStat Version 11 (VSN International Ltd, Hemel Hempstead, UK).

Results

Oxycodone experiment

This was an exploratory experiment with the goal of identifying an appropriate primary endpoint and understanding the interplay between spike reduction and assay variation. Spinal dorsal horn neurons were selected from L3-L4 when they responded predominantly to knee joint rotation. Response types were heterogeneous in their firing patterns. Figure 2 shows three distinct and common response types: high threshold cells with no baseline activity or afterdischarge following the stimulation (Figure 2A), cells with low threshold onset to a rotational force with distinct afterdischarge outlasting the stimulus (Figure 2B), and low threshold cells with ongoing baseline activity (Figure 2C). In general, threshold was not correlated with either the presence or absence of baseline firing or prolonged responses to stimulation, and there were too few cells in this study to determine whether these represented distinct cell types responding to joint rotation.

Mean spike count profiles, adjusted for baseline spike count, suggest that oxycodone reduced spike counts in all four endpoints when compared to vehicle controls (Figure 3). Comparing the two groups at the end of each infusion using ratios of geometric means for oxycodone to vehicle and 95% confidence intervals showed that these effects were statistically significant ($p<0.05$) for tonic responses at the 60 minute rotation set where the unbound plasma concentration of oxycodone reached a mean peak of 217±24 nM (mean±sem) (Figure 3A). The ratio showed an effect size of 0.15 (85% reduction) for tonic spike count. These effects were partially reversed by the addition of naloxone, with statistically non-significant differences between the vehicle and oxycodone/

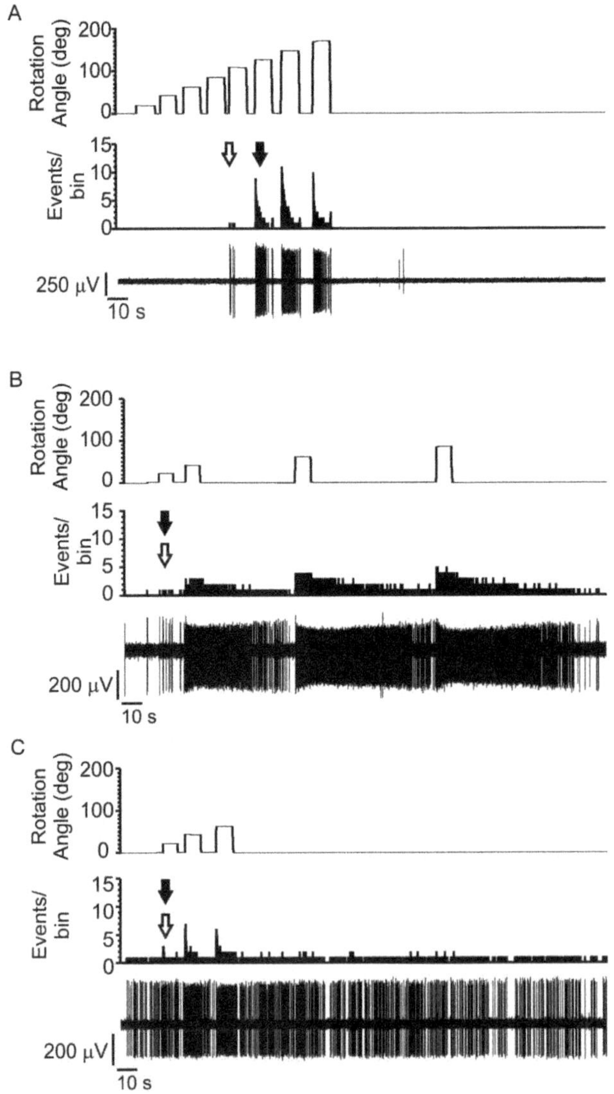

Figure 2. Spinal cord neuron responses to knee joint rotation. For each of (A), (B) and (C) the top trace shows the rotation stimulus set with rotation angle increasing in 20 degree steps and extending at least 40 degrees above the tonic firing threshold. The middle trace shows the PSTH of the response to the rotation set. White arrow denotes phasic threshold, black arrow denotes tonic threshold and bin width = 0.05 ms. The bottom trace shows the neural waveform during the joint rotation stimulus set. (A) Response from a cell showing no ongoing spike activity and high response threshold (B) A cell showing little ongoing spike activity, low threshold and extended firing after stimulus offset (C) A cell showing high ongoing spike activity with a low response threshold.

naloxone groups at the end of the naloxone infusion (90 minute time point).

Three of the 11 animals in the oxycodone group showed complete respiratory arrest before the end of the 60 minute trial where plasma levels were highest. In all cases, respiration was recovered by administering naloxone resulting in missing data points for the 60 minute trial. To determine whether the inclusion of these animals in the analysis resulted in a bias toward a larger effect size in earlier trials, we excluded all data from the three animals and reanalyzed the data. The removal of these data points did not change the effect size but the reduction in sample size did reduce statistical power and thus the 95% confidence intervals

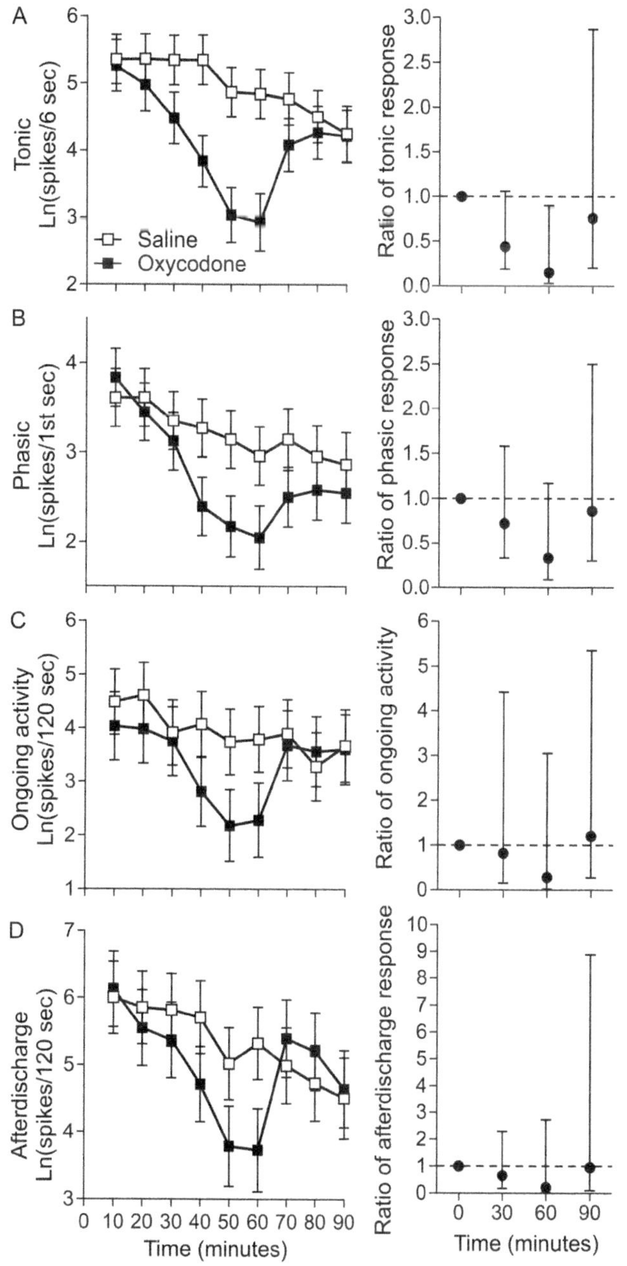

Figure 3. Effects of oxycodone on spinal dorsal horn neuronal activity. Each row shows the results for an exploratory endpoint with ANCOVA adjusted means on the left (error bars ± sem) and the ratios of adjusted means for oxycodone/saline on the right (error bars ±95%CI). Ratio graphs focus on 0, 30, 60 and 90 minutes, the time points at which a following cohort of animals was determined to have (mean±sem) 0±0 nM, 44±6 nM, 217±24 nM and 70±12 nM free plasma concentration of oxycodone respectively. The 90 minute time point is after a 30 minute infusion of 20 mg/kg/hr naloxone with no oxycodone infused. (A) tonic spike count during the six seconds following phasic spiking (B) phasic spiking during the first one second after rotation onset (C) ongoing activity quantified during the 120 seconds preceding each stimulus set (D) afterdischarge during the 120 seconds following the last rotation of each set.

were wider (data not shown). Since effect size was not impacted for earlier trials, data from these animals were included in the analysis. This study was used to estimate the within cell and between cell variability which was used to estimate the sample size required to detect oxycodone-like effects in future studies.

Naproxen experiment

This experiment followed the same methods as the oxycodone study. As with oxycodone, baseline adjusted mean spike count profiles suggest that naproxen reduced spike counts in all four endpoints when compared to vehicle controls (Figure 4), but tonic spike activity during joint rotation was designated as the primary endpoint. This was due to the observation that tonic spiking was associated with increased rotation angle into the noxious range and was the measure most affected by oxycodone treatment. Comparing the two groups at the end of each infusion using ratios of geometric means for naproxen to vehicle and 95% confidence intervals show that these effects were nearly statistically significant for the 60 minute rotation set where unbound plasma concentration of naproxen reached a mean peak of 697±45 nM (Figure 4B). When the i.v. infusion was turned off for 30 minutes, mean plasma concentration reduced to 567±34 nM and the reduced tonic spiking was statistically significant ($p<0.05$) at the 90 minute rotation set with ratios showing an effect size of 0.19 or an 81% reduction. Unlike for oxycodone, naproxen treatment significantly reduced ($p<0.05$) spike counts for all three secondary endpoints at the 90 minute rotation set (Figure 4).

Discussion

The overall objective for these experiments was to develop a high quality *in vivo* electrophysiology assay to confidently test novel compounds for efficacy against pain. Assay development is an evolving process of experimentation and refinement. The experimental methods and results presented here were developed under the guidance of a novel tool, the Assay Capability Tool (ACT), to strive for the highest possible standards of experimental conduct. The ACT was developed to guide both the development of assays and the assessment of their capability to generate reliable data. The tool is particularly useful in standardizing decision making in drug discovery but can also be applied to published experiments. This aids in the estimation of the confidence one can have in the validity of the results and guides follow-up studies.

We started by running a small pilot study with oxycodone to assess whether this model was able to detect electrophysiological changes following drug administration. This pilot study indicated that the experimental approach was viable (data not shown). We then moved on to test novel predictions about the efficacy of oxycodone and naproxen, two clinical standards of care for knee joint pain, which have differing mechanisms of action. Our next experiment was designed to further explore the role of oxycodone versus vehicle-treated controls in modulating sensitized knee joint rotation processing in the spinal cord. This provided the information to design a follow-up study to test the validity of tonic spiking activity as a primary endpoint and to test the role of naproxen.

In the oxycodone experiment, our objective was to test predictions about the role of opioid receptors in modulating four knee joint rotation response types, each with their own putative underlying physiological mechanisms. Although phasic, ongoing, and afterdischarge spiking did show reductions at 0.3 mg/kg oxycodone, the high levels of variation in the effects do not provide evidence for a strong role of opioid receptors in modulating the mechanisms underlying these responses. Tonic spike counts showed a mean reduction of 85% with 0.3 mg/kg oxycodone. Given that tonic spiking profiles in the spinal cord are consistent with the coding of stimulus intensity, these results suggest that

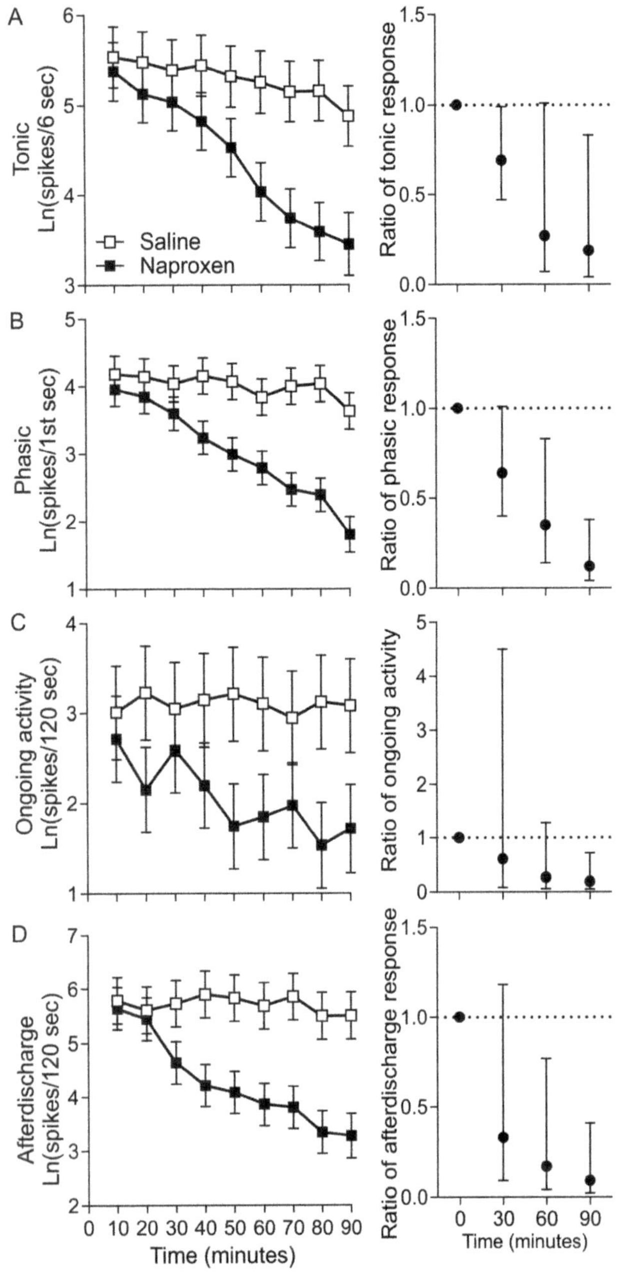

Figure 4. Effects of naproxen on spinal dorsal horn neuronal activity. Each row shows the results for an exploratory endpoint with ANCOVA adjusted means on the left (error bars ± sem) and the ratios of adjusted means for naproxen/saline on the right (error bars ±95%CI). Ratio graphs focus on 0, 30, and 60 minutes, the time points at which these animals were determined to have (mean±sem) 0±0 nM, 165±28 nM and 697±45 nM free plasma concentration of naproxen respectively and 90 minutes which is after 30 minutes of no infusion resulting in 567±34 nM free plasma concentration. (A) tonic spike count during the six seconds following phasic spiking (B) phasic spiking during the first one second after rotation onset (C) ongoing activity quantified during the 120 seconds preceding each stimulus set and (D) afterdischarge during the 120 seconds following the last rotation of each set.

opioid receptors play a strong role in modulating this coding, particularly in the noxious range. Surprisingly, no study to our knowledge has tested the effects of oxycodone against a physiological endpoint in the spinal cord, where cognitive confounds are eliminated. Nonetheless, these results are consistent with the clinical effectiveness of oxycodone in joint pain. Oxycodone is likely acting on the central nervous system as opposed to peripheral nerves since μ-opioid receptor numbers are severely reduced in sensitized rat knee joints [57]. Whether this reduction occurs in MIA sensitized joints and which opioid receptor subtypes contribute to the oxycodone effect is not known.

Comparisons between clinical and preclinical effective doses depend on differences between route of administration and potential interactions between drug effects and the anaesthetic. Despite these complications, our effective doses are either consistent with or below those in clinical and preclinical behavioral studies. For oxycodone, similar magnitude reductions have been reported in rat behavioral pain assays that require much higher doses of between 4–10 mg/kg [58–60]. Our doses, and resulting plasma concentration levels, are comparable to maximum doses administered to humans [61–63] whereas doses in most behavioral assays are much higher and overlap with severe adverse events in rats such as loss of righting reflex and catalepsy [60]. One exception is that for pain assessed by observing spontaneous behavior, such as vertical activity (rearing), other opiates show efficacy at lower doses compared to evoked behavior such as paw withdrawal [51]. This suggests that careful consideration must be made when attempting to make clinically effective dose predictions from preclinical data and that behavioral and physiological data together may better determine the validity of those predictions.

The results of this experiment also provided information to answer important questions raised in the ACT. Often in preclinical research, exploratory work must be done to adequately answer most of the questions in the ACT. At this stage, the ACT guides experimental design to incorporate components that increase confidence in the data generated in the experiments. This starts with a clearly stated scientific objective and associated experimental methods (Table 1; Q1, Q3) as well as methods to manage subjectivity in data collection and reporting, such as allocation concealment, and adhering to the ARRIVE guidelines (Q10). However, it was difficult in the oxycodone experiment to ensure that the experimenter was blind to the treatment where noticeable effects on respiratory rate were evident in some cases and respiratory rate is monitored to assess adequacy of anesthesia.

The oxycodone experiment was also designed to produce data that allowed for the first analysis of effect size for future decision-making (Q2), experimental variability (Q5), sample size calculations (Q6), primary endpoint determination (Q7) and appropriate data analysis methods (Q9, Q11, Q12). More specifically, we had evidence that tonic spiking was an appropriate primary endpoint and that an 85% reduction would resemble an oxycodone-like effect. We also determined that the statistical structure of data sets from this type of experiment require natural log transformation, analysis of covariance (ANCOVA) baseline correction and a simpler statistical model that does not rely on potentially misleading estimations (Q13).

To identify the most appropriate statistical analysis method, an initial exploratory analysis was carried out using a repeated measures linear mixed effects model. This included data from all the rotation sets to explore the shape of the response to drug over time. The mixed model was fitted using residual (or restricted) maximum likelihood (REML) with between cell (one per animal) and between repeated measures within each cell as random effects; and treatment group, time, and the treatment by time interaction as fixed effects. The values at baseline (0 minute rotation set) were included as a covariate in the model to reduce the between cell estimate of variability. A heterogeneous first order autoregressive

Table 2. Assay Capability Tool applied to the joint rotation assay.

Question:	Response		
Aligning Assay Capability with Project Objectives			
Q1: Are the scientific objectives for running the assay recorded in a protocol/SOP?	See the Introduction section		
Q2: What will a successful assay outcome look like in order to guide decision making?	For the naproxen experiment, an effect size comparable to oxycodone was set as a criteria for success		
Q3: Is the experimental design, as described in the protocol/SOP, aligned closely with the objectives?	Experiment one, testing oxycodone, was designed as an exploratory test to determine what endpoints are appropriate and what effect size should be expected. Experiment two used the selected primary endpoint to test a different mechanism against the oxycodone benchmark.		
Enabling Assay Capability by Managing Variation			
Q4: Are the assay's development and validation fully documented?	Oxycodone effects are reported for exploratory endpoints along with rationale for the primary endpoint selection		
Q5: Have the sources of variability present in the assay been explored?	Variability in baseline responses is high across cells and potentially high across experimental groups.		
Q6: Is the proposed sample size/level of replication fit for purpose?	Sample size calculation for naproxen is based on an effect size comparable to oxycodone effects		
Q7: Is there a comprehensive protocol/SOP detailing study objectives, key endpoints, experimental design, methods of analysis and timetable of activities?	See the Methods section		
Q8: How is assay performance monitored over time? What is the plan for reacting to signs of instability?	Where this experimental design is used to test novel compounds, oxycodone or naproxen effects will be monitored as positive controls to track assay stability. First response will be to investigate known sources of variability including equipment calibration and inter-experimenter reliability.		
Objectivity in Assay Conduct			
Q9: Are inclusion/exclusion criteria for the assay specified in the protocol/SOP?	Cell inclusion/exclusion is documented in the methods section and is limited to recording quality, animal health and whether they respond to joint rotation within out testable parameters.		
Q10: Is the management of subjectivity in data collection and reporting defined in the protocol/SOP?	Random allocation to experimental groups, allocation concealment and blinded outcome assessment were implemented and documented as per Sena et al. 2007.		
Q11: If the raw data are processed (e.g. by summarization or normalization) prior to analysis, is the method for doing this specified in the study protocol/SOP?	Change from baseline calculations are performed using ANCOVA and adjusted means are reported. This is documented in the methods section.		
Q12: Are rules for treating data as outliers in the analysis specified in the protocol/SOP?	Outliers are identified as part of the statistical model fitting process and documented.		
Q13: Is the analysis specified in the study protocol/SOP? Is it fit for purpose?	A detailed analysis protocol is included in the methods section		
Summary			
	Aligning Assay Capability with Project Objectives	**Enabling Assay Capability by Managing Variation**	**Objectivity in Assay Conduct**
Confidence for decision making	High	High	High
Assay Capability Tool Summary	These experiments are fit for purpose and likely to produce repeatable and reliable data upon which to base further experiments or make preclinical drug research decisions.		
Technical specification			
Target value	Both oxycodone and naproxen showed a maximum ratio of approximately 0.2 (80% reduction) for the tonic response		
Required precision	95% confidence intervals around the ratio should not overlap with a ratio value of one.		
Required replication	Sample size calculations suggest approximately 19 replications per group. The addition of future experiments will increase the confidence in this estimate.		

correlation structure was used to model the within cell correlations allowing for unequal variances across the time points. An unstructured correlation matrix was also tried but the REML failed to converge. The heterogeneous first order autoregressive structure may be reasonable due to the equally spaced time points, but the quality of the fit and the assumptions made could not be tested or checked. The complexity of this model and the potential for misleading estimates of treatment means and standard errors [68,69] meant that it was unwise to make inferences from the model. ANCOVA was preferred to the less sophisticated, and potentially biased, methods of correcting for baseline such as percent change and subtraction as it uses the data to estimate the appropriate correction to minimize the residual variability [46,47]. The estimated means from the ANCOVA represent the expected response at a typical (average) baseline response, so all comparisons of means are 'corrected' for inequalities at baseline using this method. The separate analyses at the specified time points are preferred because they are less complex and are justified based on the comparisons of interest being specified *a priori*.

The estimated effect size and level of variability were used to estimate the required sample size for future studies. Despite finding a statistically significant reduction with 12 animals per group, the sample size estimation suggested that 19 animals would be required to be confident in detecting the same effect size in a follow up study. Balancing this fact with the desire to reduce the use of animals, we chose to continue with 12 animals per group for the naproxen study. At this point in the development of an assay sample sizing should only be viewed as a guide because the estimates of both the effect size and associated variability are approximate and come with much uncertainty attached to them.

The cell selection criteria for these experiments were intentionally broad with the only requirement being sustained spiking activity in response to knee joint rotation. We made no assumptions that a particular endpoint was more likely to be affected by the pharmacological treatments. This contributed to a high level of heterogeneity in response parameters such as response threshold, presence or absence of ongoing activity and degree of afterdischarge. Heterogeneous response types across cells suggest that different classes of cells exist with different mechanisms underlying their response properties. This leaves open the possibility that compounds acting on some mechanisms may only affect a subsample of cells. This could result in a bimodal distribution in the effectiveness of a given compound across cells that could in turn result in an equivocal outcome. We have yet to see such a pattern in response to either oxycodone or naproxen in subsequent runs of this assay. The sample size chosen for these experiments would not be adequate to confidently reveal effects on only a subset of cells but, if such a pattern emerged, a follow-up study would be required to confirm cell specific effects. Such a follow-up study would likely need a larger sample size or narrower cell selection criteria. As we continue to run these experiments to test novel compounds with naproxen and oxycodone as positive controls and saline as a negative control, we will collate a larger dataset with which to investigate the effects on particular cell responses using larger sample sizes. In future studies this may allow us to set cell selection criteria and appropriate sample sizes to test if novel compounds target specific cell types or mechanisms.

We are also performing an informal interim analysis for futility halfway through the experiment. When using such experiments as assays to discover novel therapies, this approach could result in a large reduction in animal use by stopping large studies that are very unlikely to produce positive evidence to support a hypothesis. This approach is in line with the guidelines of the National Centre for the Replacement, Refinement and Reduction of Animals in Research (London, UK).

Being guided by the ACT and the answers to its questions (as summarized in Table 2) informed the design and interpretation of the follow-up experiment with naproxen.

In the naproxen experiment, our objective was to test the prediction that COX-1/COX-2 inhibition reduces the primary endpoint of tonic spiking activity in response to noxious joint rotation. Tonic spike counts showed the largest mean reduction of 81% at 90 minutes after the start of the low dose infusion. This time point is 30 minutes after reaching the peak dose of 1.5 mg/kg (mean of 697 nM free plasma exposure) suggestive of possible hysteresis in this measurement for this mechanism. As with oxycodone, the results are consistent with the clinical effectiveness of naproxen in joint pain. In humans suffering from mild to moderate osteoarthritis, a similar magnitude in the reduction in pain scores has been reported with 5–15 mg/kg oral naproxen doses [64]. Differences in blood protein binding for naproxen between humans and rats [65,66], suggests that our i.v. administered dose produces unbound concentrations within the clinical therapeutic range. Furthermore, similar magnitude effects on weight distribution in MIA treated rats can be produced by oral doses between 5–18 mg/kg [17,50] which also appear to be similar to clinical exposures [67].

Given that different pharmacological mechanisms may affect different physiological responses, it is still of value to collect secondary exploratory measures although in future experiments all positive results would require follow up experiments. For the two experiments presented here, tonic spiking activity was the only endpoint that was modulated by both oxycodone and naproxen. Naproxen also significantly reduced measures of neuronal excitability with a large reduction in afterdischarge and a moderate reduction in ongoing activity. These two measures have been of interest when testing hypotheses about neuropathic pain and central sensitization [68,69]. Since they show particularly high variation across cells, a larger sample size may be required in order to provide a repeatable result if they are identified as a primary endpoint. In the current study, both measures suggest that naproxen may have an effect of reducing the neuronal excitability seen in sensitized pain conditions that warrants further investigation.

Data generated and knowledge gained from all preceding experiments is used in the ACT to define objectives and refine the experimental design and conduct of future studies. This report constitutes the documentation of the experimental design as a foundation for future use as an assay in drug discovery (Q4). Lastly, by including in future experiments at least one of the two compounds tested here along with tests of vehicle, we can monitor assay stability over time to detect any unanticipated variability (Q8). This will ensure that the data produced from this assay in the future will be reliable and directly comparable with previous data, and decisions can be made in the context of the whole experimental system rather than a single experiment.

We would recommend following a structured ACT to gain greater insight into the capability of an assay to better inform future experiments prior to their commencement, thus leading to decisions being made with higher confidence placed on the data generated.

Supporting Information

Checklist S1 Completed "The ARRIVE Guidelines Checklist" for reporting animal data in this manuscript.
(PDF)

Dataset S1 Oxycodone dataset for all endpoints.
(CSV)

Dataset S2 Naproxen dataset for all endpoints.
(CSV)

Acknowledgments

We would like to thank John Jinks for assistance with technical development of the experiments, Chloe Brown, Robyne Hudson and Karen Townson for technical assistance and Ed Kadyszewski for collaboration on the development of the ACT.

Author Contributions

Conceived and designed the experiments: JAM HR PS KG. Performed the experiments: JAM JT HR. Analyzed the data: JAM PS. Contributed reagents/materials/analysis tools: JAM PS. Contributed to the writing of the manuscript: JAM PS KG HR RD.

References

1. Seok J, Warren HS, Cuenca AG, Mindrinos MN, Baker HV, et al. (2013) Genomic responses in mouse models poorly mimic human inflammatory diseases. Proc Natl Acad Sci U S A 110: 3507–3512.
2. van der Worp HB, Howells DW, Sena ES, Porritt MJ, Rewell S, et al. (2010) Can animal models of disease reliably inform human studies? PLoS Med 7: e1000245.
3. Smith ES, Lewin GR (2009) Nociceptors: a phylogenetic view. J Comp Physiol A Neuroethol Sens Neural Behav Physiol 195: 1089–1106.
4. Walters ET (1996) Comparative and evolutionary aspects of nociceptor function. In: C Belmonte and F Cervero, editors. Neurobiology of Nociceptors Oxford, UK: Oxford University Press. pp. 92–114.
5. Malfait AM, Little CB, McDougall JJ (2013) A commentary on modelling osteoarthritis pain in small animals. Osteoarthritis Cartilage 21: 1316–1326.
6. Gregory MH, Capito N, Kuroki K, Stoker AM, Cook JL, et al. (2012) A review of translational animal models for knee osteoarthritis. Arthritis 2012: 764621.
7. Zhang RX, Ren K, Dubner R (2013) Osteoarthritis pain mechanisms: basic studies in animal models. Osteoarthritis Cartilage 21: 1308–1315.
8. Salo PT, Theriault E (1997) Number, distribution and neuropeptide content of rat knee joint afferents. J Anat 190 (Pt 4): 515–522.
9. Hanesch U, Heppelmann B, Schmidt RF (1991) Substance P- and calcitonin gene-related peptide immunoreactivity in primary afferent neurons of the cat's knee joint. Neuroscience 45: 185–193.
10. O'Brien C, Woolf CJ, Fitzgerald M, Lindsay RM, Molander C (1989) Differences in the chemical expression of rat primary afferent neurons which innervate skin, muscle or joint. Neuroscience 32: 493–502.
11. Michaelis M, Habler HJ, Jaenig W (1996) Silent afferents: a separate class of primary afferents? Clin Exp Pharmacol Physiol 23: 99–105.
12. Schuelert N, McDougall JJ (2009) Grading of monosodium iodoacetate-induced osteoarthritis reveals a concentration-dependent sensitization of nociceptors in the knee joint of the rat. Neurosci Lett 465: 184–188.
13. Chu KL, Chandran P, Joshi SK, Jarvis MF, Kym PR, et al. (2011) TRPV1-related modulation of spinal neuronal activity and behavior in a rat model of osteoarthritic pain. Brain Res 1369: 158–166.
14. Schuelert N, Johnson MP, Oskins JL, Jassal K, Chambers MG, et al. (2011) Local application of the endocannabinoid hydrolysis inhibitor URB597 reduces nociception in spontaneous and chemically induced models of osteoarthritis. Pain 152: 975–981.
15. Combe R, Bramwell S, Field MJ (2004) The monosodium iodoacetate model of osteoarthritis: a model of chronic nociceptive pain in rats? Neurosci Lett 370: 236–240.
16. Guingamp C, Gegout-Pottie P, Philippe L, Terlain B, Netter P, et al. (1997) Mono-iodoacetate-induced experimental osteoarthritis: a dose-response study of loss of mobility, morphology, and biochemistry. Arthritis Rheum 40: 1670–1679.
17. Rashid MH, Theberge Y, Elmes SJ, Perkins MN, McIntosh F (2013) Pharmacological validation of early and late phase of rat mono-iodoacetate model using the Tekscan system. Eur J Pain 17: 210–222.
18. Schuelert N, McDougall JJ (2008) Cannabinoid-mediated antinociception is enhanced in rat osteoarthritic knees. Arthritis Rheum 58: 145–153.
19. Coggeshall RE, Hong KA, Langford LA, Schaible HG, Schmidt RF (1983) Discharge characteristics of fine medial articular afferents at rest and during passive movements of inflamed knee joints. Brain Res 272: 185–188.
20. Richter F, Natura G, Ebbinghaus M, von Banchet GS, Hensellek S, et al. (2012) Interleukin-17 sensitizes joint nociceptors to mechanical stimuli and contributes to arthritic pain through neuronal interleukin-17 receptors in rodents. Arthritis Rheum 64: 4125–4134.
21. Grubb BD, Riley RC, Hope PJ, Pubols L, Duggan AW (1996) The burst-like firing of spinal neurons in rats with peripheral inflammation is reduced by an antagonist of N-methyl-D-aspartate. Neuroscience 74: 1077–1086.
22. Kim JH, Kim HY, Chung K, Chung JM (2011) Responses of spinal dorsal horn neurons to foot movements in rats with a sprained ankle. J Neurophysiol 105: 2043–2049.
23. Rahman W, Bauer CS, Bannister K, Vonsy JL, Dolphin AC, et al. (2009) Descending serotonergic facilitation and the antinociceptive effects of pregabalin in a rat model of osteoarthritic pain. Mol Pain 5: 45.
24. Prochazkova M, Zanvit P, Dolezal T, Prokesova L, Krsiak M (2009) Increased gene expression and production of spinal cyclooxygenase 1 and 2 during experimental osteoarthritis pain. Physiol Res 58: 419–425.
25. Im HJ, Kim JS, Li X, Kotwal N, Sumner DR, et al. (2010) Alteration of sensory neurons and spinal response to an experimental osteoarthritis pain model. Arthritis Rheum 62: 2995–3005.
26. Ferland CE, Laverty S, Beaudry F, Vachon P (2011) Gait analysis and pain response of two rodent models of osteoarthritis. Pharmacol Biochem Behav 97: 603–610.
27. Ferland CE, Pailleux F, Vachon P, Beaudry F (2011) Determination of specific neuropeptides modulation time course in a rat model of osteoarthritis pain by liquid chromatography ion trap mass spectrometry. Neuropeptides 45: 423–429.
28. Lee Y, Pai M, Brederson JD, Wilcox D, Hsieh G, et al. (2011) Monosodium iodoacetate-induced joint pain is associated with increased phosphorylation of mitogen activated protein kinases in the rat spinal cord. Mol Pain 7: 39.
29. Miller TR, Wetter JB, Jarvis MF, Bitner RS (2013) Spinal microglial activation in rat models of neuropathic and osteoarthritic pain: an autoradiographic study using [3H]PK11195. Eur J Pain 17: 692–703.
30. Orita S, Ishikawa T, Miyagi M, Ochiai N, Inoue G, et al. (2011) Pain-related sensory innervation in monoiodoacetate-induced osteoarthritis in rat knees that gradually develops neuronal injury in addition to inflammatory pain. BMC Musculoskelet Disord 12: 134.
31. Sagar DR, Burston JJ, Hathway GJ, Woodhams SG, Pearson RG, et al. (2011) The contribution of spinal glial cells to chronic pain behaviour in the monosodium iodoacetate model of osteoarthritic pain. Mol Pain 7: 88.
32. Thakur M, Rahman W, Hobbs C, Dickenson AH, Bennett DL (2012) Characterisation of a peripheral neuropathic component of the rat mono-iodoacetate model of osteoarthritis. PLoS One 7: e33730.
33. Harvey VL, Dickenson AH (2009) Behavioural and electrophysiological characterisation of experimentally induced osteoarthritis and neuropathy in C57Bl/6 mice. Mol Pain 5: 18.
34. Currie GL, Delaney A, Bennett MI, Dickenson AH, Egan KJ, et al. (2013) Animal models of bone cancer pain: Systematic review and meta-analyses. Pain 154: 917–926.
35. Button KS, Ioannidis JP, Mokrysz C, Nosek BA, Flint J, et al. (2013) Power failure: why small sample size undermines the reliability of neuroscience. Nat Rev Neurosci, 10.1038/nrn3475.
36. Vesterinen HM, Egan K, Deister A, Schlattmann P, Macleod MR, et al. (2011) Systematic survey of the design, statistical analysis, and reporting of studies published in the 2008 volume of the Journal of Cerebral Blood Flow and Metabolism. J Cereb Blood Flow Metab 31: 1064–1072.
37. Sena ES, van der Worp HB, Bath PM, Howells DW, Macleod MR (2010) Publication bias in reports of animal stroke studies leads to major overstatement of efficacy. PLoS Biol 8: e1000344.
38. Macleod MR, O'Collins T, Howells DW, Donnan GA (2004) Pooling of animal experimental data reveals influence of study design and publication bias. Stroke 35: 1203–1208.
39. Ioannidis JP (2005) Why most published research findings are false. PLoS Med 2: e124.
40. Sena E, van der Worp HB, Howells D, Macleod M (2007) How can we improve the pre-clinical development of drugs for stroke? Trends Neurosci 30: 433–439.
41. Landis SC, Amara SG, Asadullah K, Austin CP, Blumenstein R, et al. (2012) A call for transparent reporting to optimize the predictive value of preclinical research. Nature 490: 187–191.
42. Kilkenny C, Browne WJ, Cuthill IC, Emerson M, Altman DG (2010) Improving bioscience research reporting: the ARRIVE guidelines for reporting animal research. PLoS Biol 8: e1000412.
43. Peers IS, South MC, Ceuppens PR, Bright JD, Pilling E (2014) Can you trust your animal study data? Nat Rev Drug Discov, 10.1038/nrd4090-c1.
44. Hirschhorn JN, Lohmueller K, Byrne E, Hirschhorn K (2002) A comprehensive review of genetic association studies. Genet Med 4: 45–61.
45. Moonesinghe R, Khoury MJ, Janssens AC (2007) Most published research findings are false-but a little replication goes a long way. PLoS Med 4: e28.
46. Senn S (2006) Change from baseline and analysis of covariance revisited. Stat Med 25: 4334–4344.
47. Vickers AJ (2001) The use of percentage change from baseline as an outcome in a controlled trial is statistically inefficient: a simulation study. BMC Med Res Methodol 1: 6.
48. Allen EA, Erhardt EB, Calhoun VD (2012) Data visualization in the neurosciences: overcoming the curse of dimensionality. Neuron 74: 603–608.
49. Nature (2013) Reducing our irreproducibility. Nature 496: 398.
50. Bove SE, Calcaterra SL, Brooker RM, Huber CM, Guzman RE, et al. (2003) Weight bearing as a measure of disease progression and efficacy of anti-inflammatory compounds in a model of monosodium iodoacetate-induced osteoarthritis. Osteoarthritis Cartilage 11: 821–830.
51. Nagase H, Kumakura S, Shimada K (2012) Establishment of a novel objective and quantitative method to assess pain-related behavior in monosodium iodoacetate-induced osteoarthritis in rat knee. J Pharmacol Toxicol Methods 65: 29–36.
52. Just S, Pawlak M, Heppelmann B (2000) Responses of fine primary afferent nerve fibres innervating the rat knee joint to defined torque. J Neurosci Methods 103: 157–162.
53. Lalovic B, Kharasch E, Hoffer C, Risler L, Liu-Chen LY, et al. (2006) Pharmacokinetics and pharmacodynamics of oral oxycodone in healthy human subjects: role of circulating active metabolites. Clin Pharmacol Ther 79: 461–479.
54. Jurna I (1988) Dose-dependent inhibition by naloxone of nociceptive activity evoked in the rat thalamus. Pain 35: 349–354.
55. Kayser V, Guilbaud G (1981) Dose-dependent analgesic and hyperalgesic effects of systemic naloxone in arthritic rats. Brain Res 226: 344–348.
56. Davies NM, Anderson KE (1997) Clinical pharmacokinetics of naproxen. Clin pharmacokinet 32: 268–293.
57. McDougall JJ, Barin AK, McDougall CM (2004) Loss of vasomotor responsiveness to the mu-opioid receptor ligand endomorphin-1 in adjuvant monoarthritic rat knee joints. Am J Physiol Regul Integr Comp Physiol 286: R634–641.

58. Meert TF, Vermeirsch HA (2005) A preclinical comparison between different opioids: antinociceptive versus adverse effects. Pharmacol Biochem Behav 80: 309–326.
59. Nielsen CK, Ross FB, Lotfipour S, Saini KS, Edwards SR, et al. (2007) Oxycodone and morphine have distinctly different pharmacological profiles: radioligand binding and behavioural studies in two rat models of neuropathic pain. Pain 132: 289–300.
60. Poyhia R, Kalso EA (1992) Antinociceptive effects and central nervous system depression caused by oxycodone and morphine in rats. Pharmacol Toxicol 70: 125–130.
61. Staahl C, Christrup LL, Andersen SD, Arendt-Nielsen L, Drewes AM (2006) A comparative study of oxycodone and morphine in a multi-modal, tissue-differentiated experimental pain model. Pain 123: 28–36.
62. Kalso E, Vainio A, Mattila MJ, Rosenberg PH, Seppala T (1990) Morphine and oxycodone in the management of cancer pain: plasma levels determined by chemical and radioreceptor assays. Pharmacol Toxicol 67: 322–328.
63. Glare PA, Walsh TD (1993) Dose-ranging study of oxycodone for chronic pain in advanced cancer. J Clin Oncol 11: 973–978.
64. Schiff M, Minic M (2004) Comparison of the analgesic efficacy and safety of nonprescription doses of naproxen sodium and Ibuprofen in the treatment of osteoarthritis of the knee. J Rheumatol 31: 1373–1383.
65. Brogden RN, Heel RC, Speight TM, Avery GS (1979) Naproxen up to date: a review of its pharmacological properties and therapeutic efficacy and use in rheumatic diseases and pain states. Drugs 18: 241–277.
66. Satterwhite JH, Boudinot FD (1995) Effects of age on the pharmacodynamics of naproxen in the rat. Exp Gerontol 30: 505–515.
67. Patiño-Camacho SI, Moreno MGL, Flores-Murrieta FJ, Déciga-Campos M (2013) The pharmacokinetic profile of the combination of naproxen and tizanidine in rat. Drug Dev Res 74: 31–37.
68. Campbell JN, Meyer RA (2006) Mechanisms of neuropathic pain. Neuron 52: 77–92.
69. Li J, Simone DA, Larson AA (1999) Windup leads to characteristics of central sensitization. Pain 79: 75–82.

13

Effects of Danshensu on Platelet Aggregation and Thrombosis: *In Vivo* Arteriovenous Shunt and Venous Thrombosis Models in Rats

Chen Yu[1]*[⁹], Dong Qi[2⁹], Wei Lian[3], Qing-Zhong Li[1], Hong-Juan Li[1], Hua-Ying Fan[4]*

1 School of Pharmacy, Binzhou Medical University, Yantai, Shandong, China, **2** Department of Nephrology, Yantai Yu-Huang-Ding/Qingdao University Hospital, Yantai, Shandong, China, **3** Yantai Yan-Tai-Shan Hospital, Yantai, Shandong, China, **4** School of Pharmacy, Yantai University, Yantai, Shandong, China

Abstract

Danshensu, a type of dihydroxyphenyl lactic acid, is one of the most abundant active phenolic acids in the dried root of *Salvia miltiorrhizae* (Lamiaceae)—widely used traditional Chinese medicine. The effects of danshensu on platelet aggregation and thrombus formation in rats were examined using various methods. It was found that danshensu significantly reduced thrombus weight in 2 experimental thrombosis models; dose-dependent inhibition of adenosine diphosphate (ADP) and arachidonic acid (AA)-induced platelet aggregation occurred in normal and blood stasis-induced rats; Danshensu also significantly mitigated blood viscosity, plasma viscosity and hematocrit levels. Moreover, danshensu significantly inhibited venous thrombosis-induced expression of cyclooxygenases-2 (COX-2) rather than cyclooxygenases-1(COX-1) in the venous walls, down regulated thromboxane B_2 (TXB_2) and up regulated 6-keto prostaglandin $F_{1\alpha}$ (6-keto-$PGF_{1\alpha}$), normalizing the TXB_2/6-keto-$PGF_{1\alpha}$ ratio. In addition, danshensu did not induce gastric lesions and even had protective effects on aspirin-induced ulcer formation at doses as high as 60 mg/kg. These findings suggest that the antithrombotic and antiplatelet aggregation effects of danshensu are attributed to its highly selective inhibition of COX-2 and ability to normalize the thromboxane A_2(TXA_2)/prostacyclin(PGI_2) balance. These findings suggest that danshensu have great prospects in antithrombotic and antiplatelet therapy.

Editor: Pablo Garcia de Frutos, IIBB-CSIC-IDIBAPS, Spain

Funding: This study was supported by the Project of National Natural Science Foundation of China (Grant No. 81303259), URL: http://www.nsfc.gov.cn/, Shandong Province Natural Science Foundation (No. ZR2010HL065), URL: http://www.sdnsf.gov.cn/portal/, Research Award Fund for Outstanding Young and Middle-aged Scientists of Shandong Province of China (project No. BS2013YY046), URL: http://www.sdstc.gov.cn/, and the Programs for Science and Technology Development and Plan of Yanta (No. 2013WS262), URL: http://www.ytstc.gov.cn/. The funders had no role in study design, data collection and analysis, decision to publish, or preparation of the manuscript.

Competing Interests: The authors have declared that no competing interests exist.

* Email: yuchen810624@163.com (CY); katiefhydong@sina.com (HYF)

⁹ These authors contributed equally to this work.

Introduction

Thrombus formation accelerates the progression of various cardiovascular and cerebrovascular disorders. Thromboembolic complications of arteriosclerosis, heart attack, stroke and peripheral vascular disease are the principal causes of death in developed countries. Arterial and venous thrombi comprises primarily platelet aggregates.

Platelets mediate the initiation of thrombosis through platelet adhesion, activation and aggregation [1]. A collaborative meta-analysis of randomized trials has demonstrated that antiplatelet therapy is beneficial in treating thromboembolic diseases and preventing serious vascular events, arterial occlusion and venous thromboembolism in a wide range of patients who are at high risk for occlusive vascular events [2]. Thus, the inhibition of platelet function has the potential to treat circulatory diseases, spurring the development of many antiplatelet and antithrombotic agents and prompting an examination of their effects in preventing thrombosis.

Danshen, the dried root of *Salvia miltiorrhizae* (Lamiaceae), is one of the most widely used traditional herbal medicines against various cardiovascular and cerebrovascular diseases, including coronary heart disease, myocardial infarction, stroke and hypertension. Danshen contains hydrophilic phenolics and lipophilic quinones, which have many pharmacological and therapeutic properties [3].

Increasing data have demonstrated that danshensu is an abundant and representative phenolic acid in danshen [4]. Danshensu (chemical structure shown in Fig. 1)—known as β-3,4-dihydroxyphenyl-lactic acid—has several mechanisms by which it elicits its therapeutic effects. Danshensu can mitigate cardiovascular and cerebrovascular disturbances [5] by improving microcirculation, increasing blood flow, relaxing the coronary arteries and promoting anticoagulation [6].

However, the antithrombotic and antiplatelet effects and mechanisms of danshensu are unknown. The purpose of this study was to determine the effects and mechanisms of danshensu with regard to platelet aggregation, thrombus formation and blood circulation so as to provide pharmacological evidence that supports its clinical application.

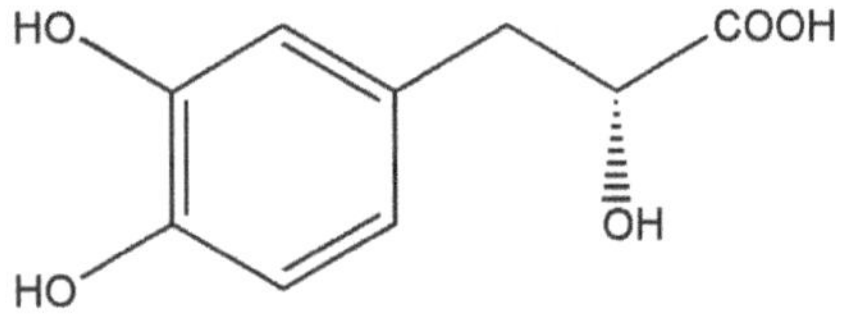

Figure 1. Chemical structure of danshensu ($C_9H_{10}O_5$, molecular weight = 198.17).

Results

Effects on platelet aggregation *in vivo*

To assess the effect of danshensu on platelet aggregation, we measured the inhibition of platelet aggregation on danshensu induced by ADP and AA in normal rats.As shown in Fig. 2, compared with the control group, ADP and AA-induced platelet aggregation was altered by pretreatment with danshensu and aspirin. Danshensu dose-dependently inhibited AA-induced platelet aggregation by approximately 13.9% at 15 mg/kg, 17.9% at 30 mg/kg and 21.5% at 60 mg/kg, respectively. This result showed that similar inhibition in the ADP-induced platelet aggregation.The inhibition of platelet aggregation induced by ADP was 10.5%, 14.6% and 23.5% at doses of 15, 30, and 60 mg/kg, respectively.

Further, we determined effect of danshensu on platelet aggregation in blood stasis rats induced by AA. Blood stasis increased platelet aggregation compared with the control group as shown in Fig. 3, which was also modified by pretreatment with danshensu in a dose-dependent manner. This inhibitory effect of danshensu at dose of 60 mg/kg was comparable with that of aspirin at 20 mg/kg in blood stasis rats.

Effect on thrombus formation

Two rat models of thrombosis were developed by installing an arteriovenous shunt and ligating the inferior vena cava to study the antithrombotic activity and mechanism of danshensu *in vivo*. Pretreatment with danshensu (15 to 60 mg/kg) decreased thrombus formation dose-dependently in the arteriovenous shunt model.The inhibition of thrombus formation was about 12.6%, 18.2% and 29.6% respectively (Fig. 4).

As shown in Fig. 5, this result was confirmed by inferior vena cava model. Residual thrombi from the occlusive vessels of all rats were measured. Compared with the thrombotic control group, aspirin at 20 mg/kg decreased the thrombus weight from 35.37±3.03 mg to 24.14±4.23 mg versus 29.65±5.62 mg with 15 mg/kg, 25.78±3.95 mg with 30 mg/kg and 23.84±2.26 mg with 60 mg/kg of danshensu, respectively. Antithrombotic activity of danshensu at dose of 60 mg/kg is comparable with that of aspirin at 20 mg/kg.

Effects on COX and possible mechanisms

Inhibitory effects of danshensu and aspirin against 2 cyclooxygenases (COX) isoforms were first examined *in vitro* using enzymatic assays. While danshensu had little inhibitory effect on COX-1, danshensu decreased COX-2 activity at 20 to 200 μM even at 200 μM yielding an IC_{50} value of approximately 44 μM (Fig. 6 A vs B).

In contrast, aspirin inhibited COX-1 and COX-2, with geometric mean IC_{50} values of 39.8 and 60.7 μM, respectively. The IC_{50} ratios of COX-1 to COX-2 for danshensu and aspirin exceeded 10 and 0.67 respectively, it is demonstrated that danshensu selectively inhibits COX-2 over COX-1 by approximately 20-fold.

The effects of danshensu on COX-1 and COX-2 levels were examined using western blot technique. As shown in Fig. 7, the expression of COX-1 and COX-2 induced by inferior vena cava ligation was significantly elevated when compared with control group. It is clear that aspirin significantly inhibited both COX-1 and COX-2 expression while danshenu only significantly inhibited COX-2 but not COX-1 expression (Fig. 7B vs D). This observation indicates that danshensu exerts its antiplatelet effect by selectively targeting on COX-2.

Next, we measured the serum concentrations of TXB_2 and 6-keto-PGF1α in the rats. TXB_2 and 6-keto-$PGF_{1\alpha}$ levels increased significantly, accompanying a rise in the TXB_2/6-keto-$PGF_{1\alpha}$

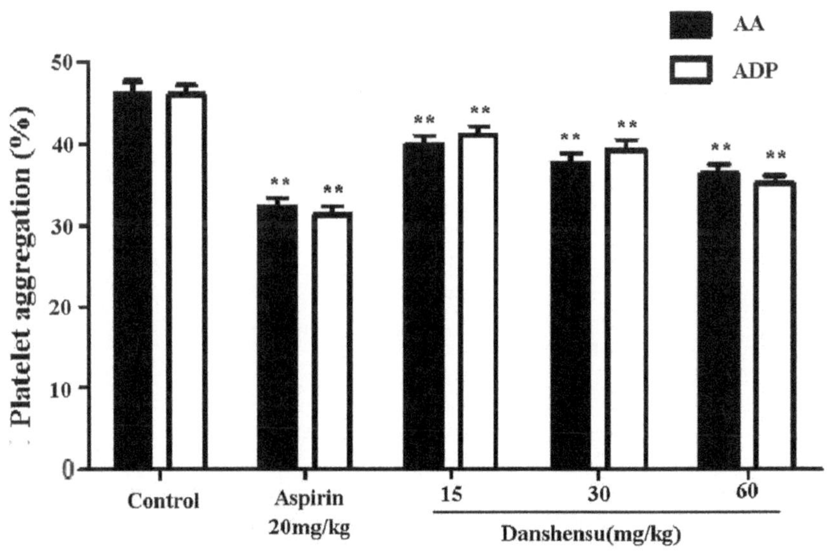

Figure 2. Effect of danshensu on platelet aggregation in normal rats. Blood was drawn 60 min after intragastric danshensu administration. Platelet aggregation was induced by diphosphate (ADP) and arachidonic acid (AA). Data are expressed as mean ± SEM (each group, n = 10). $^{**}P<0.01$ with control group.

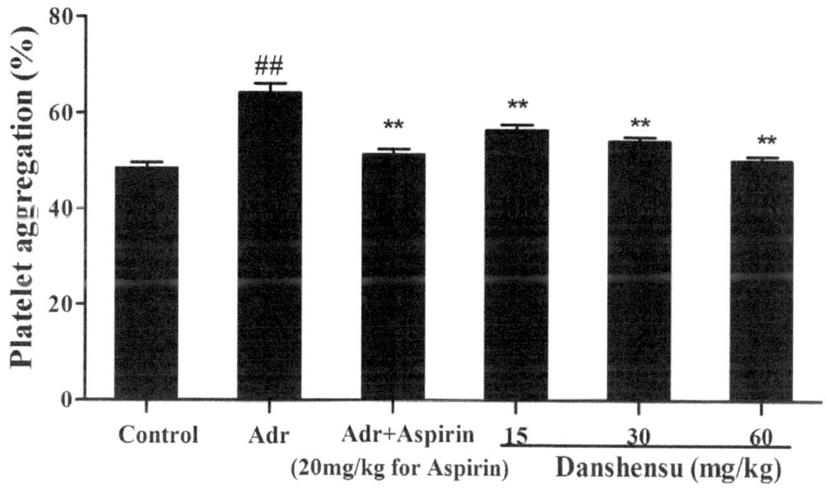

Figure 3. Effect of danshensu on platelet aggregation in blood stasis rats. Blood was drawn 60 min after intragastric danshensu administration. Platelet aggregation was induced by arachidonic acid (AA). Data are expressed as mean ± SEM (each group, n = 10). The blood stasis model was built during the interval between when 2 injections of adrenaline hydrochloride (Adr) were given to rats placed in ice-cold water. ##$P<$ 0.01 compared with normal control. *$P<0.05$ **$P<0.01$ compared with Adr control.

ratio in the 2 thrombosis models. Aspirin significantly reduced TXB_2 and 6-keto-$PGF_{1\alpha}$ levels, decreasing the TXB_2/6-keto-$PGF_{1\alpha}$ ratio. Danshensu downregulated TXB_2 and increased 6-keto-$PGF_{1\alpha}$ levels, especially at 30 and 60 mg/kg, normalizing the TXB_2/6-keto-$PGF_{1\alpha}$ ratio better than aspirin (Tables 1 and 2).

Effect on hemorheology

whole blood viscosity (WBV) at all shear rates, plasma viscosity (PV) and hematocrit values (Hct) significantly rose in blood stasis rats, but danshensu significantly reduced blood viscosity, plasma viscosity and hematocrit, particularly at 30 and 60 mg/kg (Table 3).

Protective effects of danshensu on gastric mucosa

We examined the gastrointestinal (GI) effects of oral administration of danshensu and aspirin in rats for 7 days. The ulcer index for all groups is summarized in Fig. 8. Aspirin resulted in gastric lesions and the ulcer index was significantly higher than the control group. In contrast, danshensu did not induce gastric lesions, even at as high as 60 mg/kg.

We also investigated the effect of danshensu on aspirin-induced gastric lesions. The macroscopic findings of open stomachs are shown in Fig. 9A, we found that oral administration of aspirin (200 mg/kg body weight) induced severe mucosal damage in the gastric corpus of mice. Danshensu had no damaging effects on the stomach. In addition co-administration of danshensu with aspirin could inhibit aspirin-induced ulcer formation. Fig. 9B shows the ulcer score of gastric hemorrhagic ulcers in each group. These data suggest that danshensu has gastroprotective activities and it also prevents aspirin-induced gastric ulcer formation.

Discussion

Many life-threatening diseases, such as atherosclerosis, cerebrovascular thrombosis, coronary artery disease, stroke and tumor metastasis are related with platelet dysfunctions [7]. Many

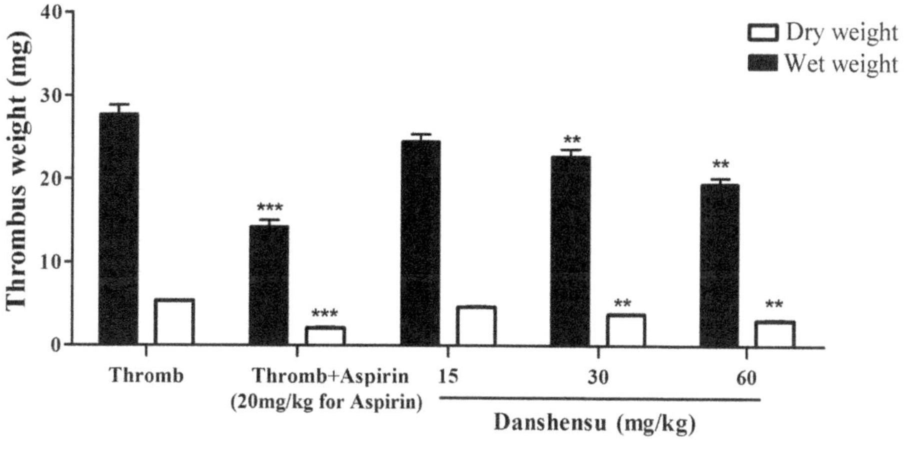

Figure 4. Antithrombotic activity of danshensu in the rat model of arteriovenous shunt. The drug or solvent was administered orally 60 min before thrombogenic challenge. Data are expressed as mean ± SEM (each group, n = 10). Thromb: thrombosis. *$P<0.05$, **$P<0.01$, ***$P<$ 0.001 compared with thrombotic control group.

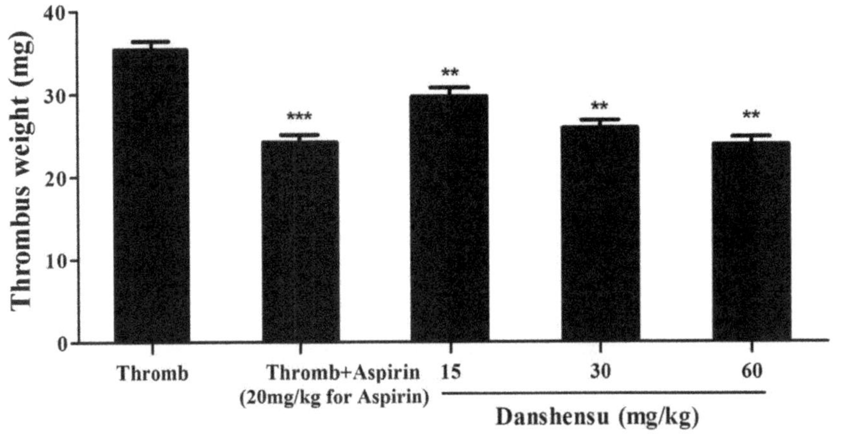

Figure 5. Antithrombotic activity of danshensu in the rat model of ligating inferior vena cava. The drug or solvent was administered orally 60 min before the thrombogenic challenge. Data are expressed as mean ± SEM (each group, n = 10). Thromb: thrombosis. $^{*}P<0.05$, $^{**}P<0.01$, $^{***}P<0.001$ compared with thrombotic control group.

available antiplatelet agents interfere with platelet function at various levels of activation, which results in several clinical disadvantages, including gastrointestinal side effects and hemorrhage. For this reason, a search for safer and more effective antiplatelet agents without these adverse effects would be highly desirable. In recent years, new therapeutic agents have been derived from Chinese herbs and there is growing interest in this area.

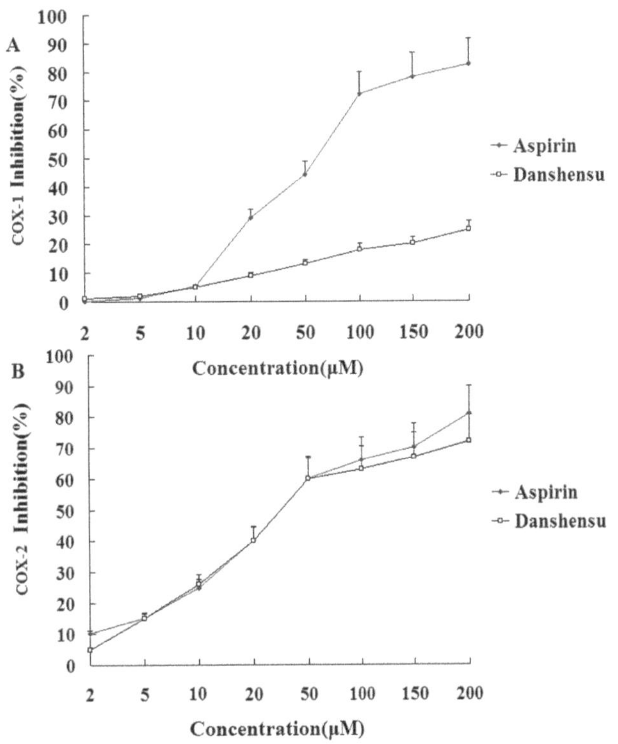

Figure 6. Direct effect of various concentrations of danshensu and aspirin on the enzymatic activities of COX-1 and COX-2. Danshensu and aspirin (water, as a control) were incubated with COX-1 (A) or COX-2 (B) for 10 min and then AA was added. COX enzyme activities are reflected by the amount of PGE_2 produced. PGE_2 production was measured by ELISA. Enzyme activity in the sample without treatment (water alone) served as control and results are expressed as inhibitory rate of COX-1 and COX-2 activity compared with solvent control.

In this study, we examined the antiplatelet and antithrombotic effects of danshensu and the pharmacological mechanisms. We determined effects of danshensu on platelet function by measuring ADP and AA-induced platelet aggregation. Our results showed that danshensu produced marked antiplatelet effect on ADP and AA platelet agonists ex vivo aggregation. This inhibitory effect of danshensu at dose of 60 mg/kg was comparable with aspirin at 20 mg/kg in blood stasis-induced rats.

The effects of danshensu on thrombus formation were studied in arteriovenous shunt model and inferior vena cava model; these models simulate arterial and venous thrombosis observed in humans [8]. Our results demonstrated that danshensu has potent antithrombotic effects against arterial and venous thrombosis.

To assess the effect of danshensu on microcirculation, we evaluated hemorheologic parameters in blood stasis model. Blood stasis can result in platelet aggregation and hemorheological abnormalities. Hemorheological disorders mediate the pathogenesis and development of many cardiovascular and cerebrovascular diseases [9]. In this study, rats were injected subcutaneously with adrenaline hydrochloride (Adr) and treated with cold stress. As a result, blood viscosity, plasma viscosity and hematocrit increased significantly compared with the control group. Our results suggest that Adr combined with exposure to ice-cold water induces blood stasis resulting in hemorheological abnormalities. Platelet aggregation is believed to be a factor that determines blood viscosity [10], consistent with our results that danshensu improves hemorheologic parameters, ameliorates blood stasis and promotes circulation by decreasing whole blood viscosity, secondary to the inhibitory effect on platelet aggregation.

In our study, Danshensu exhibited apparent antiplatelet and antithrombotic activity. In order to explore the further mechanisms of antiplatelet and anti-thrombosis, the activity and expression of COXs were measured. We also evaluated the levels of TXB_2 and 6-keto-$PGF_{1\alpha}$ in both arterial and venous thrombosis models. Our results indicated that danshensu could selectively inhibit COX-2 rather than COX-1 to regulate the balance of TXA_2/PGI_2. Therefore, danshensu exhibited superior antiplatelet and antithrombotic effects compared with aspirin.

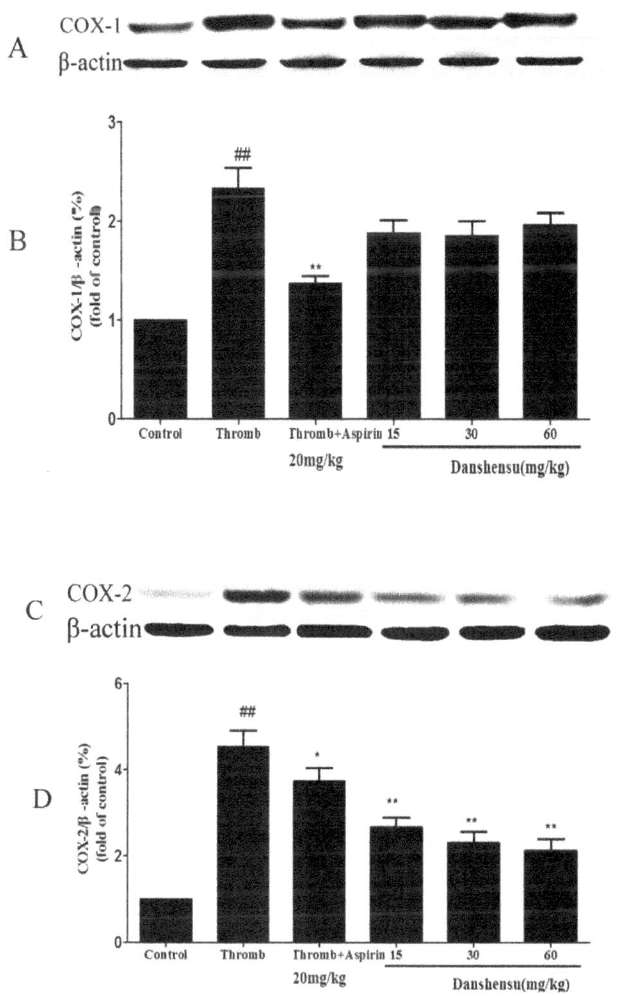

Figure 7. The effects of danshensu on COX expression. Rats were given 15, 30 and 60 mg/kg danshensu intragastrically and 20 mg/kg aspirin for 7 days. Venous thrombus formation was induced by inferior vena cava (IVC) ligation to produce thrombus after last administration.Vein walls were harvested from venous thrombosis and the expression of COX-1 and COX-2 was assessed by western analysis (A and C). β-actin was measured to confirm equal loading of proteins. Densitometric analysis of COX-1 (B) and COX-2 (D) expression is represented by the mean from 3 separate experiments. Data were normalized to β-actin levels. Thromb: thrombosis. ##$P<0.01$ compared with normal control. *$P<0.05$, **$P<0.01$ compared with thrombotic control group.

Disruption of the TXA_2-PGI_2 balance increases the risk of thrombosis [11]. TXA_2 and PGI_2 are metabolites of arachidonic acid, which is hydrolyzed by COXs and transformed into endoperoxides, prostaglandins (PGs) and TXA_2 [12]. COXs exist as 2 distinct isoforms: COX-1 and COX-2. COX-1 which is constitutively expressed in most tissues and has high levels of activity in the the gastrointestinal tract, is thought to exert homeostatic properties that are crucial for gastric physiologic function, including mucosal protectionwhereas COX-2 is absent from most healthy tissues but is induced by proinflammatory and proliferative stimuli after exposure to cytokines, immunological stimuli and growth factors [13,14]. TXA_2 is a potent inducer of platelet aggregation and vasoconstriction and its levels rise in thrombus models. In contrast, PGI_2 is a potent platelet inhibitor. An increase in TXA_2 results in the adhesion, aggregation and release of platelets. However, PGI_2 inhibits platelet aggregation [15,16]. In our study, aspirin significantly decreased both TXB_2 and 6-keto-$PGF_{1\alpha}$ levels due to its non-selective and irreversible COX inhibition. Aspirin exerts its antiplatelet activity through inhibition of both COX-1 and COX-2, therefore inhibits not only the production of TXA_2 in platelets, but also the production of anti-aggregatory PGI_2 in vessel walls. This phenomenon is referred to as the "aspirin dilemma"[17] and is considered to be a reason underlying the insufficient efficacy and unclear dose-response effects of aspirin [18,19]. Compared with aspirin, danshensu with higher selectivity for COX-2 is able to normalize the TXA_2/PGI_2 balance better, by upregulating 6-keto-$PGF_{1\alpha}$ and downregulating TXB_2 simultaneously.

Finally, we evaluated the protective effects of danshensu on gastric mucosa. We compared the ulcerogenic effects of danshensu and aspirin on gastric mucosa and demonstrated that danshensu did not cause any apparent ulceration of the gastric mucosa in rats, even at a dose of 60 mg/kg. In contrast, aspirin had a potent ulcerogenic effect at the antithrombotic dose(20 mg/kg) and produced severe hemorrhagic necrotic lesions in the gastric mucosa even at a dose of 200 mg/kg Aspirin-induced gastric lesion was completely inhibited by the coadministration of danshensu. The observed differences in gastric ulcerogenic properties between danshensu and aspirin may be related with the difference in COX-1 selectivity. COX-1-derived PGs are thought to play a dominant role in gastric mucosal defense and cytoprotection and it has been confirmed that selective inhibition of COX-1 alone may not cause ulcers, but inhibition of both COX-1 and COX-2 is required for the development of gastric lesions [20,21]. Thus, danshensu by selectively inhibit COX-2 only, is considered to be potentially less damaging to the gastrointestinal tract than aspirin that also block COX-1.

In conclusion, our findings suggest that danshensu has potent antithrombotic effects and antiplatelet aggregation activity without inducing GI adverse events. This might be attributed to danshensu's mechanism of its functions as a highly selective COX-2 inhibitor with an ability to normalize TXA_2/PGI_2 balance superior to aspirin. Thus, Danshensu may have good prospects in antithrombotic and antiplatelet therapy.

Materials and Methods

Chemicals and reagents

Danshensu (purity 98%) was provided by Nanjing Zelang Medical Biological Technology Co. Ltd (Nanjing, China). Aspirin (purity 98%) was produced by Anhui Fengyuan Pharmaceutical Co. Ltd (Anhui, China). Arachidonic acid (AA) was purchased from Sigma-Aldrich Chemical Co. (USA). Heparin sodium was purchased from Jiangsu Wanbang Biochemical Medicine Co. Ltd. (Jiangsu, China). Adrenaline hydrochloride was purchased from Tianjin Jinyao Amino Acids Co. Ltd. (Tianjin, China). COX inhibitor screening assay kits were purchased from Cayman Chemical Company (Ann Arbor, MI, USA). Primary antibodies against COX-1, COX-2, β-actin and horseradish peroxidase (HRP)-conjugated secondary antibody were purchased from Santa Cruz Biotechnology, Inc. The thromboxane B_2 (TXB_2) and 6-keto prostaglandin $F_{1\alpha}$ (6-keto-$PGF_{1\alpha}$) radioimmunoassay kits were produced by Tianjin Jiuding Engineering of Medicine and Biology Co. Ltd. (Tianjin, China).

Animals and treatments

Male Sprague-Dawley rats (weight approximately 300 g, 3–4 months each) were purchased from Shandong Lvye Pharmaceu-

Table 1. Effects of danshensu on plasma TXB_2 and 6-keto-$PGF_{1\alpha}$ levels and TXB_2-6-keto-$PGF_{1\alpha}$ ratio in rats in the arteriovenous shunt model.

Group	Dose(mg/kg)	TXB_2 (pg/mL)	6-keto-$PGF_{1\alpha}$ (pg/mL)	TXB_2/6-keto-$PGF_{1\alpha}$
Normal		180.0±8.3	487.3±16.6	0.38±0.01
Thromb		552.2±18.9##	602.5±20.4##	0.93±0.03##
Thromb+Aspirin	20	56.5±1.9***	190.5±7.5***	0.30±0.01***
Thromb +Danshensu	15	258.1±10.2**	621.7±19.8*	0.40±0.01**
	30	228.7±11.5**	638.3±22.1**	0.37±0.02**
	60	206.4±8.9**	649.2±15.8**	0.35±0.02**

Blood was drawn from the abdominal aorta at the end of arteriovenous shunt test period and anticoagulated with indomethacin-EDTA-Na_2. Plasma samples were prepared by centrifugation and analyzed by radioimmunoassay. Data are expressed as mean±SEM (each group, n = 10). #$P<0.05$, ##$P<0.01$ compared with normal group, *$P<0.05$, **$P<0.01$, ***$P<0.001$ compared with thrombotic control group.

tical Co. Ltd., China (certificate No. SCXK (Lu) 20030008). Male ICR mice (weight approximately 25 g, 8–9 weeks each) were purchased from the Animal Department of the College of Medicine, Beijing University (certificate no. SCXK (Jing) 2006–0008).

Animals were acclimated for at least 1 week to a temperature of 24±1°C and humidity of 55±5%. The animals were maintained with free access to standard diet and tap water. The experimental procedures were approved by the Office of Experimental Animal Management.

Committee of Shandong Province, China (certificate No. SYXK (Lu) 20090015). Rats were given 15, 30 and 60 mg/kg danshensu and 20 mg/kg aspirin intragastrically (i.g.). All drugs were dissolved in 0.9% normal saline as vehicle. The control rats were given 0.9% normal saline. All drugs and saline were administered orally to rats once daily at 9 AM for 7 days. All *in vivo* experiments were conducted 60 min after the treatment.

Assay of *ex vivo* Platelet Aggregation in Rats

Blood was collected after the last administration of danshensu and saline. All rats were anesthetized with 10% chloral hydrate and blood was collected from the abdominal aorta and anticoagulated with citrate (3.8%; 1 vol anticoagulant: 9 vol blood). Platelet-rich plasma (PRP) was prepared by centrifuging the blood at 1000 rpm for 8 min and at 3000 rpm for 15 min to prepare platelet-poor plasma (PPP). The platelet concentration was adjusted to $1.8-2\times10^9$/mL with PPP. Then, 0.3 mL of PRP was placed in a cuvette and stirred with a rotor at 37°C for 5 min, after which 6 μM ADP and 100 μM AA was added. Aggregation was measured with a platelet aggregometer (LBY-NJ4, Pulisheng Instrument Co. Ltd. China). Results were recorded as light transmission at maximal aggregation after the addition of an aggregating agent. Data are expressed as percentage of maximal aggregation.

In vivo arteriovenous shunt thrombosis

Rat arterial-venous shunts (silk thread model) were prepared with 2 2-cm-long polyethylene tubes (1 mm i.d.), linked by a central section (8 cm long; 2 mm i.d.) that contained a 5-cm piece of silk thread and was filled with saline solution that contained heparin 50 U/kg. Rats were anesthetized with chloral hydrate (350 mg/kg, i.p.) and an arterial-venous shunt was placed between the right carotid artery and left jugular vein [22,23]. After blood was circulated through the shunt for 15 minutes, both ends of the tube were pinched, the silk thread was removed from the shunt tube and the wet and dry weights were measured by subtracting the pre-experiment weight of the 5-cm silk thread.The rate of inhibition of thrombosis formation was calculated as inhibition (%) = $(A-A_1)/A\times100\%$, where A is the thrombus weight of the thrombosis control group and A_1 is the weight after treatment with the agents. The sham group did not undergo the surgery. All rats fasted overnight before the operation.

Venous thrombosis model

Venous thrombus formation was induced by inferior vena cava (IVC) ligation to produce a stasis thrombus as described [24,25].

Table 2. Effects of danshensu on plasma TXB_2 and 6-keto-$PGF_{1\alpha}$ levels and TXB_2-6-keto-$PGF_{1\alpha}$ ratio in rats the venous thrombosis model.

Group	Dose(mg/kg)	TXB_2 (pg/mL)	6-keto-$PGF_{1\alpha}$ (pg/mL)	TXB_2/6-keto-$PGF_{1\alpha}$
Normal		197.0±8.2	528.3±16.8	0.37±0.03
Thromb		605.2±21.9##	652.5±24.6##	0.95±0.03##
Thromb+Aspirin	20	106.5±4.2***	395.0±14.5***	0.29±0.01***
Thromb +Danshensu	15	358.1±12.8**	663.7±24.2*	0.50±0.02**
	30	328.7±10.6**	684.3±25.1**	0.45±0.02**
	60	306.4±8.2***	719.2±20.9**	0.40±0.02**

Blood was drawn from the abdominal aorta at the end of venous thrombus formation period and anticoagulated with indomethacin-EDTA-Na_2. Plasma samples were prepared by centrifugation and analzyed by radioimmunoassay. Data are expressed as mean±SEM (each group, n = 10). #$P<0.05$, ##$P<0.01$ compared with normal group, *$P<0.05$, **$P<0.01$, ***$P<0.001$ compared with thrombotic control group.

Table 3. The effect of danshensu on the hemorheological parameters in rats.

Group	WBV(mPa.s)			PV(mPa.s)	Hct(%)
	Low shear rate	Medium shear rate	High shear rate		
Normal Control	22.72±1.21	5.88±0.25	4.44±0.11	1.41±0.08	0.41±0.02
Adr Control	39.55±1.35##	9.01±0.32##	6.52±0.23##	2.06±0.06##	0.45±0.02##
Adr Aspirin 20 mg/kg	26.59±0.87**	6.82±0.21**	5.02±0.19**	1.66±0.06*	0.44±0.04
Adr Danshensu 15 mg/kg	35.36±2.25*	8.64±0.51*	6.28±0.31*	1.89±0.08*	0.45±0.02*
Adr Danshensu 30 mg/kg	31.24±1.08**	7.74±0.23**	5.65±0.18**	1.67±0.09*	0.44±0.02*
Adr Danshensu 60 mg/kg	27.12±1.05**	6.65±0.19**	4.78±0.12**	1.45±0.42**	0.43±0.02*

Rats were treated by subcutaneous injection of adrenaline hydrochloride and cold stress. The normal control rats received only saline. Next, blood was collected 30 min after drug administration. Hemorheologic parameters were analyzed by routine laboratory assays. Data are expressed as mean±SEM (each group, n = 10). #P<0.05, ##P<0.01 compared with normal control. *P<0.05 **P<0.01 compared with Adr control. Adr: adrenaline hydrochloride, WBV: whole blood viscosity, PV: plasma viscosity, Hct: hematocrit.

Rats were anesthetized with chloral hydrate (350 mg/kg, i.p.). After the rats were fixed on a temperature-controlled heating pad (38°C) to maintain body temperature, the abdomen was opened surgically. The intestines were moved gently to one side and covered with saline-moistened gauze and the vena cava was exposed by blunt dissection. One millimeter above the bifurcation of the vena iliaca and vena cava, the free vein was ligated by tightening the proximal and distal segments using 4-0 suture (Shinva Medical, China) to induce blood stasis. The abdominal cavity was closed provisionally and blood stasis was maintained for 4 h. After the abdomen was reopened, the ligated venous segment was excised and opened longitudinally to remove the thrombus. The vein wall and thrombus were divided by blunt or sharp dissection. The isolated thrombus was blotted of excess blood and weighed immediately. Harvested vein samples were homogenized for subsequent biochemical analysis. Sham operation was performed in the control group.

Measurement of plasma TXB_2 and 6-keto-$PGF_{1\alpha}$

Blood was drawn from the abdominal aorta at the end of the arteriovenous shunt test period or venous thrombosis model. Plasma was prepared by centrifuging blood at 4000 rpm for 5 min. TXA_2 and PGI_2 levels were estimated by measuring their stable hydrolysis products—TXB_2 and 6-keto-$PGF_{1\alpha}$, respectively—per standard procedures using EIA kits (Cayman Chemical) and expressed as pg/mL.

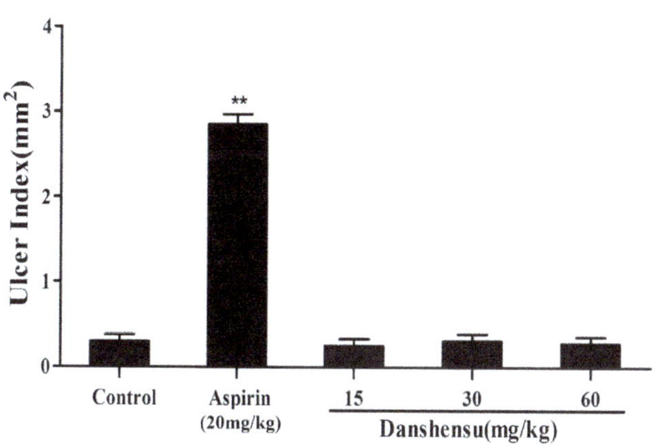

Figure 8. Gastric ulcerogenic response induced by danshensu and aspirin in rats. The test compounds were administered orally at the indicated dose (mg/kg) to rats for 7 days. The animals were sacrificed after the last drug administration and the total length of mucosal lesions in each stomach was used to create an ulcer index. Data are presented as the mean ± SEM (each group, n = 10). **P<0.01 versus the control group.

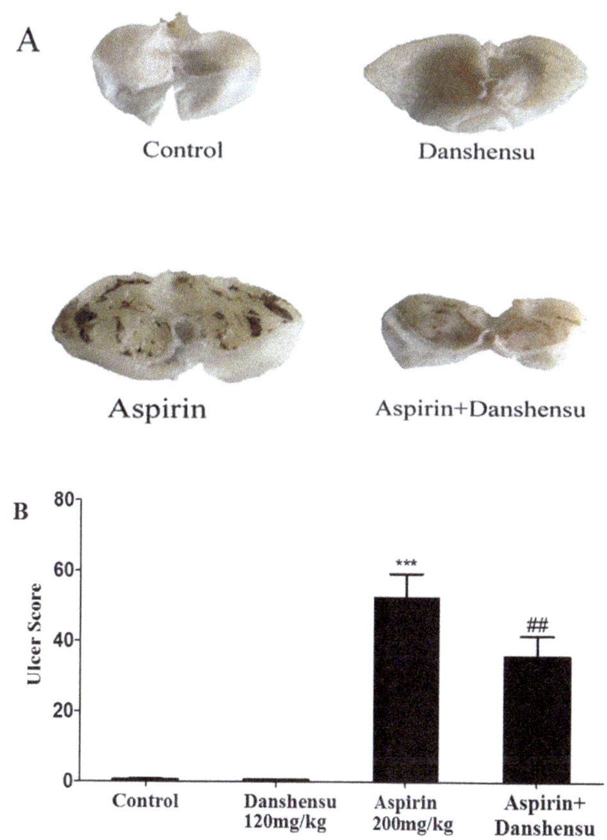

Figure 9. Effects of danshensu on aspirin-induced gastric lesions in mice. A: Photographs of gastric mucosa in the control group and danshensu, aspirin and aspirin + danshensu treatment groups are shown. B: The hemorrhagic ulcer index (mm^2) for each condition. Values are shown as the mean ± SEM(each group, n = 10). **P<0.01 compared with the control rats. ##P<0.01 compared with the aspirin-treated rats.

Effects of Danshensu on COX activity and expression

The inhibition of COX-1 and COX-2 by danshensu and aspirin was determined using COX inhibitor screening assay kits per the manufacturer's instructions. Danshensu and aspirin (with the same volume of water serving as control) were incubated directly with COX-1 or COX-2 in reaction buffer for 10 min. Then, AA was added as substrate and the reaction continued for another 2 min. Then, 0.1 N HCl and saturated stannous fluoride solution were added immediately to stop the enzymatic reaction. The amount of prostaglandin E_2 (PGE_2) that was generated by COX was measured using Cayman ELISA kits. The effects of danshensu and aspirin on COX activity were evaluated by comparing the amounts of PGE_2 production between reactions with and without the drugs. Inhibitory rates were calculated, based on PGE_2 production, as follows: Inhibitory rate (%) = (PGE_2 in Control groups-PGE_2 in drug-treated groups) ×100/PGE_2 in Control groups.

To measure COX-1 and COX-2 expression, venous walls from the venous thrombosis were analyzed by western blot. Venous samples were homogenized mechanically on ice and centrifuged at 4500 g for 10 minutes at 4°C; total proteins were then collected from the supernatants and the protein content was measured using a BCA protein assay kit.

Samples were separated by SDS-PAGE for immunoblot analysis. After the electrophoresis running for 60 min, proteins were transferred onto polyvinylidenedifluoride (PVDF) membranes. The membranes were blocked with 3% skim milk and saturated in Tris-buffered saline with 1% Tween 20 for 1 h at room temperature. Then, the membrane was incubated with primary anti-COX-1 and anti-COX-2 (1:300; Cayman Chemical) overnight at 4°C. The membranes were washed 3 times for 5 min each and incubated in horseradish peroxidase (HRP)-conjugated secondary antibody solution for 1 h at room temperature. The blots were washed again and visualized by using an enhanced chemiluminescence (ECL) detection kit (Beyotime Institute of Biotechnology) and exposure to photographic film. Images were collected and the respective bands were quantitated by densitometric analysis using the DigDoc100 program.

Effects of danshensu on blood stasis

The blood stasis model was established per previous reports [26]. The rats were divided randomly into 6 groups of 10 rats each: normal control, model group given 0.9% normal saline, aspirin (20 mg/kg) and Danshensu (15, 30 and 60 mg/kg). All drugs and saline were administered orally to the rats once per day at 9 AM for 7 days. After the sixth administration, blood stasis was induced by placing the rats in ice-cold water between 2 injections of adrenaline hydrochloride (Adr). All other rats were injected subcutaneously with Adr (0.8 mg/kg), except the control rats, which were injected with 0.9% (w/v) NaCl saline solution. Two hours after the first injection, all rats except the control group were soaked in ice water (0–2°C) for 5 min and reinjected with Adr (0.8 mg/kg) subcutaneously 2 h later to effect blood stasis. Afterward, the rats were placed into cages and fed freely.

Blood samples were collected and anticoagulated with heparin 30 min after the last administration of drugs or saline on the following day. Hemorheologic parameters, including WBV at various shear rates, PV and Hct, were measured by routine laboratory assays. Another aliquot of blood was collected into plastic tubes that contained 3.8% citrate and prepared PRP and PPP as described in *Assay of ex Vivo Platelet Aggregation in Rats*. Platelet aggregation was measured by arachidonic acid-induced.

Ulcerogenic Effects of Danshensu on Gastric Mucosa

Rats were sacrificed by cervical dislocation and the stomachs were removed immediately to determine the gastric ulcer index after the platelet aggregation assayas described with modifications [27,28]. The stomach tissues were split longitudinally and opened along the greater curvature. The total length (mm) of visible mucosal lesions in each stomach sample was measured and used to establish an ulcer index. An independent observer scored the macroscopic appearance of the gastric mucosa. The ulcer area was calculated as $\pi/4 \times a \times b$ mm^2, where a is the long axis and b is the short axis. The ulcer area was expressed as an ulcer index.

Effects of danshensu on aspirin-induced gastric lesion in mice

To investigate the effect of danshensu on aspirin-induced gastric lesions, male ICR mice were randomly divided into 4 groups. Group 1 received 1% carboxymethylcellulose in water as vehicle, Group 2 received danshensu treatment (120 mg/kg body weight), Group 3 received aspirin treatment (200 mg/kg body weight, suspended in 1% carboxymethylcellulose in water) and Group 4 received treatment of aspirin and danshensu. All drugs were administered orally once per day at 9 AM for 7 days. The mice were anesthetized with ether and sacrificed. One hour after the last administration, the isolated stomach was ligated at pylorus and cardia ends, filled with 1.5 mL of 2% formalin and immersed in 2% formalin for 15 min. Then, the stomach was cut along the greater curvature and the lengths of lesions on the stomach wall were measured as described [29].

Statistical analysis

Data were analyzed using SigmaStat 3.1 (SPSS Inc.; Chicago, IL) and expressed as mean±standerd error of means (SEM). $P<0.05$ was considered to be statistically significant.

Acknowledgments

Chen Yu and Dong Qi contributed equally to this work.

Author Contributions

Conceived and designed the experiments: CY DQ. Performed the experiments: CY DQ. Analyzed the data: WL QZL HJL. Contributed reagents/materials/analysis tools: HJL HYF. Wrote the paper: CY DQ.

References

1. Ruggeri ZM, Loredana Mendolicchio G (2007) Adhesion Mechanisms in Platelet Function Circulation Research. 100: 1673–1685.
2. Antithrombotic Trialists' Collaboration. (2002) Collaborative meta-analysis of randomisedtrials of antiplatelet therapy for prevention of death, myocardial infarction and stroke in high risk patients. BMJ; 324: 71–86.
3. Kang DG, Oh H, Sohn EJ, Hur TY, Lee KC, et al. (2004) Lithospermic acid B isolated from Salviae miltiorrhiza ameliorates ischaemia/reperfusion-induced renal injury in rats. Life Sci. 75: 1801–1816.
4. Chan K, Chui SH, Wong DY, Ha WY, Chan CL, et al (2004) Protective effects of Danshensu from the aqueous extract of Salvia miltiorrhiza (danshen) against homocysteine-induced endothelial dysfunction, Life Sci. 75: 3157–3171.
5. Zhao GR, Zhang HM, Ye TX, Xiang ZJ, Yuan YJ, et al (2008) Characterization of the radical scavenging and antioxidant activities of Danshensu and salvianolic acid B. Food and Chemical Toxicology. 46: 73–81.
6. Chan K, Chui SH, Wong DY, Ha WY, Chan CL, et al (2004) Protective effects of Danshensu from the aqueous extract of Salvia miltiorrhiza (Danshen) against homocysteine-induced endothelial dysfunction. Life Sciences; 75: 3157–3171.

7. Tran H, Anand SS (2004) Oral antiplatelet therapy in cerebrovascular disease, coronary artery disease and peripheral arterial disease. J Am Med Assoc. 292: 1867–1874.
8. Damiano BP, Mitchell JA, Giardino E, Corcoran T, Haertlein BJ, et al (2001) Antiplatelet and Antithrombotic Activity of RWJ-53308, A Novel Orally Active Glycoprotein IIb/IIIa Antagonist. Thromb Res. 104: 113–126.
9. Nosal' R, Jancinova V (2002) Cationic amphiphilic drugs and platelet phospholipase A2 (cPLA2). Thromb Res. 105: 339–345.
10. Ryu KH, Han HY, Lee SY, Jeon SD, Im GJ, et al (2009) Ginkgo biloba extract enhances antiplatelet and antithrombotic effects of cilostazol without prolongation of bleeding time. Thrombosis Research 124: 328–334.
11. Baskurt OK, Meiselman HJ (2003) Blood Rheology and Hemodynamics. Semin Thromb Hemost. 29: 435–450.
12. Takeuchi K (2012) Pathogenesis of NSAID-induced gastric damage: importance of cyclooxygenase inhibition and gastric hypermotility. World J Gastroenterol18(18).: 2147–2160.
13. Halter F, Tarnawski AS, Schmassmann A (2001) Cyclooxygenase 2-implications on maintenance of gastric mucosal integrity and ulcer healing: controversial issues and perspectives. Gut. 49: 443–453.
14. Masferrer JL, Zweifel BS, Seibert K (1990) Selective regulation of cellular cyclooxygenase by dexamethasone and endotoxin in mice. J Clin Invest. 86: 1375–1379
15. Lechi C, Andrioli G, Gaino S, Tommasoli R, Zuliani V, et al (1996). The antiplatelet effects of a new nitroderivative of acetylsalicylic acid–an in vitro study of inhibition on the early phase of platelet activation and on TXA2 production. Thrombosis and Haemostasis. 76(5): 791–798.
16. Weiss HJ, Turitto VT (1979) Prostacyclin (prostaglandin I2, PGI2) inhibits platelet adhesion and thrombus formation on subendothelium. Blood. 53(2): 244–250
17. Patrono C, Garcia Rodriguez LA, Landolfi R, Baigent C (1979) Low-dose aspirin for the prevention of atherothrombosis. N Engl J Med. 353(22): 2373–83.
18. Collaboration AT (2002). Collaborative meta-analysis of randomised trials of antiplatelet therapy for prevention of death, myocardial infarction and stroke in high risk patients. BMJ. 324 (7329): 71–86.
19. Sakata C, Kawasaki T, Kato Y, Abe M, Suzuki K, et al (2013) ASP6537, a novel highlcy selective cyclooxygenase-1 inhibitor, exerts potent antithrombotic effect without "aspirin dilemma". Thrombosis Research 132: 56–62.
20. Wooten JG, Blikslager AT, Ryan KA, Marks SL, Law JM, et al (2008) Cyclooxygenase expression and prostanoid production in pyloric and duodenal mucosae in dogs after administration of nonsteroidal anti-inflammatory drugs. Am J Vet Res. 69(4): 457–64.
21. Wallace JL, McKnight W, Reuter BK, Vergnolle N (2000) NSAID-induced gastric damage in rats: Requirement for inhibition of bothe cyclooxygenase 1 and 2. Gastroenterology. 119: 706–14.
22. Umar A, Boisseau M, Yusup Az, Upur H, Bégaud B, et al (2004). Interactions between aspirin and COX-2 inhibitors or NSAIDs in a rat thrombosis model. Fundam Clin Pharmacol. 18(5): 559–563.
23. Umoisseau M, Garreau C, Begaud B, Molimard M, Moore N (2003) Effects of armagnac extracts on human platelet function *in vitro* and on rat arteriovenous shunt thrombosis *in vivo*. Thromb Res. 110, 135–140.
24. Henke PK, Varga A, De S, Deatrick CB, Eliason J, et al (2004). Deep vein thrombosis resolution is modulated by monocyte CXCR2-mediated activity in a mouse model. Arterioscler Thromb Vasc Biol. 24: 1130–1137.
25. Henke PK Varma MR, Deatrick KB, Dewyer NA, Lynch EM, et al (2006) Neutrophils modulate post-thrombotic vein wall remodeling but not thrombus neovascularization. Thromb Haemost 2006; 95: 272–281.
26. Chen XP, Wang XW, Zhang YY, Xu XF, Ke WB, et al (2007) Effect of ethanol extract of terminalia chebula on microrheological characteristics in acute blood stasis model rat. Chin J Hemorh. 17(4): 525–528.
27. Sakata C, Kawasaki T, Kato Y, Abe M, Suzuki K, et al (2013) ASP6537, a novel highly selective cyclooxygenase-1 inhibitor, exerts potent antithrombotic effect without"aspirin dilemma" Thrombosis Research. 132: 56–62
28. Mei XT, Xu DH, Xu SK, Zheng YP, Xu SB (2013) Zinc(II)-curcumin accelerates the healing of acetic acid-induced chronicgastric ulcers in rats by decreasing oxidative stress and downregulationof matrix metalloproteinase-9, Food and Chemical Toxicology. 60: 448–454
29. Guth PH, Aures D, Paulsen G (1989) Topical aspirin plus HCl gastric lesion in the rat. Gastroen-terology. 76–88.

14

Systematic Regional Variations in Purkinje Cell Spiking Patterns

Jianqiang Xiao[1], Nadia L. Cerminara[2], Yuriy Kotsurovskyy[1], Hanako Aoki[4], Amelia Burroughs[2], Andrew K. Wise[3], Yuanjun Luo[4], Sarah P. Marshall[1], Izumi Sugihara[4,5], Richard Apps[2]*¶, Eric J. Lang[1]*¶

1 Department of Neuroscience & Physiology, New York University School of Medicine, New York, New York, United States of America, **2** School of Physiology and Pharmacology, University of Bristol, Bristol, United Kingdom, **3** The Bionics Institute, East Melbourne, Victoria, Australia, **4** Department of Systems Neurophysiology, Graduate School of Medicine, Tokyo Medical and Dental University, Tokyo, Japan, **5** Center for Brain Integration Research, Tokyo Medical and Dental University, Tokyo, Japan

Abstract

In contrast to the uniform anatomy of the cerebellar cortex, molecular and physiological studies indicate that significant differences exist between cortical regions, suggesting that the spiking activity of Purkinje cells (PCs) in different regions could also show distinct characteristics. To investigate this possibility we obtained extracellular recordings from PCs in different zebrin bands in crus IIa and vermis lobules VIII and IX in anesthetized rats in order to compare PC firing characteristics between zebrin positive (Z+) and negative (Z−) bands. In addition, we analyzed recordings from PCs in the A2 and C1 zones of several lobules in the posterior lobe, which largely contain Z+ and Z− PCs, respectively. In both datasets significant differences in simple spike (SS) activity were observed between cortical regions. Specifically, Z− and C1 PCs had higher SS firing rates than Z+ and A2 PCs, respectively. The irregularity of SS firing (as assessed by measures of interspike interval distribution) was greater in Z+ bands in both absolute and relative terms. The results regarding systematic variations in complex spike (CS) activity were less consistent, suggesting that while real differences can exist, they may be sensitive to other factors than the cortical location of the PC. However, differences in the interactions between SSs and CSs, including the post-CS pause in SSs and post-pause modulation of SSs, were also consistently observed between bands. Similar, though less strong trends were observed in the zonal recordings. These systematic variations in spontaneous firing characteristics of PCs between zebrin bands in vivo, raises the possibility that fundamental differences in information encoding exist between cerebellar cortical regions.

Editor: Alain Chédotal, Institut de la Vision, France

Funding: This work was supported by grants to EJL from the National Science Foundation, United States of America (www.NSF.gov) (Grant: IOS-1051858) and National Institute of Neurological Disorders and Stroke (www.ninds.nih.gov) (Grant: NS-37028), to RA and NLC from the Medical Research Council, United Kingdom (www.mrc.ac.uk/index.htm) (Grant: G1100626), and to IS from the Japan Society for the Promotion of Science (JSPS) (www.jsps.go.jp/english/) (Grants-in-Aid for Scientific Research-KAKENHI, 25430032). The funders had no role in study design, data collection and analysis, decision to publish, or preparation of the manuscript.

Competing Interests: IS is a PLOS ONE Editorial Board member and this does not alter the authors' adherence to PLOS ONE Editorial policies and criteria.

* Email: eric.lang@nyumc.org (EJL); r.apps@bristol.ac.uk (RA)

¶ RA and EJL are joint senior authors on this work.

Introduction

The circuitry and the physiological properties of a brain region's cellular constituents constrain its computational properties. The cerebellar cortex offers what appears to be perhaps a unique opportunity for deriving structure-function correlations, because, with few exceptions, it is an essentially anatomically uniform structure whose few morphologically distinct cell types are interconnected according to relatively simple geometric rules. This uniformity is not absolute; for example, unipolar brush cells are limited primarily to so-called vestibulocerebellar regions [1]; nevertheless, the microcircuitry of most cerebellar cortical regions appears to be quite alike, suggesting that most cortical regions perform similar computations, and indeed, theories of cerebellar function have tended to be global in nature and based largely on a generic anatomical circuit diagram [2–7].

Belying this apparent uniformity, it has become increasingly clear that cerebellar cortical regions vary considerably on a genetic/molecular level [8–11]. A number of genes are expressed only in specific areas, and, indeed, the differential expression patterns of various molecules have been used to subdivide the cortex into discrete compartments [8,11].

Among the various gene expression patterns that can be used to compartmentalize the cerebellar cortex that of zebrin II (aldolase C) is the most well-characterized. In mammals and birds, regions in which Purkinje cells (PCs, the sole output neurons of the cerebellar cortex) express zebrin (Z+) alternate with ones that do not (Z−), subdividing much of the cerebellar cortex into longitudinally running alternating Z+ and Z− bands [11–15].

This zebrin banding pattern is particularly useful as a frame of reference because it shows at least some correspondence with the topographies of the afferent (particularly the olivocerebellar zonal system) and efferent projections to and from the cortex [8,16–24]. Moreover, the expression patterns of a number of other genes can be straightforwardly mapped onto that of zebrin, and many of these likely affect neuronal activity. For example, excitatory amino acid transporter 4 (EAAT4), which is preferentially localized to perisynaptic regions of the PC dendritic plasma membrane, is much more highly expressed in Z+ than Z− PCs [25,26], and loss of its activity significantly enhances both parallel fiber and climbing fiber evoked EPSCs [27–32].

Such results suggest that the spiking patterns of PCs could vary significantly between cerebellar cortical regions, which, in turn, could lead to differences in the integrative/computational properties between local cortical regions, and potentially to differences in the functional states of the targets of these local cortical regions. Yet, the issues of whether the spontaneous spiking patterns of cerebellar cortical regions vary systematically between molecularly-defined compartments, and the behavioral consequences of such variation, remain unknown. Here we focus on the first part of this issue, and show that spontaneous PC activity varies systematically between Z+ and Z− bands of the cerebellar cortex.

Zones defined on the basis of physiological responses to stimulation of cerebellar afferents represent a second well-established scheme for compartmentalizing the cerebellar cortex [33–35]. Thus, we also looked for differences in PC firing patterns between such zones. A large degree of overlap between physiologically-defined zones and zebrin bands exists, and so, a priori, similar results should be found using both compartmentalization criteria. Yet, although the physiological zones and zebrin bands overlap extensively, they are not congruent, and thus comparisons between these two schemes could reveal fundamental organizational principles of cerebellar function.

In sum, a significant number of differences in the molecular and physiological properties of Z+ and Z− bands have been described. Such differences make it plausible that PC spiking activity should also vary between Z+ and Z− bands. Here, we report on the differences in spontaneous in vivo firing patterns of PCs between Z+ and Z− bands, and compare them with similar findings between different physiological zones.

Methods

Experiments were performed in accordance with the NIH's *Guide for the Care and Use of Laboratory Animals* and the UK Animals (Scientific Procedures) Act 1986. Experimental protocols were approved by the Institutional Animal Care and Use Committees of New York University School of Medicine and the institutional Ethical Review Group at the University of Bristol.

General surgical procedures

In most experiments in which the zebrin band of the recorded PCs was determined, female Sprague-Dawley rats (225–300 g) were initially anesthetized with ketamine (100 mg/kg) and xylazine (8 mg/kg) intraperitoneally. Supplemental anesthetic was given via a femoral catheter (ketamine, ~260 μg/kg/min; xylazine, ~50 μg/kg/min) to maintain a constant depth of anesthesia. In the other experiments urethane was used as the anesthetic and an initial dose of 1.2–1.5 g/kg (i.p.) was given with supplemental doses given if needed. In experiments where PCs were assigned to physiologically-identified cerebellar cortical zones, recordings were obtained from male Wistar rats anesthetized with ketamine (100 mg/kg) and xylazine (5 mg/kg) intraperitoneally, and supplementary doses of anesthetic were administered as required. In all experiments, the depth of anesthesia was regularly assessed by a paw pinch to monitor reflex muscle tone. Rectal temperature was maintained at 37°C. To gain access to the cerebellum, animals were placed in a stereotaxic frame, and a craniotomy performed to expose the posterior lobe of the cerebellum.

Recording and localization of PCs

Zebrin band experiments. Following removal of the dura, the cortical surface was stabilized and protected by covering it with an electron microscope grid pre-embedded in a thin sheet of silicone rubber. The grid was cemented onto the skull surrounding the craniotomy. Extracellular recordings of PC activity at the somatic level were obtained from the apices of crus II and vermis lobule VIII using glass microelectrodes filled with 2.0 M NaCl solution and mounted on a motorized 3D manipulator (MCL-3, Lang GmbH & Co. KG). A 3 to 5-min continuous recording of spontaneous activity was made when simple spikes (SSs) and complex spikes (CSs) were both observed, usually at a depth between 200 and 300 μm. The presence of SSs and the initial positivity of the CS waveform indicated that the recordings were made at or close to the PC soma. Neural activity was recorded using a multichannel recording system (MultiChannel Systems, Germany) with a 25 kHz/channel sampling rate, gain of 1000x, and band pass filters set at 0.2–8.0 kHz.

Recordings of dendritic CSs from a dataset that was used for other purposes in a previous study were also analyzed [36]. In these experiments a multielectrode recording approach was used in which CS activity was obtained from arrays of crus 2a PCs simultaneously. The surgical procedures were essentially identical to those just described for the somatic recordings. The electrodes used in the multielectrode experiments were filled with a 1:1 mixture of 2.0 M NaCl and glycerin (the addition of glycerin slowed evaporation of the internal electrode solution). Details of the construction and implantation of the electrodes can be found in [37]. In brief, individual electrodes were generally implanted to depths of 100–150 μm below the brain surface, corresponding to mid-molecular layer levels, and then were released from the micromanipulator. Once all electrodes in the array have been implanted CSs were recorded simultaneously from all electrodes for a 20-min period. It should be noted that SSs are not observed when recording CS activity from the middle molecular layer. This is consistent with the poor back propagation of somatic sodium spikes into the dendrites [38].

At the end of every experiment, the recording pipette was drained of the NaCl solution, refilled with alcian blue solution, and connected to a pressure-injection system, while the pipette remained in place on the microdrive. Injections were then made either at the corners of the recording platform, or, when only a few PCs were recorded in the experiment, to the location of each recorded PC based on its coordinates relative to an origin point defined on the surface of the lobule. To make the injection, the pipette was lowered into the cortex to a depth of 200–300 μm and pressure applied to eject a small amount of the dye solution. The animal was then intracardially perfused with phosphate buffered saline (PBS) followed by 4% paraformaldehyde. The brains were embedded in gelatin and cut in the plane parallel to the cerebellar surface of the recording area into 80 μm-thick serial sections. This thickness (unusually large for immunostaining) was used to locate the injection marks in a small number of sections. All serial sections were then processed for zebrin staining as previously described [12,13]. Briefly, sections were incubated with the biotinylated rabbit anti-Aldoc antibody (#69076, immunogen:

amino acids 322–344 of rat Aldoc; produced in one of the laboratories and tested for specificity with Western blot [12]; 320 ng/ml) for 48 hours, then with biotinylated peroxidase-avidin complex (PK6100 Elite ABC kit; Vector Laboratories, Burlingame, CA) for 8–12 hr, and finally incubated with diaminobenzidine (0.5 mg/ml), glucose oxidase (0.01 mg/ml; type II, G-6125; Sigma, St. Louis, MO), ammonium chloride (4 mg/ml), and beta-D(+)-glucose (2 mg/ml) in phosphate-buffered saline for 60 min. Sections were mounted on glass slides, dried and coverslipped with Permount (Fisher Scientific, Fair Lawn, NJ). Serial sections were photographed with 4x objective. Image files of photos were trimmed at the cerebellar surface and superimposed by referring to the folial contour and the labeled zebrin bands by using graphics software (Illustrator, Adobe, San Jose, CA, U.S.A.). The location of the recording sites relative to zebrin bands in crus II or lobule VIII was determined based on the stained zebrin bands and recovered dye marks, which emerged in the superimposed assembly of photographs, and the coordinates of the recording sites (Fig. 1). Due to uneven shrinkage of the tissue, and the narrowness of some zebrin bands, not all cells could be confidently localized to a specific zebrin band. Only cells located with high confidence were included in the analyses.

Zonal experiments. Recordings of PCs in this study were from a dataset that was used previously [39]. Glass-insulated tungsten microelectrodes (Alpha-Omega, Israel) were used to record PC activity extracellularly. The recordings of individual PCs lasted approximately 30 min on average. Waveforms were filtered between 0.3–5.0 kHz. Recordings were digitized on-line (sampling rate, 21 kHz) using a Cambridge Electronic Design (CED, Cambridge, UK) 1401 analog-to-digital converter and Spike2 software (CED).

Climbing fiber fields were first evoked by peripheral stimulation and recorded using a surface electrode in order to map the approximate positions of the physiologically-identified A2 and C1 zones as a guide for the single unit recordings (for details see [40]). In brief, bipolar percutaneous stimulating electrodes were inserted into the contralateral whisker pad and the ipsilateral forelimb. Stimuli were given (single pulse; 0.1 ms duration, 1 Hz) at an intensity sufficient to evoke a small but visible muscle twitch from the stimulated body part.

The criteria used to classify individual PCs as located within a particular cerebellar cortical zone were as follows: (i) If the recording track was located no more than 0.6 mm lateral from the paravermal vein, (ii) less than 2.5 mm from the cortical surface, and (iii) the cell responded to contralateral face stimulation with an increase in CSs with an onset latency <30 ms, then it was classified as located in the A2 zone. Similarly, if the recording track was (i) between 0.6–1.3 mm lateral from the paravermal vein, (ii) less than 2.5 mm from the cortical surface, and (iii) the cell responded to ipsilateral forelimb stimulation with an increase in CSs with an onset latency <25 ms, then the PC was classified as located in the neighboring C1 zone.

Data Analysis

In zebrin band experiments, spikes were detected and sorted offline using Igor Pro (Wavemetrics, Lake Oswego). For PCs recorded in the zonal experiments, SS and CS activity was discriminated independently via a template matching algorithm (Principal component analysis, Spike2). In all experiments cross-correlation between the firing time of SSs and CSs was performed to ensure that they were recorded from the same PC, based on the presence of a post-CS pause in SS firing. The pause was measured as the latency from the onset of a CS to the first SS that occurred

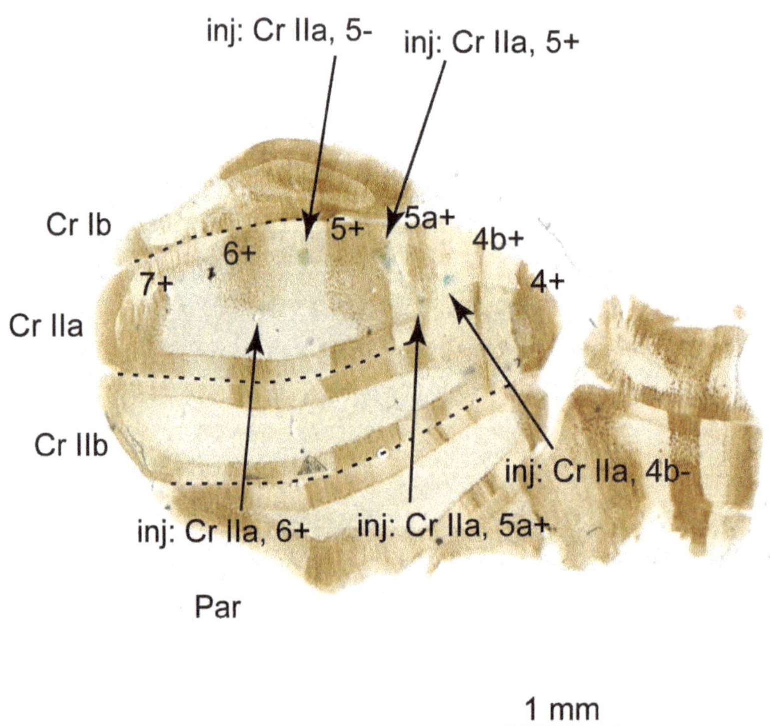

Figure 1. Zebrin staining of the hemisphere of the rat cerebellum viewed in coronal section. Sulci between lobules indicated by dashed lines. The alcian blue dye spots used to locate the PC recording sites are marked with arrows (location of spot indicated by label at tail end of arrow). Z bands 4+ to 7+ are labeled. Abbreviations: Cr= crus; Par, paramedian; and inj = injection site.

following that CS. Subsequent analyses of zebrin band experiments were performed using custom routines in Igor Pro, Matlab (Mathworks, Natick), and Excel (Microsoft). Analysis of zonal experiments was performed using Neuroexplorer (Nex Technologies, Madison, AL) and Prism (Graphpad, La Jolla).

Some of the data were found to be normally distributed, but others were not. Thus, for the sake of simplicity and consistency, a non-parametric Mann–Whitney U-test was used for testing the statistical significance and medians are presented. In rare cases, which are noted in the text, when the data were normally distributed and the parametric t-test gave a different result than the non-parametric test, the results of the t-test (and mean ±s.d.) are also presented and took precedence.

The duration of the post-CS pause in SSs is different in Z+ and Z- bands (see Results). To investigate how much of this difference was due to differences in baseline SS firing rates between bands we first calculated the expected pause duration as if it were simply a function of SS firing rate; that is, under the assumption that CSs and SSs occur independently. Deviations from this value could then be used as a measure of the active suppression that was present.

The expected pause value under the assumption of independence equals one half the mean SS interspike interval (ISI_{SS}), which can be shown as follows. Take two successive SSs (SS_k and SS_{k+1}) separated by the time interval, t_i, with a CS occurring between them. Since the CSs and SSs are independent, the CS occurs with equal probability at any point in the interval t_i. Thus, the probability of the CS occurring at time t is $Pr(t) = 1/t_i$ and the average time of the CS in the interval is given by

$$E_{CS}(t) = \int_0^{t_i} \Pr(t) * t dt$$

which evaluates to $t_i/2$. The expected pause is then the difference from the average time of the CS to the second SS, $t_i - t_i/2 = t_i/2$. In general, the ISI_{SS} will vary between SSs so that the average pause for a SS train will be given by:

$$\frac{1}{N}\sum_{i=1}^{N} E_{pause}(i) = \frac{1}{N}\left(\frac{t_1}{2} + \frac{t_2}{2} + \ldots \frac{t_N}{2} +\right) = \frac{1}{2}\left(\frac{1}{N}(t_1 + t_2 + \ldots + t_N)\right)$$

This sum, however, is simply half the mean of all ISI_{SS} that contain a CS. Given the assumption of independence these ISIs should represent a random sample of all ISI_{SS}, and thus be an unbiased estimate of the mean ISI_{SS} of the complete SS population. The ratio of the SS pause to the mean ISI_{SS} is therefore 0.5.

Results

Database

This study presents results related to differences in PC activity between Z+ and Z− bands using four specific datasets, the first three consist of recordings of PC activity under ketamine/xylazine anesthesia. The first set consists of crus IIa and vermis lobule VIII PCs whose locations were verified histologically using reconstructed zebrin maps (n = 38 PCs, 11 animals) (see Methods, 'Recording and localization of PCs'). A second dataset of recordings of SS and CS activity were analyzed from PCs whose locations were physiologically identified to be in the A2 or C1 zones (n = 26 PCs, 14 animals). Although the physiological zones and zebrin bands are not entirely congruent in the posterior lobe of the rat cerebellum, the A2 zone comprises mainly Z+ bands whereas the C1 zone comprises mainly Z− ones [17]. Because these zones are not fully equivalent to the zebrin bands, we present the data from the zebrin and zonally-identified PCs separately for each analysis. Furthermore, later we present anatomical and statistically analyses in support of the validity of using the A2 and C1 zones as surrogates for Z+ and Z− bands (see later Results subsection *'Degree of overlap of physiologically-defined zones with zebrin bands'*). The third dataset consists of multielectrode recordings from a prior study [36], which, because of electrode placement in the mid to upper molecular layer (see Methods), consists only of CS activity. In this dataset PC locations with respect to the zebrin bands were verified histologically as described in the Methods. The fourth dataset consists of PC activity from lobules VIII and IX that was recorded and identified in exactly the same manner as described for the first dataset, except that urethane was used as the anesthetic.

The specific locations of all recordings are listed in Table 1. Examples of the recordings in each dataset are shown in figure 2. In the presentation below we describe the results from the ketamine/xylazine recordings (data sets 1, 2 and 3). In the final Results subsection we compare these results with those from the urethane recordings.

PCs in Z− bands show higher SS firing rates

Comparison of SS average firing rates (total number of SSs divided by recording duration) between PCs in Z+ and Z− bands revealed a significant difference between these populations. Under ketamine, Z− cells fire at rates that are 92% higher, on average, than Z+ cells (Z− = 44.8 Hz, n = 18; Z+ = 22.5 Hz, n = 20; p = 0.0006). Figure 3A plots the entire distribution of SS firing rates of somatically-recorded, zebrin-identified PCs, and shows that while the distributions of the two PC populations overlap, the Z− distribution is shifted toward higher firing rates.

We also examined PCs recorded in the A2 and C1 zones in medial aspects of crus II, paramedian lobule, and copula pyramidis, and found a similar difference in the average SS firing rates of PCs between the two zones. SS rates for C1 (mainly Z−) were significantly higher (67%) than for A2 (mainly Z+), consistent with our first dataset (Fig. 3B; medians: C1 = 34.9 Hz, n = 8; A2 = 20.2 Hz, n = 16; p = 0.0537, Mann–Whitney U-test; means: C1 = 33.2±11.9 Hz, n = 8; A2 = 19.9±13.2 Hz, n = 16; p = 0.022, t-test; note that in two cells from the A2 zone only CSs were recorded and so these PCs were not included in this analysis).

If the two datasets are combined, the difference between the Z+/A2 and Z−/C1 groups remains highly statistically significant (Z−/C1: 40.1 Hz, n = 26; Z+/A2: 20.2 Hz, n = 36; p~0). In sum, the results as a whole indicate that SS rates are higher in Z− bands than in Z+ ones throughout much, if not all, of the posterior lobe.

The regularity of SS activity varies between Z+ and Z− bands

Regularity of SS activity may be a critical parameter governing the efficacy of transmission of information to the cerebellar nuclei, particularly if PCs use a rate code, as is often assumed (e.g., see [5]). Thus, we investigated whether the regularity of SS activity varied between Z+ and Z− bands, as any differences might point to differences in the way Z+ and Z− cortical bands interact with their target cerebellar nuclear regions.

We measured the absolute and relative regularity of the SS trains using the standard deviation and coefficient of variation

Table 1. Spatial distribution of the recorded cells.

A.	Zebrin bands	Somatic	Dendritic	All
	Ketamine/Xylazine			
	Crus IIa 4−	1	3	4
	Crus IIa 4b−	2	4	6
	Crus IIa 4b+	1		1
	Crus IIa 5−	10	13	23
	Crus IIa 5+	5	20	25
	Crus IIa 5a−	2		2
	Crus IIa 5a+	3		3
	Crus IIa 6−		8	8
	Crus IIa 6+	4	15	19
	Crus IIa 7+		2	2
	Lobule VIII 1−	2		2
	Lobule VIII 1+	1		1
	Lobule VIII 2+	3		3
	Urethane			
	Lobule VIII 1−	2		2
	Lobule VIII 2+	2		2
	Lobule VIII 2−	1		1
	Lobule VIII 3+	1		1
	Lobule VIII 3−	1		1
	Lobule VIII 4−	1		1
	Lobule IX 2+	11		11
	Lobule IX 3+	4		4
	Sum	57	65	122

B.	Physiological zones	Somatic
	Crus II A2	13
	Crus II C1	1
	Paramedian A2	5
	Paramedian C1	4
	Copula Pyramidis C1	3
	Sum	26

A) The zebrin bands for all PCs were histologically identified. Some of the cells were somatically recorded; others dendritically. B) The zonal locations of an additional sample of PCs were physiologically determined. All cells were somatically recorded. A2 zone comprises mainly Z+ bands while the C1 zone comprises mainly Z− bands. Two cells recorded in Crus II A2 zone did not fire SSs and were not included in the analysis of SS firing rate.

(CV = SD/mean), respectively, of the interspike interval (ISI) distribution. The spike trains of Z+ PCs were more irregular in both absolute and relative terms (Fig. 4A, B; SDs: Z− = 14.2 ms, n = 18; Z+ = 54.3 ms, n = 20; $p = 0.0018$; CVs: Z− = 0.57, n = 18; Z+ = 0.97, n = 20; $p = 0.0172$).

For the zonal data, trends consistent with the zebrin data were found, although these differences were not statistically significant (Fig. 4C, D; SDs: C1 = 53.6 ms, n = 8; A2, 101.0 ms, n = 16; $p = 0.0708$; CVs: mainly Z− C1 = 1.54, n = 8, mainly Z+ A2 = 2.08, n = 16, $p = 0.4812$).

CS firing rate relationship to Z bands

It is known that CS and SS rates can influence each other, leading to either an inverse or a direct correlation in rates, depending on the experimental manipulation [41–47]. Thus, given the observed differences in SS firing rates between Z+ and Z− bands we next investigated whether CS firing rates also varied. In contrast to the SS results, those for CSs were not consistent between datasets. For the somatic recordings from PCs in zebrin-identified locations, the distribution of firing rates overlapped substantially with no statistical difference in the medians (Fig. 5A; Z− = 1.15 Hz; n = 18; Z+ = 1.16 Hz, n = 20; $p = 0.92$). In contrast, in recordings from zonally-identified PCs, A2 cells showed significantly higher CS firing rates than did C1 cells (Fig. 5B; C1 = 0.24 Hz, n = 8; A2 = 0.66 Hz, n = 18; $p = 0.0083$).

It is perhaps not surprising that the results from these two datasets differ with regard to CS firing rates, as CSs are generated in response to activity arising in inferior olivary neurons rather than by local cerebellar cortical network activity, and thus CS firing rates may be less completely determined by factors related to the molecular make up of zebrin bands than are SS rates. In particular, CS firing rates not only are influenced by GABAergic inhibitory inputs from the cerebellar nuclei (whose activity is indeed modulated by PC activity), but also by non-GABAergic,

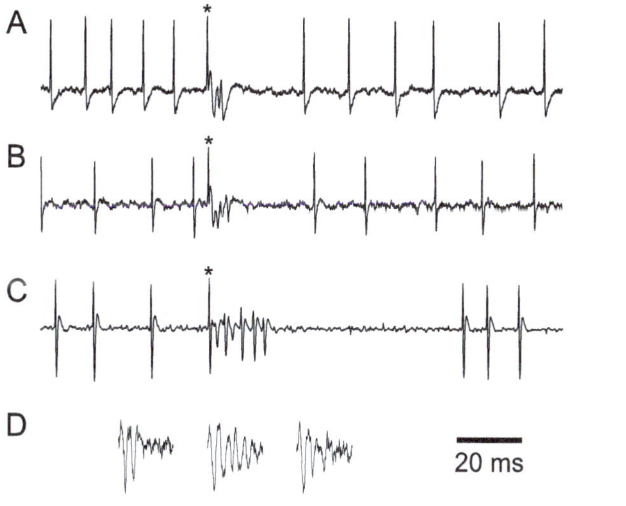

Figure 2. Extracellular recordings of PC activity. (A–B) Sample recordings from zebrin localized PCs recorded under ketamine/xylazine (A) and urethane (B) that show both SSs and a CS (indicated by '*'). Note the pause in SSs following the CS. (C) Recording of PC from the zonal database displaying both SSs and a CS (indicated by '*'). Again note the pause in SSs following the CSs. The recording in C was filtered with a higher cutoff frequency for the high pass filter, eliminating the slower potential that can be seen in the recordings in (A and B), and on which the spikelets ride. (D) Extracellular traces showing three CSs from recorded from a PC with the electrode in the molecular layer, approximately 100 μm below the folial surface of crus 2a. Note how the number and size of the spikelets varies between CSs, but that the size and shape of the initial spike are nevertheless relatively constant, indicating that a single unit is being recorded.

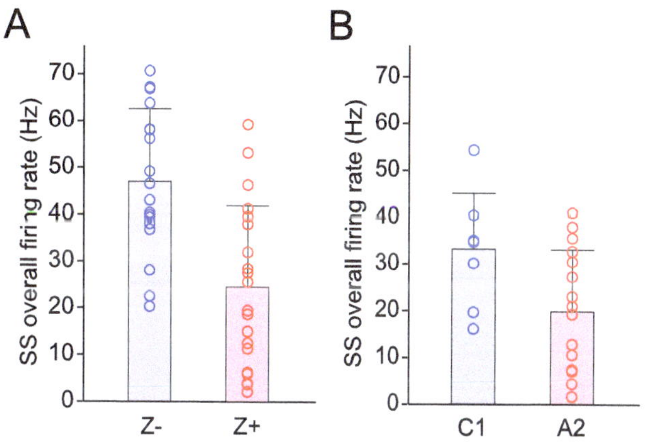

Figure 3. Z− PCs have higher SS firing rates. The difference in SS firing rate is consistent for both histologically (A) and physiologically (B) located PCs. Circles represent the overall firing rates of individual PCs in Z− bands or C1 zone (blue) and in Z+ bands or A2 zone (red). In each distribution, the bar indicates the mean. Error bars indicate one SD of the distribution.

presumably glutamatergic inputs from extra-cerebellar regions [48].

Thus, to determine the relationship between CS firing rates and zebrin, if any, it would be ideal to hold these other potential variables constant. While we could not do that, we examined CS activity recorded from PCs that were recorded simultaneously, and hence under an identical brain state (dataset 3) [36]. The CS firing rates in this larger dataset overlapped substantially with those of the somatically recorded CSs, with median CS firing rates that fell in between those of the two somatic datasets (Fig. 5C; Z+ = 0.62 Hz, n = 37; Z− = 0.81 Hz, n = 28). A small but statistically significant difference in CS average firing rates between Z+ and Z− PCs was found ($p = 0.0499$); however, in this case it was the Z− PCs that showed the higher rates. Although the difference was small, it was generally consistent across experiments, as shown by comparing the median CS firing rates for pairs of Z+ and Z− PCs obtained in the same experiment (Fig. 5D). In five of six experiments rates were higher for Z− cells ($p = 0.018$, paired t-test).

In sum, there were mixed findings relating to CS firing rates in relation to zebrin bands. However, CSs also have a profound influence on subsequent SS activity and the following sections consider this aspect of CS activity in more detail.

Differences in the post-CS pauses in SS activity between Z+ and Z− bands

One of the distinctive interactions between SSs and CSs is the pause in SS activity following most CSs [49–51]. The post-CS pause has also been suggested to be a potentially important mechanism for distinguishing CS and SS activity by the cerebellar nuclei [52]. Thus, we investigated whether the characteristics of the pause varied between Z+ and Z− bands.

The interval between each CS and the SS immediately following it was measured and the median pause duration was calculated for each cell. The population median pause duration of PCs in Z+ bands were found to be 56.5% longer than those in Z− bands (Z− = 21.9 ms, n = 18; Z+ = 34.2 ms, n = 20; $p = 0.0068$; Fig. 6A). In addition, as a population, PCs from Z+ bands showed a much wider distribution in the cell-to-cell variation of pause duration than did PCs from Z− bands, even when this variation was normalized to account for the differences in the mean pause duration of the Z+ and Z− populations (CV: Z+ = 0.554; Z− = 0.288).

Analysis of the zonal dataset showed results consistent with the zebrin data. A2 PCs (mainly Z+) showed longer pauses than did C1 PCs (mainly Z−) (C1 = 28.2 ms, n = 8; A2 = 37.2 ms, n = 16); however, the difference in medians did not reach statistical significance ($p = 0.0922$, Mann–Whitney U-test). Nevertheless, as shown in Fig. 6B, the difference in the distribution of pause durations between A2 and C1 cells shows good agreement with the Z+ and Z− data, respectively. Also consistent with the zebrin data, was the finding that the normalized variation in pause duration among A2 PCs was higher than that among C1 PCs (CV: A2, 0.747; C1, 0.396).

For the zebrin data, we next analyzed factors that could contribute to the significant difference in pause duration. First we investigated the effect of the slower SS firing rates of Z+ PCs. With a slower average firing rate the duration of the time between a CS and the immediately succeeding SS will be greater on average. Specifically, assuming that the occurrences of SSs and CSs are independent, the expected latency of a SS following a CS is equal to half the mean SS ISI (see Methods). Secondly, we investigated whether any of the difference in post-CS pause duration between Z+ and Z− bands involved differences in active suppression of SS activity.

To separate the contribution of these two factors to the difference in pause duration between Z+ and Z− bands, we normalized the mean SS pause duration of each PC by the mean SS ISI. This ratio should equal 0.5 (pause = ISI/2, so pause/ISI = 1/2) if the entire pause in SSs is simply a function of SS firing rate. The majority of PCs in both Z+ and Z− bands show ratios

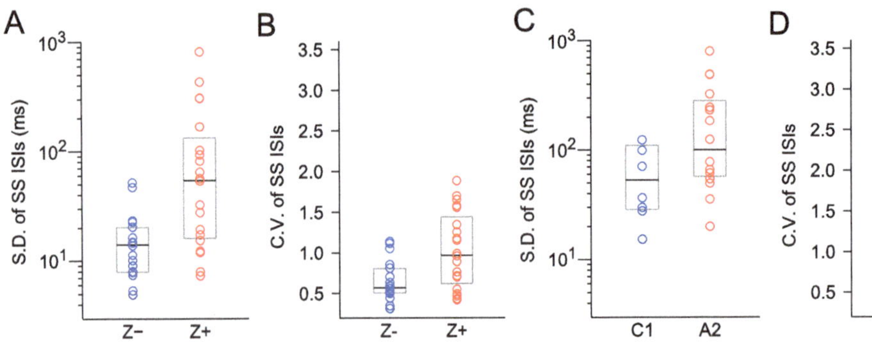

Figure 4. Z− PCs have more regular SS trains than do Z− PCs. Plots of the SD (A) and CV (B) of the ISI distributions for SS trains from Z+ and Z− PCs. Analogous plots for the zonal data are shown in (C) and (D). In each plot data the circles represent values from individual PCs, the horizontal lines show the medians of the various distributions, and the boxes indicate the interquartile ranges.

that are higher than 0.5 (Fig. 7), which indicates that the pause in SSs is longer than would be expected if the pause duration is based solely on SS firing rate. Thus, there is active suppression of SSs following a CS in both Z+ and Z− bands. However, the ratios of the Z− PCs are significantly higher than those of the Z+PCs (Z− = 1.51, n = 18; Z+ = 1.14, n = 20; p = 0.0317), indicating a greater active suppression of SSs by CSs in Z− bands.

In sum, although the absolute pause duration is greater in Z+ PCs, this is largely attributable to the lower SS firing rates (i.e., longer mean ISIs) in those PCs, because when mean ISI is controlled for, Z− PCs show a greater relative pause in SS activity following a CS.

PCs in Z+ bands have a stronger increase in SS local activity after CS

After the initial pause in SSs following a CS, there is often a longer latency modulation in SSs, which may take the form of a delayed return to baseline activity or a transient overshoot in activity [53]. To test whether the post-pause modulation differs between Z+ and Z− PCs, we measured the average firing rate of SS in a 100-ms time window that started at the onset of each CS. This post-CS firing rate was normalized by the overall SS firing rate of the same cell to provide a ratio that reflected the post-CS change in SS firing rate relative to the overall spiking level of the cell. This ratio was significantly different between Z+ and Z- cells (Fig. 8A; Z− = 1.05, n = 18; Z+ = 1.16, n = 20; p = 0.0065).

Thus, in Z+ bands there is a stronger positive modulation of SS activity following each CS; this relative increase in activity occurred despite the longer initial pause of PCs in Z+ bands. Furthermore, the CV of the distribution of ratio values was much wider for Z+ cells than for Z− cells (Z− = 0.160, Z+ = 0.437; or 1:2.7), indicating that PCs in Z+ bands are more heterogeneous with regard to how SSs and CSs interact.

PCs in the A2 and C1 zones showed a similar differential in their post-pause modulation of SSs to the Z+ and Z− PCs (Fig. 8B). That is, A2 PCs had a relatively higher modulation of SS levels than did C1 PCs, but the difference in the modulation ratios was not statistically significant (C1 = 1.22, n = 8; A2 = 1.26, n = 16; p = 0.8303). The CV of the ratio value for the A2 cell population was larger than that for the C1 population (C1 = 0.31, A2 = 1.04; or 1:3.4), consistent with the zebrin data.

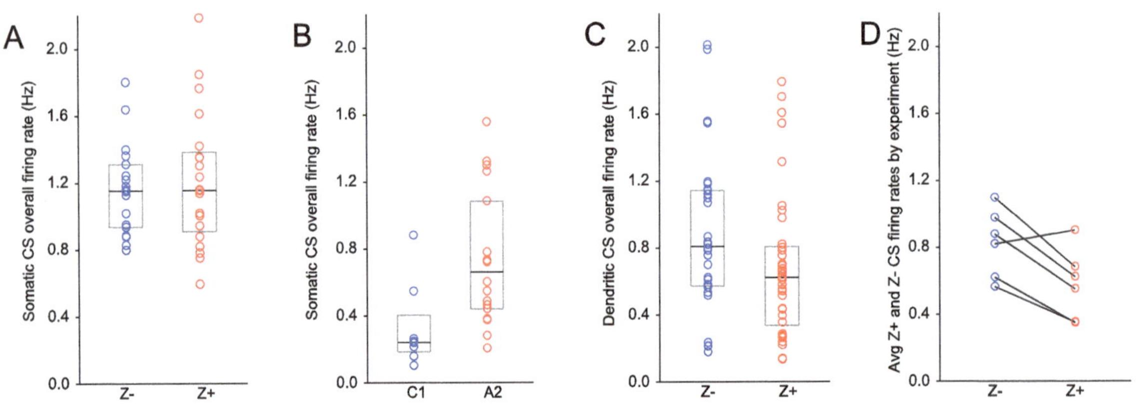

Figure 5. Variable relationship of CS firing rate to Z+ and Z− bands. (A–C) Distribution of CS firing rates for Z− (or C1) and Z+ (or A2) cells. Circles represent the firing rates of individual PCs. In each distribution, the box indicates the 1st and 3rd quartile and the black line represents the median of the distribution. (A) Somatically recorded Z+/− PCs show comparable CS firing rate. (B) Somatically recorded PCs in C1 zone show significantly lower firing rates than those in A2 zones. (C) Dendritically recorded PCs in Z− bands had a higher median rate than Z+ bands despite the wide scatter of values within each type of band. (D) Median firing rates compared between Z+ and Z− bands within individual experiments. Each circle represents median CS firing rate for all Z− (blue) or Z+ (red) PCs from an individual experiment. Lines connect the Z+ and Z− cells obtained in the same experiment.

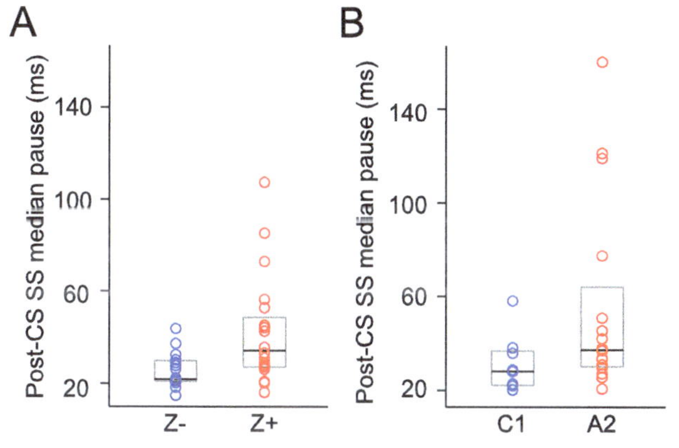

Figure 6. PCs in Z+ bands show longer absolute post-CS pauses in SS than those in Z− bands. The difference is consistent for both histologically (A) and physiologically (B) located PCs. Each circle represents the median duration of the pause of individual PCs in Z− bands or C1 zone (blue) and in Z+ bands or A2 zone (red). The black lines indicate the overall median across each group, and the grey boxes indicate the range from 25% to 75% of each distribution. Note that Z+ bands and A2 zone also consistently show higher variation than Z− bands and C1 zone.

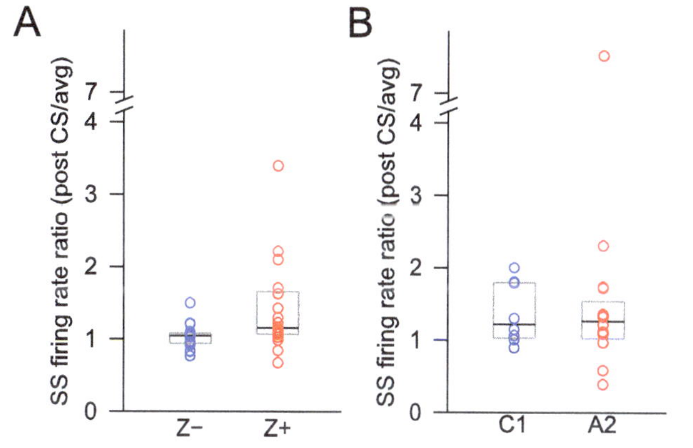

Figure 8. Stronger increase in SS activity after CS in Z+ than Z− bands. The difference is consistent for both histologically (A) and physiologically (B) located PCs. Each circle represents the median ratio of the SS firing rate for the 100-ms period after a CS to the overall SS firing rate for the individual PCs in the Z− bands or the C1 zone (blue) and in the Z+ bands or the A2 zone (red). The black lines indicate the overall median across each group, and the grey boxes indicate the range from 25% to 75% of each distribution.

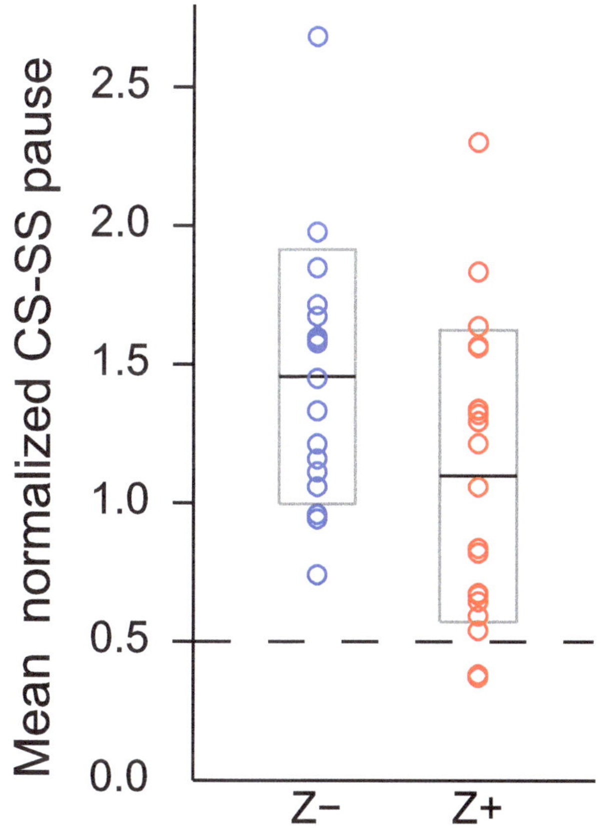

Figure 7. CSs in Z− bands cause a relatively stronger active suppression of SSs. The mean SS pause duration of each PC was normalized by dividing by its mean SS ISI. The distribution of ratio is shown for Z+ and Z− PCs. Dashed line indicates the expected ratio if the latency from a CS to the first succeeding SS is solely a function of SS firing rate. The solid black lines indicate the overall median across each group, and the grey boxes indicate the range from 25% to 75% of each distribution.

Differences in Z+ and Z− PC activity under urethane

To rule out the possibility that the observed differences between Z+ and Z− PCs reflect the particular anesthetic state in which the recordings were obtained we investigated whether similar differences between Z+ and Z− PCs existed under urethane, an anesthetic that acts via different mechanisms than ketamine/xylazine. Recordings were obtained of Z+ and Z− PCs from vermis lobules VIII and IX (Z−, $n = 5$; Z+, $n = 18$; for details on lobular and zebrin band distribution see Table 1). With one exception, all of the parameters that showed significant differences between Z+ and Z− under ketamine/xylazine showed identically-directed differences under urethane. Specifically, under urethane, statistically significant differences were found for SS firing rate (Z− = 44.2 Hz; Z+ = 21.0 Hz; $p = 0.0009$), the SD of the SS ISI (Z− = 6.67 ms; Z+ = 14.47 ms; $p = 0.0041$), and the post-CS pause in SSs (Z− = 40.9 ms; Z+ = 82.4 ms; $p = 0.0279$). For the CV of the SS ISI distribution, the difference between Z+ and Z− cells was not significant (Z− = 0.272; Z+ = 0.370; $p = 0.1679$). The post-pause modulation of SS activity in the 100 ms post-CS period could not be compared with the values under ketamine/xylazine because the pause duration under urethane was longer than half of this period in most PCs (hence no spikes were present for at least the first half of the period). The differences in the various parameters between Z+ and Z− PCs are summarized in the top halves of Tables 2A and B (labeled 'Global'), and show the consistency of the results the three data sets where SS activity was recorded. That is, for each parameter analyzed (except CS firing rate), the inequality sign points in the same direction for all three datasets (Table 2B, Global).

Zebrin-related differences are present in multiple regions

The above results suggest that the differences between Z+ and Z− PC firing patterns are a general phenomena, at least throughout much of the posterior lobe of the cerebellar cortex. To test the generality of the results further, we analyzed the differences between Z+ and Z− bands for individual lobules. For the zebrin experiments enough Z+ and Z− PCs were present in crus IIa and vermis lobule VIII to make comparisons. For the zonal recordings this was the case for the paramedian lobule.

Table 2. Comparison of differences between Z− and Z+ regions by region and anesthetic.

(A)

	N	SS FR (Hz)	SD (ms)	CV	CS FR (Hz)	Pause (ms)	NPause	PPause
Global								
Zebrin K/X	18/20	44.8/22.5	14.2/54.3	0.57/0.97	1.15/1.16	21.9/34.2	1.51/1.14	1.05/1.16
Zebrin U	5/18	44.2/21.0	6.7/14.5	0.27/0.37	0.36/0.88	40.9/82.4	1.96/1.47	n/a
Zonal K/X	8/16[a]	34.9/20.2	53.6/101.0	1.54/2.08	0.24/0.66	28.2/37.2	2.47/1.38	1.22/1.26
Regional								
cIIA K/X	15/13	49.2/32.0	13.7/19.1	0.56/0.71	1.13/1.14	21.7/27.7	1.59/1.29	1.04/1.15
VIII K/X	3/7	28.1/5.9	22.4/165.1	0.63/1.34	1.22/1.35	32.1/56.2	1.16/0.67	1.08/1.62
VIII U	5/3	44.2/29.8	6.7/12.8	0.27/0.41	0.36/0.77	40.9/83.0	1.96/2.63	n/a
PM K/X	5/4	37.4/10.7	32.2/231.8	1.34/2.57	0.2/0.72	97.3/159.8	2.47/1.38	1.10/1.32

(B)

	N	SS FR	SD	CV	CS FR	Pause	NPause	PPause
Global								
Zebrin K/X	18/20	**>	**<	*<	≈	**<	*>	**<
Zebrin U	5/18	**>	**<	<	*<	*<	>	n/a
Zonal K/X	8/16[a]	*[b]>	[T]<	<	**<	[T]<	>	<
Regional								
cIIa K/X	15/13	*>	[T]<	<	≈	<	*>	*<
VIII K/X	3/7	*>	*<	*<	<	*<	>	<
VIII U	5/3	*>	*<	<	<	*<	<	n/a
PM K/X	5/4	[T]>	[T]<	<	<	<	>	<

(A) Summary of values for each parameter that was analyzed. The format is Z−/Z+. Global section gives the medians for the entire populations for the three data sets where somatic recordings were obtained. The Regional section provides data for each of the lobules where enough Z+ and Z− cells were recorded to make a comparison. K/X: ketamine/xylazine, U: urethane. cIIa: crus IIA, VIII: vermis lobule VIII, PM: paramedian lobule. SS FR = SS average firing rate; SD, CV = SD and CV of the SS ISI distribution; Pause: the median post CS-pause in SS activity; NPause = the normalized pause in SS activity (mean Pause/mean SS ISI); PPause = increase in SS firing rate within 100 ms post-PC; a: 16 A2 cells included for most of the measurements except CS FR, for which 18 A2 cells were included, because 2 PCs in the A2 zone had no SS activity; (B) Summary of the direction and significance of the difference in parameter values between Z− and Z+ bands. The > and < symbols indicate cells in Z− regions have a larger or smaller value for each parameter, respectively. **: $P<0.01$; *: $0.01<P<0.05$; T: $0.05<P<0.1$; b: based on t-test instead of non-parametric test, see Methods.

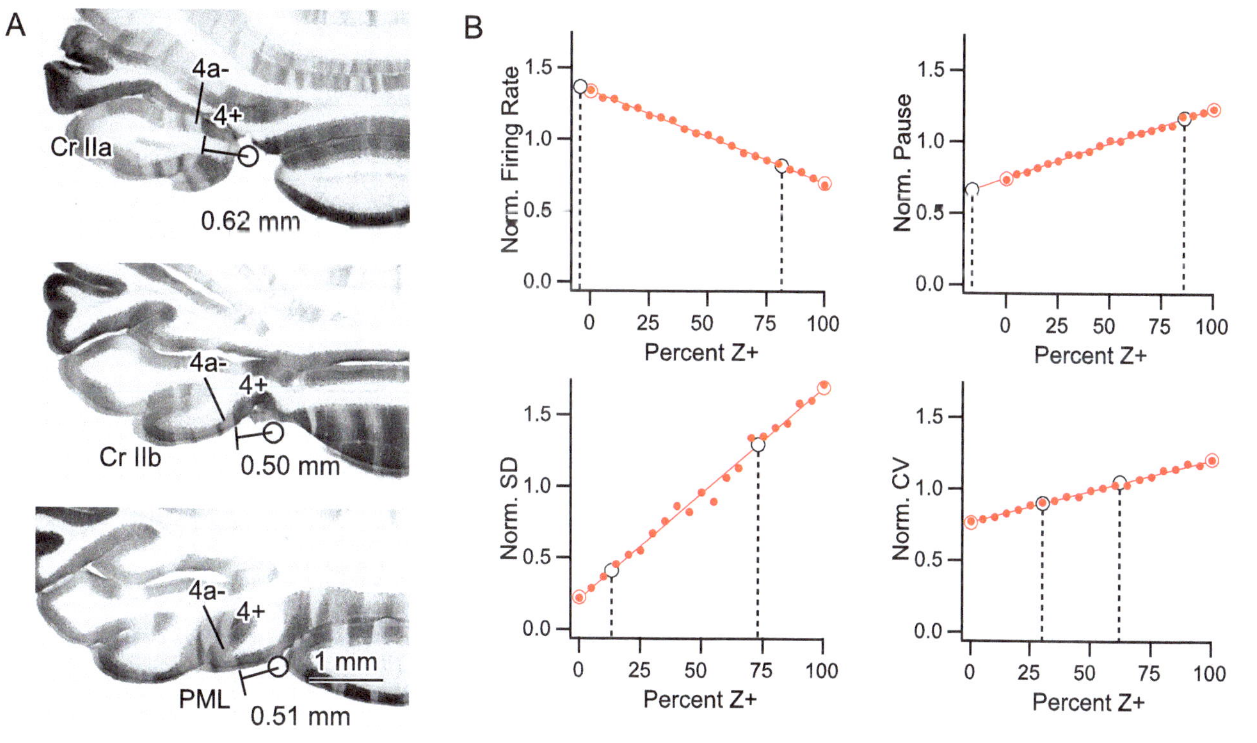

Figure 9. Zebrin composition of A2 and C1 zones. (A) Anatomical estimate of zebrin bands for A2 and C1 zones in crus II and paramedian lobule. In horizontal sections on which the apical area of crus IIa, crus IIb, and paramedian lobules were seen, the distance between the putative position of the paravermal vein and the boundary between Z+ band 4+ and Z− band 4a− was measured. Circle indicates the putative position of the paravermal vein. This boundary roughly corresponded to the physiological boundary between A2 and C1 zones (0.6 mm, Methods). (B) Plots of normalized spike train parameters (firing rate, SS pause, SD of ISI, and CV of ISI) for populations consisting of different percentages of Z+ PCs. Simulated population averages indicated by filled small red circles. Values for experimental zebrin datasets indicated by large unfilled red circles (Z− at 0%, Z+ at 100%). Lines are least squares fits to the simulated population data. Large unfilled black circles show zonal data (C1 shown by left circle in each plot, A2 by right circle). Placement of black circles along x-axis was determined using the experimental parameter value in the corresponding regression equation, and thus provided an estimate of the percentage of Z+ PCs in the population (indicated by dashed black lines).

In almost all cases, each individual lobule showed the same trends as were observed in the combined population (Table 2A,B, bottom halves labeled 'Regional'). That is, relative to their Z+ counterpart, each Z− region had higher SS firing rates, greater absolute and relative regularity, shorter absolute but longer relative pauses, and a less positive post-CS modulation of SSs following the initial pause. In most cases these differences were statistically significant (indicated by * or ** in Table 2B). There was just one exception other than CS firing rate: the normalized pause duration in vermis VIII under urethane. Thus, the general consistency in the results across lobules and anesthetics suggests that the observed differences between PC activity in Z+ and Z− bands is a common organizational principle of the cerebellar posterior lobe, and possibly the entire cerebellum.

Degree of overlap of physiologically-defined zones with zebrin bands

To validate the use of the A2 and C1 zones, respectively, as surrogates for Z+ and Z− bands, we estimated the zebrin composition of these zones for the regions of cortex where PC activity was recorded. In zebrin (aldolase C) immunostained brains, Z+ band 4+ is generally located under the paravermal vein and extends up to 0.5–0.6 mm laterally in crus IIa, crus IIb and paramedian lobule (Fig. 9A). Since fixed tissue for immunostaining is slightly shrunken from the physiological brain, the boundary between 4+ and 4a- (0.5–0.6 mm lateral to the center of the paravermal vein) is likely to correspond to the physiological boundary between the A2 and C1 zones (i.e. 0.6 mm from the paravermal vein, see Methods). As our A2 recordings were located no more than 0.6 mm lateral from the paravermal vein (see Methods), we can therefore safely assume that the PCs we recorded in the A2 zone were all Z+.

The Z− band 4a− (~0.18 mm wide, measured in crus IIb in the center panel of Fig. 9A) is located immediately lateral to 4+, followed by a very narrow Z+ band (4b+, ~0.08 mm wide), a Z− band (4b−, ~0.33 mm wide), a very narrow Z+ band (5a+, ~0.05 mm wide) and a Z- band (5a−, ~0.21 mm wide; making a total of 0.85 mm and Z+: Z− ratio of 0.13: 0.72). These measures were variable among lobules (crus IIa, IIb and paramedian lobule) and among individuals to some extent. As our C1 recordings were located within the range 0.6–1.3 mm lateral to the paravermal vein, we can assume that C1 zone mostly corresponds to the series of Z−/Z+ bands between 4a− and 5a− or the medial part of these series. Then, assuming a random positional sampling of PCs, we can estimate that a PC in the C1 zone in the areas of cortex under study has an 85% (=0.72/(0.13+0.72)) chance of being Z−.

Although the anatomical estimate indicates that random samples of PCs from the A2 and C1 zones from the lobules we recorded should be good surrogates for Z+ and Z− PC populations, respectively, it does not necessarily imply that the PCs in the actual dataset represent random samples. Thus, to test further whether the A2 and C1 data were Z+ and Z− surrogates, we generated mixed populations of Z+ and Z− PCs from the zebrin dataset by randomly sampling with replacement the Z+ and Z− identified PC populations. Each population had a total of 20 PCs. For each ratio of Z+ to Z− PCs (Z+/Z−: 20/0, 19/1, …, 0/20) 100 populations were generated, and the average value of a normalized spiking parameter (SS firing rate, SD and CV of the SS firing rate, and absolute pause duration) was calculated. The parameters were normalized such that the overall mean of each parameter was equal to one for the entire zonal and zebrin populations, which was done to eliminate the absolute differences in these parameters between the zonal and zebrin datasets. Thus, only the relative differences between Z+ and Z− cells, and correspondingly, A2 and C1 cells, remained.

The average value of each parameter from the simulated populations was then plotted as a function of the percentage of Z+ cells in the population (Fig. 9B, small red filled circles). The true experimental populations are indicated by large unfilled red circles at 0% (Z−) and 100% (Z+) on the plots, and closely match the averages of the corresponding simulated populations. A line was then fit (least squares) to the simulated data for each parameter. The parameter values for the A2 and C1 datasets were then entered into the linear regression equations to calculate an estimate of the percentage of Z+ cells in each zonal population.

Firing rate was the parameter showing the most robust difference between Z+ and Z− PCs and it provided estimates that most closely matched that of the anatomical estimates for the A2 (81.5% Z+) and C1 (−4.3% Z+, physically one cannot have less than 0% but the value of the zonal data falls slightly above that of the regression line at 0% leading to the negative percentage estimate) zones. Based on the four parameters the average estimate of the percentage of Z+ PCs for the C1 zone was 5.7±20.5%, and that for the A2 zone was 76.4±11.6%, both of which are close to that of the anatomical estimates.

In sum, both anatomical and statistical analyses suggest that our C1 zone recordings consisted of a pure or nearly pure Z− population of PCs. These analyses also support the use of our A2 zone recordings as a good, though not perfect, surrogate for a Z+ population because the large majority of the recordings are likely Z+.

Discussion

The principal finding of this paper is that consistent differences exist in the spontaneous activity of PCs in different regions of the cerebellar cortex, which implies that the cerebellar cortex is functionally heterogeneous despite its uniform circuitry. In particular, SSs were found to have higher firing rates and less variable spike trains in Z− compared to Z+ bands. Significant differences in the basic interactions between SSs and CSs were also found. The PC recordings covered a significant amount of the cerebellar posterior lobe, suggesting that the observed differences in firing pattern between Z+ and Z− regions likely reflects a general organizational principle of the cerebellar cortex. Moreover, essentially the same findings were obtained for most of the parameters under two distinct types of anesthesia, indicating that the observed differences between the spontaneous firing patterns in Z+ and Z− bands are robust, and therefore that they likely will be observed in other physiological brain states.

Methodological Issues

Most of the experiments were done under ketamine/xylazine anesthesia, which raises the issue of how applicable the results are to the awake brain state, in particular. The possibility that the observed differences in activity between Z+ and Z− PCs are specific to the ketamine anesthesia state was ruled out by finding similar differences using urethane anesthesia. Moreover, there are additional reasons to believe that the results have general validity. Specifically, the SS results appear to be robust in that similar differences between Z+ and Z− regions in SS firing rates and patterns, and in SS-CS interactions, were observed in two independent laboratories even though recordings were obtained from different rat strains using different (albeit similar) anesthetic and recording protocols, and the recorded PCs were located in different cerebellar regions. (Differences in CS firing rates were not consistent, but possible reasons for this are discussed later.) Furthermore, other aspects of cerebellar cortical physiology (e.g., CS synchrony patterns) are similar in ketamine/xylazine anesthetized preparations and in awake animals [54–59], suggesting that many of the parameters governing the cerebellar cortical network are similar in both the waking and ketamine-anesthetized conditions, though the specific activity patterns in the anesthetized animal almost certainly do not precisely match those that occur in the awake animal, and some parameters of activity can differ significantly [60]. Finally, while this paper was under review, similar findings were reported in awake mice, extending the generality of the findings of zebrin-related differences in spike activity [61]. In particular, the two studies found similar differences in SS firing rates and absolute SS pause duration between Z+ and Z− bands. Regarding CS activity Zhou et al. found higher rates in Z− cells whereas our datasets were not fully consistent.

Possible mechanisms underlying differences in SS activity between Z+ and Z− bands

A number of mechanisms exist that potentially could explain the difference in SS firing rates between zebrin compartments observed here. The most straightforward is the possibility that there are systematic differences in the intrinsic excitability between PCs. Specifically, PCs have an intrinsic spike generator that allows them to fire spontaneously in the absence of synaptic drive [45,62–64], and systematic variations in this generator between Z+ and Z− band PCs could lead to differences in SS firing patterns. Indeed, such a systematic regional variation has been described for the depolarization-induced slow current (DISC), which increases PC excitability, and which is expressed more strongly in posterior vermis PCs [65,66], but posterior vermis is largely Z+, and thus DISC expression appears to be the opposite of what would explain the differences in SS rates found here. However, evidence has just been reported that differences related to the activity of TRPC3 (transient receptor potential cation channel type C3) in PCs contribute to differences in spiking characteristics between Z+ and Z− bands [61].

Alternatively, or in combination with any differences in PC intrinsic excitability, variations in the synaptic input to PCs could exist, either because of differences in the activity levels of the mossy fiber/granule cell input pathway to Z+ and Z− regions or because of differences in synaptically-related conductances between zebrin compartments. Differences in the activity levels of mossy fiber/granule cell input pathway to Z+ and Z− regions seems less plausible as a general mechanism, because the great diversity of mossy fiber sources makes it less likely for there to be a consistent matching of low and high activity levels to the Z+ and Z− bands, respectively. Also, while some mossy fiber systems align well with specific zebrin bands [8,18,24], in other cases the relationship is more complex [16].

Thus, a more likely possibility is that the synaptic efficacy of the parallel fiber-PC synapse varies between zebrin bands. Indeed, differences in the expression levels of several molecules exist between Z+ and Z− PCs that could lead to differences in synaptic transmission that could, in turn, explain the differences in SS rates we found. In particular, excitatory amino acid transporters (EAATs) act to limit EPSCs at parallel fiber synapses onto PCs [29–31]. One of these transporters, EAAT4, is found predominantly at perisynaptic regions on the PC dendritic membrane, and is highly expressed in Z+ PCs but not Z− PCs [25,26,67]. Given this differential expression of EAAT4, the excitatory drive from parallel fibers could be weaker in Z+ PCs, thereby leading to lower SS rates.

Another possible mechanism that could underlie the differences in overall SS firing rates is differential activation of molecular layer interneurons (MLIs; i.e., basket and stellate cells) in Z+ and Z− bands by parallel fiber activity [68]. Activation of a beam of parallel fibers leads to a traveling wave of excitation of the PCs and MLIs contacted by the parallel fibers [69,70]. The activation of the MLIs then produces a wave of inhibition that travels in the wake of the excitatory wave to PCs directly underneath the parallel fiber beam, and to PCs located on either side of the parallel fiber beam [70,71]. However, the amplitude of the evoked inhibition on PCs is not constant, but rather waxes and wanes as this second wave travels along the parallel fiber beam, such that strong activation of MLIs occurs in Z+ bands and weak activation in Z− bands [68]. Thus, parallel fiber drive to PCs would be more strongly countered by inhibition in the Z+ bands, which potentially would lead to lower SS firing rates.

The relative contributions of these and other possible mechanisms to the differences in SS activity we reported here will require study of synaptic currents and the intrinsic properties of PCs at the single and network level.

Variations in CS firing rates between zebrin bands

We obtained mixed results when comparing CS activity across zebrin bands obtained from our different datasets. Nevertheless, that differences were found in two of three datasets suggests that CSs may also vary systematically between cerebellar cortical regions. However, multiple factors may underlie this variation, only some of which are correlated with zebrin expression. In fact, several factors that are known to contribute to CS firing rates can have opposite effects, and which one dominates may vary between different behavioral contexts, leading to a differing relationship between SS and CS activity levels.

For example, in the case of zonal recordings of CS firing rates, these were higher in the A2 zone, and thus varied inversely with SS rates. This inverse relationship is consistent with the well-known observation that changes in CS rates induced by direct manipulation of inferior olive excitability produce an inverse effect on SS rates [41–44,72]. This inverse correlation of SS and CS is driven, at least in part, by climbing fiber activation of cerebellar cortical interneurons [43,50,73,74] (however, see, [41,42]), and is likely mediated via spillover of glutamate from climbing fiber-PC synapses [75–77].

In contrast, in the zebrin dataset a positive correlation of CS and SS firing rates was found across Z+ and Z− bands (i.e., both were higher in the Z− band). Such a relationship could be driven by the difference in SS activity that feeds into the disynaptic PC-cerebellar nucleo-inferior olivary pathway. Given the closed loop nature of the pathways interconnecting the cerebellar cortex, cerebellar nuclei and inferior olive, and that Z+ and Z− PCs project to separate cerebellar nuclear regions [23,78], this raises the possibility that the relatively higher SS activity in Z− bands would more strongly inhibit the cerebellar nuclei. This, in turn, could lead to a relatively stronger disinhibition of the inferior olivary regions projecting back to the Z− bands, resulting in increased CS activity. Support for the significance of this mechanism comes from studies showing manipulation of SS levels in discrete cortical regions produces correlated changes in CS activity [46,47].

During behavior, examples of both positive and negative correlation of SSs and CSs exist [79,80]. In sum, the inconsistency with regard to CS firing rate we observed may be attributable to the fact that CSs are evoked by inferior olivary activity, which is not part of the cerebellar cortex. As a result CSs, are likely to be subject to more factors uncorrelated with the pattern of zebrin expression than is the case for the cerebellar cortical neurons responsible for generating and modulating SS activity.

CS-SS interactions

Although the absolute duration of the pause in SSs following a CS was longer in Z+ bands, a greater active suppression of SS activity was found for Z− regions when SS firing rate differences were controlled for. Evidence indicates that the pause in SSs is at least partly caused by activation of MLIs and GABA release [46,50,73,74]. However, MLIs appear not to receive climbing fiber synapses [81], but instead are activated by climbing fiber activity via glutamate spillover from climbing fiber-PC synapses [75,76,82]. EAAT4 is found in the perisynaptic membrane of climbing fiber-PC synapses [25,67], and controls glutamate spillover at those synapses [27,83], raising the possibility that the differing EAAT4 expression levels may also underlie the observed differences in active suppression of SSs between Z+ and Z− bands. That is, the relatively weak expression of EAAT4 in Z− band PCs could allow climbing fiber activity to cause greater MLI activation, leading to greater active inhibition of SSs following each CS.

The post-CS pause in SSs is generally followed by a subsequent modulation of SSs [53], which was found to be more pronounced in Z+ regions, although this effect was subtle. This difference may also be ascribable to variations in EAAT4 expression. This is because the post-pause SS modulation is also likely mediated by MLIs, as local block of GABA-A receptors reduces this modulation, for both negative and positive directions [46]. Moreover, glutamate spillover has recently been shown to cause not only activation of MLIs but also to lead to feed-forward inhibition of MLIs, which can last on the order of 100 ms [82], the same timescale as the duration of the modulation. Thus, in Z− bands the lower EAAT4 level allows the CS to activate more strongly the MLI network, which can then more strongly modulate SS activity.

Implications for cerebellar function

The differences in spontaneous PC activity between Z+ and Z− bands observed here are raise the possibility that information arriving via different cerebellar afferent systems could be transformed by networks characterized by quite distinct operational states. Moreover, it may be more complex than a simple binary choice (Z+ versus Z−), because not all afferent systems respect the zebrin-defined compartments. In this regard it is interesting to compare the band and zone results, because while the bands and zones are closely aligned in the cortical regions we recorded, they are not congruent, and although the zebrin and zonal datasets showed the same trends (except for CS firing rates), the stronger, more statistically significant results were always found for the zebrin dataset. This suggests that the observed firing pattern differences are a reflection of the intrinsic organization of the cerebellar cortex, and that differences in the spiking patterns between zones are likely a secondary consequence of the close spatial alignment between zones and bands from the recorded regions. However, since the degree of alignment between bands and zones varies among afferent systems and cerebellar cortical regions, the Z+/Z− ratio of an afferent's target region will vary among afferents, and thus may be an important functional parameter for determining the type of information processing that different input signals undergo.

Finally, the difference in the regularity of the firing patterns between Z+ and Z− PCs may have important implications for the transmission of information from the cerebellar cortex to the cerebellar nuclei. This is because Z+ and Z− PCs target distinct regions in the cerebellar nuclei [23,78]. PCs are often assumed to use rate coding, and if this is the case, the greater variability in the ISI distribution of Z+ PCs raises the possibility that information transmission from Z+ bands to the cerebellar nuclei is less efficient, as the efficiency of a rate code depends strongly on the regularity of the firing pattern [84].

The functional significance of this difference in SS regularity is difficult to gauge, because of uncertainties about the actual code used by PCs and about the exact convergence ratio of PCs to nuclear neurons. For example, a large degree of convergence in the PC-cerebellar nuclear projection, as suggested by anatomical results [85], could minimize the importance of differences in regularity by allowing averaging across the converging PC population, assuming that the "noise" in the SS activity in different PCs is independent. However, several physiological studies have suggested that the convergence in the PC-cerebellar nuclear projection may be relatively small (on the order of 10's:1 rather than 100's:1) [4,86], in which case the differing noise levels may have a significant impact on coding efficiency. Regardless of what the exact convergence ratio turns out to be, if PCs really only use rate coding, it seems surprising to have approximately half of them generate significantly more irregular spike trains. Thus, the present results suggest that SSs use additional coding mechanisms, consistent with other reports (for review see [87].

Increased irregularity in SS activity has been proposed as a cause of motor coordination disorders including ataxia and dystonia [88–90]. However, recent theoretical and experimental findings have questioned the association of irregular SS firing patterns and motor coordination deficits [91,92]. Our finding that PCs can display differing levels of firing regularity under normal physiological conditions would also argue against irregular firing patterns necessarily being pathological. Instead, as suggested above, this variation in regularity suggests that the cerebellar cortex employs multiple coding schemes, and that the specific code(s) used may vary between cerebellar regions. These results need to be verified in awake animals, but the demonstration of regularity differences in spiking between Z+ and Z− bands under two distinct anesthetic states raises the likelihood of this being an important characteristic of cerebellar activity that needs to be taken into account in future hypotheses of cerebellar function.

Author Contributions

Conceived and designed the experiments: NLC RA IS EJL. Performed the experiments: JX NLC YK HA AKW SPM RA EJL. Analyzed the data: JX NLC YK HA AB AKW YL SPM IS RA EJL. Contributed reagents/materials/analysis tools: JX AB EJL. Contributed to the writing of the manuscript: JX NLC RA IS EJL.

References

1. Dino MR, Willard FH, Mugnaini E (1999) Distribution of unipolar brush cells and other calretinin immunoreactive components in the mammalian cerebellar cortex. J Neurocytol 28: 99–123.
2. Marr D (1969) A theory of cerebellar cortex. J Physiol (Lond) 202: 437–470.
3. Albus JS (1971) A theory of cerebellar function. Math Biosci 10: 25–61.
4. Eccles JC, Ito M, Szentágothai J (1967) The Cerebellum as a Neuronal Machine. Berlin: Springer-Verlag.
5. Eccles JC (1973) The cerebellum as a computer: patterns in space and time. J Physiol (Lond) 229: 1–32.
6. Braitenberg V (2002) In defense of the cerebellum. Ann N Y Acad Sci 978: 175–183.
7. Bloedel JR (1992) Functional heterogeneity with structural homogeneity: How does the cerebellum operate? Behavioral Brain Science 15: 666–678.
8. Apps R, Hawkes R (2009) Cerebellar cortical organization: a one-map hypothesis. Nat Rev Neurosci 10: 670–681.
9. Hawkes R, Gravel C (1991) The modular cerebellum. Prog Neurobiol 36: 309–327.
10. Hawkes R (1997) An anatomical model of cerebellar modules. Prog Brain Res 114: 39–52.
11. Voogd J, Ruigrok TJH (1997) Transverse and longitudinal patterns in the mammalian cerebellum. Prog Brain Res 114: 21–37.
12. Sugihara I, Shinoda Y (2004) Molecular, topographic, and functional organization of the cerebellar cortex: a study with combined aldolase C and olivocerebellar tracing. J Neurosci 24: 8771–8785.
13. Sugihara I, Quy PN (2007a) Identification of aldolase C compartments in the mouse cerebellar cortex by olivocerebellar labeling. J Comp Neurol 500: 1076–1092.
14. Brochu G, Maler L, Hawkes R (1990) Zebrin II: a polypeptide antigen expressed selectively by Purkinje cells reveals compartments in rat and fish cerebellum. J Comp Neurol 291: 538–552.
15. Hawkes R, LeClerc N (1987) Antigenic map of the rat cerebellar cortex: the distribution of parasagittal bands as revealed by monoclonal anti-Purkinje cell antibody mabQ113. J Comp Neurol 256: 29–41.
16. Ji Z, Hawkes R (1994) Topography of Purkinje cell compartments and mossy fiber terminal fields in lobules II and III of the rat cerebellar cortex: spinocerebellar and cuneocerebellar projections. Neuroscience 61: 935–954.
17. Voogd J, Pardoe J, Ruigrok TJH, Apps R (2003) The distribution of climbing and mossy fiber collateral branches from the copula pyramidis and the paramedian lobule: Congruence of climbing fiber cortical zones and the pattern of zebrin banding within the rat cerebellum. J Neurosci 23: 4645–4656.
18. Quy PN, Fujita H, Sakamoto Y, Na J, Sugihara I (2011) Projection patterns of single mossy fiber axons originating from the dorsal column nuclei mapped on the aldolase C compartments in the rat cerebellar cortex. J Comp Neurol 519: 874–899.
19. Pijpers A, Apps R, Pardoe J, Voogd J, Ruigrok TJ (2006) Precise spatial relationships between mossy fibers and climbing fibers in rat cerebellar cortical zones. J Neurosci 26: 12067–12080.
20. Pakan JM, Graham DJ, Wylie DR (2010) Organization of visual mossy fiber projections and zebrin expression in the pigeon vestibulocerebellum. J Comp Neurol 518: 175–198.
21. Sugihara I, Shinoda Y (2007c) Molecular, topographic, and functional organization of the cerebellar nuclei: analysis by three-dimensional mapping of the olivonuclear projection and aldolase C labeling. J Neurosci 27: 9696–9710.
22. Sugihara I (2011) Compartmentalization of the deep cerebellar nuclei based on afferent projections and aldolase C expression. Cerebellum 10: 449–463.
23. Chung SH, Marzban H, Hawkes R (2009) Compartmentation of the cerebellar nuclei of the mouse. Neuroscience 161: 123–138.
24. Cerminara NL, Aoki H, Loft M, Sugihara I, Apps R (2013) Structural basis of cerebellar microcircuits in the rat. J Neurosci 33: 16427–16442.
25. Dehnes Y, Chaudhry FA, Ullensvang K, Lehre KP, Storm-Mathisen J, et al. (1998) The glutamate transporter EAAT4 in rat cerebellar Purkinje cells: a glutamate-gated chloride channel concentrated near the synapse in parts of the dendritic membrane facing astroglia. J Neurosci 18: 3606–3619.
26. Nagao S, Kwak S, Kanazawa I (1997) EAAT4, a glutamate transporter with properties of a chloride channel, is predominantly localized in Purkinje cell dendrites, and forms parasagittal compartments in rat cerebellum. Neuroscience 78: 929–933.
27. Otis TS, Kavanaugh MP, Jahr CE (1997) Postsynaptic glutamate transport at the climbing fiber-Purkinje cell synapse. Science 277: 1515–1518.
28. Brasnjo G, Otis TS (2001) Neuronal glutamate transporters control activation of postsynaptic metabotropic glutamate receptors and influence cerebellar long-term depression. Neuron 31: 607–616.
29. Barbour B, Keller BU, Llano I, Marty A (1994) Prolonged presence of glutamate during excitatory synaptic transmission to cerebellar Purkinje cells. Neuron 12: 1331–1343.
30. Takahashi M, Kovalchuk Y, Attwell D (1995) Pre- and postsynaptic determinants of EPSC waveform at cerebellar climbing fiber and parallel fiber to Purkinje cell synapses. J Neurosci 15: 5693–5702.
31. Takayasu Y, Iino M, Ozawa S (2004) Roles of glutamate transporters in shaping excitatory synaptic currents in cerebellar Purkinje cells. Eur J Neurosci 19: 1285–1295.
32. Tzingounis AV, Wadiche JI (2007) Glutamate transporters: confining runaway excitation by shaping synaptic transmission. Nat Rev Neurosci 8: 935–947.
33. Ruigrok TJ (2011) Ins and outs of cerebellar modules. Cerebellum 10: 464–474.
34. Voogd J (2012) A note on the definition and the development of cerebellar Purkinje cell zones. Cerebellum 11: 422–425.

35. Cerminara NL, Apps R (2011) Behavioural significance of cerebellar modules. Cerebellum 10: 484–494.
36. Sugihara I, Marshall SP, Lang EJ (2007b) Relationship of complex spike synchrony to the lobular and longitudinal aldolase C compartments in crus IIA of the cerebellar cortex. J Comp Neurol 501: 13–29.
37. Sasaki K, Bower JM, Llinas R (1989) Multiple Purkinje cell recording in rodent cerebellar cortex. Eur J Neurosci 1: 572–586.
38. Llinas R, Sugimori M (1980b) Electrophysiological properties of in vitro Purkinje cell dendrites in mammalian cerebellar slices. J Physiol (Lond) 305: 197–213.
39. Wise AK, Cerminara NL, Marple-Horvat DE, Apps R (2010) Mechanisms of synchronous activity in cerebellar Purkinje cells. J Physiol (Lond) 588: 2373–2390.
40. Atkins MJ, Apps R (1997) Somatotopical organisation within the climbing fibre projection to the paramedian lobule and copula pyramidis of the rat cerebellum. J Comp Neurol 389: 249–263.
41. Colin F, Manil J, Desclin JC (1980) The olivocerebellar system. I. Delayed and slow inhibitory effects: an overlooked salient feature of cerebellar climbing fibers. Brain Res 187: 3–27.
42. Rawson JA, Tilokskulchai K (1981) Suppression of simple spike discharges of cerebellar Purkinje cells by impulses in climbing fibre afferents. Neurosci Lett 25: 125–130.
43. Montarolo PG, Palestini M, Strata P (1982) The inhibitory effect of the olivocerebellar input on the cerebellar Purkinje cells in the rat. J Physiol (Lond) 332: 187–202.
44. Demer JL, Echelman DA, Robinson DA (1985) Effects of electrical stimulation and reversible lesions of the olivocerebellar pathway on Purkinje cell activity in the flocculus of the cat. Brain Res 346: 22–31.
45. Cerminara NL, Rawson JA (2004) Evidence that climbing fibers control an intrinsic spike generator in cerebellar Purkinje cells. J Neurosci 24: 4510–4517.
46. Marshall SP, Lang EJ (2009) Local changes in the excitability of the cerebellar cortex produce spatially restricted changes in complex spike synchrony. J Neurosci 29: 14352–14362.
47. Chaumont J, Guyon N, Valera AM, Dugue GP, Popa D, et al. (2013) Clusters of cerebellar Purkinje cells control their afferent climbing fiber discharge. Proc Natl Acad Sci USA 110: 16223–16228.
48. Lang EJ (2002) GABAergic and glutamatergic modulation of spontaneous and motor-cortex-evoked complex spike activity. J Neurophysiol 87: 1993–2008.
49. Granit R, Phillips CG (1956) Excitatory and inhibitory processes acting upon individual Purkinje cells of the cerebellum in cats. J Physiol (Lond) 133: 520–547.
50. Bloedel JR, Roberts WJ (1971) Action of climbing fibers in cerebellar cortex of the cat. J Neurophysiol 34: 17–31.
51. Ebner TJ, Bloedel JR (1981a) Temporal patterning in simple spike discharge of Purkinje cells and Its relationship to climbing fiber activity. J Neurophysiol 45: 933–947.
52. Aizenman CD, Linden DJ (1999) Regulation of the rebound depolarization and spontaneous firing patterns of deep nuclear neurons in slices of rat cerebellum. J Neurophysiol 82: 1697–1709.
53. McDevitt CJ, Ebner TJ, Bloedel JR (1982) The changes in Purkinje cell simple spike activity following spontaneous climbing fiber inputs. Brain Res 237: 484–491.
54. Lang EJ, Sugihara I, Welsh JP, Llinás R (1999) Patterns of spontaneous Purkinje cell complex spike activity in the awake rat. J Neurosci 19: 2728–2739.
55. Ozden I, Sullivan MR, Lee HM, Wang SS (2009) Reliable coding emerges from coactivation of climbing fibers in microbands of cerebellar Purkinje neurons. J Neurosci 29: 10463–10473.
56. Lang EJ (2009) Functional imaging confirms principles of cerebellar functioning found with multisite recording [electronic response to Ozden, I., Sullivan, M.R., Lee, H.M., Wang, S.S.H. Reliable coding emerges from coactivation of climbing fibers in microbands of cerebellar Purkinje neurons. J. Neurosci. 29, 10463–10473.]. J Neurosci 29.
57. Mukamel EA, Nimmerjahn A, Schnitzer MJ (2009) Automated analysis of cellular signals from large-scale calcium imaging data. Neuron 63: 747–760.
58. Armstrong DM, Rawson JA (1979) Activity patterns of cerebellar cortical neurones and climbing fibre afferents in the awake cat. J Physiol (Lond) 289: 425–448.
59. Shin SL, Hoebeek FE, Schonewille M, De Zeeuw CI, Aertsen A, et al. (2007) Regular patterns in cerebellar Purkinje cell simple spike trains. PLoS One 2: e485.
60. Schonewille M, Khosrovani S, Winkelman BH, Hoebeek FE, De Jeu MT, et al. (2006) Purkinje cells in awake behaving animals operate at the upstate membrane potential.Nat Neurosci 9: 459–461; author reply 461.
61. Zhou H, Lin Z, Voges K, Ju C, Gao Z, et al. (2014) Cerebellar modules operate at different frequencies. eLife 3: e02536.
62. Llinas R, Sugimori M (1980a) Electrophysiological properties of in vitro Purkinje cell somata in mammalian cerebellar slices. J Physiol (Lond) 305: 171–195.
63. Häusser M, Clark BA (1997) Tonic synaptic inhibition modulates neuronal output pattern and spatiotemporal synaptic integration. Neuron 19: 665–678.
64. Raman IM, Bean BP (1999) Ionic currents underlying spontaneous action potentials in isolated cerebellar Purkinje neurons. J Neurosci 19: 1663–1674.
65. Kim YS, Shin JH, Hall FS, Linden DJ (2009) Dopamine signaling is required for depolarization-induced slow current in cerebellar Purkinje cells. J Neurosci 29: 8530–8538.
66. Shin JH, Kim YS, Linden DJ (2008) Dendritic glutamate release produces autocrine activation of mGluR1 in cerebellar Purkinje cells. Proc Natl Acad Sci USA 105: 746–750.
67. Tanaka J, Ichikawa R, Watanabe M, Tanaka K, Inoue Y (1997) Extra-junctional localization of glutamate transporter EAAT4 at excitatory Purkinje cell synapses. Neuroreport 8: 2461–2464.
68. Gao W, Chen G, Reinert KC, Ebner TJ (2006) Cerebellar cortical molecular layer inhibition is organized in parasagittal zones. J Neurosci 26: 8377–8387.
69. Eccles JC, Llinas R, Sasaki K (1966b) The inhibitory interneurones within the cerebellar cortex. Exp Brain Res 1: 1–16.
70. Eccles JC, Llinas R, Sasaki K (1966c) Parallel fibre stimulation and the responses induced thereby in the Purkinje cells of the cerebellum. Exp Brain Res 1: 17–39.
71. Eccles JC, Sasaki K, Strata P (1966h) The profiles of physiological events produced by a parallel fibre volley in the cerebellar cortex. Exp Brain Res 2: 18–34.
72. Savio T, Tempia F (1985) On the Purkinje cell activity increase induced by suppression of inferior olive activity. Exp Brain Res 57: 456–463.
73. Latham A, Paul DH (1971) Spontaneous activity of cerebellar Purkinje cells and their responses to impulses in climbing fibres. J Physiol (Lond) 213: 135–156.
74. Burg D, Rubia FJ (1972) Inhibition of cerebellar Purkinje cells by climbing fiber input. Pflügers Arch 337: 367–372.
75. Szapiro G, Barbour B (2007) Multiple climbing fibers signal to molecular layer interneurons exclusively via glutamate spillover. Nat Neurosci 10: 735–742.
76. Mathews PJ, Lee KH, Peng Z, Houser CR, Otis TS (2012) Effects of climbing fiber driven inhibition on Purkinje neuron spiking. J Neurosci 32: 17988–17997.
77. Jorntell H, Ekerot CF (2003) Receptive field plasticity profoundly alters the cutaneous parallel fiber synaptic input to cerebellar interneurons in vivo. J Neurosci 23: 9620–9631.
78. Sugihara I, Fujita H, Na J, Quy PN, Li BY, et al. (2009) Projection of reconstructed single Purkinje cell axons in relation to the cortical and nuclear aldolase C compartments of the rat cerebellum. J Comp Neurol 512: 282–304.
79. Simpson JI, Belton T, Suh M, Winkelman B (2002) Complex spike activity in the flocculus signals more than the eye can see. Ann N Y Acad Sci 978: 232–236.
80. Winkelman BH, Belton T, Suh M, Coesmans M, Morpurgo MM, et al. (2014) Nonvisual complex spike signals in the rabbit cerebellar flocculus. J Neurosci 34: 3218–3230.
81. Hámori J, Szentágothai J (1980) Lack of evidence of synaptic contacts by climbing fibre collaterals to basket and stellate cells in developing rat cerebellar cortex. Brain Res 186: 454–457.
82. Coddington LT, Rudolph S, Vande Lune P, Overstreet-Wadiche L, Wadiche JI (2013) Spillover-mediated feedforward inhibition functionally segregates interneuron activity. Neuron 78: 1050–1062.
83. Brasnjo G, Otis TS (2004) Isolation of glutamate transport-coupled charge flux and estimation of glutamate uptake at the climbing fiber-Purkinje cell synapse. Proc Natl Acad Sci USA 101: 6273–6278.
84. Stein RB (1967) The information capacity of nerve cells using a frequency code. Biophys J 7: 797–826.
85. Palkovits M, Mezey E, Hamori J, Szentagothai J (1977) Quantitative histological analysis of the cerebellar nuclei in the cat. I. Numerical data on cells and on synapses. Exp Brain Res 28: 189–209.
86. Person AL, Raman IM (2012) Purkinje neuron synchrony elicits time-locked spiking in the cerebellar nuclei. Nature 481: 502–505.
87. Heck DH, De Zeeuw CI, Jaeger D, Khodakhah K, Person AL (2013) The neuronal code(s) of the cerebellum. J Neurosci 33: 17603–17609.
88. Walter JT, Alvina K, Womack MD, Chevez C, Khodakhah K (2006) Decreases in the precision of Purkinje cell pacemaking cause cerebellar dysfunction and ataxia. Nat Neurosci 9: 389–397.
89. Hoebeek FE, Stahl JS, van Alphen AM, Schonewille M, Luo C, et al. (2005) Increased noise level of Purkinje cell activities minimizes impact of their modulation during sensorimotor control. Neuron 45: 953–965.
90. Alvina K, Khodakhah K (2010) The therapeutic mode of action of 4-aminopyridine in cerebellar ataxia. J Neurosci 30: 7258–7268.
91. Glasauer S, Rossert C, Strupp M (2011) The role of regularity and synchrony of cerebellar Purkinje cells for pathological nystagmus. Ann N Y Acad Sci 1233: 162–167.
92. Stahl JS, Thumser ZC (2013) 4-aminopyridine does not enhance flocculus function in tottering, a mouse model of vestibulocerebellar dysfunction and ataxia. PLoS One 8: e57895.

15

Spinal fMRI Reveals Decreased Descending Inhibition during Secondary Mechanical Hyperalgesia

Torge Rempe[1,2]*, Stephan Wolff[1], Christian Riedel[1], Ralf Baron[2,3], Patrick W. Stroman[4], Olav Jansen[1], Janne Gierthmühlen[1,3]

1 Dept of Neuroradiology, University Hospital of Kiel, Arnold-Heller-Strasse 3, Haus 41, 24105 Kiel, Germany, **2** Dept of Neurology, University Hospital of Kiel, Arnold-Heller-Strasse 3, Haus 41, 24105 Kiel, Germany, **3** Division of Neurological Pain Research and Therapy, University Hospital of Kiel, Arnold-Heller-Strasse 3, Haus 41, 24105 Kiel, Germany, **4** Centre for Neuroscience Studies, Dept of Diagnostic Radiology, Dept of Physics, 228 Botterell Hall, Queen's University, Kingston, Ontario, Canada

Abstract

Mechanical hyperalgesia is one distressing symptom of neuropathic pain which is explained by central sensitization of the nociceptive system. This sensitization can be induced experimentally with the heat/capsaicin sensitization model. The aim was to investigate and compare spinal and supraspinal activation patterns of identical mechanical stimulation before and after sensitization using functional spinal magnetic resonance imaging (spinal fMRI). Sixteen healthy subjects (6 female, 10 male, mean age 27.2±4.0 years) were investigated with mechanical stimulation of the C6 dermatome of the right forearm during spinal fMRI. Testing was always performed in the area outside of capsaicin application (i.e. area of secondary mechanical hyperalgesia). During slightly noxious mechanical stimulation before sensitization, activity was observed in ipsilateral dorsolateral pontine tegmentum (DLPT) which correlated with activity in ipsilateral spinal cord dorsal gray matter (dGM) suggesting activation of descending nociceptive inhibition. During secondary mechanical hyperalgesia, decreased activity was observed in bilateral DLPT, ipsilateral/midline rostral ventromedial medulla (RVM), and contralateral subnucleus reticularis dorsalis, which correlated with activity in ipsilateral dGM. Comparison of voxel-based activation patterns during mechanical stimulation before/after sensitization showed deactivations in RVM and activations in superficial ipsilateral dGM. This study revealed increased spinal activity and decreased activity in supraspinal centers involved in pain modulation (SRD, RVM, DLPT) during secondary mechanical hyperalgesia suggesting facilitation of nociception via decreased endogenous inhibition. Results should help prioritize approaches for further in vivo studies on pain processing and modulation in humans.

Editor: Theodore J. Price, University of Texas at Dallas, United States of America

Funding: The study was supported by the German Federal Ministry of Education and Research (BMBF, 01EM05/04). However, the authors received no specific funding for this work. The funders had no role in study design, data collection and analysis, decision to publish, or preparation of the manuscript.

Competing Interests: Ralf Baron reported grant/research support by: Pfizer, Genzyme, Grünenthal. Member of the IMI "Europain" collaboration and industry members of this are: Astra Zeneca, Pfizer, Esteve, UCB-Pharma, Sanofi Aventis, Grünenthal, Eli Lilly and Boehringer Ingelheim. German Federal Ministry of Education and Research (BMBF): German Research Network on Neuropathic Pain, Modelling Pain Switches. German Research Foundation (DFG). He received honoraria as a speaker from Pfizer, Genzyme, Grünenthal, Mundipharma, Sanofi Pasteur, Medtronic, Eisai, UCB BioSciences, Lilly, Boehringer Ingelheim, Astellas, Desitin and as a consultant from Pfizer, Genzyme, Grünenthal, Mundipharma, Allergan, Sanofi Pasteur, Medtronic, Eisai, UCB BioSciences, Lilly, Boehringer Ingelheim, Astellas, Novartis, Bristol-Myers Squibb, Biogenidec, AstraZeneca. Olav Jansen received honoraria as a speaker from Penumbra and as a consultant from Strykker, Philips and Boehringer Ingelheim. Janne Gierthmühlen received honoraria as a speaker from Pfizer and travel grants from Grünenthal. There are no conflicts of interests relevant to this article and none of the competing interests alter the authors' adherence to PLOS ONE policies on sharing data and materials.

* Email: t.rempe@neurologie.uni-kiel.de

Introduction

Mechanical pinprick hyperalgesia is a very distressing symptom presented by approximately 29% of neuropathic pain patients [1]. During a state of hyperalgesia, an already nociceptive stimulus is perceived as even more painful [1]. Secondary hyperalgesia develops in the uninjured area surrounding a nerve injury and is caused by central sensitization, i.e. by modulation of the spinal and supraspinal nociceptive system [2,3]. It can be induced experimentally in healthy humans by the heat/capsaicin model [4].

Anatomically, the vast majority of the nociceptive second order neurons is located in the dorsal gray matter (dGM) of the spinal cord. From there they project to supraspinal nuclei in the brainstem and the thalamus before these afferent nociceptive impulses are transferred to further subcortical and cortical structures [5]. The nociceptive neurons in the spinal cord and in the brainstem have an important contribution in the transmission and modulation of pain. This knowledge is based mostly on animal experiments, observation of the effects of injury and disease as well as postmortem anatomical studies [3,6,7].

With the emergence of functional magnetic resonance imaging of the brain (fMRI) [8] and, to a lesser extent, of the brainstem [9,10], non-invasive methods have become available to provide insight into human pain processing in vivo. To investigate pain processing on the spinal level and in the brainstem, spinal fMRI is of great interest, however, its utilization is limited because of significant technical challenges such as cerebro-spinal fluid-pulsations, breathing/swallowing-motions, and the spinal cord's small cross-sectional dimension.

In order to address these challenges, recent spinal fMRI studies use a turbo spin-echo sequence with a relatively short echo time rather than the more conventional gradient echo imaging sequence sensitive to the blood oxygenation level-dependent (BOLD) effect [11–14]. It demonstrates BOLD contrast but also reveals a second contrast mechanism and important source of neuronal activity-related signal change in spinal fMRI termed "signal enhancement by extravascular water protons" (SEEP). This functionally induced signal is thought to originate from cellular swelling and thus changed extravascular water content due to increased intravascular pressure at sites of activity. This new technique is believed to localize sites of neuronal activity more precisely than conventional T_2*-weighted gradient echo imaging sequences, which have rather poor field homogeneity [11–14].

However, spinal fMRI studies of human pain processing are still rare [15–17]. While spinal fMRI has recently been used successfully to demonstrate signal intensity changes in the spinal cord and brainstem during innocuous and noxious thermal stimulation and heat allodynia/hyperalgesia [18], there is still no spinal fMRI study that examines spinal and supraspinal changes in activity during secondary mechanical hyperalgesia up to this point.

Therefore, the aims were (A) to investigate spinal and supraspinal processes occurring as a consequence of mechanical stimulation and (B) to compare activation patterns of identical mechanical stimuli before and after induction of sensitization with the heat/capsaicin model in healthy subjects in order to investigate the specific pain-related components of secondary mechanical hyperalgesia. Within this study we could successfully demonstrate (A) increased activity in ipsilateral dGM after induction of hyperalgesia, (B) decreased activity in nociceptive regions of the brainstem and (C) a correlation between these supraspinal deactivations and activations of ipsilateral dGM during secondary mechanical hyperalgesia suggesting a facilitation of nociception via decreased descending endogenous inhibition.

Materials and Methods

Subjects

Sixteen right-handed [19] healthy volunteers (6 females, 10 males, mean age 27.2±4.0 years, range 23–32 years) were included in the study. All subjects were free of any acute or chronic pain conditions. Comorbidities such as diseases of the peripheral or central nervous system were ruled out. None of the subjects were on drugs that might have interfered with itch or pain sensations and flare responses. The study was in accordance with the Declaration of Helsinki and was approved by the Ethical Committee of the Faculty of Medicine at Christian-Albrechts-University of Kiel. Written informed consent was obtained from all participants.

Psychophysics

On the right (= ipsilateral) lateral volar forearm approximately 3 cm distal to the elbow in the C6 dermatome a 3×3 cm square area [area A, site of sensitization] and an adjacent 2×5 cm area directly distal to it [area B, for mechanical stimulation] were marked (figure 1).

Experimental set-up

All subjects underwent two identical MRI sessions back-to-back on the same day with mechanical stimulation in the same area before and after sensitization.

fMRI data acquisition. All scans were performed in a 3T human MRI scanner (Philips Achieva 3T). For acquisition of functional image data, a half-Fourier, single-shot turbo spin-echo sequence with a phased-array head-neck receiver coil (TE = 38 ms, TR = 9000 ms, 288×144×20 mm FOV, 192×96 matrix) was used [17,21]. At TE = 38 ms, this sequence is about equally sensitive to contributions of both BOLD and SEEP [14,22,23]. With this configuration 10 contiguous 2 mm thick sagittal slices were acquired, spanning from above the thalamus to below the C7/T1 intervertebral disc with a resulting voxel size of $1.5\times1.5\times2$ mm^3. To reduce sources of motion artefacts (e.g. heart, lungs and throat), a spatial saturation pulse was applied to the region anterior to the vertebral column.

Mechanical stimulation. In order to enable the stimulation of a larger dermatomal area (possibly leading to a higher signal in the spinal cord) mechanical stimulation was performed using a self-made brush consisting of 15 stiff von-Frey-hairs (166 mN). Care was taken that the site of stimulation was always within the area of secondary hyperalgesia [area B]. The mechanical stimulation paradigms consisted of 8 stimulation periods of 40 seconds alternating with eight baseline periods (64 volumes). After each session, subjects were asked to rate the stimulus intensity on the numerical rating scale (NRS, ranging from 0 to 10 with 0 representing "no pain" and 10 being the "maximum pain that can be imagined") by verbal response.

Heat/Capsaicin sensitization model. The heat/capsaicin sensitization model was used to induce secondary mechanical hyperalgesia [4]. Therefore, area A was stimulated with a computer-controlled Peltier thermode (Medoc TSA-2001, Haifa, Israel) at 45°C for 5 minutes. Afterwards a gauze pad with 1 ml solution of 0.6% capsaicin in 45% ethanol was placed on area A for 30 minutes. During capsaicin-application, the subjects were asked once a minute for NRS ratings of perceived pain intensity and temperature sensation at the application site. The temperature sensation was quantified on the NRS with 0 representing "neutral temperature" and −10/+10 representing "the maximum cold/warmth that can be imagined". After patch removal and at the end of the second fMRI block the borders of the area of punctate mechanical hyperalgesia were assessed by a stiff von-Frey-hair (166 mN). The dimensions of flare and mechanical hyperalgesia were then determined by the calculation: $(D/2)\times(d/2)\times\pi$ (D = horizontal diameter, d = vertical diameters of the area) to assess the stability of the pain model throughout the experiment.

Analysis and Statistics

For the analysis of the resulting 3D fMRI image data a general linear model (GLM) was used. The basis set consists of a boxcar model paradigm convolved with the tissue response function [12] and models of cardiac-related spinal cord motion as confounds [17,21]. Its results demonstrate the weighting factors β1 (magnitude of the pattern matching the stimulation paradigm convolved with the tissue response function) and β0 (average voxel intensity). Corrections for bulk motion and a normalization to a consistent coordinate space of the brainstem and spinal cord were then performed as described previously [21]. A random-effects analysis by McGonigle et al. was used to determine combined group results [24]. This consists of the calculation of the mean and standard deviation of the ratio of β1/β0 representing the relative signal intensity response across studies. T values of >2.5 or <−2.5 were assumed as significant activity as they correspond with $p<0.0075$ [17]. Contrast calculations between mechanical stimulation before and after sensitization were performed on a voxel-by-voxel basis by the partial least squares (PLS) method [25]. A bootstrap ratio of

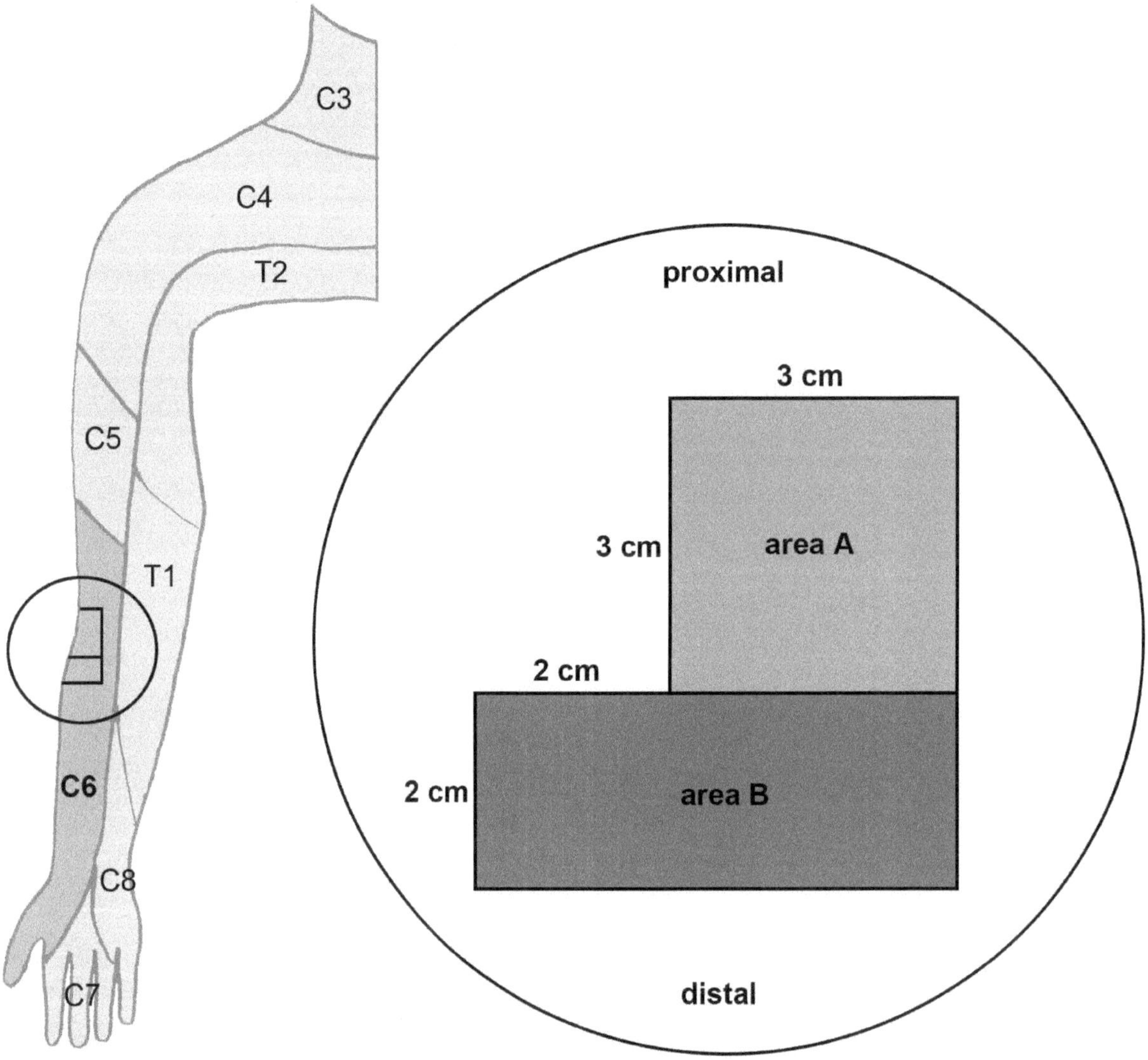

Figure 1. Areas of sensitization and stimulation on the right lateral volar forearm. For orientation, the schematic drawing on the left shows a dermatome map of the right upper extremity (redrawn and modified from [20]). The area of testing (marked by the circle) is situated on the right lateral volar forearm in the C6 dermatome. *Area A:* Site of sensitization with the heat/capsaicin model (3×3 cm square area 3 cm distal to the elbow in the C6 dermatome). *Area B:* Site of mechanical stimulation corresponding to the area of secondary mechanical hyperalgesia (2×5 cm area distal to area A).

≥5 was chosen for differences between two contrasted responses to be significant [17].

Spinal cord segments adjacent to C6 were included in the analysis since (A) primary afferent fibers split up into longitudinal collaterals innervating the bordering segments and (B) slightly individual anatomical dermatome-borders with a coincidental stimulation of surrounding dermatomes (i.e. C5, T1) were respected.

Psychophysical data are presented as mean ± standard deviation (SD) unless otherwise specified. Wilcoxon matched pairs test was used for calculation of psychophysical intragroup differences and Spearman rank test for correlation calculations using the numbers of voxels ($n_{(v)}$), signal change ($\Delta_{(S)}$) and % signal change ($\Delta_{(S/S)}$) across all volunteers provided by the fMRI data. P values <0.05 were considered to be statistically significant.

Results

Psychophysics

Capsaicin-application induced painful and warm sensations in all subjects (figure 2A). The capsaicin-induced flare decreased in size throughout testing (82.0 ± 18.8 cm^2 after patch removal vs. 67.0 ± 16.8 cm^2 at the end of testing, $p=0.002$). However, the dimension of secondary mechanical hyperalgesia was stable (77.1 ± 24.5 cm^2 after removal of capsaicin vs. 89.5 ± 35.7 cm^2 at the end of scanning, $p=0{,}125$) and included the area of stimulation [area B] at all times, thus ensuring the stability of the pain model throughout the experiment. Corresponding to mechanical hyperalgesia, the subjects' mean ratings of pain intensity for the mechanical stimulus were higher compared to those before sensitization (3.4 ± 2.2 vs. 2.1 ± 1.8, $p=0.003$; figure 2B).

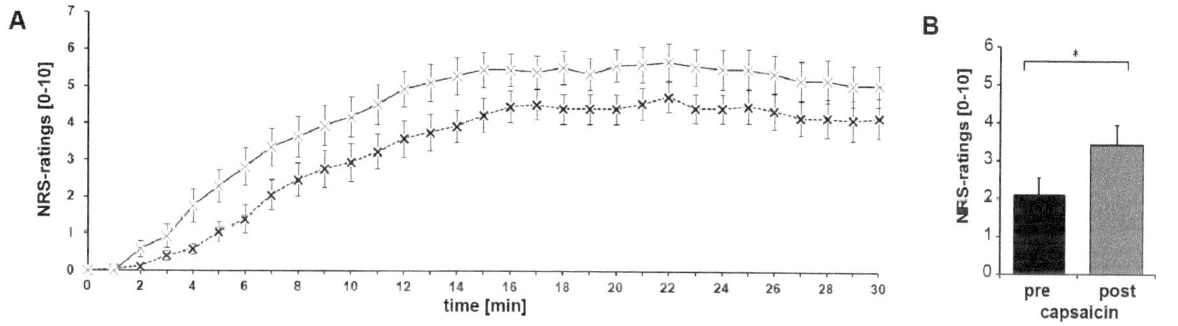

Figure 2. Psychophysical data. (A) Mean ratings of pain intensity (dashed line) and temperature perception (solid line) during capsaicin application. Capsaicin was applied at time 0. Mean ± standard error of the mean (SEM). (B) Mean pain ratings for the mechanical stimulus before and after application of capsaicin. Capsaicin induced secondary mechanical hyperalgesia. Mean ± SEM. *: $p<0.05$.

fMRI

Spinal group activation patterns and contrast maps. During mechanical stimulation prior to sensitization, spinal deactivations i.e. decreased signal intensity during stimulation were observed in deep dGM layers of C6 and C8 bilaterally and C7 contralaterally. After capsaicin exposure, mechanical stimulation in the area of secondary hyperalgesia lead to activations (increased signal intensity during stimulation) in T1 and deactivations in C7 in ipsilateral superficial dGM. Ventral activations were observed in ipsilateral ventral gray matter (vGM) of C4 before and after sensitization (figures 3, 4).

Activations in ipsilateral vGM of C7 correlated positively to the subjects' NRS-ratings before ($\Delta_{(S)}$: $R=0.513$; $p=0.042$) and after sensitization ($\Delta_{(S)}$: $R=0.533$; $p=0.041$), i.e. the higher the perceived pain intensity, the higher were activations in vGM of C7.

Contrast calculations between mechanical stimulation before and after sensitization with the heat/capsaicin model revealed activations in superficial ipsilateral (C7, C8) dGM. The observed lateral deviation of superficial dGM-activations might arise from BOLD-contributions in signal change located in superficial draining veins [14]. Contralateral activations were observed in deep dGM of C8 and vGM of C7. Deactivations were found in C4 in ipsilateral vGM and contralateral dGM (figures 3, 4).

Supraspinal group activation patterns and contrast maps. Prior to sensitization, supraspinal activity was observed in the ipsilateral dorsolateral pontine tegmentum (DLPT) (figure 5A). The activity in the ipsilateral dorsal pons correlated positively to activity in ipsilateral dGM of C4 ($n_{(v)}$: $R=0.611$; $p=0.012$) and C5 ($n_{(v)}$: $R=0.613$; $p=0.012$).

In contrast to measurements prior to sensitization, deactivations in contralateral DLPT were observed during secondary mechanical hyperalgesia (figure 5A). These deactivations correlated with activations in ipsilateral dGM of C5 ($n_{(v)}$: $R=0.546$; $p=0.035$) and T1 ($n_{(v)}$: $R=0.621$; $p=0.012$). Deactivations in the ipsilateral pons correlated with activations in ipsilateral dGM of C4 ($n_{(v)}$: $R=0.595$; $p=0.019$) and T1 ($n_{(v)}$: $R=0.555$; $p=0.039$; $\Delta_{(S/S)}$: $R=-0.538$; $p=0.047$), i.e. the higher the deactivations in the dorsal pons, the higher were activations in ipsilateral dGM (note that R in $n_{(v)}$ is positive because $n_{(deactivated\ voxels)}$ correlates positively to $n_{(activated\ voxels)}$ while $\Delta_{(S/S)}$ is negative because activations, i.e. positive $\Delta_{(S/S)}$-values are correlating to deactivations, i.e. negative $\Delta_{(S/S)}$-values).

After sensitization, deactivations were also visible in the ipsilateral and median caudal pons/rostral medulla most likely corresponding to the area of the rostral ventromedial medulla (RVM, figure 5A). Deactivations in the ipsilateral rostral ventral medulla correlated with ipsilateral dGM activations (C4: $n_{(v)}$: $R=0.699$; $p=0.004$; $\Delta_{(S)}$: $R=-0.827$; $p<0.001$; $\Delta_{(S/S)}$: $R=-0.770$; $p=0.001$; C6: $\Delta_{(S)}$: $R=-0.537$; $p=0.039$). Deactivations in midline RVM correlated with deactivations in ipsilateral dGM (C5: $n_{(v)}$: $R=0.556$; $p=0.031$; C7 = $n_{(v)}$: $R=0.599$; $p=0.018$; $\Delta_{(S)}$: $R=0.608$; $p=0.016$). Visible deactivations in the caudo-dorsal contralateral medulla corresponded to the localization of the subnucleus reticularis dorsalis (SRD, figure 5B) and correlated with spinal activations in ipsilateral dGM (C4: $\Delta_{(S/S)}$: $R=-0.560$; $p=0.030$; C8: $\Delta_{(S/S)}$: $R=-0.578$; $p=0.024$; T1 = $n_{(voxels)}$: $R=0.554$; $p=0.040$).

Supraspinal calculations of contrast maps showed deactivations in the RVM (figure 5A).

Discussion

The present study shows spinal and supraspinal signal intensity changes during mechanical stimulation and secondary mechanical hyperalgesia in healthy subjects. The main findings are (A) increased activity in ipsilateral dGM after induction of hyperalgesia, (B) decreased activity in supraspinal centers of pain processing and modulation (DLPT, RVM, SRD) and (C) a correlation between supraspinal deactivations and activations of ipsilateral dGM during secondary mechanical hyperalgesia induced by the heat/capsaicin model. Results suggest a facilitation of nociception via decreased descending endogenous inhibition during secondary mechanical hyperalgesia.

Spinal cord

Ipsilateral dGM. Anatomically, the vast majority of primary nociceptive afferent fibers projects to the ipsilateral dGM. Therefore, application of noxious stimuli should lead to activation of projection neurons located in the marginal layer of the dorsal horn [27]. Supportingly, this study showed superficial dGM-activations during painful stimulation after sensitization. Animal experiments suggest a higher activation of spinal nociceptive projection neurons by the same noxious stimulus during experimental pain states [3,6]. For example, Simone et al. showed an increase of monkey spinothalamic tract neuron responses to punctate mechanical stimuli during capsaicin-induced secondary hyperalgesia [2]. The current study is now the first one to reproduce such findings from animal experiments in human subjects in vivo as contrast maps revealed activations in superficial dGM that may correspond with increased activity during central sensitization.

Mechanical hyperalgesia and increased dGM activity can also be due to deficient inhibitory interneuron (ININ)-mediated

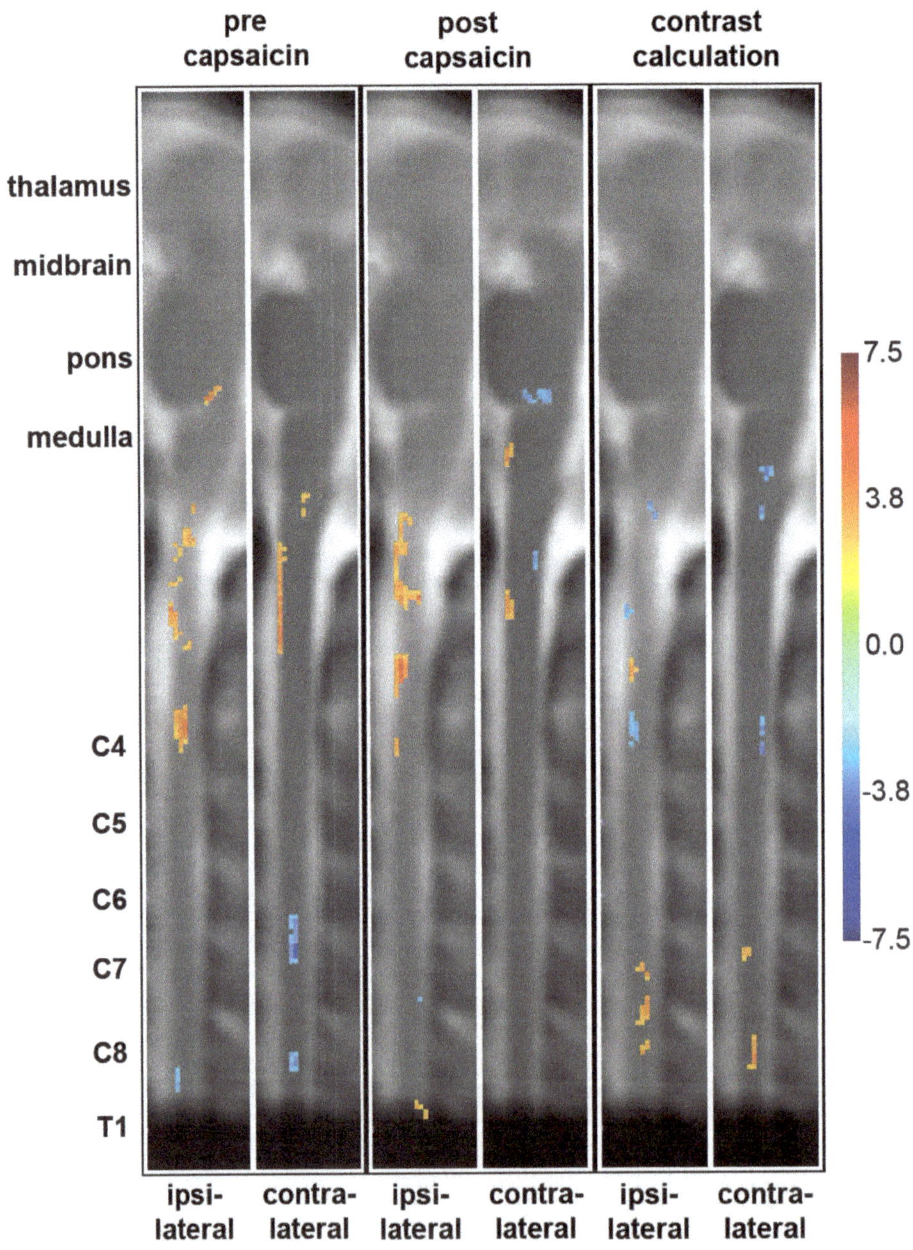

Figure 3. Sagittal slices of group activation patterns and contrast maps. Columns 1 to 4 show areas of activity across brain stem and cervical spinal cord before (1st and 2nd column) and after (3rd and 4th column) sensitization with the heat capsaicin model representing the significance (T-value) of each active voxel across the 16 subjects. Columns 5 and 6 show partial-least squares (PLS) results of contrast calculations on a voxel-by-voxel basis. The left column of each 2 columns (e.g. 1st, 3rd and 5th) corresponds to the ipsilateral side of the stimulus, the right column to the contralateral side. The color bar on the right indicates the corresponding significance, i.e. T-value (columns 1–4) or bootstrap-ratio (columns 5–6) for each color.

inhibition of projection neurons [28,29]. Interestingly, deactivations in deep dGM in C6 and C8 were observed prior to sensitization but disappeared during secondary mechanical hyperalgesia.

Contralateral dGM. Signal intensity changes were also observed in contralateral dGM during both conditions, consistent with a previous study using tactile stimuli [16]. These observations could be explained by primary afferent fibers ending in the contralateral dorsal horn [30] as well as by interneurons of ipsilateral dGM that cross the midline [17]. Our results also show differences during mechanical hyperalgesia compared to mechanical stimulation prior to sensitization suggesting a participation of the contralateral dGM in the development of central sensitization. It would be important for future studies to focus on such changes in contralateral dGM as contralateral somatosensory abnormalities have been observed in human unilateral neuropathic pain states [31].

vGM. Pain stimuli lead to withdrawal reflexes, i.e. the activation of ipsilateral motor neurons via spinal interneurons or supraspinal reticular nuclei [32]. Because mechanical stimuli were perceived as (slightly) painful, vGM-activity can be expected and was accordingly observed in both fMRI sessions. The positive correlation between the subjects' NRS-ratings and the activity in ipsilateral vGM of C7 suggests that stronger pain stimuli lead to

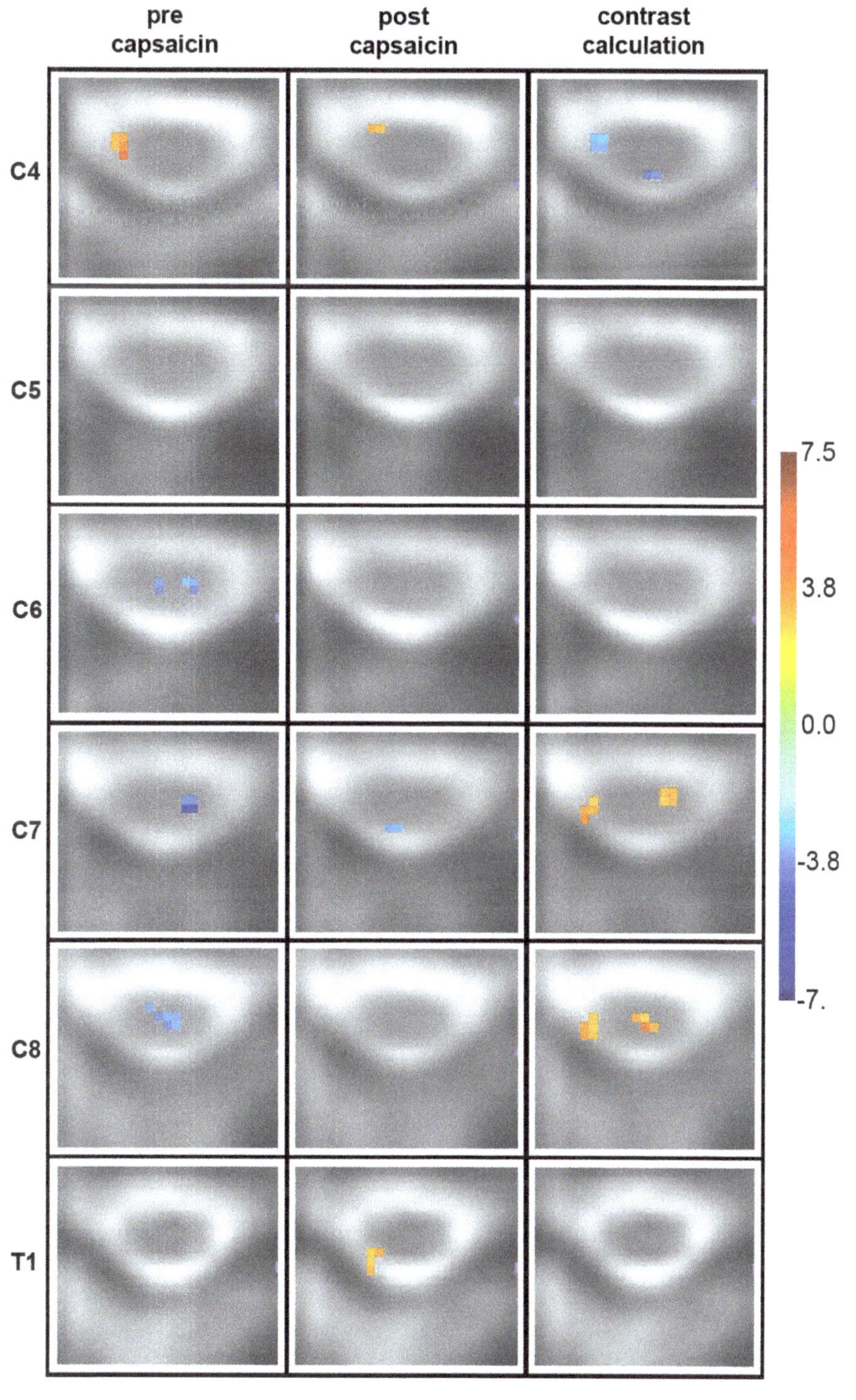

Figure 4. Spinal group activation patterns before (left column) and after (middle column) sensitization and contrast maps (right column). The transverse slices are in radiological orientation with the left side corresponding to the right body side and approximate the corresponding spinal cord segment for a rostral-caudal span from C4 to T1. They show spinal regions of signal intensity change before (left column) and after (middle column) sensitization with the heat/capsaicin model representing the significance (T-value) of each active voxel across the 16 subjects. The right column shows partial-least squares (PLS) results of contrast calculations on a voxel-by-voxel basis. The color bar in figure 3 indicates the corresponding significance, i.e. T-value (left and middle column) or bootstrap-ratio (right column) for each color. *Left Column:* Activations in ipsilateral vGM of C4. Deactivations in bilateral deep dGM of C6 and C8 and contralateral deep dGM of C7. *Middle column:* Ipsilateral activations in superficial dGM of T1 and vGM of C4. Deactivations in ipsilateral superficial dGM of C7. *Right column:* Activations in ipsilateral superficial dGM (C7, C8) and in contralateral vGM (C7) and deep dGM (C8). Deactivations in ipsilateral vGM and contralateral dGM of C4.

higher reflex answers. The C7 segment innervates both M. pronator teres and M. pronator quadratus. As the arm was held in a supine position throughout noxious stimulation, the activation of these muscles would be needed to escape the stimulus.

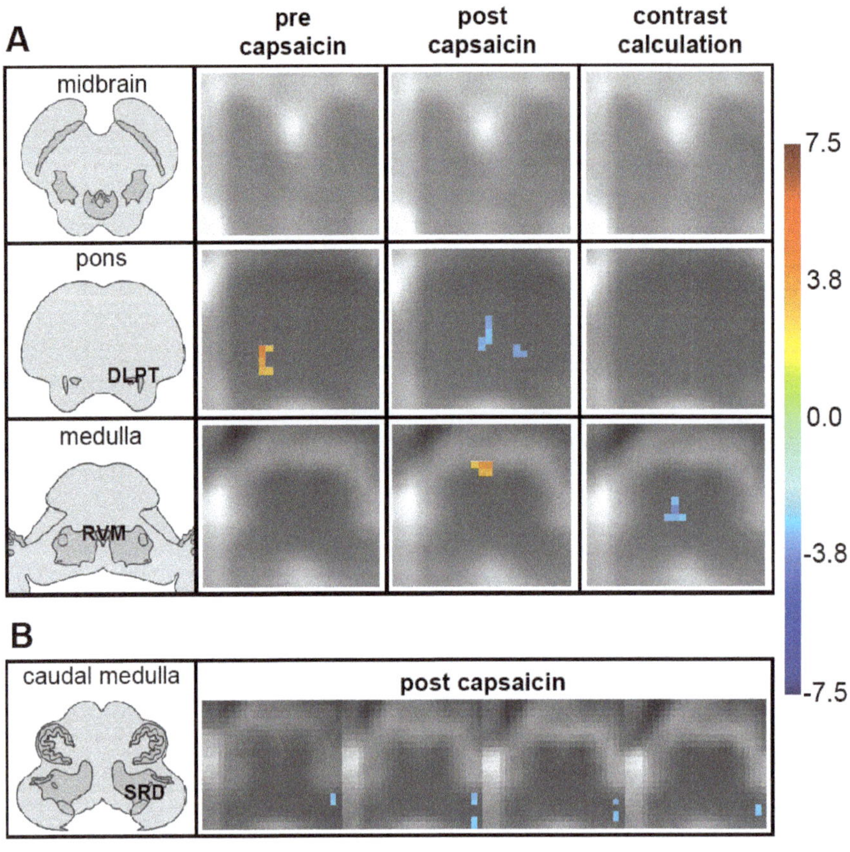

Figure 5. Supraspinal group activation patterns and contrast maps. Slices are in radiological orientation with the left side corresponding to the right body side. The color bar in figure 3 indicates the corresponding significance, i.e. T-value (combined group results pre/post capsaicin) or bootstrap-ratio (contrast calculation) for each color. Anatomical transverse sections on the left were modified from [26]. (A) The transverse slices approximate the corresponding brainstem region (midbrain, pons, medulla) for a rostral-caudal span. They show supraspinal regions of signal intensity change before (left column) and after (middle column) sensitization with the heat/capsaicin model representing the significance (T-value) of each active voxel across the 16 subjects. The right column shows partial-least squares (PLS) results of contrast calculations on a voxel-by-voxel basis. *Left column:* Activations in the ipsilateral DLPT (dorsolateral pontine tegmentum) during mechanical stimulation prior to application of capsaicin. *Middle column:* Deactivations in the contralateral DLPT and in the RVM (rostral ventromedial medulla) during secondary mechanical hyperalgesia (note that visible medial pontine deactivations are situated in the caudal pons/rostral medulla and therefore most likely correspond to the location of the RVM). *Right column:* Deactivations in the RVM. (B) The adjacent 1 mm thick transverse slices in consecutive arrangement located in the medulla show signal intensity changes during secondary mechanical hyperalgesia. Deactivations are observed in contralateral subnucleus reticularis dorsalis (SRD).

Brainstem

DLPT. Animal testing shows that the DLPT plays a central role in the modulation of nociception. With its noradrenergic fibers to the dGM, it mediates a negative feedback loop triggered by noxious stimuli to prevent excessive pain sensation [7,33]. This descending inhibition is for the most part mediated by the ipsilateral DLPT [34]. Accordingly, this study showed activations in the ipsilateral DLPT during painful mechanical stimulation prior to sensitization. Moreover these activations correlated with activations in ipsilateral dGM, possibly reflecting either an augmented activation of endogenous inhibition by higher activation of projection neurons [7] or a noradrenergic activation of spinal ININs (indirect inhibition of projection neurons) as it has been shown in animal studies [35]. Similarly, previous fMRI studies also showed activations of the DLPT during painful stimuli in healthy humans [15,36].

An absence of this noradrenergic inhibition by the DLPT is thought to be a mechanism for the development of neuropathic pain [3,37]. Interestingly, a bilateral decrease of DLPT-activation was seen during secondary mechanical hyperalgesia which correlated with ipsilateral dGM-activations. Compatibly, Becerra et al. showed bilaterally decreased DLPT-activity during mechanical hyperalgesia/allodynia in neuropathic pain patients [38]. Our results could thus correspond to a reduced descending noradrenergic inhibition with consecutive higher activation of spinal projection neurons.

Besides decreased inhibition, central sensitization is also thought to be mediated by coexisting excitatory descending facilitation [3,6,39]. Two earlier fMRI studies investigating secondary mechanical hyperalgesia demonstrated activity in rostral brainstem regions (midline-periaqueductal gray, contralateral cuneiform nucleus [10], contralateral mesencephalic pontine reticular formation [9]) that could be a correlate for excitatory nociceptive facilitation. Why did the current study not show these activations? Possible explanations could be overlapping processes of activation and simultaneous suppression of anti-nociceptive descending pathways in the very limited space of these brainstem nuclei or the different experimental set ups (MRI sequences or devices).

RVM. Based on current concepts of pain modulation, OFF-cells, a specific cell-type of the RVM, physiologically mediate antinociception [39,40]. In the condition of central sensitization, this OFF-cell activity is decreased [41]. Compatibly, this study shows decreased activity in the RVM during secondary mechanical hyperalgesia. A deactivation of OFF-cells would lead to a decreased inhibition of spinal projection neurons. Supportingly, this study shows correlations between deactivation of ipsilateral RVM and activations in ipsilateral dGM during secondary mechanical hyperalgesia. However, it has to be kept in mind that spinal inhibition can also be caused by the activation of ININs [29]. The observed correlation between deactivations in median RVM and ipsilateral dGM could therefore correspond to decreased OFF-cell mediated activation of ININs during secondary mechanical hyperalgesia.

SRD. The SRD is believed to play a major role in the mechanism of diffuse noxious inhibitory control (DNIC) [42]. An absence of this control is thought to be a reason for the development of neuropathic pain [39]. Accordingly, this study shows deactivations in contralateral SRD during secondary mechanical hyperalgesia which correlated with activations in the ipsilateral dGM. This could correspond to a facilitation of nociception via decreased endogenous inhibition by SRD and consequently higher dGM-activations - a similar and additional mechanism to nociceptive modulation by DLPT and RVM.

Limitations

Even though spin-echo spinal cord fMRI is a new reliable and non-invasive method to show functional processes in the spinal cord [15–18], its spatial resolution is still limited. Thus, an exact localization of the anatomical area corresponding to the observed activity is extremely difficult and can sometimes be only speculative. Furthermore, interpretation of results is complicated due to interconnections and often dichotomous roles of areas involved in pain processing/modulation, i.e. excitatory and inhibitory roles.

Conclusion

Using spin-echo spinal cord fMRI, it was possible to investigate pain modulatory processes during secondary mechanical hyperalgesia in the brainstem and spinal cord of healthy subjects. This study is the first one to show an increase of ipsilateral dGM-activity during secondary mechanical hyperalgesia in human subjects in vivo. Furthermore, this study succeeds in showing decreased activity in areas of the brainstem that have been proven important for processes of central sensitization in animal experiments (DLPT, RVM, SRD). Moreover, those deactivations correlated with dGM-activity. With these findings, this study gives new insights in human pain processing in vivo. Since findings of animal experiments and results of previous fMRI studies could be reproduced, spin-echo spinal cord fMRI has been shown to be a reliable method for the examination of spinal and supraspinal pain processing and modulation. Herewith, it qualifies for further investigations including treatment of neuropathic pain.

Acknowledgments

We are indebted to the subjects who participated in the study for their consent and co-operation.

Author Contributions

Conceived and designed the experiments: JG. Performed the experiments: TR SW. Analyzed the data: TR PWS JG. Contributed reagents/materials/analysis tools: PWS. Contributed to the writing of the manuscript: TR CR RB PWS OJ JG.

References

1. Baron R, Binder A, Wasner G (2010) Neuropathic pain: diagnosis, pathophysiological mechanisms, and treatment. Lancet Neurol 9: 807–819.
2. Simone DA, Sorkin LS, Oh U, Chung JM, Owens C, et al. (1991) Neurogenic hyperalgesia: central neural correlates in responses of spinothalamic tract neurons. J Neurophysiol 66: 228–246.
3. Westlund KN (2006) The dorsal horn and hyperalgesia. In: Cervero F, Jensen TS, editors. Handbook of Clinical Neurology, Vol 81 (3rd series): Pain. Amsterdam: Elsevier B.V. pp. 178–186.
4. Petersen KL, Rowbotham MC (1999) A new human experimental pain model: the heat/capsaicin sensitization model. Neuroreport 10: 1511–1516.
5. Villanueva L, Lopez-Avila A, Le Bars D (2006) Ascending nociceptive pathways. In: Cervero F, Jensen TS, editors. Handbook of Clinical Neurology, Vol 81 (3rd series): Pain. Amsterdam: Elsevier B.V. pp. 93–102.
6. Ossipov MH, Porreca F (2006) Descending excitatory systems. In: Cervero F, Jensen TS, editors. Handbook of Clinical Neurology, Vol 81 (3rd series): Pain. Amsterdam: Elsevier B.V. pp. 193–210.
7. Pertovaara A, Almeida A (2006) Descending inhibitory systems. In: Cervero F, Jensen TS, editors. Handbook of Clinical Neurology, Vol 81 (3rd series): Pain. Amsterdam: Elsevier B.V. pp. 179–192.
8. Baron R, Baron Y, Disbrow E, Roberts TP (1999) Brain processing of capsaicin-induced secondary hyperalgesia: a functional MRI study. Neurology 53: 548–557.
9. Lee MC, Zambreanu L, Menon DK, Tracey I (2008) Identifying brain activity specifically related to the maintenance and perceptual consequence of central sensitization in humans. J Neurosci 28: 11642–11649.
10. Zambreanu L, Wise RG, Brooks JC, Iannetti GD, Tracey I (2005) A role for the brainstem in central sensitisation in humans. Evidence from functional magnetic resonance imaging. Pain 114: 397–407.
11. Stroman PW (2005) Magnetic resonance imaging of neuronal function in the spinal cord: spinal FMRI. Clin Med Res 3: 146–156.
12. Stroman PW, Kornelsen J, Lawrence J, Malisza KL (2005) Functional magnetic resonance imaging based on SEEP contrast: response function and anatomical specificity. Magn Reson Imaging 23: 843–850.
13. Stroman PW, Krause V, Malisza KL, Frankenstein UN, Tomanek B (2002) Extravascular proton-density changes as a non-BOLD component of contrast in fMRI of the human spinal cord. Magn Reson Med 48: 122–127.
14. Stroman PW, Wheeler-Kingshott C, Bacon M, Schwab JM, Bosma R, et al. (2014) The current state-of-the-art of spinal cord imaging: methods. Neuroimage 84: 1070–1081.
15. Cahill CM, Stroman PW (2011) Mapping of neural activity produced by thermal pain in the healthy human spinal cord and brain stem: a functional magnetic resonance imaging study. Magn Reson Imaging 29: 342–352.
16. Ghazni NF, Cahill CM, Stroman PW (2010) Tactile sensory and pain networks in the human spinal cord and brain stem mapped by means of functional MR imaging. AJNR Am J Neuroradiol 31: 661–667.
17. Stroman PW (2009) Spinal fMRI investigation of human spinal cord function over a range of innocuous thermal sensory stimuli and study-related emotional influences. Magn Reson Imaging 27: 1333–1346.
18. Rempe T, Wolff S, Riedel C, Baron R, Stroman PW, et al. (2014) Spinal and supraspinal processing of thermal stimuli: An fMRI study. J Magn Reson Imaging DOI:10.1002/jmri.24627.
19. Oldfield RC (1971) The assessment and analysis of handedness: the Edinburgh inventory. Neuropsychologia 9: 97–113.
20. Trepel M (2008) Neuroanatomie: Struktur und Funktion. Munich: Elsevier GmbH, Urban & Fischer Verlag.
21. Stroman PW, Figley CR, Cahill CM (2008) Spatial normalization, bulk motion correction and coregistration for functional magnetic resonance imaging of the human cervical spinal cord and brainstem. Magn Reson Imaging 26: 809–814.
22. Figley CR, Stroman PW (2012) Measurement and characterization of the human spinal cord SEEP response using event-related spinal fMRI. Magn Reson Imaging 30: 471–484.
23. Stroman PW, Bosma RL, Beynon M, Dobek C (2012) Removal of synergistic physiological motion and image artefacts in functional MRI of the human spinal cord. 20th Annual Meeting of the International Society for Magnetic Resonance in Medicine. Melbourne, Australia.
24. McGonigle DJ, Howseman AM, Athwal BS, Friston KJ, Frackowiak RS, et al. (2000) Variability in fMRI: an examination of intersession differences. Neuroimage 11: 708–734.
25. McIntosh AR, Lobaugh NJ (2004) Partial least squares analysis of neuroimaging data: applications and advances. Neuroimage 23 Suppl 1: S250–263.
26. Naidich TP, Duvernoy HM, Delman BN, Sorensen AG, Kollias SS, et al. (2009) Duvernoy's Atlas of the Human Brain Stem and Cerebellum. Wien New York: Springer. pp. 53–93.

27. Millan MJ (1999) The induction of pain: an integrative review. Prog Neurobiol 57: 1–164.
28. Meisner JG, Marsh AD, Marsh DR (2010) Loss of GABAergic interneurons in laminae I–III of the spinal cord dorsal horn contributes to reduced GABAergic tone and neuropathic pain after spinal cord injury. J Neurotrauma 27: 729–737.
29. Millan MJ (2002) Descending control of pain. Prog Neurobiol 66: 355–474.
30. Light AR, Perl ER (1979) Spinal termination of functionally identified primary afferent neurons with slowly conducting myelinated fibers. J Comp Neurol 186: 133–150.
31. Huge V, Lauchart M, Forderreuther S, Kaufhold W, Valet M, et al. (2008) Interaction of hyperalgesia and sensory loss in complex regional pain syndrome type I (CRPS I). PLoS One 3: e2742.
32. Morgan MM (1998) Direct comparison of heat-evoked activity of nociceptive neurons in the dorsal horn with the hindpaw withdrawal reflex in the rat. J Neurophysiol 79: 174–180.
33. Fields HL, Basbaum AI (1994) Central nervous system mechanisms of pain modulation. In: Wall PD, Melzack R, editors. Textbook of Pain. 3 ed. Edinburgh: Churchill Livingstone. pp. 243–257.
34. Clark FM, Proudfit HK (1991) The projection of noradrenergic neurons in the A7 catecholamine cell group to the spinal cord in the rat demonstrated by anterograde tracing combined with immunocytochemistry. Brain Res 547: 279–288.
35. Gassner M, Ruscheweyh R, Sandkuhler J (2009) Direct excitation of spinal GABAergic interneurons by noradrenaline. Pain 145: 204–210.
36. Dunckley P, Wise RG, Fairhurst M, Hobden P, Aziz Q, et al. (2005) A comparison of visceral and somatic pain processing in the human brainstem using functional magnetic resonance imaging. J Neurosci 25: 7333–7341.
37. Xu M, Kontinen VK, Kalso E (1999) Endogenous noradrenergic tone controls symptoms of allodynia in the spinal nerve ligation model of neuropathic pain. Eur J Pharmacol 366: 41–45.
38. Becerra L, Morris S, Bazes S, Gostic R, Sherman S, et al. (2006) Trigeminal neuropathic pain alters responses in CNS circuits to mechanical (brush) and thermal (cold and heat) stimuli. J Neurosci 26: 10646–10657.
39. Ossipov MH, Dussor GO, Porreca F (2010) Central modulation of pain. J Clin Invest 120: 3779–3787.
40. Gebhart GF (2004) Descending modulation of pain. Neurosci Biobehav Rev 27: 729–737.
41. Kincaid W, Neubert MJ, Xu M, Kim CJ, Heinricher MM (2006) Role for medullary pain facilitating neurons in secondary thermal hyperalgesia. J Neurophysiol 95: 33–41.
42. Villanueva L, Bouhassira D, Le Bars D (1996) The medullary subnucleus reticularis dorsalis (SRD) as a key link in both the transmission and modulation of pain signals. Pain 67: 231–240.

The Conditioned Place Preference Test for Assessing Welfare Consequences and Potential Refinements in a Mouse Bladder Cancer Model

John V. Roughan[1]*, Claire A. Coulter[1], Paul A. Flecknell[1], Huw D. Thomas[2], Kenneth J. Sufka[3]

1 Comparative Biology Centre, The Medical School, University of Newcastle, Newcastle upon Tyne, United Kingdom, **2** Northern Institute for Cancer Research, The Medical School, University of Newcastle, Newcastle upon Tyne, United Kingdom, **3** Research Institute of Pharmaceutical Sciences and Departments of Psychology and Pharmacology, Peabody Building, University of Mississippi, Oxford, Mississippi, United States of America

Abstract

Most pre-clinical analgesic efficacy assays still involve nociceptive testing in rodents. This is despite concerns as to the relevance of these tests for evaluating the pain-preventative properties of drugs. More appropriate methods would target pain rather than nociception, but these are currently not available, so it remains unknown whether animal pain equates to the negatively affective and subjective/emotional state it causes in humans. Mouse cancer models are common despite the likelihood of substantial pain. We used Conditioned Place Preference (CPP) testing, assessments of thermal hyperalgesia and behaviour to determine the likelihood that MBT-2 bladder cancer impacts negatively on mouse welfare, such as by causing pain. There was no CPP to saline, but morphine preference in tumour bearing mice exceeded that seen in tumour-free controls. This occurred up to 10 days before the study end-point alongside reduced body weight, development of hyperalgesia and behaviour changes. These effects indicated mice experienced a negative welfare state caused by *malaise* (if not pain) before euthanasia. Due to the complexity of the assessments needed to demonstrate this, it is unlikely that this approach could be used for routine welfare assessment on a study-by-study basis. However, our results show mice in sufficiently similar studies are likely to benefit from more intensive severity assessment and re-evaluation of end-points with a view to implementing appropriate refinements. In this particular case, a refinement would have been to have euthanased mice at least 7 days earlier or possibly by provision of end-stage pain relief. CPP testing was found to be a helpful method to investigate the responses of mice to analgesics, possibly on a subjective level. These findings and those of other recent studies show it could be a valuable method of screening candidate analgesics for efficacy against cancer pain and possibly other pain or disease models.

Editor: Bradley Taylor, University of Kentucky Medical Center, United States of America

Funding: The study was funded by the UK National Centre for the 3Rs (NC3Rs): http://www.nc3rs.org.uk/, Grant Number G0900763, PI: JV Roughan. The funder had no role in study design, data collection and analysis, decision to publish, or preparation of the manuscript.

Competing Interests: The authors have declared that no competing interests exist.

* Email: j.v.roughan@ncl.ac.uk

Introduction

An array of nociceptive tests are used to determine the potential efficacy of new analgesics, and laboratory rats and mice are overwhelmingly the most widely used test subjects. These tests are typically classified according to the duration and intensity of the noxious stimulus and the nature of the response. Acute or phasic nociceptive assays that apply heat or mechanical stimulation (e.g. the tail-flick and Hargreaves tests; von Frey, respectively), due to the largely reflexive nature of the responses obtained, are considered less appropriate than tonic or sub-chronic tests (e.g. formalin or carrageenan) that elicit significant and persistent inflammation [1]. However, the inadequacies of both are well known [2]. Despite the development of animal simulations of persistent pain syndromes (e.g. arthritic or neuropathic pain), concerns prevail as to their clinical relevance. These ultimately stem from a continuing lack of understanding of how animal pain equates to the human experience; being a multidimensional phenomenon including both sensory and affective emotional state changes (collectively termed 'life quality' changes). Theoretically at least, animal pain and analgesic assays that inform on changes in these states should afford greater translational validity. This need has driven recent calls for the development of more clinically relevant *in-vivo* models [3,4] providing a more systems-based approach [5]. This rationale explains why affective (subjective) state assessment is increasingly being considered as a more relevant approach to establishing the welfare consequences of models where animals could be exposed to pain [6–8]. Cancer models are one research area where considerably more knowledge on how extensively pain impacts on welfare may be long overdue.

A large and steadily increasing number of animals (mainly mice) are used in cancer testing (471,000 in the UK in 2012; a 16% increase on the previous year [9]) with only minimal knowledge regarding potentially negative impacts on welfare. However, the guidelines that are meant to minimise suffering in these studies [10,11] do not incorporate any evaluation of changes in underlying subjective state, and obtaining evidence of cancer pain in rodents has relied heavily on assessing underlying nociceptive changes [12–15], and it seems this is still the case today [16–19]. Our group has extensively assessed changes in naturalistic behaviours as a means of assessing post-operative pain in rodents and other species using both manual [20–26] and automated methods [27–30], or used a combination of both types of analysis [31]. However, such behaviour analysis has rarely been used to assess the effects of cancer, and those few studies that cite 'pain behaviour' actually mean nociceptive or nocifensive behaviours (i.e. withdrawal or guarding) rather than true spontaneous (e.g. home-cage) behaviour (see for example [14,32]). Whichever method of data collection is used, establishing links between outcome and causation in behavioural studies is difficult because many factors can contribute to the observed changes. Changes could occur as an indirect result of procedural influences (e.g. anaesthesia, hypothermia, dehydration) or factors linked to these such as fear and associated anxiety. Nevertheless, establishing whether and when pain arises in cancer studies would have significant consequences. Firstly it would encourage a more rigorous approach to ethical decision making by enabling researchers to apply more effective cost-benefit analyses when determining if end-points are justified. Improving welfare standards in this manner would also be beneficial to studies because unalleviated pain may also jeopardise model validity. Preventing pain has been shown to be beneficial to validity in at least one cancer trial [33] and possibly other *in-vivo* research applications [34]. Cancer pain is also an area where advances in human treatments are urgently required. Pain is the most common and feared consequence of cancer and between 30–60% of oncology patients continue to report pain prior to, throughout and following treatment [35]. Indeed, it seems the outlook remains bleak despite 40 years of attempts to address the problem [36]. Clearly, cancer pain management needs to be refined, and animal cancer models provide an ideal platform for parallel progress on welfare advancement and drug discovery. Despite this, cancer models are not generally used to screen potential analgesics, with only rare exceptions [13,37]. This may be because most cancer studies have alternative aims, but could also be due to a lack of appropriate assessment methods; i.e. those that accommodate subjective aspects.

Conditioned Place Preference (CPP) testing is widely used to evaluate the psychoactive (affective) properties of drugs in animals [38], but usually to identify abuse liability by humans. Animals are conditioned by being confined in one 'place' and pairing that with drug treatment, whereas in another place they are given only a placebo. As the 'places' have distinctly different cues (usually in colour or texture) animals progressively associate the drugs' affect with the place where they experienced it. If this is a rewarding experience, either due to the drugs' positively or negatively reinforcing (analgesic) effects, animals typically spend longer in, or visit the drug-paired place more frequently. Provision of analgesia is a positive experience in painful humans, so if the same applies to animals then CPP studies have potential for evaluating both the aversive properties of pain and the analgesic effects of drugs. The approach has increasingly been applied to research on pain following the first demonstration that arthritis causes enhanced CPP to morphine and the N-methyl-D-aspartate antagonist MK-801 [39]. It was subsequently shown that a bradykinin B_1 receptor antagonist has therapeutic potential against chronic inflammatory pain [40]. A considerable time later, King et al. showed CPP is also an effective method for assessing analgesics against neuropathic pain [41]. Qu et al. illustrated the relevance of CPP to assessing subjective aspects of neuropathic pain in rats by showing that the rostral anterior cingulate cortex is essential to mediating pain affect [42]. Rutten et al. were also able to use CPP to dissociate between the positively and negatively rewarding consequences of analgesics with opioid-like affects compared to other mechanisms in a rat inflammatory (carrageenan) model [43]. Davoody et al. then showed increased CPP to clonidine (an α-2 agonist) in rats using spinal cord injury as a centralised pain model [44]. Okun et al. utilised a similar approach to show CPP to several different drugs in an osteoarthritic model [45], and most recently, Park et al. showed absence of positive reinforcement (reward) to gabapentin in normal mice, but CPP in a polyneuropathic pain model caused by antineoplastic (cisplatin) treatment [46]. Collectively, these findings clearly demonstrate that the CPP paradigm is capable of providing animals with a means to report on their awareness of pain, and so could offer a more appropriate method of evaluating its centralised (affective/subjective) as opposed to nociceptive (effective) properties.

The notion that pain could be as complex in animals (at least in mammals) as it is in humans is underlined by the fact that no single measurement criterion can (so far) effectively evaluate it. Bateson et al. originally applied a multiple measures approach to scientific problem solving (later termed 'triangulation') [47], citing that although "evidence obtained by different approaches was ambiguous", "when the whole body of evidence was considered, much greater confidence could be placed on a particular meaning". In addressing the problem of animal suffering, and accepting that "we cannot directly observe an animals' feelings", Bateson recommended that "we should use a variety of tasks to gain confidence in conclusions" [48]. Accordingly, studies are now increasingly applying several different measures in an attempt to characterise pain more reliably [49,50]. In this study we adopted a comparable approach by assessing a standard welfare parameter (body weight) alongside peripheral hypersensitivity testing, monitoring spontaneous exploratory behaviour and conducting CPP testing. Despite several limitations, hyperalgesia (hypersensitivity) testing still provides a valuable secondary indicator of pain of various different modalities including cancer [12,16,19]. Behaviour changes are also a common response to pain, but data collection and analyses are often time consuming, especially if applied in studies that typically last several weeks; as is usually the case in cancer studies. Interpretation of these data can also be problematic because, as has already been described, there are always alternative explanations for any behavioural changes that are detected. One often cited possibility is that signs of incapacity in rodents could be hidden as an adaptive response to reduce the likelihood of predation; although to our knowledge this has never been shown unequivocally. To at least partly overcome the time limitation we used automated behaviour registration software (HomeCageScan; Clever Systems Inc., VA, USA (HCS)). This recognises a range (>20) mouse behaviours with comparable accuracy to manual analysis by a trained observer [27,28]. In this study we contrasted findings on hyperalgesia and behaviour changes with the results of CPP testing to assess the consequences of bladder cancer on the welfare of mice; applying the concept of triangulation. So far as we are aware, no previous attempt has been made to evaluate the CPP approach as described here during tumour development; with consecutive conditioning and testing cycles. We also sought to gauge (at least hypothetically) whether this could be a useful approach to screening candidate drugs for the treatment of cancer pain in humans. We found tumour mice gained less weight, developed hyperalgesia and showed behaviour changes that were time-linked to enhanced morphine seeking in tumour-bearing mice in the 7 days preceding euthanasia. We concluded that the most likely explanation for these changes was pain. If not due to pain, at the very least the results indicated negative impacts on welfare, possibly including *malaise*. Ordinarily mice would only be removed from studies after this time, indicating a likely need for end-point refinement in this mouse model of bladder cancer. Our method of applying CPP testing could also be a potentially useful method of testing the effectiveness of analgesics intended for cancer and other conditions, especially those where pain can escalate over time.

Methods

Ethics Statement

All work was conducted in accordance with the Animals (Scientific Procedures) Act 1986 and was subject to local ethical review. The experiments also adhered to the guidelines of the Committee for Research and Ethical Issues of the International Association for the Study of Pain (IASP). All procedures were approved by the UK Home Office (Project Licence PPL 60/4431).

Subjects and Husbandry

All mice were female C3H/HeN, weighed 25 to 30 g on delivery (Charles River Laboratories Inc., UK) and had free access to a commercial pelleted diet (R&M no.3 SDS LTD., Whitham, UK) and tap water in groups of 10 for one week of acclimation. They were then housed singly (Macrolon 2 cages; North Kent Plastics, UK) for another week prior to enrolment. Sawdust and wood shavings were used as bedding and cages were supplemented with 'Sizzle Nest', an aspen chew-block and a cardboard tube (B & K Universal). Room temperature was maintained at 21 ± 1°C with 15–20 air changes per hour under a 12-hour light cycle (lights off at 19:00 h). All testing was conducted between 10 am and 3 pm.

Data Collection

The results of 3 studies using separate groups of mice are described; (1) Hargreaves (nociceptive testing) study, (2) Behaviour study and (3) Conditioned Place Preference (CPP) testing consisting of a Pilot dose ranging investigation and then a main study. The data obtained on studies 1 and 2 were from exploratory trials undertaken by colleagues of the Northern Institute for Cancer Research (NICR) using syngeneic MBT-2 (Mouse Bladder Tumour) cells derived from C3H/HeN/J mice (cells donated by Prof. Michael O'Donnell (University of Iowa, Iowa City, IA, USA) and Dr. William A. Larchian (EMH/Cleveland Clinic Prostate Centre, Cleveland, OH, USA)). The CPP data were obtained from mice specifically obtained for testing. Our colleague's objectives were; initially to characterise the growth profile of orthotopically implanted bladder tumours (Study 1) and then to refine the implant methodology (Study 2). However, both studies were an opportunity to collect supplemental data on pathological effects (possibly including pain) that would help in the design of the main (CPP) study; thereby reducing animal use to as low a level as possible.

Hargreaves Study

This was a pilot study undertaken to establish the growth characteristics of orthotopically implanted MBT-2 cells that would inform on the eventual design of the CPP study. Group sizes were determined by NICR colleagues based on their study requirements. Mice were randomly allocated to three groups of 5 that underwent laparotomy for orthotopic implantation of 100 µl of Dulbecco's Phosphate Buffered Saline (DPBS), or the same volume of DPBS containing 2×10^4 or 2×10^5 MBT-2 cells. A fourth group of 5 mice were anaesthesia only controls. Eight mice that underwent surgery were randomly chosen to receive 5 mg/kg meloxicam (subcutaneously; s/c) to alleviate post-surgical pain [27], while the remainder received saline (0.3 mls s/c; $n = 7$). Anaesthesia was induced with 5% isoflurane in oxygen (5 l/min.) in a Perspex chamber. Mice then lay in dorsal recumbency on a heating blanket to maintain body temperatures between 34.5 and 37.5°C and anaesthesia was maintained with 1.5–2% isoflurane in oxygen (500 ml/min.). Depth was monitored by observing respiratory rates and regularly assessing toe-pinch reflexes. Simple eye ointment (Pliva Pharma Ltd., UK) was used to prevent corneal drying. Surgery was a 0.5 cm midline incision in the skin and muscles overlying the bladder. Once exposed, 0.1 ml of saline or the appropriate tumour cell suspension was injected intramuscularly into the bladder wall using an insulin syringe. The abdominal muscles and skin were closed separately using 5/0 polyglactin 910 ('Vicryl', Ethicon Ltd, Edinburgh, UK) and tissue glue ('Nexaband', Abbott laboratories, Chicago). Anaesthesia lasted approximately 10 minutes.

Thermal withdrawal latencies were obtained at baseline, and at 1 hour and 1 day (24 hours) following surgery, and then on days; 3, 7, 10, 14, 17, 21 and 24 using the Plantar Test (Model 37370; Ugo Basile, Italy) according to the method of Hargreaves [51]. Animals were placed in clear acrylic chambers on a glass floor and habituated for 10 minutes. An infra-red heat source was alternately applied to the mid-plantar area of each hind paw (70% of maximum heating capacity; equivalent to 253 ± 7 mW/cm^2; 30 second cut-off). This provided a suitable range of response latencies in normal mice (~between 3 and 8 seconds). Three responses were obtained from each hind paw with a minimum interval of 1 minute between ipsilateral recordings. Data were only obtained from the anaesthesia control mice until day 3 when they were required elsewhere. Body weights were recorded daily until day 4, and then on nociceptive test days. As tumours were internal, growth stage was estimated by daily palpation by an experienced technician who graded tumours on a 3 point scale; from 1 (barely present) to 3 (obvious without handling). These inspections also included a record of activities associated with abdominal pain in rodents [21,31] and other signs of ill-health such as haematuria, lethargy, dehydration and poor coat and body condition.

Behaviour Study

The behaviour data were collected as part of a follow-up study (again without additional animal use) to assess a potentially more refined (non-surgical) method of cell implantation [52]. Our colleagues sought to establish if tumour engraftment could be improved with this method, whereas we wished to evaluate the longer term effects of cancer growth on behaviour. As before, group sizes were pre-determined; 20 mice were allocated to the DPBS group and 20 to the tumour group. Anaesthesia was induced as previously described but in batches of 5 mice using a custom-made open-mask gas delivery system. The implant procedure has already been described, but briefly, the bladder of each mouse was accessed via a 27 gauge paediatric cannula placed in the urethra. Urine was voided by gentle supra-pubic pressure and aspiration, and the bladder mucosa conditioned with a mild acid rinse (50 µl of 0.1 M HCl) for 20 seconds. This was also aspirated and then neutralised with 50 µl 0.1 M KOH, and three DPBS washes. The bladder was emptied before instilling 50 µl of 5×10^6 MBT-2 cells or the same volume of DPBS via a syringe tied to the tail. The greater cell concentration was in anticipation of an unknown cell fraction being voided in urine following recovery. Cells were left *in-situ* for 30 minutes, following which the mice were placed in an incubator at 37°C for 20 minutes. Daily tumour development was monitored as before and body weights were also recorded daily. Mice were filmed individually for 10 minutes using a video camera (Sony DCR-HC96, Sony, Japan) positioned on a tripod 30 cm from the front of clear '1284'cages ($35 \times 20 \times 14$ cm; Techniplast, UK Ltd) containing only bedding (Aspen sawdust). The procedure for behaviour data collection was as previously

	Block 1			Block 2			Block 3.....
Baseline	Day 1	Day 2	Day 3	Day 4	Day 5	Day 6	Day 7......
Initial Preference Testing (15mins)	Conditioning 1 (am) Saline, S-	Conditioning 3 (am) Saline, S-	Preference 1 Drug Free	Conditioning 5 (am) Saline, S-	Conditioning 7 (am) Saline, S-	Preference 2 Drug Free	Repeat (am)...
	Conditioning 2 (pm) Saline/Mor2, S+	Conditioning 4 (pm) Saline/Mor2, S+		Conditioning 6 (pm) Saline/Mor2, S+	Conditioning 8 (pm) Saline/Mor2, S+		Repeat (pm)....

Figure 1. Timeline of CPP testing. Successive blocks were each of two conditioning days where mice underwent morning S− (saline) and then afternoon S+ (morphine or saline) treatments and were confined for 45 minutes in the black or white chamber. The third day of each block was a drug free preference test, and 3 day cycle was repeated until euthanasia.

described [28] except that it was on alternate days before tumour detection, and then daily. Filming was always during the light phase but the time of day each mouse was filmed was randomised within the tumour and control groups.

Conditioned Place Preference Studies

The CPP work was conducted in 2 stages. The first was a pilot study to explore development of CPP to morphine under repetitive conditioning and testing cycles, and to identify a morphine dose for the main CPP study. The chosen dose would be one that supported only modest place preference but retained sufficient analgesic properties to elicit negative reinforcement in tumour bearing mice. Numbers were determined using a retrospective power analysis on previous morphine CPP results across a range of dose rates in normal mice (1 and 5 mg/kg s/c) [53] that should also elicit significant analgesic effects [54,55]. Sample sizes of 8 or 10 were retrospectively found to achieve 79% or 91% power in detecting significant CPP to a drug (3 or 5 mg/kg morphine) versus placebo-paired compartment. The CPP apparatus consisted of black (steel rod floored) and white (steel grid floored) compartments separated by a grey (solid floored) start chamber. We used 4 identical testing units (Med Associates, St Albans, VT, USA; Model CPP-3013AT) equipped with automatically controlled guillotine doors and lights. Compartments housed infra-red arrays to automatically record compartment residence times and movements within and between the 3 compartments. An initial trial was used to determine the baseline compartment preference of each animal. For this they were placed into the central (grey) start chamber for 1 minute prior to turning on the lights and opening the guillotine doors. Preference testing was always conducted between 10 am and 2 pm. The relative time spent exploring the black and white compartments over a subsequent 15 minute trial was calculated as a proportion of the total test time (see CPP data analysis section). The mice were assigned for S+ (saline or morphine) conditioning in the compartment in which they spent proportionately the least amount of time (i.e. their non-preferred chamber), but no mice showed proportionate initial compartment preferences exceeding 0.6 (the CPP analysis section details the preference calculation method). The design was then counter-balanced such that the initial relative group preference approximated as closely as possible to 0.5 (i.e. equal numbers were assigned per group to the black (B) or white (W) S+ chambers). On this basis eight mice were allocated to each of 2 morphine groups spanning the likely range of effective analgesic dose rates (1 or 5 mg/kg s/c) and a representative group of 4 mice were saline controls. Once we reached the stage of cancer testing we knew the traditional CPP approach of repetitive conditioning trials followed by a single preference test would not be appropriate. This was because if pain occurred; we also wished to capture its onset. Informed by this, all CPP testing (including in the pilot study) consisted of repetitive 3 day blocks, with each block comprising 2 days of conditioning before a drug-free preference test each subsequent day (shown in Figure 1). For the pilot study the 4 controls received only saline (0.03 mls s/c) under both the S− and S+ conditions. Because of possible morphine 'carry-over' to afternoon S+ trials it was necessary that vehicle (S−) injections were always given in the morning and S+ (morphine or saline) in the afternoon. Morphine was obtained as morphine sulphate solution (30 mg/ml; NHS Supplies, UK) and was appropriately diluted with water for injection (wfi) to be administered subcutaneously in a volume of 0.03 mls. All injections were given immediately before placement into the allocated B or W compartment for a 45 minute conditioning period with the guillotine doors closed. Mice were returned to their home-cages immediately following each conditioning session. Four consecutive preference tests were undertaken for the pilot study (4 test blocks; Figure 1) precisely following the method used to determine the initial compartment preference.

The main CPP investigation began with a repeat of initial preference testing. Each mouse was assigned a B or W compartment for subsequent S−/S+ conditioning in the previously described manner (balancing numbers initially preferring the B or W compartment across the control and tumour groups). As before, mice were assigned to their initially non-preferred compartment as far as possible. Tumour mice were again implanted via the urethra with 50 µl DPBS containing 5×10^6 MBT-2 cells. Thirty mice were orthotopically implanted with tumour cells and ten were saline controls. These numbers were informed by our previous findings on numbers of graft failures following urethral implantation. We planned to balance the design (and further conserve animal usage) by assigning any such failures to control groups, but only if there were no palpable or other signs of tumour development after 21 days. Tumour absence was also confirmed *post-mortem*. Once the clinical inspections confirmed tumour growth, each mouse began CPP conditioning and a treatment matched non-tumour control entered the study simultaneously. The 3 day series of conditioning and test sessions then continued until mice were euthanased (see section on end-point determination). Experimental groups therefore formed a 2 (Drug)×2 (Treatment) factorial design that combined conditioning to morphine or 0.9% Saline in tumour or non-tumour mice. We selected an intermediate dose of morphine (2 mg/kg s/c) for the main study based on the findings of the pilot study. In the main CPP study preference tests were also 45 instead of 15 minutes, but the methodology was otherwise identical to that used in the pilot study. Due to time constraints and the potential confound of placement into other unfamiliar environments (effectively other 'places'), behaviour and hyperalgesia assessments were not undertaken as the CPP study progressed. However, the effect of late-stage analgesic treatment on behaviour was assessed as a potential refinement option. This meant that on euthanasia days mice were filmed for 20 minutes before and after injection of the conditioning dose of morphine (2 mg/kg s/c) and identical recordings were made from an equal number of controls on the last day of the study.

End-point determination

Clinical inspections were conducted in all studies to determine if tumour-bearing mice needed to be withdrawn. These were in accordance with published guidelines [10,11] and with the advice of highly experienced animal care staff. Euthanasia was unavoidable once animals had a large palpable tumour or more than 15% body weight loss, and if either of these coincided with significant haematuria (indicated by blood stained fur and/or bedding). All mice including the controls underwent palpation. They were restrained in the manner that is usual for an intraperitoneal injection. The bladder region was then gently palpated between the thumb and forefinger, but with sufficient pressure to determine the earliest time of onset of tumour development as reliably as possible.

Data Analysis

Hargreaves study. As response latencies were initially similar between the left and right hind-paws, all values were averaged to calculate the overall mean response latency at each recording time. The data met the requirements for parametric analysis so were examined using repeated measures ANOVA with 'Time' (10 levels) and 'Group' (4 levels; 2×tumour; 1×placebo and anaesthesia only) as within and between-subject's factors respectively. *Post-hoc* individual time and group comparisons were made and probability levels adjusted accordingly (*Bonferroni*). The body weight changes were also calculated as change from baseline and the same statistical methods applied. For greater clarity, the weight changes are depicted as absolute values at each time-point. Due to absence of nociceptive data in the non-surgery control mice after day 3 and body weight data after day 4 all analyses following these times included the surgery groups only. Finally, the effects of pre-surgery meloxicam were examined by comparing baseline response latencies to the 1 hour time point in the ANOVA; but with 'pre-treatment' (meloxicam or saline) as a between subject's factor ($n=7$ (Saline) versus $n=8$ (meloxicam)).

Behaviour study. The behaviour data were processed using HCS automated analysis software. The measures used were total distance travelled and five behaviour classes comprising different elements of the 20 individual behaviours the system recognised. These were: 1) Rearing (comprising 'Rear Up' (both partial and full bipedal extension) & the reciprocal activity 'Come Down'); 2) Active behaviour (including walking, running, jumping and climbing); 3) Abdominal Grooming, and 5) Resting (inactive periods). We summed the occurrences of behaviours within each class as the relative magnitude of class elements was sufficiently uniform. The mean frequency of each class was calculated for each mouse on each filming day. The relative duration of each class (duration/frequency) was also calculated to investigate the possibility that time spent engaging in each type of activity changed independently of its total occurrence. All behaviour data were tested and met the assumptions necessary for parametric analysis. Repeated measures ANOVA was used with 'Time' (Days) and 'Group' (Tumour versus Control) as the within and between subject's factors for each measurement. Calculations of body weight change from baseline following non-surgical tumour implantation were evaluated again with 'Time' and 'Group' (saline or tumour) as within and between subjects factors, also using repeated measures ANOVA. Multiple comparisons between individual times were again probability corrected (*Bonferroni*).

Conditioned Place Preference Studies. In both the pilot study and main CPP study the initial black or white compartment preferences were calculated as the proportionate time spent in each compartment. Where t = time, the Black (B) compartment preference (Bpref) was therefore calculated as tB/(tB+tW), and the White (W) compartment preference (Wpref) as tW/(tW+tB). Thus, a proportionate score of >0.5 indicated a greater preference for that chamber and this became the S+ condition. All subsequent calculations of chamber preference were made in the same way, and the proportion of time spent exploring the S+ chamber relative to S−(tS+/((tS+)+(tS−)) was the dependent measure over successive preference tests. We again used repeated measures ANOVA to compare S+ preference scores over successive tests in the pilot and main study with 'Time' and 'Group' as respective within and between subject's factors. The source of any individual group differences was again determined using *post-hoc* analyses and applying *Bonferroni* correction of probability levels.

Results

All results are expressed as mean±1SEM. The electronic files pertaining to all analyses are publicly available at Dryad (http://datadryad.org/), or can be accessed by contacting the lead author.

Hargreaves Study

Three mice in the 20 K group had palpable tumours (graded 1–2) at day 14, and three in the 200 K group reached this stage by day 10. Thereafter tumour burden gradually increased, and by day 21 tumours were apparent in all animals such that in several cases tumours could be identified without need for palpation. There was no indication of a need to euthanase any mice before the pre-scheduled study end-point on day 24. As expected, the anaesthesia controls showed no adverse effects, and aside from the first day following surgery the saline/surgery controls also appeared 'normal'. Figure 2a shows the mean change in Hargreaves withdrawal latencies (threshold to respond) in the tumour and control groups over the time course of the study. Thresholds were initially similar across the 4 groups; between 4.5 and 5.5 seconds; indicating equivalent nociceptive status initially. Although withdrawal occurred significantly earlier at the 1 hour time-point in the surgery groups (5±0.4 vs 3±0.3 seconds; ($F(1,13)=16.6$, $p=0.001$), by 24 hours these showed thresholds that were no longer significantly different from baseline. This was also the case in in the anaesthesia controls over their 3 post-treatment recording days. The surgery controls had also apparently recovered by day 3, and over the time course of the study their response thresholds remained relatively consistent; from 4.3±1.4 at baseline compared to 4.3±1.2 s on day 24. By contrast, mice implanted with tumours showed an overall increase in thermal sensitivity (thresholds/latency to respond reduced). These effects led to a significant overall '|Group' effect (Tumour vs Control; ($F(1,12)=12.2$, $p=0.001$) and 'Group x Time' interaction ($F(18,108)=2.6$, $p=0.001$). *Post hoc* analyses showed both tumour groups had significantly reduced thresholds compared to DPBS controls arising on day 14 ($p=0.019$, 0.001, 20 K and 200 K vs. DPBS, respectively). This was maintained until day 21 in both groups, but by day 24 only the 200 K group showed significantly reduced response latencies relative to controls ($p=0.002$). There were no significant effects of meloxicam (positive or otherwise) on either withdrawal thresholds or body weight (data therefore not shown).

As shown in Figure 2b Surgery/Saline mice were somewhat lighter initially, but not significantly so (~1.5 g). To account for this ANOVA with individual (*post-hoc*) comparisons was conducted on calculations of weight change from baseline over the first 3 days. Post-surgery losses averaged 1.7±0.3 g overall ($F(1,13) = 32.4$, $p<0.001$). Weights were maintained in the non-surgery mice. Both tumour (surgery) groups showed this weight loss from 1 to 3 days, with the greatest mean loss being 2.2±0.8 g in the 200 K tumour group on day 1. The 20 K and 200 K tumour groups both lost significantly more weight than the anaesthesia controls on post-surgical days 1 and 2 (p = 0.01, 0.003 (day 1); 0.01, 0.04 (day 2), 20, 200 K groups respectively). The same comparison between the surgery and anaesthesia controls was not significant, probably because the surgery controls were initially lighter. The surgery controls therefore lost seemingly less weight immediately, and had recovered more weight by day 3 than either the 20 K (p = 0.038) or 200 K tumour groups (p = 0.018). By day 4 there were no significant group differences. The pattern was then of increased weight until the end of the study. This resulted in a significant effect of 'Time' ($F(6,72) = 7.1$, $p = 0.002$). Groups showed only a modest (~1.5–2 g) increase in weight, although by the end of the study (days 17 to 24) there was evidence that weight gain slowed more in the high cell density group than the other surgery groups. This greater overall reduction in weight in the last week in the high density (200 K) tumour group, and over the last 3 days in the 20 K group resulted in a significant 'Group×Time' interaction ($F(2,12) = 4$, $p = 0.045$).

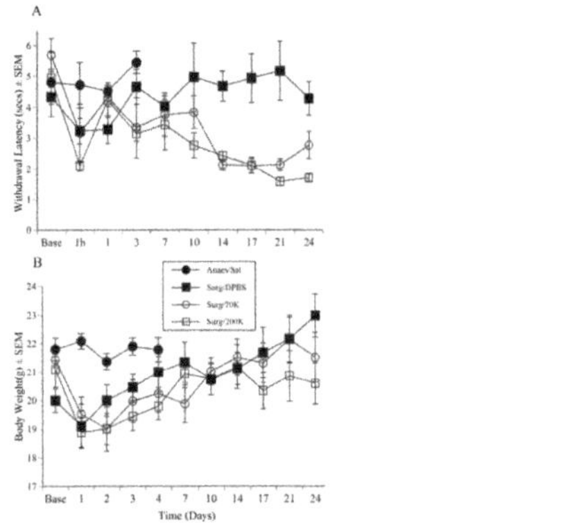

Figure 2. Hargreaves study results. The results of nociceptive testing (A) and recording weight changes (B) (mean±SEM) in mice that underwent anaesthesia only (Anaes), or anaesthesia followed by laparotomy for orthotopic implantation of DPBS (100 µl) or MBT-2 bladder tumour cells (2×10^4 or 2×10^5; 20 K or 200 K, respectively) (n = 5 per group)). (A) Hargreaves recordings were at baseline (Base), 1 hour (1 h), and then on the days indicated by the *abscissa.* Mice implanted with the highest cell concentration showed lower Hargreaves response thresholds (p = 0.02) than the anaesthesia only controls over the first 3 days (indicating hyperalgesia). Also, beginning on day 14, mice with tumours developed significant hyperalgesia compared to surgery/saline controls (p = 0.019, 0.001 (2×10^4 or 2×10^5 groups respectively)). (B) Tumour groups lost significantly more weight over the first 3 days than either the anaesthesia only or surgery controls (p≤0.04), but mean baseline body weight was recovered in these mice by post-operative day 4.

Behaviour Study

Of the 20 mice implanted for the behaviour study (non-surgically) 12 (60%) developed tumours. The implant procedure caused only marginal weight loss (0.8±0.1 g), and all mice fully recovered their starting weights by day 2. The time to detect a solid tumour mass was relatively uniform (28±1.7 days), but subsequent tumour development was considerably more varied. The time from tumour detection to reaching end-point criteria ranged from 10 to 23 days (mean 13.6±3.5). The first mouse was euthanased on day 37 following implantation and 2 mice survived without obvious concerns for 50 days (when the study ended). An inverse relationship was predicted between *ex-vivo* tumour wet weights and survival time (days from detection to euthanasia), but no such relationship was found; average tumour mass was 1.1±0.17 g, range 0.4 to 2 g. The net effect of the varied tumour growth rate was that numbers in the tumour groups were progressively depleted, so aside from immediately following implantation, plotting results on a conventional ascending timescale was not helpful. For both the behaviour and body weight data we therefore examined the results in reverse of the time (day) mice were euthanased; predicting this would be the time when the tumour and control groups would be most distinct. The data were first standardised by matching those from the tumour group to equivalent control data (in terms of elapsed study time). Figure 3 shows the behaviour results from the last 15 days before each mouse was euthanased, with data from an equivalent elapsed study time in controls mice. Panels 3a–d respectively show distance travelled, active, rearing and grooming behaviour frequency. The ANOVA showed tumour bearing mice travelled significantly less overall (Figure 3a; $F(1,22) = 6.65$, $p = 0.017$), and the group difference widened as time progressed. This was especially obvious from 7 days prior to euthanasia when the tumour mice began a marked decline in activity, whereas the opposite effect was observed in controls, leading to a significant 'Group×Time' interaction ($F(14, 308) = 4.1$, $p = 0.001$). There were less obvious group differences in active behaviour (Figure 3b). The groups were not significantly different overall, but the pattern of increasing activity in controls versus a decline in tumour mice was maintained, but was only marginally significant ('Group×Time'; $F(14,308) = 2.3$, $p = 0.04$). The last 7 days was again the time when group differences were most apparent, however, there was a noticeable spike in active behaviour in tumour mice 3 days prior to euthanasia that partially impacted on the distance measure. Rearing behaviour showed the most obvious group separation, with the tumour mice rearing less during the entire 2 weeks prior to euthanasia (Figure 3c; $F(1,22) = 14.3$, $p = 0.001$). There was no particularly obvious decline in tumour versus control mice over the terminal 7 days, but rearing was maintained at a markedly greater

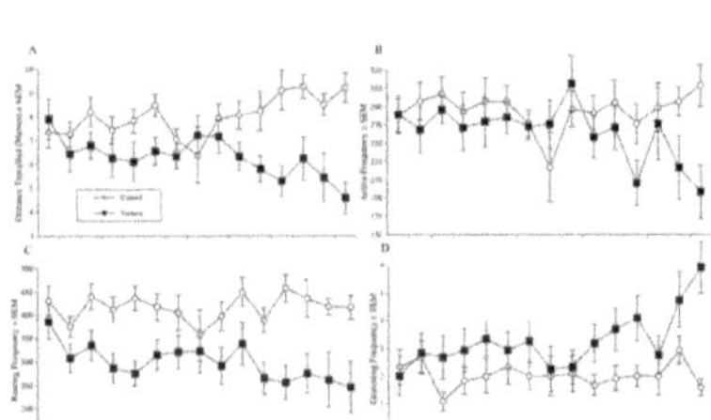

Figure 3. Behaviour study results – Changes preceding euthanasia. Results of automated behaviour analysis (HCS) during the period 15 to 1 day prior to euthanasia in the Hargreaves study (mean±SEM). (A) Tumour mice travelled significantly less distance overall ('Group', p = 0.017) and showed a pronounced decline over the 8 days before euthanasia ('Group×Time', p = 0.001). (B) Active behaviour showed a decline during the days preceding euthanasia (−3 to −1). (C) Tumour mice reared less over the entire 2 weeks prior to euthanasia than controls ('Group', p = 0.001) and (D) groomed more overall ('Group', p = 0.038), but more intensively so over the final 7 study days ('Group×Time', p = 0.048).

frequency in controls (416±90 vs. 245±189). Grooming showed a slight overall increase in both groups over time ('Time' factor significant; $F(14,308) = 2.1$, $p = 0.05$; Figure 3d). The tumour mice also groomed more frequently overall ($F1,22) = 4.9$, $p = 0.038$), but again, the major effect in tumour mice was an increase in grooming frequency over the final 7 days (significant 'Group x Time' interaction; $F(14,308) = 2.1$, $p = 0.048$). This result was rendered only modestly significant due to another incongruous effect 3 days prior to euthanasia when grooming frequency fell in tumour mice. Rest periods (inactive behaviour) were no more frequent in control or tumour mice until the final 3 days when tumour mice tended to show a reduction compared to only a very slight increase in controls (not shown).

The body weight data on the day each mouse was euthanased were matched as previously described: with results in tumour mice matched to data from an equivalent elapsed study time in a randomly chosen non-tumour control. This was repeated for each day prior to euthanasia. Figure 4 shows the mean body weights of the control and tumour groups from 37 days prior to euthanasia. The pre-study weights of the 2 groups were not significantly different. Both groups were gaining weight 37 days prior to the eventual study end, however, the tumour group stopped gaining weight 2 weeks later (22 days before euthanasia). ANOVA showed a significant 'Group×Time' interaction 12 days prior to euthanasia ($F(1,23) = 8.55$, $p = 0.008$). *Post-hoc* analyses (independent samples t-tests) showed that by this time the mean weight of tumour bearing mice was 25±1.1 g, compared to 26±1.3 g in controls ($p = 0.015$). The control mice then steadily increased in weight whereas the reverse occurred in the tumour group (or at least they continued to fail to gain weight). By the end of the study (on day −1) the mean weight of control mice was 27±1.8 g compared to 24.5±2.5 g in the tumour group ($p = 0.009$). In the tumour mice this amounted to a proportional weight loss of 4.6% compared to the time when they were heaviest (Day 24 prior to euthanasia). We tried to minimise any masking effect of underlying tumour burden on this weight estimate by subtracting *ex-vivo* tumour wet weights, but did not find mice with larger tumours lost significantly more weight.

Conditioned Place Preference Studies

The results of the CPP pilot study are shown in Figure 5 according to mean S+ preference scores of the groups given saline and each morphine dose. ANOVA indicated a significant overall 'Group' difference ($F(1,2) = 5.6$, $p = 0.013$). The *post-hoc* analysis showed mice given 5 mg/kg morphine had significantly elevated S+ scores over tests 2 to 4 compared to the saline controls ($p = 0.005$) or the mice given the lower morphine dose ($p = 0.041$). Saline was predictably ineffective, but as 1 mg/kg morphine was also not different from saline an intermediate morphine dose of 2 mg/kg was chosen for the main CPP study.

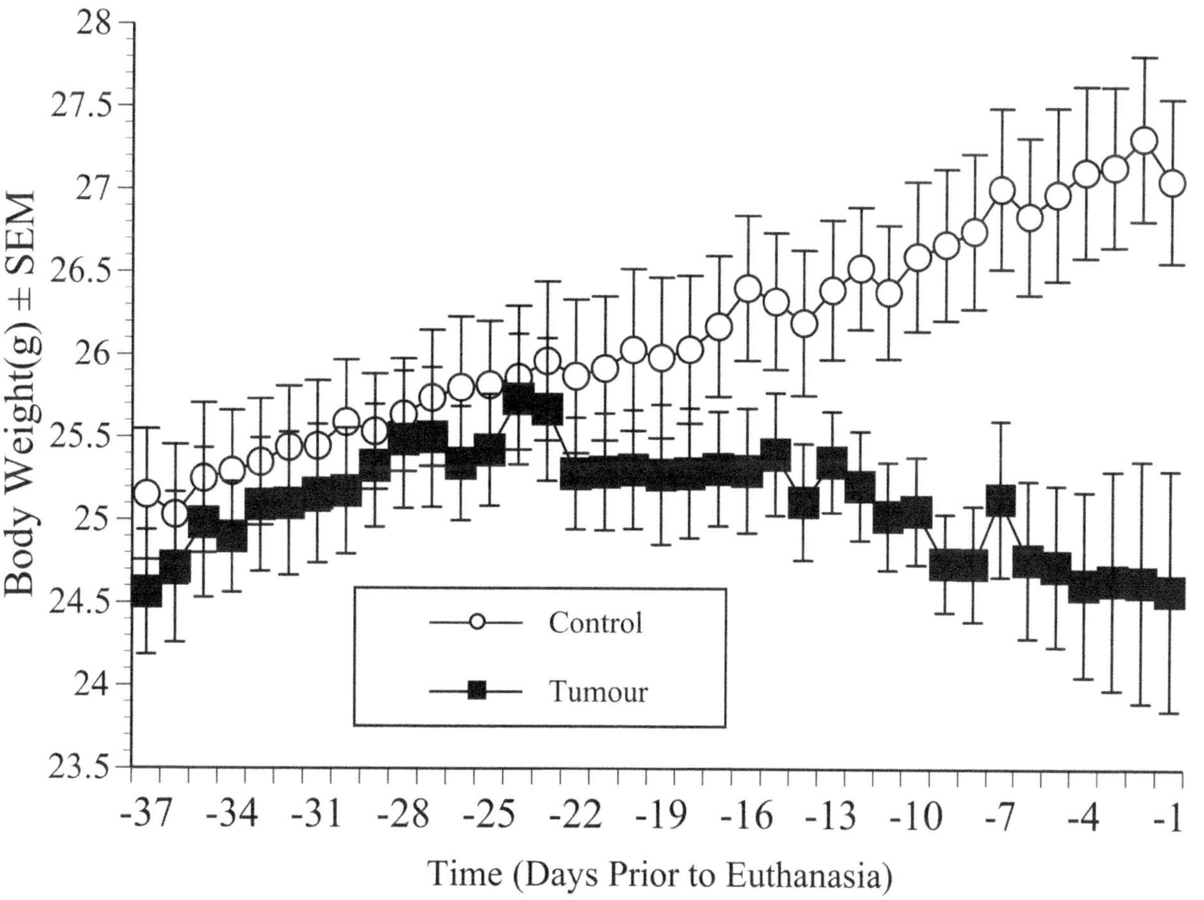

Figure 4. Body weight in catheterised mice (implanted non-surgically). The mean (±SEM) body weight of groups of mice implanted orthotopically with either MBT-2 tumours (5×10^6 cells/mouse; 50 μl) or an equal volume of saline, and used to collect behaviour data (n = 12 per group; graft successes only). As in Figure 3, data on days prior to euthanasia are shown following time matching (equivalent elapsed study time). Tumour-bearing mice were significantly lighter than controls from day 12 ('Group'; p = 0.008) and progressively lost more weight until the study end.

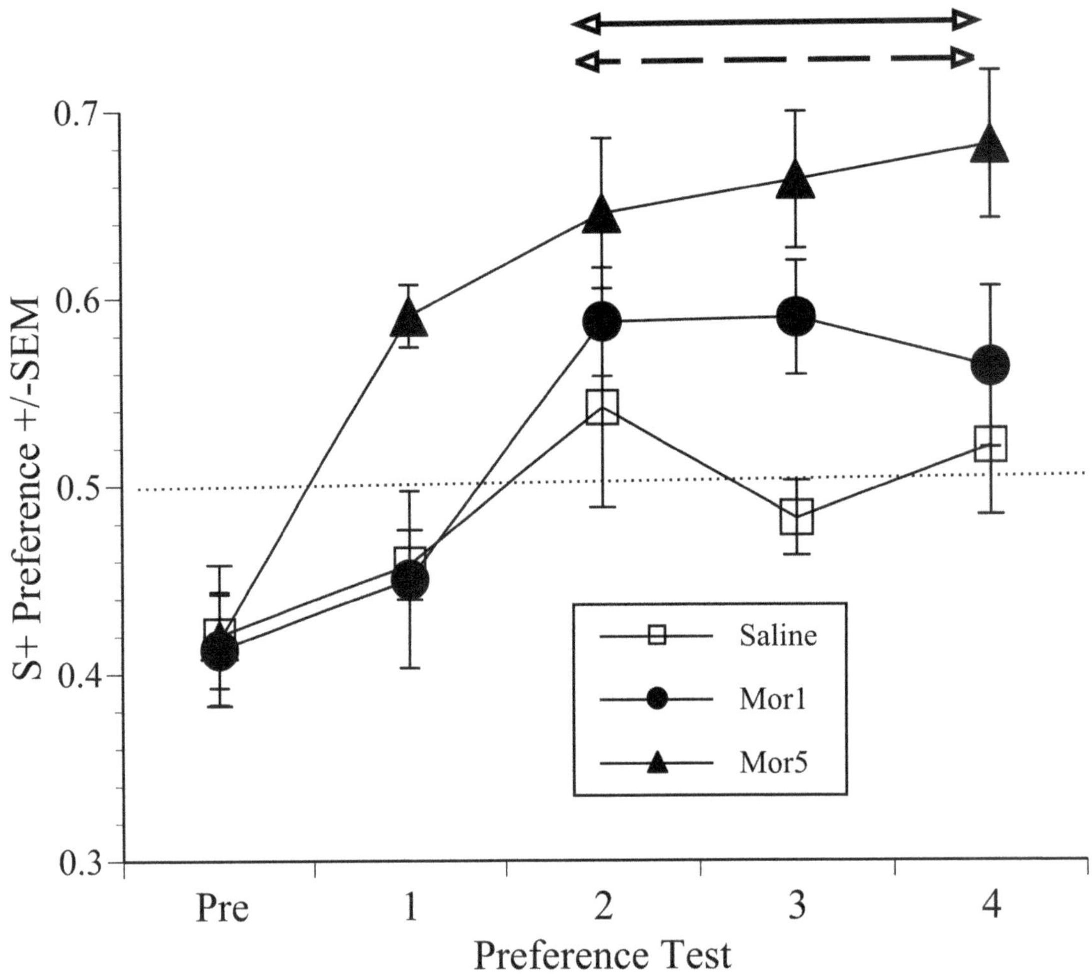

Figure 5. CPP pilot study results. Mean S+ chamber preference scores (±SEM) across 4 successive tests in mice conditioned to saline (0.03 mls; n = 4) or morphine (Mor) at 1 or 5 mg/kg (n = 8/group). Mice were conditioned in their initially non-preferred chamber (Pre). Scores above 0.5 (dotted line) indicate enhanced S+ (morphine or saline) chamber preference. Arrowed lines at the top of the chart denote the time period over which the preference for 5 mg/kg morphine exceeded 1 mg/kg ($p < 0.05$; dashed arrowed line) or saline ($p < 0.01$; solid arrowed line).

Implant success in the main CPP study was 70% with 21 of the 30 implanted mice developing tumours. As planned, four non-growth mice were randomly assigned to control groups, one of which subsequently developed a tumour (so data were rejected). Although overall engraftment was improved from that seen in the behaviour study, the time from implantation to detection of a solid tumour mass over the bladder was more varied. Of the mice where grafts were successful, 75% presented tumours within 14–21 days. Subsequent rates of tumour development were also varied, leading to a broad range of times from tumour detection to the time that mice were euthanased (13–46 days). This meant the number of tests conducted in tumour mice before they reached the endpoint criteria ranged from only 4 to 15 CPP trials (mean ± SD; 8.4±2.73). To minimise the impact of this variation we re-applied the selection procedure to focus on the times likely to reveal group differences; where tumour-bearing mice should show an enhanced morphine preference if they were experiencing pain. As the minimum number of tests was four, the results of the last 4 tests prior to euthanasia were examined (i.e. CPP tests −4, −3, −2 & −1); equivalent to days 10, 7, 4 and 1 day before the study ended. As in the behaviour analysis, data from the non-tumour control (saline or morphine) groups were time-matched as far as was possible to the total number of cycles of conditioning/preference testing undergone by individuals in the equivalent tumour groups.

There were no significant differences in S+ scores between the morphine and saline treated mice on the 3 test days after tumour detection, and both the normal and tumour bearing mice trained only to saline displayed essentially equal preference to the S+ and S− chambers over these trials (i.e. preference scores close to 0.5; data not shown). This illustrated that the apparatus and study design were unbiased. As predicted, the responses to morphine were clearer over the last 4 preference trials (Figure 6). From 10 to 4 days before euthanasia (preference tests −4 to −1) there was little change in morphine preference in controls, but the morphine-treated tumour mice displayed the highest S+ place preference scores of all four groups; the combined effect being an overall significant effect of drug treatment ($F(1,29) = 4.9$, $p = 0.035$). The morphine preference in the tumour group increased over the final 3 preference tests (7 days). Mean S+ preference over this time was calculated and results compared between groups using ANOVA. This also showed a significant overall treatment effect ($F(3,29) = 6.74$, $p = 0.001$). *Post-hoc* tests showed tumour mice conditioned to morphine had significantly elevated S+ scores in comparison to both the saline controls

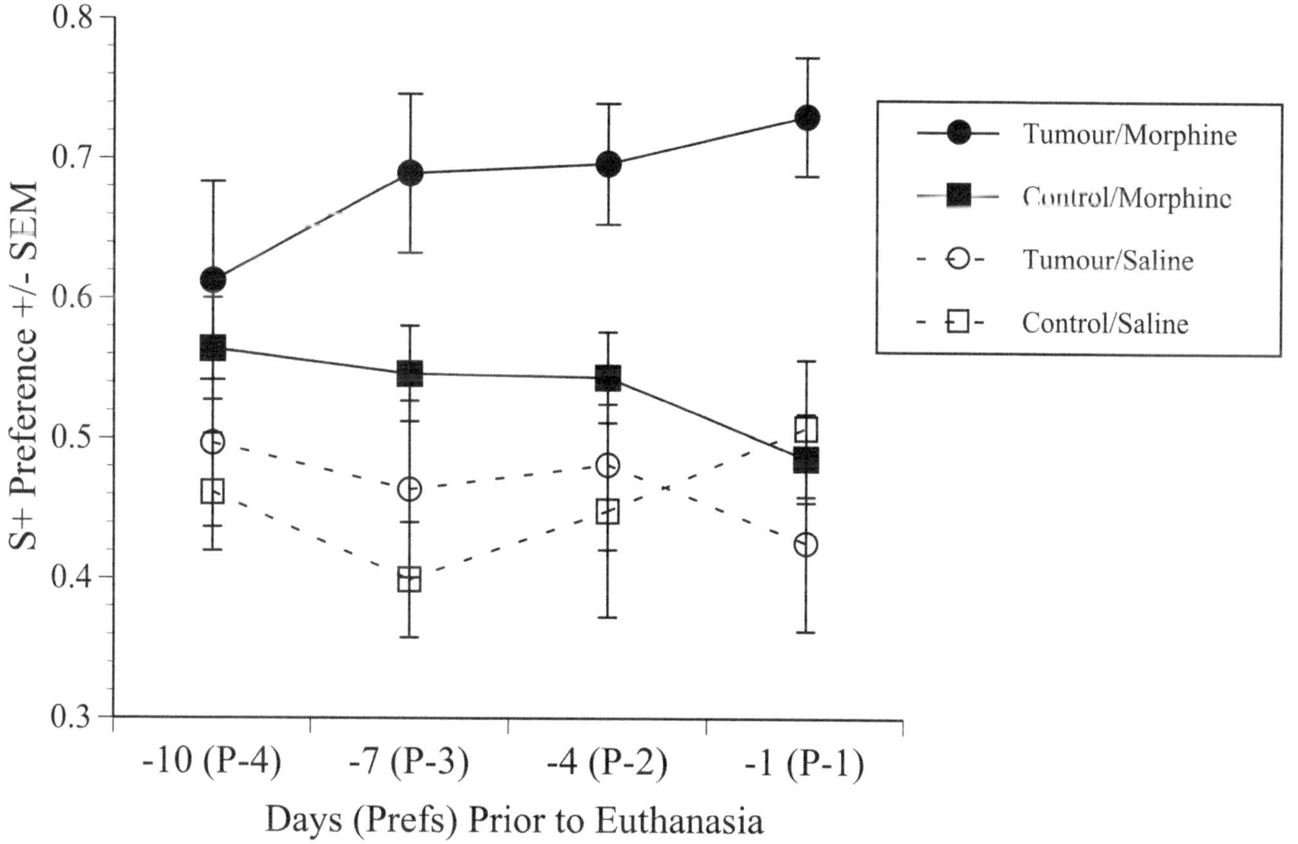

Figure 6. CPP morphine preference scores preceding euthanasia. Mean S+ chamber preference scores (±SEM) during the last 4 preference tests (actual days in brackets) prior to euthanasia (Day −1(1)) in normal (Control) and tumour bearing (Cancer) groups conditioned to Saline or Morphine (2 mg/kg; s/c). Scores above 0.5 indicate an enhanced S+ chamber preference. Note especially the cancer mice conditioned to morphine show enhanced morphine seeking (higher CPP S+ score) than either the saline or tumour control groups ($p = 0.005$; $p < 0.001$, respectively), but from days −7 to −1 prior to euthanasia their morphine chamber preference also significantly exceeded the morphine preference of controls conditioned to morphine ($p = 0.02$).

($p = 0.005$) and the saline tumour mice ($p < 0.001$). The key comparison, however, was between the morphine preference scores of the tumour and control mice. Mice with tumours had a significantly greater preference for the morphine paired chamber than the morphine controls ($p = 0.02$). These findings were consistent with the notion that mice in pain will show a place preference to a compartment paired with an analgesic drug over one paired with only saline, but crucially, more so than the drug preference shown by normal mice.

Analysis of the body weight data indicated there were no significant group differences at baseline (before cell implantation). Body weights from the time period over which the CPP results indicated was the most important phase of the study were then assessed; the final 4 preferences tests (Figure 7). We used calculations of change in weight from before the previous test day (14 days prior to euthanasia). Repeated measures ANOVA was used with 'Time' (4 levels) as a within-subjects factor, and both 'Drug' (morphine or saline) and 'Treatment' (cancer or control) as between subject's factors. Over the final 10 days of the study the tumour bearing mice showed a small but nevertheless significant reduction in weight (1.6±0.8) compared to non-cancer mice. The non-cancer groups either maintained body weight or showed a marginal weight increase during this period (0.6±1 g) (significant 'Time×Treatment' interaction; $F(2,50) = 11$, $p < 0.001$). Morphine had no significant effects on body weight.

There was only a marginal difference in mean tumour burden between the saline and morphine groups; tumour wet-weight at *post-mortem* was 1.04±0.75 in the saline group versus 0.83±0.45 g in mice conditioned to morphine. An independent samples t-test showed morphine was unlikely to be responsible for this very slight difference ($t(16) = 0.91$, $p = 0.4$). We initially explored whether tumour burden was a significant contributor to morphine chamber preference on the last CPP test (Preference test P-1). Pearson's correlation showed no significant relationship between S+ preference scores and tumour burden in the saline group ($r = -0.19$; $p = 0.64$; Figure 8a), however, tumour burden was significantly positively correlated with preference for the morphine paired chamber ($r = 0.70$; $p = 0.034$; Figure 8b). The same relationship between tumour burden and morphine seeking was also apparent at 4 days (Preference test P-2) before euthanasia ($r = 0.72$; $p = 0.029$ (not shown)). However, the same comparison at the P-2 time point in mice conditioned to saline was not significant ($r = 0.22$; $p = 0.59$) (P-2 data not drawn)). These results therefore showed that increasing tumour burden made a positive contribution to morphine chamber preference.

The final phase of data collection in the CPP study was to determine whether we could recognise any behaviour-based evidence of reduced pain following terminal morphine treatment. We assessed the effect of the training dose of morphine given on the last study day on grooming, rearing and inactive behaviour

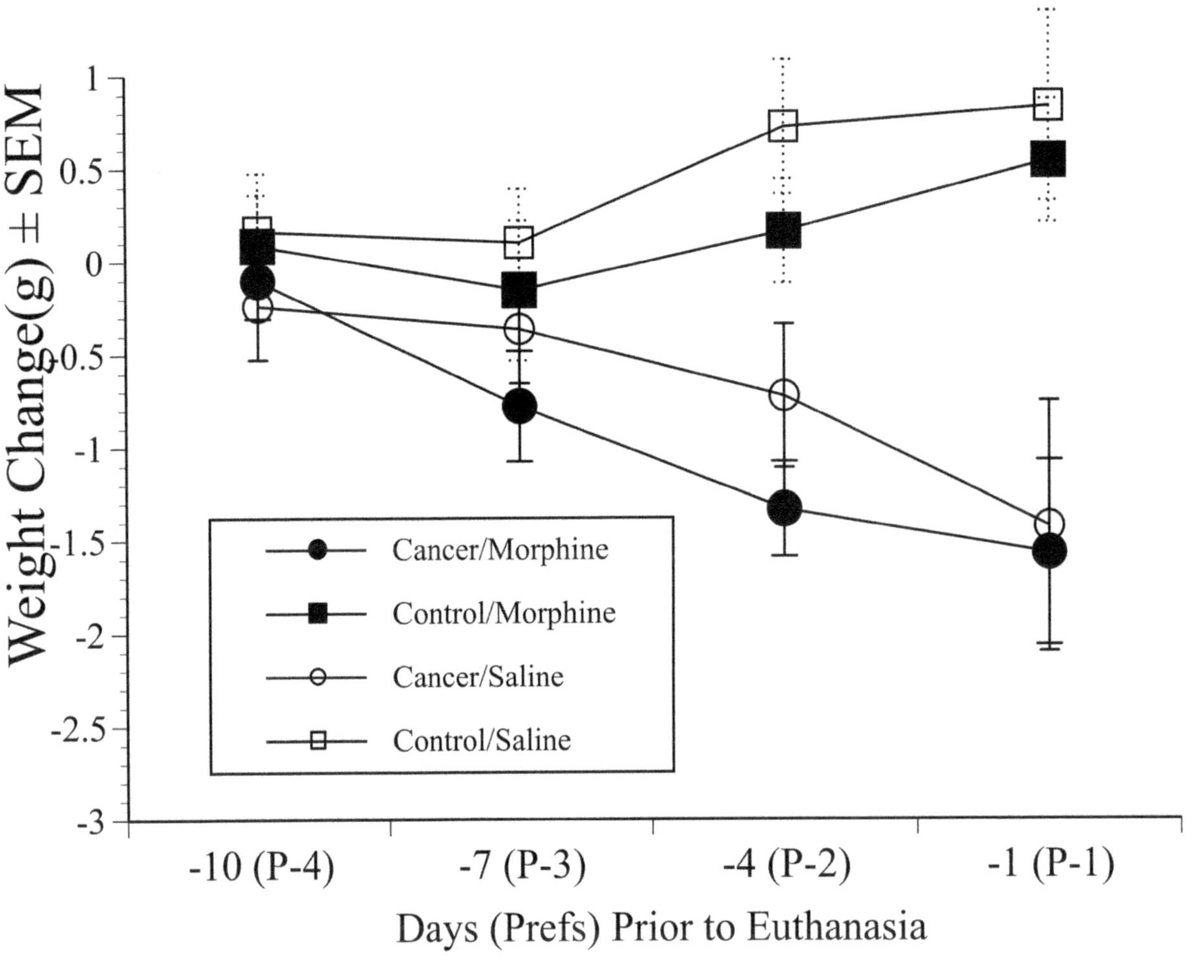

Figure 7. Body weight change in mice used in CPP testing. Mean weight (±SEM) on days −10 to −1 prior to euthanasia relative to weight observed on day −14 in mice in the main CPP study. Weights in tumour-bearing mice significantly declined over the final 7 study days compared to control groups ('Group (Cancer vs Control)×Time', p = 0.001), with no apparent effect of morphine.

frequency (Figure 9). For reasons previously given, total distance travelled was the only measure needed to evaluate changes in active behaviour. The analysis used 'Time' (pre and post-morphine) and 'Group' (tumour vs. non-tumour) as within and between subject's factors, and *post-hoc* analyses (Bonferroni) identified individual group differences. Prior to morphine the tumour-bearing mice travelled significantly less distance than controls ($F(1.28) = 6.4$, $p = 0.017$; Figure 9a). This increased in all mice following morphine ('Time' factor significant; $F(1, 28) = 9.2$, $p = 0.005$). Rearing frequency was similar across all groups initially, and all groups showed significantly reduced rearing behaviour following morphine ('Time' factor significant; $F(1,27) = 83$, $p<0.001$; Figure 9b). The mice with tumours initially groomed more than controls ($F(1,28) = 104$, $p = 0.001$), and morphine had no significant effect on this in either control group, and no significantly greater effect in tumour mice irrespective of whether they had previously been exposed to morphine (Figure 9c). Inactive behaviour was significantly more frequent in the controls versus the tumour groups prior to morphine ($F(1,28) = 11.2$, $p = 0.002$; Figure 9d), but all mice rested more frequently following drug treatment ($F(1,28) = 36.7$, $p<0.001$).

Discussion

The work had two main aims. The first was to determine whether a relatively common mouse bladder cancer model had negative impacts on welfare, including effects caused by *malaise*, anxiety and ultimately pain. If there were any such effects we hoped to highlight these and provide information on potential refinements to prevent possible suffering in similar studies in the future. A second aim was to determine whether the Conditioned Place Preference (CPP) test provides a potentially more relevant alternative to testing analgesics against cancer pain than other presently available methods. The work consisted of a series of studies where in addition to CPP testing, we investigated the development of hyperalgesia, behaviour changes and potential prophylactic effects of morphine in terminal-stage cancer-bearing mice.

In the first study the Hargreaves method was used to evaluate any development of thermal hyperalgesia over a 24 day period following surgical implantation of bladder tumour cells. We found withdrawal thresholds reduced between 10 to 14 days prior to euthanasia, and this hyperalgesic effect was maintained until the end of the study. This increase in peripheral sensitisation provided our first evidence that this type of cancer might progressively impact negatively on welfare. A subsequent investigation exam-

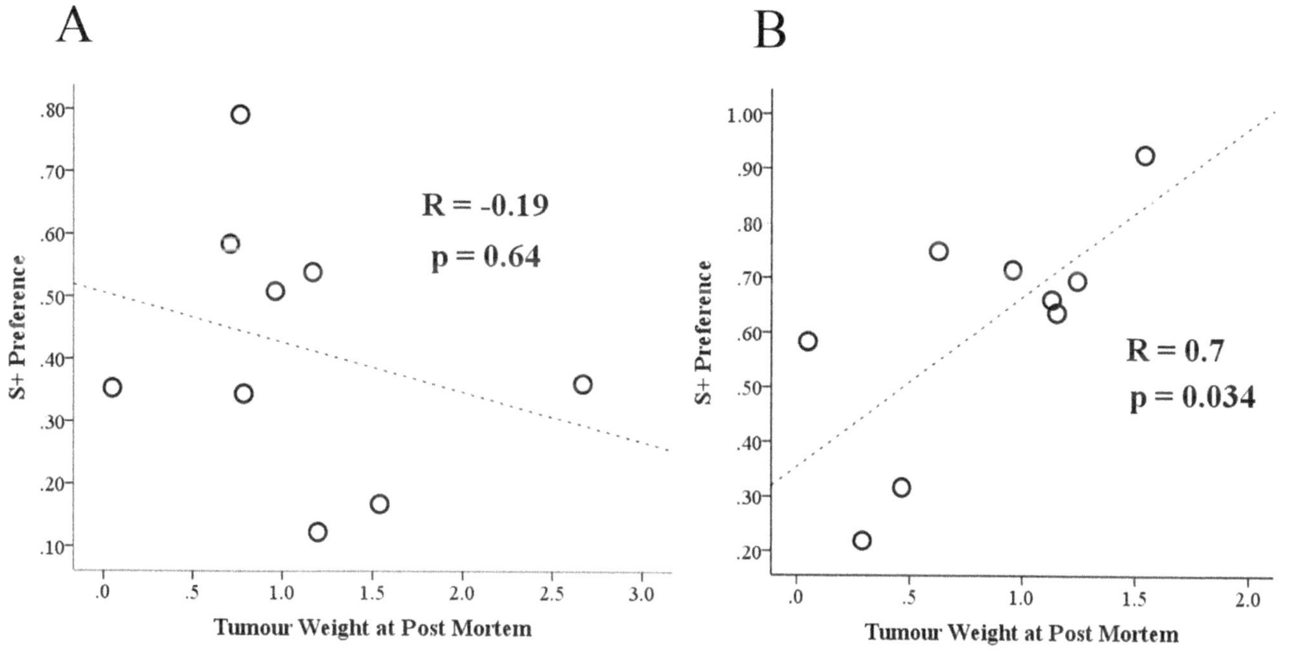

Figure 8. Relationship between morphine seeking (CPP score) and tumour burden. Scatterplots showing: (A) the relationship between relative S+ preference scores for saline on the day immediately prior to euthanasia versus post-mortem (wet) tumour weights (day P-1; Pearson's Correlation); and (B) the same relationship between tumour weight and S+ chamber preference on day P-1 for mice exposed to morphine. Tumour mass bore no significant relationship with saline chamber preference, but as panel B shows, morphine seeking significantly increased with increasing tumour burden.

ined changes in the behaviour of mice implanted with tumours via a potentially more refined non-surgical approach. Recordings of behaviour were processed using an automated system. This showed abnormal behaviour changes began between 7 and 10 days before the study ended, with the most notable effects being reduced distance travelled, reduced active and rearing behaviour and increased abdominal grooming. Changes to behaviours such as these have previously been attributed to abdominal pain in mice [30,31,56] and are similar to those that occur post-operatively in rats [21]. However, the most conclusive evidence that the mice actually experienced pain came from the CPP study. Morphine seeking was found to be significantly positively linked to tumour burden, but most importantly, tumour bearing mice developed a greater preference for the morphine-paired chamber than any other group. They may also have found the placebo-paired chamber aversive, but the pattern of drug seeking strongly indicated the change in compartment preference was due to the negatively reinforcing (pain relieving) properties of morphine. As with the nociceptive and behaviour changes, the changes in morphine-seeking primarily emerged during the last 10 days of the study (4 preference tests). This not only indicated the presence of pain, but showed CPP testing could be a potentially effective and relevant means of evaluating analgesics against cancer and other types of pain.

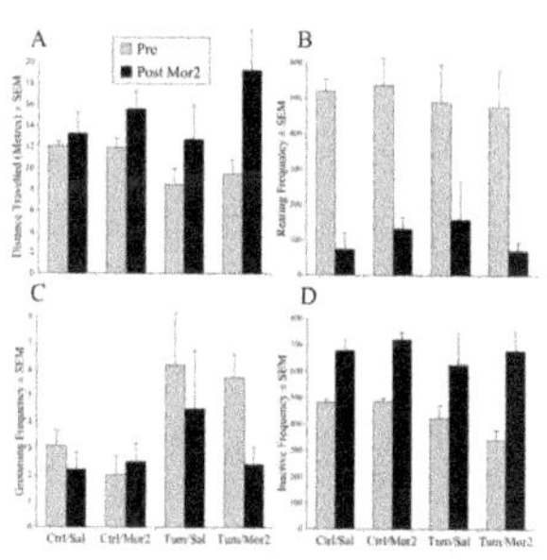

Figure 9. Behaviour changes following terminal morphine. Behaviour results showing the mean (±SEM) frequency before and 30 minutes after terminal-stage treatment with morphine (2 mg/kg s/c) in tumour (Tum) or control (Ctrl) mice that underwent CPP testing and were conditioned to morphine (Mor2) or saline (Sal). (A) Distance travelled; (B) Rearing; (C) Grooming; (D) Inactive periods (Pre) and following (Post) morphine treatment (2 mg/kg s/c). Morphine significantly increased overall activity, indicated by increased distance travelled and reduced rearing ('Time'; $p = 0.005$; $p = 0.001$, Distance and Rearing respectively). Grooming was reduced by morphine but not significantly, and inactive frequency increased ('Time', $p < 0.001$, respectively).

Our findings were obtained despite a number of challenges, mainly the variable success of implanting tumours and the subsequent rates of cancer growth. Although engraftment was 100% using the surgical approach, it dropped to only 60% on our first attempt to implant via the urethra, then improved to 70% in the CPP study. There were several reasons why we persisted with non-surgical implantation of tumours despite the lower graft success. This method initially offered the possibility of being less costly, both financially and in terms of welfare. Conditioning of the bladder epithelium using a mild acid rinse and subsequent buffering was meant to maintain graft success but be less invasive. Non-surgical implantation also meant there was a reduced likelihood of needing to provide peri-operative analgesics; an issue that often concerns researchers who wish to rule out non-specific influences on tumour development. Potential welfare benefits were indicated by an absence of post-procedural weight loss compared to the effects of surgery. Mice that underwent surgical implantation also showed reduced thermal response thresholds, both immediately following surgery and during the latter stage of cancer growth; albeit unfortunate that we had no comparable nociceptive data from the catheterised mice. Finally, stress such as caused by surgery is a known tumour growth promoter [33,57], and any more rapid development could have been detrimental to the eventual timescale for CPP testing. Although tumour seeding was lower and subsequent growth slower via the urethral route, a positive aspect was that this allowed more time for CPP conditioning and also accommodated our preferred approach of only recruiting mice once tumours were detected. Establishing the most appropriate time to begin CPP testing was important since conditioning disease/pain-free mice to morphine could have had other unwanted consequences; e.g. tolerance issues or opioid-induced hyperalgesia. Avoiding these may have been important in our eventual ability to illustrate greater morphine seeking in tumour mice. Directly incorporating nociceptive testing was initially considered in determining when to begin conditioning (i.e. when thresholds reduced), but would have added a further unknown and potentially confounding variable; effectively a third compartment/place to which mice would have been exposed for relatively long periods. From an oncology perspective, however, implanting mice via the urethra may not have been the best option. This is because there are also valid welfare arguments in favour of surgical implantation, especially when tumour growth is more varied. Such variation could increase the number of animals needed to achieve adequate statistical power; making it even more challenging to determine an appropriate study end-point. The longer study duration would also increase facility (housing/husbandry) costs; an obviously important factor in overall cost-benefit analyses.

The behaviour study was meant to establish if bladder cancer impacted on aspects of behaviour in a similar way to other sources of abdominal pain in mice (e.g. vasectomy [31]), and thus required extensive collection of video footage for automated analysis using HCS software. We have previously used this system to assess the behaviour of mice, and shown it can provide precision equivalent to manual scoring [27,28]. However, this was where the varied tumour growth had its first major impact; forcing us to apply the data matching procedure to meaningfully analyse the results. We evaluated responses across 5 behaviour categories during the 2 weeks before euthanasia. This was the period of tumour growth considered most likely to encompass the time of development of any tumour-related pain. Abdominal grooming was more frequent in tumour-bearing mice, whereas distance travelled was reduced, and active behaviour and rearing all occurred substantially less frequently than in controls, especially over the final 7 days prior to euthanasia (Figure 3). There were, however, some unexpected findings. There was an increase in active behaviour and reduced grooming in tumour mice 3 days before euthanasia (Figures 3b and d), and another decline in active behaviour in controls on day −8. We looked for some unplanned event as a possible explanation (e.g. unscheduled husbandry), but the laboratory records held no clues. An adverse reaction to palpation was also unlikely as this was repeated on each of the 2 days that followed without any apparent impact. The effects were also unlikely to have been due to the data manipulation procedure as the period over which matching was conducted spanned 2 weeks and 7 separate dates. Indeed, we cannot offer a more rational explanation, and can only state that some mice were prone to some unusual activity patterns. Nevertheless, the clear disparity between the control and tumour mice over the period preceding euthanasia highlighted this as a key period for later evaluation in the CPP study.

The morphine doses chosen for the CPP pilot study (1 and 5 mg/kg) was another key decision. This was based on evidence of significant anti-nociceptive effects in both phasic (thermal) and tonic (abdominal writhing) tests in mice [54,55]. The larger dose had also previously been shown to elicit relatively robust CPP in rats, whereas 1 mg/kg was only marginally effective [39]. As non-tumour mice in the pilot study developed CPP to 5.0 or 1.0 mg/kg morphine in as a few as two to four conditioning trials (Figure 5) an intermediate dose of 2 mg/kg was chosen for the main study. However, the apparent speed of development of CPP, even in mice given 1 mg/kg, necessitated extending the amount of time used for later preference trials. Exploration time was increased to 45 minutes in the main study, however, only the first 15 minutes served as the dependent measure of preference. This was done in an attempt to minimise CPP development in non-tumour control mice as drug-free tests of this length can serve to facilitate extinction. The design of the main CPP experiment was informed by the original studies where the potential of CPP for evaluating the negatively reinforcing (i.e. analgesic) properties of drugs. Initially, arthritic rats showed an enhanced choice preference to a morphine paired chamber relative to drug treated controls [39] and it was concluded that this was because morphine was more rewarding in the context of pain. However, this interpretation was somewhat obscured in that non-inflamed rats showed an equivalent chamber time preference, and only the choice measure was significant. Sufka [39] describes some possible reasons; one being that choice testing could be a more relevant measure of response strength, whereas time could be influenced by factors unrelated to reinforcement. The intrinsically rewarding properties of morphine also presented challenges of interpreting unconditioned responding (the animals' subjective state), and why choice was superior to time. Then, however, a series of 6 discrete trials was used over 3 days of testing. Although we could not conduct similar choice trials due to a greater burden of conditioning and testing, we investigated the surrogate measure of entrances to each compartment over the first 60 s of each preference test. This, however, did not prove more informative than time preference so the results were not presented. Sufka's original conclusion regarding the value of the CPP methodology in the context of negative reinforcement was ultimately strengthened when a Bradykinin B_1 antagonist was used, which unlike morphine, had no intrinsically rewarding effects but was also preferred by formalin treated versus control rats [40]. This highlighted CPP as a method that could be applied outside of its usual domain for testing the abuse liability of drugs, and it has since been applied in several neuropathic and inflammatory pain models, all of which have successfully used 'time' as the dependent measure of unconditioned responding [41–43,45,46]. These studies, and the results presented here show CPP testing is one of the very few methods with potential for effectively differentiating between the sensory (nociceptive) and affective dimensions of pain. We know of only one previous study where the CPP methodology has been used to assess cancer pain [58], and this failed to show CPP to morphine 24 days after development intra-plantar melanoma. Notably, they used a much higher morphine dose than in our study (10 mg/kg), so the lack of effects may have been due to tolerance issues or drug-induced hyperalgesia; both very common effects of repetitive opioid treatment. There was little evidence for either in our study since there were no differential behavioural responses to terminal morphine treatment in pre-exposed or drug naïve mice. Additionally, the morphine preference of controls changed relatively little from 10 to 4 days before euthanasia, whereas drug-seeking significantly increased over the same time period in the tumour mice. Tolerance would presumably have increased drug seeking in controls, and conversely, hyperalgesia should have prevented this in cancer mice. In reality, however, we may actually have underestimated when pain began because the first time that the cancer-bearing morphine group showed significantly elevated morphine seeking was 7 days (3 preference tests) before euthanasia. As learning this association could conceivably have required several conditioning cycles, the actual time when pain (and its relief) became salient cues may have been at some earlier time point.

Since the tumour model described by Betourne et al. [58] should still have caused localised pain, another possible explanation of their negative findings could be that the mice were so incapacitated that they were insufficiently motivated make a chamber choice. However, other design differences could also offer an explanation. As in Sufka's original study [39], all other studies where the CPP paradigm has been applied to pain have used the traditional approach of conditioning (using one or several drug exposures) followed by preference testing. We applied CPP testing where there could be severe, but slowly developing pain, but additionally, we wished not only to assess its presence but capture its onset. This meant applying a radical design change, incorporating repeated sets of conditioning trials interspersed with multiple preference tests (see Figure 1). So far as we are aware this approach has not been used previously and our positive result may, at least in part, have been due to the more frequent conditioning trials consolidating the association between pain and drug treatment. Our method of processing results by matching mice according to the total number of conditioning and test cycles undertaken, though again unconventional, may also have helped clarify the main effects. As in the behaviour study, this was needed to minimise the impact of the variable tumour growth. This variation meant mice were enrolled in the study at different times, with the net consequence that we could not be certain that animals entered the study at equivalent stages of cancer development. Using the data matching procedure we only examined CPP scores during the likely critical study time of the 10 days before euthanasia. Although this method of processing the data was not ideal, it does not detract from our main conclusion that the increased preference for morphine in cancer mice relative to controls indicated the emergence of pain.

Another study objective was to investigate the need for refinements if there was evidence of pain following tumour implantation. To this end we tested if a pre-procedural dose of meloxicam (5 mg/kg) was an appropriate method of controlling post-surgical in the Hargreaves study. Mice seem to require relatively high doses of NSAIDs [26,59] compared to the recommended rates for pain prevention in rats [23]. This was therefore a comparatively low pre-procedural dose, and was based on investigators' concerns over possible later impacts on tumour development. Although a relatively common reason for excluding analgesics from cancer studies [60] there was no such effect here. In agreement with behavioural and other physiological evidence [23,26] 5 mg/kg meloxicam also did not prevent post-surgical hyperalgesia, so switching to an alternative (e.g. buprenorphine) could be a refinement option, and is one that has already been shown to be less likely to interact with cancer study results [33] than other NSAIDs or opioids.

The effects of morphine were also assessed on euthanasia days when tumours were at an advanced stage. This delayed euthanasia by 75 minutes, but was justifiable since any positive effects could establish if the conditioning dose of morphine was analgesic. If so, this would provide further evidence of pain and establish if this was a refinement option in studies with a strong case for prolonging data collection. Although tumour-bearing mice travelled less and groomed more before morphine, our ability to detect any positive effects was confounded by several non-specific effects of drug treatment. Despite the pre-treatment differences, morphine increased the distance travelled and the frequency of bouts of inactivity and rearing in all mice including the controls (Figure 9). Such non-specific effects of opioids on behaviour are well documented [1,61–64], and we continue to find these can subvert attempts to confirm beneficial effects in studies of post-operative pain in rats in mice [31,65,66]. However, morphine had little influence on grooming in normal mice, and there were indications of post-treatment reductions in grooming in the cancer groups (Figure 9c). Grooming behaviour has previously been concluded to be important for assessing effects due to abdominal surgery or other manipulation likely to induce acute visceral discomfort [30,31,56,67], cancer [68], arthritis [69] and also shows pattern alterations during stress [70]. Perhaps consistent with stress, the cancer-bearing mice were less frequently inactive (unable to rest) prior to morphine (Figure 9d), but again, post-treatment effects were similar in all mice so no positive outcomes were detectable.

To maximise the welfare of mice used in cancer studies the refinements resulting from this work would ideally be widely applicable; such as to soft tissue cancers in general. Present results support this, at least for bladder cancer, since we implanted cells via 2 very different approaches (one surgical, one not) yet still found a commonality in pain symptoms over the final 7–10 study days. An obvious general recommendation would be to monitor animals as closely as possible during this time, possibly adding hyperalgesia and/or behaviour assessments to standard end-point determinations. We cannot state the extent to which behaviour or nociceptive changes should necessitate euthanasia, but increased grooming and the highly significant effects on rearing during cancer development indicate both could be useful. Although the effects on rearing could be also have been caused by *malaise* or some associated lethargy, they still indicated compromised welfare. Nociceptive assessments, however, require specialised equipment (e.g. Hargreaves apparatus) and routine CPP testing would obviously be implausible. The simplest alternative is to rely on weight changes, and accordingly, current model-specific guidelines suggest animals with solid internalised tumours and showing 'severe' cachexia (amounting to between 15 to 20% of baseline body weight) should be euthanased [11]. However, all cancer-bearing mice presently remained within these limits, with the greatest weight loss in the behaviour study being in the tumour group (4.6%). In the CPP study we found the greatest loss was 5 g in a tumour bearing mouse during the final 10 study days. We predicted that the repeated morphine treatments might minimise differences between the tumour and control groups, but seemingly not. One possible explanation is that although both the control and tumour groups were palpated daily, those with tumours may have experienced additional discomfort. We have previously shown that palpation adversely affects the behaviour of rats with bladder cancer [71]. Whether this was currently the case is speculative, but it is nevertheless advisable to be cautious in the manner and frequency of palpation. Body weight assessments should also be adjusted for increased mass due to progression of cancer. Although this was attempted it was found to be difficult, as in any model where tumours are internalised. In any event there was no effective relationship between body weight changes, *ex-vivo* tumour burden and survival (measured by study days from detection to euthanasia). Thus, even if palpation was an effective measure of burden, this would not have been useful in forecasting the need for euthanasia. A more likely scenario was that pain severity and survival were more closely governed by the tissues impacted on during cancer growth rather than burden *per se*. A better approach would be to use more sophisticated methods such as imaging tumours. We plan to use this in future studies to investigate relationships between tumour morphology and welfare, and the general applicability of the CPP and other findings where tumours grow in tissues where they are differentially likely to cause pain. As the majority of evidence indicated the mice were painful despite only moderate weight loss, we suggest protocols relying on this as a primary welfare indicator might consider a more conservative end-point; such as *any* consistent weight loss over a 2 to 3 day period in an otherwise healthy mouse. In studies where more consistent tumour growth is achieved and study duration can be estimated more accurately, our results suggest end-points might be brought forward by at least one week. The precise time is obviously still difficult to identify, but experienced care staff can be exceptionally capable in estimating survival.

A fundamental 3Rs principle is to obtain maximum from the least number of animals, but without compromising scientific integrity. By applying several different assessment methods we hoped to detect cancer pain or other negative impacts on welfare as reliably as possible. Using separate study groups, although a possible weakness, had the major advantage of minimising the burden of testing on individual mice. Indeed, the impact of high intensity testing may be the reason that at least one report has emerged where a range of different 'quality of life' assessments failed to demonstrate negative consequences in a rat neuropathic pain model [50]. We believe the present series of experiments achieved a good level of precision due to the consistency of findings despite some substantial methodological variations. Overall, our studies were conducted in a manner that closely complied with the 3Rs principle of reduction; the majority of data being collected in mice already undergoing cancer trials. However, this meant studying the female mice our colleagues routinely use; due to the greater ease of implanting tumours via the urethra. Oestrus stage could therefore have impacted on our results depending on what stage coincided with conditioning, such as by altering the sensitivity of the mice to morphine. The mice were singly housed, but not isolated. They were also fully acclimated and never in contact with male mice, thus over the course of the study the mice would have undergone several oestrus cycles. It was not feasible to attempt to determine the impact of this on results due to the additional sampling that would have been required. We could have implemented measures to disrupt or halt oestrus, however, the relatively frequent morphine treatments may have caused this already. Determining oestrus stage would also have been very time consuming, and could also have been counterproductive to results. There is extensive literature on sex and strain differences in response to pain and to drug treatment [72–76], so ideally we would repeat the work to establish if the CPP findings generalise to male mice also. However, this would necessitate either surgical tumour implantation, or the more invasive approach of catheterising the urethra of males, both of which could render results questionable. Overall, we argue that it is unlikely that only using female mice significantly weakened our main findings. It could also have been advantageous had we been able to apply the mouse grimace scale (MGS) as an adjunct to the various other measurement parameters [59,77,78]. However, the work was completed prior to its development, and the quality of video recording in the behaviour study, together with the method of filming for analysis by HCS meant the data were not suitable for retrospective analysis using this approach.

Conclusions

The essence of this work was to address a recently highlighted need for more appropriate (systems-based) methods of analgesic drug screening, and the development of more relevant translational pain models. We used a common mouse cancer model and multiple test methods to simultaneously address a second but no less important aim. This was to establish if cancer has a negative impact on the welfare of mice (predictably caused by pain), as this would demand greater effort in refining present end-point guidelines. The work constitutes the most comprehensive series of studies so far undertaken to determine whether bladder cancer is painful to mice. We showed reduced body condition and weight, changes in spontaneous behaviour, and the development of peripheral sensitivity (hyperalgesia) as tumours developed. Added to this we used the CPP paradigm as a means of offering mice the opportunity to self-report on any awareness of pain. Those with cancer spent longer in an environment where they previously experienced the effects of morphine than mice conditioned to morphine alone. Another critical finding was that morphine seeking was closely linked (increased) with tumour burden. However, the validity of our conclusion that these effects indicated pain hinges on whether mice sought morphine as a result of its association with pain relief. It also assumes that the various other changes provide complementary evidence of this. We argue that according to the triangulation principle these results collectively provide convincing evidence of the presence of clinical-type pain in this mouse cancer model. If not pain, there was at least very strong evidence of negative impacts on welfare highlighting a need for a range of possible refinements. Mice in this bladder cancer model could benefit from removal at least 7, and possibly even 10 days prior to the scheduled end-point. Relying only on weight changes or other model-specific signs may not be sufficient to ensure mice do not experience pain before they are euthanased. Rearing deficits may be a useful early indicator of the onset of adverse effects. We found no evidence that provision of morphine was detrimental either to cancer development or to the welfare of mice. In mice implanted surgically there were also no obvious effects of a pre-surgery dose of meloxicam either on post-surgery nociception or tumour development. A more refined surgical protocol might be one using a more appropriate dose of an NSAID for pain prevention, but this would require preliminary work to determine how these or other pharmacological candidates might impact on result validity. However, depending on the sensitivity of required outcomes, future studies of this type might involve buprenorphine; where it has been shown in at least one cancer study to have negligible or even beneficial effects in terms of both welfare refinement and result validity [33]. In light of the numerous other examples where CPP testing has now been applied to assess centralised pain in models other than cancer, we also conclude that CPP testing offers a method of increasing the translational relevance of the results of analgesic screening studies.

Acknowledgments

We wish to thank our colleagues of Newcastle University's Northern Institute for Cancer Research (NICR) for help with cell culturing, developing the implant methodology and for providing access to their animals. The manuscript was prepared according to the ARRIVE guidelines [79] recommended by the UK NC3Rs and others.

Author Contributions

Conceived and designed the experiments: JVR CC PAF HT KS. Performed the experiments: JVR CC PAF HT KS. Analyzed the data: JVR CC PAF HT KS. Contributed reagents/materials/analysis tools: JVR CC PAF HT KS. Wrote the paper: JVR CC PAF HT KS.

References

1. Cowan A, Doxey JC, Harry EJ (1977) The animal pharmacology of buprenorphine, an oripavine analgesic agent. Br J Pharmacol 60: 547–554.
2. Dennis SG, Melzack R (1979) Comparison of phasic and tonic pain in animals. In: Bonica JJ, editor. Advances in pain research and therapy. New York: Raven Press. 747–760.
3. Mogil JS, Crager SE (2004) What should we be measuring in behavioral studies of chronic pain in animals. Pain 112: 12–15.
4. Sufka K (2011) Translational challenges and analgesic screening assays. Pain 152: 1942–1943.
5. Mao J (2012) Current challenges in translational pain research. Trends Pharmacol Sci 33: 568–573.
6. Duncan IJH (1996) Animal welfare defined in terms of feelings. Acta Agriculturae Scandinavica Section A-Animal Science Supplementum 27: 29–35.
7. Flecknell P, Leach M, Bateson M (2011) Affective state and quality of life in mice. Pain 152: 963–964.
8. Mendl M, Burman OHP, Parker RMA, Paul ES (2009) Cognitive bias as an indicator of animal emotion and welfare: Emerging evidence and underlying mechanisms. Appl Anim Behav Sci 118: 161–181.
9. HMSO (2012) Statistics of Scientific Procedures on Living Animals (Great Britain). London: Her Majesty's Stationary Office.
10. UKCCCR (1998) United Kingdom Co-ordinating Committee on Cancer Research (UKCCCR) Guidelines for the Welfare of Animals in Experimental Neoplasia (Second Edition). Br J Cancer 77: 1–10.
11. Workman P, Aboagye EO, Balkwill F, Balmain A, Bruder G, et al. (2010) Guidelines for the welfare and use of animals in cancer research. Br J Cancer 102: 1555–1577.
12. Asai H, Ozaki N, Shinoda M, Nagamine K, Tohnai I, et al. (2005) Heat and mechanical hyperalgesia in mice model of cancer pain. Pain 117: 19–29.
13. Fox A, Medhurst S, Courade JP, Glatt M, Dawson J, et al. (2004) Anti-hyperalgesic activity of the cox-2 inhibitor lumiracoxib in a model of bone cancer pain in the rat. Pain 107: 33–40.
14. Lee BH, Seong J, Kim UJ, Won R, Kim M (2005) Behavioral characteristics of a mouse model of cancer pain. Yonsei Med J 46: 252–259.
15. Zhang HW, Iida Y, Andoh T, Nojima H, Murata J, et al. (2003) Mechanical hypersensitivity and alterations in cutaneous nerve fibers in a mouse model of skin cancer pain. J Pharmacol Sci 91: 167–170.
16. Calixto-Campos C, Zarpelon AC, Correa M, Cardoso RDR, Pinho-Ribeiro FA, et al. (2013) The Ehrlich tumor induces pain-like behavior in mice: a novel model of cancer pain for pathophysiological studies and pharmacological screening. BioMed Res Int 2013: 624815.
17. Hang L-H, Shao D-H, Chen Z, Chen Y-F, Shu W-W, et al. (2013) Involvement of spinal CC chemokine ligand 5 in the development of bone cancer pain in rats. Basic Clin Pharmacol Toxicol 113: 325–328.
18. Liu M, Yang H, Fang D, Yang J-J, Cai J, et al. (2013) Upregulation of P2×3 receptors by neuronal calcium sensor protein VILIP-1 in dorsal root ganglions contributes to the bone cancer pain in rats. Pain 154: 1551–1568.
19. Zhao J, Zhang H, Liu SB, Han P, Hu S, et al. (2013) Spinal interleukin-33 and its receptor ST2 contribute to bone cancer-induced pain in mice. Neurosci 253: 172–182.
20. Leach MC, Allweiler S, Richardson C, Roughan JV, Narbe R, et al. (2009) Behavioural effects of ovariohysterectomy and oral administration of meloxicam in laboratory housed rabbits. Res Vet Sci 87: 336–347.
21. Roughan JV, Flecknell PA (2001) Behavioural effects of laparotomy and analgesic effects of ketoprofen and carprofen in rats. Pain 90: 65–74.
22. Roughan JV, Flecknell PA (2003) Validation of a behaviour-based postoperative pain-scoring system in rats. Proceedings of the Association of Veterinary Anaesthetists Spring Meeting, Dublin 2002. Vet Anaesth Analg 30: 54.
23. Roughan JV, Flecknell PA (2003) Evaluation of a short duration behaviour-based post-operative pain scoring system in rats. Eur J Pain 7: 397–406.
24. Roughan JV, Flecknell PA (2006) Training in behaviour-based post-operative pain scoring in rats - An evaluation based on improved recognition of analgesic requirements. Appl Anim Behav Sci 96: 327–342.
25. Roughan JV, Flecknell PA, Orr HE (2003) Behavioural assessment of post-operative pain and analgesic effects of carprofen in the domestic rabbit. 8th World Congress of Veterinary Anaesthesia. Knoxville, USA. 143.
26. Wright-Williams SL, Courade J-P, Richardson CA, Roughan JV, Flecknell PA (2007) Effects of vasectomy surgery and meloxicam treatment on faecal corticosterone levels and behaviour in two strains of laboratory mouse. Pain 130: 108–118.
27. Roughan JV, Wright-Williams SL, Flecknell PA (2009) Automated analysis of postoperative behaviour: assessment of HomeCageScan as a novel method to rapidly identify pain and analgesic effects in mice. Lab Anim 43: 17–26.
28. Miller AL, Flecknell PA, Leach MC, Roughan JV (2011) A comparison of a manual and an automated behavioural analysis method for assessing post-operative pain in mice. Appl Anim Behav Sci 131: 138–144.
29. Dickinson AL, Leach MC, Flecknell PA (2009) The analgesic effects of oral paracetamol in two strains of mice undergoing vasectomy. Lab Anim 43: 357–361.
30. Miller AL, Wright-Williams SL, Flecknell PA, Roughan JV (2012) A comparison of abdominal and scrotal approach methods of vasectomy and the influence of analgesic treatment in laboratory mice. Lab Anim 46: 304–310.
31. Wright-Williams S, Flecknell PA, Roughan JV (2013) Comparative effects of vasectomy surgery and buprenorphine treatment on faecal corticosterone concentrations and behaviour assessed by manual and automated analysis methods in C57 and C3H mice. PLoS ONE [Electronic Resource] 8: e75948.
32. Vermeirsch H, Nuydens RM, Salmon PL, Meert TF (2004) Bone cancer pain model in mice: evaluation of pain behavior, bone destruction and morphine sensitivity. Pharmacol Biochem Be 79: 243–251.
33. Franchi S, Panerai AE, Sacerdote P (2007) Buprenorphine ameliorates the effect of surgery on hypothalamus-pituitary-adrenal axis, natural killer cell activity and metastatic colonization in rats in comparison with morphine or fentanyl treatment. Brain Behav Immun 21: 767–774.
34. Martucci C, Panerai AE, Sacerdote P (2004) Chronic fentanyl or buprenorphine infusion in the mouse: similar analgesic profile but different effects on immune responses. Pain 110: 385–392.
35. Valeberg BT, Rustoen T, Bjordal K, Hanestad BR, Paul S, et al. (2008) Self-reported prevalence, etiology, and characteristics of pain in oncology outpatients. Eur J Pain 12: 582–590.
36. van den Beuken-van Everdingen MHJ, de Rijke JM, Kessels AG, Schouten HC, van Kleef M, et al. (2007) Prevalence of pain in patients with cancer: a systematic review of the past 40 years. Ann Oncol 18: 1437–1449.
37. Medhurst S, Bowes M, Kidd BL, Glatt M, Muller M, et al. (2001) Antinociceptive effects of the bisphosphonate, zoledronic acid, in a novel rat model of bone cancer pain. Brit J Pharmacol 134.
38. Bardo MT, Bevins RA (2000) Conditioned place preference: what does it add to our preclinical understanding of drug reward? Psychopharmacology 153: 31–43.
39. Sufka KJ (1994) Conditioned place preference paradigm: a novel approach for analgesic drug assessment against chronic pain. Pain 58: 355–366.
40. Sufka KJ, Roach JT (1996) Stimulus properties and antinociceptive effects of selective bradykinin B1 and B2 receptor antagonists in rats. Pain 66: 99–103.
41. King T, Vera-Portocarrero L, Gutierrez T, Vanderah TW, Dussor G, et al. (2009) Unmasking the tonic-aversive state in neuropathic pain.[Erratum appears in Nat Neurosci. 2010 Aug;13(8):1033]. Nat Neurosci 12: 1364–1366.
42. Qu C, King T, Okun A, Lai J, Fields HL, et al. (2011) Lesion of the rostral anterior cingulate cortex eliminates the aversiveness of spontaneous neuropathic pain following partial or complete axotomy. Pain 152: 1641–1648.
43. Rutten K, De Vry J, Robens A, Tzschentke TM, van der Kam EL (2011) Dissociation of rewarding, anti-aversive and anti-nociceptive effects of different classes of anti-nociceptives in the rat. Eur J Pain 15: 299–305.
44. Davoody L, Quiton RL, Lucas JM, Ji Y, Keller A, et al. (2011) Conditioned place preference reveals tonic pain in an animal model of central pain. J Pain 12: 868–874.
45. Okun A, Liu P, Davis P, Ren J, Remeniuk B, et al. (2012) Afferent drive elicits ongoing pain in a model of advanced osteoarthritis. Pain 153: 924–933.
46. Park HJ, Stokes JA, Pirie E, Skahen J, Shtaerman Y, et al. (2013) Persistent hyperalgesia in the cisplatin-treated mouse as defined by threshold measures, the conditioned place preference paradigm, and changes in dorsal root ganglia activated transcription factor 3: the effects of gabapentin, ketorolac, and etanercept. Anesth Analg 116: 224–231.
47. Bateson PP, Rose SP, Horn G (1973) Imprinting: lasting effects on uracil incorporation into chick brain. Science 181: 576–578.
48. Bateson P (1991) Assessment of pain in animals. Anim Behav 42: 827–839.
49. McNabb CT, Uhelski ML, Fuchs PN (2012) A direct comparison of affective pain processing underlying two traditional pain modalities in rodents. Neurosci Lett 507: 57–61.
50. Urban R, Scherrer G, Goulding EH, Tecott LH, Basbaum AI (2011) Behavioral indices of ongoing pain are largely unchanged in male mice with tissue or nerve injury-induced mechanical hypersensitivity. Pain 152: 990–1000.
51. Hargreaves K, Dubner,R, Brown F, Flores C, Joris J (1988) Basic Section - A new and sensitive method for measuring thermal nociception in cutaneous hyperalgesia. Pain 32, 77–88.
52. Chin J, Kadhim S, Garcia B, Kim YS, Karlik S (1991) Magnetic resonance imaging for detecting and treatment monitoring of orthotopic murine bladder tumor implants. J Urology 145: 1297–1301.
53. Suzuki T, Tsuji M, Mori T, Misawa M, Endoh T, et al. (1996) Effect of the highly selective and nonpeptide delta opioid receptor agonist TAN-67 on the morphine-induced place preference in mice. J Pharmacol Exp Ther 279: 177–185.
54. Dashti-Rahmatababi MH, Hejazian SH, Morshedi A, Rafati A (2007) The analgesic effect of Carum copticum extract and morphine on phasic pain in mice. J Ethnopharmacol 109: 226–228.
55. Stevenson GW, Bilsky EJ, Negus SS (2006) Targeting pain-suppressed behaviours in preclinical assays of pain and analgesia: Effects of morphine on acetic acid-suppressed feeding in C57BL/6J mice. J Pain 7: 408–416.
56. Cesarovic N, Arras M, Jirkof P (2014) Impact of inhalation anaesthesia, surgery and analgesic treatment on home cage behaviour in laboratory mice. Appl Anim Behav Sci.
57. Hasegawa H, Saiki I (2002) Psychosocial stress augments tumor development through beta-adrenergic activation in mice. Jpn J Cancer Res 93: 729–735.
58. Betourne A, Familiades J, Lacassagne L, Halley H, Cazales M, et al. (2008) Decreased motivational properties of morphine in mouse models of cancerous-

or inflammatory-chronic pain: implication of supraspinal neuropeptide FF2 receptors. Neuroscience 157: 12–21.
59. Matsumiya LC, Sorge RE, Sotocinal SG, Tabaka JM, Wieskopf JS, et al. (2012) Using the Mouse Grimace Scale to reevaluate the efficacy of postoperative analgesics in laboratory mice. J Am Assoc Lab Anim 51: 42–49.
60. Sasamura T, Nakamura S, Iida Y, Fujii H, Murata J, et al. (2002) Morphine analgesia suppresses tumor growth and metastasis in a mouse model of cancer pain produced by orthotopic tumor inoculation. Eur J Pharmacol 441: 185–191.
61. Liles JH, Flecknell PA (1993) The effects of surgical stimulus on the rat and the influence of analgesic treatment. Brit Vet J 149: 515–525.
62. Liles JH, Flecknell PA (1993) The influence of buprenorphine or bupivacaine on the post-operative effects of laparotomy and bile-duct ligation in rats. Lab Anim 27: 374–380.
63. Hayes JH, Flecknell PA (1999) A comparison of pre- and post-surgical administration of bupivacaine or buprenorphine following laparotomy in the rat. Lab Anim 33: 16–23.
64. Hayes KE, Raucci JA, Jr., Gades NM, Toth LA (2000) An evaluation of analgesic regimens for abdominal surgery in mice. Contemp Top Lab Anim 39: 18–23.
65. Roughan JV, Flecknell PA (2000) Effects of surgery and analgesic administration on spontaneous behaviour in singly housed rats. Res Vet Sci 69: 283–288.
66. Roughan JV, Flecknell RA (2004) Behaviour-based assessment of the duration of laparotomy-induced abdominal pain and the analgesic effects of carprofen and buprenorphine in rats. Behav Pharmacol 15: 461–472.
67. Craft RM, Henley SR, Haaseth RC, Hruby VJ, Porreca F (1995) Opioid antinociception in a rat model of visceral pain: systemic versus local drug administration. J Pharmacol Exp Ther 275: 1535–1542.
68. Nagahata S, Harano N, Ono K, Seta Y, Shiiba S, et al. (2007) A rat model for cancer pain in the trigemina nerve area. Eur J Pain 11: 69–69.
69. Dimitrijevic M, Laban O, Djuric VJ, Stanojevic S, Miletic T, et al. (2001) Behavior and Severity of Adjuvant Arthritis in Four Rat Strains. Brain Behav Immun 15: 255–265.
70. Kalueff AV, Tuohimaa P (2004) Grooming analysis algorithm for neurobehavioural stress research. Brain Res Protoc 13: 151–158.
71. Roughan JV, Flecknell PA, Davies BR (2004) Behavioural assessment of the effects of tumour growth in rats and the influence of the analgesics carprofen and meloxicam. Lab Anim 38: 286–296.
72. Mogil JS (2006) Sex, gender and pain. In: Cervero F, Jensen TS, editors. Handbook of Clinical Neurology. Amsterdam: Elsevier. 325–341.
73. Mogil JS (2012) Sex differences in pain and pain inhibition: multiple explanations of a controversial phenomenon. Nat Rev Neurosci 13: 859–866.
74. Sorge RE, LaCroix-Fralish ML, Tuttle AH, Sotocinal SG, Austin J-S, et al. (2011) Spinal cord Toll-like receptor 4 mediates inflammatory and neuropathic hypersensitivity in male but not female mice. J Neurosci 31: 15450–15454.
75. Mogil JS, Chesler EJ, Wilson SG, Juraska JM, Sternberg WF (2000) Sex differences in thermal nociception and morphine antinociception in rodents depend on genotype. Neurosci Biobehav R 24: 375–389.
76. Mogil JS, Wilson SG, Bon K, Lee SE, Kyungsoon C, et al. (1999) Heritaility of nociception I: Responses of 11 inbred mouse strains on 12 measures of nociception. Pain 80: 67–82.
77. Leach MC, Klaus K, Miller AL, Scotto di Perrotolo M, Sotocinal SG, et al. (2012) The assessment of post-vasectomy pain in mice using behaviour and the Mouse Grimace Scale. PLoS ONE [Electronic Resource] 7: e35656.
78. Langford DJ, Bailey AL, Chanda ML, Clarke SE, Drummond TE, et al. (2010) Coding of facial expressions of pain in the laboratory mouse. Nat Methods 7: 447–449.
79. Kilkenny C, Browne WJ, Cuthill IC, Emerson M, Altman DG (2010) Improving bioscience research reporting: The ARRIVE guidelines for reporting animal research. J Pharmacol Pharmacother 1: 94–99.

17

Practitioner Perspectives on Strategies to Promote Longer-Term Benefits of Acupuncture or Counselling for Depression: A Qualitative Study

Hugh MacPherson[1]*, Liz Newbronner[1,2], Ruth Chamberlain[2], Stewart J. Richmond[1], Harriet Lansdown[1], Sara Perren[1], Ann Hopton[1], Karen Spilsbury[1]

1 Department of Health Sciences, University of York, York, United Kingdom, **2** Firefly Research & Evaluation, North Yorkshire, United Kingdom

Abstract

Background: Non-pharmacological interventions for depression may help patients manage their condition. Evidence from a recent large-scale trial (ACUDep) suggests that acupuncture and counselling can provide longer-term benefits for many patients with depression. This paper describes the strategies practitioners reported using to promote longer-term benefits for their patients.

Methods: A qualitative sub-study of practitioners (acupuncturists and counsellors) embedded in a randomised controlled trial. Using topic guides, data was collected from telephone interviews and a focus group, altogether involving 19 counsellors and 17 acupuncturists. Data were audio recorded, transcribed verbatim and analysed using thematic content analysis.

Results: For longer-term impact, both acupuncturists and counsellors encouraged insight into root causes of depression on an individual basis and saw small incremental changes as precursors to sustained benefit. Acupuncturists stressed the importance of addressing concurrent physical symptoms, for example helping patients relax or sleep better in order to be more receptive to change, and highlighted the importance of Chinese medicine theory-based lifestyle change for lasting benefit. Counsellors more often highlighted the importance of the therapeutic relationship, emphasising the need for careful "pacing" such that the process and tools employed were tailored and timed for each individual, depending on the "readiness" to change. Our data is limited to acupuncture practitioners using the principles of traditional Chinese medicine, and counsellors using a humanistic, non-directive and person-centred approach.

Conclusions: Long-term change appears to be an important focus within the practices of both acupuncturists and counsellors. To achieve this, practitioners stressed the need for an individualised approach with a focus on root causes.

Editor: Fan Qu, Women's Hospital, School of Medicine, Zhejiang University, China

Funding: This research is supported by the National Institute for Health Research (NIHR) under Programme Grants for Applied Research (Grant No. RP-PG-0707-10186). The views expressed in this presentation are those of the author(s) and not necessarily those of the NHS, the NIHR or the Department of Health. The funders had no role in study design, data collection and analysis, decision to publish, or preparation of the manuscript.

Competing Interests: Liz Newbronner and Ruth Chamberlain worked for Firefly Research & Evaluation and were commissioned by the Department of Health Sciences, University of York, to conduct the interviews and work with the authors to analyse the data and prepare this manuscript. This does not alter the authors' adherence to PLOS ONE policies on sharing data and materials.

* Email: hugh.macpherson@york.ac.uk

Background

Depression is a common illness in primary care. Some of the optimism regarding the potential of selective serotonin re-uptake inhibitors (SSRIs) as a treatment for depression has faded in the light of concerns about effectiveness and safety. [1] A recent meta-analysis has concluded that antidepressants have only a modest advantage over placebo, with the magnitude of benefit increasing with severity of depression. [2] There is an ongoing interest, especially among patients, in the potential of non-pharmacological treatments for depression, with the hope that they might avoid some of the concerns about antidepressants regarding safety and dependency. [3] Furthermore, for many patients, depression is a chronic and recurring illness, and non-pharmacological treatments that seek to improve longer-term outcomes are potentially of interest.

Evidence from a recent large-scale trial (ACUDep) [4] has suggested that acupuncture and counselling can provide longer-term benefits for many patients with on-going depression in primary care. The ACUDep trial recruited 755 patients with depression via 27 participating primary care practices; 302 were randomised to up to 12 acupuncture sessions; 302 to up to 12 counselling sessions; and 151 to usual care alone. The counselling was delivered within a recognised, manualised competency framework developed by Roth et al. at the University College of London's Centre for Outcomes Research and Effectiveness. [5] The acupuncture diagnosis and treatment, including selection of points, was based on the principles of traditional Chinese medicine, the details of which are reported elsewhere. [6]

Both acupuncture and counselling were found to be effective in reducing the symptoms of depression when compared to usual care, and these differences were significant at the 3 and 6 month time points, as well as when averaged over the 12 month period. [4][7] The trial focused on the effectiveness and cost effectiveness of the interventions. However, we were keen to understand the experiences of those providing treatments (acupuncture or counselling) within the trial, and in particular the aspects of these interventions that practitioners perceived to be associated with their longer-term benefit. In doing so, these insights will help understanding of the interventions and help inform both clinical practice and any future research design.

Underreported within randomised controlled trials are qualitative analyses of strategies employed by acupuncturists and counsellors within treatment for depression that are intended to promote longer-term change. In one qualitative study, interviews with patients receiving counselling in routine practice were used to identify the key characteristics of the intervention that were experienced as beneficial in the longer term. [8] In the authors' interpretation, a key component was the client's active engagement during and between counselling sessions. In turn this enabled a change to take place in the way they conducted their lives and relationships. We are unaware of any published qualitative studies of the processes of care associated with long-term change in the case of acupuncture for depression.

This qualitative study, embedded within a clinical trial, was designed to explore the perceptions and experiences of counsellors and acupuncturists who provided the treatment interventions within the trial. The aim was to understand better the key aspects of their work and their perceptions of the 'active ingredients' of counselling or acupuncture that were intended to promote longer-term benefits for the patients and may help in our understanding of the trial results. The study also provided an opportunity to identify important issues relating to professional practice and future policy, which are not reported here, including support needs and working arrangements; the acceptability and feasibility of different treatment options; the implications for the provision of acupuncture or humanistic counselling for treating depression within primary care settings; and related commissioning issues.

Methods

Recruitment of participants

To provide treatments for trial participants, 41 counsellors and 23 acupuncturists were recruited from across the regions of Yorkshire and the North East of England. Altogether these practitioners treated 497 (out of 604) patients participating in the intervention arms of the ACUDep trial. After the end of the trial's treatment phase, acupuncturists and counsellors who had consulted with at least two patients in the trial were invited to take part in the qualitative sub-study. They were sent an information sheet and consent form and asked to indicate whether they would prefer to be involved in a one-to-one telephone interview or a focus group. The aim was to recruit up to 30 counsellors and acupuncturists (approximately 15 in each group). Ethical approval was obtained from the York NHS Research Ethics Committee (REC ref: 09/H1311/75), which included approval for procedures that required written consent from all participants.

Interview and focus group data collection

The topic guides for the interviews and focus group were developed by the ACUDep research team to address the main research question of practitioner strategies intended to promote longer-term benefits for patients – a key finding of the trial results. The initial ideas were developed into topic guides for the interviews, one for each of the practitioner groups, and one for the focus group discussion which comprised both acupuncturists and counsellors. Along with questions, the topic guides also included prompts.These were then refined further at face-to-face meetings, such that the guides covered the practitioner's professional background and experience of working with depression, their approach to treating depression, their perceptions of working within the trial, and their thoughts on the implications for policy and professional practice. These issues were considered important for interpretation of the qualitative data.

All participants provided written consent. Those who agreed to take part in a telephone interview were contacted (either by telephone or email) to arrange a convenient time for the one-to-one interview. Arrangements were confirmed by email and the topic guide to be used in the interview was attached. Only small numbers of practitioners expressed a preference for a focus group discussion and so only one group discussion was held. Many issues covered in the group discussion were similar to those expressed in the individual interviews. However, the group discussion provided an opportunity for therapists to explore together any differences and similarities in their perceptions and experiences. This added to the richness of the data. The interviews and focus group were conducted by two experienced health services researchers from the research team who were not involved in the conduct of the trial itself (LN and RC). The interviews commonly lasted around 45 minutes (range 40 to 90) and the focus group 90 minutes. They were all audio-recorded (with participants' permission) and transcribed verbatim.

Data analysis

The transcripts were analysed thematically. [9] The main areas of inquiry covered in the topic guides were used for a framework approach to thematic content analysis, which involved analysing the data across the two groups of practitioners contributing to the study. [10] The framework was created in an Excel spreadsheet and coded and populated with data from the transcripts by the two researchers who had conducted the interviews (LN and RC). An inductive process was used to identify themes, drawing on shared experiences or points of difference identified from the data. As this study was intended to broaden our understanding of practice in relation to the treatment of patients with depression, the analysis also sought to draw out findings which might inform the practice of acupuncturists and counsellors.

Results

Practitioner characteristics

Forty-one therapists consented to be involved in the study but five therapists later withdrew or didn't respond when the fieldwork was being set up. The sub-study included individual telephone interviews with15 counsellors and13 acupuncturists (n = 28) and one focus group with 4 counsellors and 4 acupuncturists (n = 8) (Table 1). The sample for the qualitative sub-study included over half (56%) of the total number of therapists involved in the main trial.

The 17 participating acupuncturists were registered members of the British Acupuncture Council with at least three years' post-qualification experience and practising with the theoretical

Table 1. Breakdown of study participants.

	Number involved in main trial	Number involved in one-to-one interviews	Number involved in the focus group	Total number participating
Counsellors	41	15	4	19
Acupuncturists	23	13	4	17
Total	64	28	8	36

approach of traditional Chinese medicine. [6] The acupuncturists were predominantly male (39% were female), with an average duration of practice of 12 years. In the trial they treated on average 9 patients, who attended on average for 10 sessions. The 19 counsellors were members of the British Association for Counselling and Psychotherapy, who were accredited or were eligible for accreditation having completed 400 supervised hours post-qualification, and provided clients a humanistic style of counselling based on competences developed for Skills for Health. [11] They were predominantly female practitioners (79%), with an average duration of practice of 7 years. In the trial they treated on average 7 patients, who attended on average for 9 sessions.

Trial patient characteristics

Practitioners were treating patients in the trial who had ongoing depression for at least 3 months and a score of 20 or more on the Beck Depression Inventory (BDI-II), with 38% having depression categorised as "moderate" and 62% "severe". [4] The mean age was 44 years and 73% were female. They were (on average) 25 years old when they experienced their first episode of depression. In terms of prescribed medication, 69% were on anti-depressants and 48% were on analgesics.

Overview of the findings from thematic analysis

A cluster of eight themes emerged from the framework analysis. Almost all of the acupuncturists and counsellors stressed the importance they attached to promoting longer-term benefits. To achieve this, practitioners commonly reported on the need to focus on the root causes, to address treatment for each individual patient, and to value small incremental changes from one session to the next as precursors to sustained benefit over the longer term. Acupuncturists more commonly reported on the need to address concurrent physical symptoms, for example helping patients relax or sleep better in order to be more receptive to change. Most also highlighted the importance of Chinese medicine theory-based lifestyle change as an approach to promoting more lasting benefit. Counsellors more often highlighted the importance of the therapeutic relationship, emphasising the need for careful "pacing" such that the process and tools employed were tailored and timed for each individual, depending on the "readiness" to change. These findings are presented in more detail below.

Importance of a long-term focus

Long-term change appears to be an important focus within the practices of both acupuncturists and counsellors. Almost all of the practitioners mentioned the long-term perspective as inherent to the way they worked.

> *with something like depression, longer term for me, longer term approach is very fundamental.*(acupuncturist1)

For acupuncturists, this perspective was drawn from the theoretical approach of traditional Chinese medicine, in which long-term change needed to be facilitated by lifestyle changes related to acupuncture theory. For counsellors it was drawn from the humanistic approach, which many contrasted with what was perceived as the "quick fix" of cognitive behavioural therapy (CBT).

> *I would like to think that the whole approach is based on longer term change, in terms of the client learning ways of coping. Not just with the present crisis, whatever it might be, but hopefully that they would take something from it that they could apply in the future.*(counsellor1)

When comparing acupuncturists and counsellors, the reported long-term focus involved some differences in approach, as described above, as well as some similarities, especially with regard to encouraging insight into root causes on an individual basis and seeking small incremental changes as important precursors of overall benefit.

Identifying root causes

The commitment to identifying and addressing the root causes of depression within the treatment process was a commonly expressed factor among both acupuncturists and counsellors. Acupuncturists commonly used the theoretical concept of "root" (ben) and "branch" (biao).

> *Within Chinese Medicine we talk about treating the root and the branch. And there is merit in treating both.*(acupuncturist2)
>
> *Looking for underlying causes. Obviously there's some symptomatic stuff, but always looking at the root causes and using that as where I would start to work out my treatment principles.*(acupuncturist3)

The counsellors were more interested in "going deeper" and "further back (in time)" with their clients as a way of getting to the root causes.

> *From my experience generally, you've got to get to the root causes of depression, so it's much deeper than a CBT approach, so I think if people don't do that when clients present depression, then perhaps they are failing the clients at some level.*(counsellor2)
>
> *I suppose for me the long term change generally stems from a clear understanding of just what's been at the root of it all.*(counsellor3)

The implications of this approach, as reported by several practitioners, are that unless the underlying causes are addressed, then it is likely that there will not be the sustained long-term change that is desired.

Individualisation

When practised within the theoretical framework of traditional Chinese medicine, acupuncture treatment has been customised to the individual, such that treatment varies not only between patients but also, for the same patient, it varies over time. Likewise for the counsellors in the trial, all of whom were committed to working within the humanistic tradition, a person-centred approach was provided.

> *Everybody's different, so whenever a patient comes in, obviously, you take their full medical history. And quite often there will be other key characteristics, so not everybody gets the same points diagnosis, because of the different underlying features of their condition.*(acupuncturist4)
> *That the reason for depression for individuals and how it's processed is unique and therefore the process focuses on how the client experiences it. I also think it's useful to bear in mind the possible causes and theories to be shared with the client.*(counsellor4)

Valuing incremental change

Practitioners reported a certain amount of caution about expecting sudden or cathartic changes in their patients. More common was a sense that positive benefit required a series of small incremental changes that when combined with self-help approaches would hopefully build a more sustained improvement.

> *Well long term change can even come about from even small changes, really. If somebody can just sleep all night, it's surprising.*(acupuncturist5)
> *I think to try almost to help people take responsibility and realise that there maybe is something that they can do. I think sometimes people get trapped in feeling depressed and feeling unable to do anything. So almost helping empower them to find changes that they can start to make, to make those improvements for themselves, which over time build up and help them move forward.*(counsellor5)

Addressing concurrent physical symptoms

Acupuncturists generally stressed the importance of addressing concurrent physical symptoms, for example helping patients relax or sleep better in order to be more receptive to change.

> *What I find really interesting about working on the trial is that a lot of time people came with depression but in reality there was a host of other signs and symptoms that they were not happy in their life. Just kind of bowel, musculoskeletal, anything. So when they got a sense that I was treating them as a whole person, rather than just treating the depression........ When I'd sorted out their back, their stomach, ulcers, bad knees, you know, suddenly their depression got better. To me, that's how Traditional Chinese Medicine should be – it works with everything. Rather than, you know, like depression as a standalone thing.*(acupuncturist2)

By contrast, the counsellors were less focused on the physical symptoms, and worked more on the assumption that by treating the underlying causes of depression there should be a knock-on effect in terms of reducing physical symptoms.

> *I'm not particularly interested in just treating symptoms, but what I'm usually interested in and what people are usually asking for is that they want to understand why they're feeling the way that they are. If you can deal with that issue, then it should help them to rid themselves of the symptoms really.*(counsellor6)

Lifestyle changes

Almost all of the acupuncturists highlighted the importance of giving advice about lifestyle change that was relevant to the Chinese medicine perspective.

> *Yeah, it's overall sort of aimed at the long-term and I think people, you know, if they get further along with the acupuncture, they realise that it's all to do with lifestyle change as well and that those things are going to be the ones that bring them lasting benefit. Because often people start to feel better after a few treatments and then when they build in the lifestyle thing, when they actually start to think, oh, this acupuncture seems to be working for me, maybe I'll follow some of the advice as well.* (acupuncturist6)

Those acupuncturists who reported on the role of lifestyle change tended to stress the importance of tailoring the advice to the patient, both in terms of content related to acupuncture theory (e.g. diet, relaxation, exercise, etc) as well as likely acceptability.

The counsellors worked within a trial protocol that had a strong emphasis on working within the humanistic tradition, which included being non-directive. [11] The protocol therefore limited the extent that they could offer lifestyle advice within the trial. Some counsellors, who typically worked more eclectically elsewhere, said they might normally include lifestyle advice, especially when working with people with addictions.

Therapeutic relationship

Counsellors consistently stressed the importance of the therapeutic relationship.

> *I tend to think that lasting change requires a greater degree of insight [than CBT]. But I think the change often comes – I suppose this is what puts me very squarely in the humanistic camp, the existential camp, I think it's often the relationship itself – it's actually having a new experience of a relationship for some people can be transformative.*(counsellor3)
> *But the essence of my approach is the relationship and building good levels of rapport and trust and helping the client to feel okay with you. So it's an okay space at the start and if that forms well, that's a springboard, hopefully, for sort of therapeutic practice and change for people.*(counsellor2)

However for some acupuncturists, this was also reported as a component of the treatment process that helped engender longer-term gains.

And it's kind of like a trust relationship – if they believe in the acupuncture, they believe in what you're telling them. And that kind of gives them the impetus to carry on in the longer term.(acupuncturist6)

Careful "pacing" based on "readiness to change"

Many of the counsellors emphasised the need for careful "pacing" such that the process and tools employed were tailored and timed for each individual, depending on the "readiness" to change.

And what I'm very aware of in counselling is that people will come to therapy at different stages of readiness to change. And it's very difficult to measure how useful it's been. So for example, with one client I can think of in the trial, I think he would have – I think it was probably a first experience for him, from being listened to and from being taken seriously and I think that was huge. He was very stuck. In terms of how much that was going to affect outcomes, in terms of was he going to make the necessary changes, he might have been able to begin to identify, or briefly identify, what it was in his life that was making him depressed – in terms of outcomes he wasn't at the stage where he was going to make any massive changes. But I think just having that experience, that first experience. That kind of thing is so hard to measure, isn't it?(counsellor6)

I tend to go with the speed of the client. However, if I can – my personal approach would be to help them in as short a sessions as possible to get them to feel better. However, I'm very careful to work with their speed. So am I short or long term.(counsellor7)

A number of acupuncturists identified issues related to timing, expressing the point that as patients improve, ideally appointments should be spread out towards the end of the course of treatment and beyond, as a way of sustaining benefit over the longer term.

In summary, the themes capture both similarities and differences in approaches between acupuncture and counselling, with most practitioners of both interventions having a shared sense of the prerequisites for sustained long-term benefit. The impression formed from the interviews is that the various approaches do not operate in isolation. Although the emphasis may vary, the themes appear to be integrated into a coherent combination that uniquely informs the practice of each practitioner.

Generalisability issues

With regard to the extent that these findings are transferable to other settings, the majority of counsellors said that the severity of the depression amongst trial patients was not markedly dissimilar to the people they routinely saw. By contrast, the acupuncturists were generally less used to dealing with patients with moderate to severe depression, and many said that they less commonly saw patients who consulted primarily because of a diagnosis of depression. Several of the therapists reported that the trial patients had a different attitude towards treatment compared to their private patients, particularly a more limited knowledge of the therapeutic intervention and a lower level of motivation to help themselves. Therapists also noted that there were a greater proportion of patients in lower income brackets, with more long-standing depression, or with unmanaged drug/alcohol addictions.

Discussion

Principal findings

Both acupuncturists and counsellors generally delivered treatments with an eye to encouraging longer-term change with the intention that, ideally, any putative benefit would be sustained well beyond the 12 sessions that were provided within the trial. While both types of practitioners reported on the need to address the root causes, the approach differed. For the acupuncturists there was a focus drawn from Chinese medicine theory on treating the root cause (the *ben*) as well as the manifesting symptoms (the *biao*) with the precise details of the intervention customised to their patients at an individual level. Meanwhile the approach of the counsellors was to get below the surface of the clients' problems and to "go deeper" and "further back (in time)" as a way of getting a handle on the root cause and, as with the acupuncturists, this required an individualised approach.

There were further differences in approach to facilitating more sustained benefits. Acupuncturists were more focussed on physical symptoms, on whether these could be resolved by acupuncture in order to speed up the improvements in the symptoms of depression, and on providing lifestyle advice linked to the Chinese medicine diagnosis. Meanwhile counsellors were more explicit on the importance of a strong therapeutic relationship accompanied by a careful consideration of what might be a manageable pace of change.

Strengths and limitations

The sub-study is nested within the largest trial to date of acupuncture or counselling for depression, and provides unique access to clusters of practitioners who have reported here on the treatments that they provided. The patient group is clearly defined, all with "moderate" to "severe" depression as categorised by the Beck Depression Inventory (BDI-II). The methods used, involving interviews, verbatim transcripts, and thematic analysis, are consistent with many of the markers of quality in qualitative research. [12] We have helped establish the credibility and dependability of the results through involving an independent research team (LN and RC) to help conduct the study, by arranging meetings of stakeholders to review the research questions and the methods used, and by discussing the emerging themes and refining these through debate to agreement. A substantive report emerged from this process, from which a component is reported here. With regard to the transferability of the results, we have provided details of the practitioners as well as the patients who were the focus of our sub-study, such that readers can draw conclusions regarding relevance for other areas. In terms of limitations, our data is limited to patients receiving acupuncture as practised by those using the theories of traditional Chinese medicine and to clients receiving counselling as provided in the humanistic and non-directive and person-centred style.

Relationship to the wider literature

There is limited evidence in the literature for longer-term benefits associated with acupuncture for depression. [13] In a systematic review of RCTs, counselling for depression has been reported to be no better than GP care in the long term [14], though in a review of pre-post comparisons of client outcomes, benefits have been reported to last a year or more. [15] The trial, within which this sub-study was nested, provided some further evidence on longer-term effects beyond the period of treatment. [4] Within the wider literature there is a dearth of evidence on the acupuncture treatment factors that might be associated with longer-term change in the symptoms of depression. The findings from a small study involving interviews with six practitioners in a trial of acupuncture for back pain found that these acupuncturists had a goal of a positive long-term outcome, and developed a therapeutic partnership to support the active engagement of patients in their own recovery. [16] Consistent with many of the findings we report here, the authors reported that the key elements were: establishing rapport, using an interactive diagnostic process, matching treatment to the patient, and using explanatory models from Chinese medicine to aid a shared understanding and motivate lifestyle changes to reinforce the potential recovery.

In the counselling literature, a qualitative study reported on the long-term effects of counselling, with data drawn from 15 clients who had received counselling from between one and three years previously. [8] The authors' interpretation of the client interview data led them to describe a model of the change process and mechanisms that were perceived as essential to produce lasting benefit. They identified as key elements of the counselling process the active engagement of the client during and between sessions, and the acquisition of a "box of skills" to be built on further after the counselling was finished. Unlike in the current study, in which all clients of counsellors received humanistic counselling, the authors did not identify the counselling approach provided. Another difference between this study and ours, is that all patients in our study had been diagnosed with depression.

Implications for clinical practice and research

One implication for clinical practice is that, while both acupuncture and counselling for depression appear to be associated with longer-term benefits, the interventions seem to work in different ways. Further research is needed from the perspective of patients and clients on their experiences of treatment from these two modalities. To assist referral, a clearer understanding is needed of which type of person with depression would benefit from acupuncture and which from counselling. While taking into account patient preference, such a typology would provide referring clinicians with valuable guidance on suitability for referral.

Another question is in regard to the nature of depression, and the extent to which physical symptoms are also present. Evidence suggests that 69% of people experiencing depression in primary care initially present with physical symptoms [17] and 50% of people with depression are also in pain. [18] Our study has found that acupuncturists are interested in the physical symptoms that may accompany depression, and will routinely address these symptoms as part of the treatment.

One can speculate that this focus on physical symptoms may in part explain why the acupuncturists in this trial, who reported being less experienced in treating moderate to severe depression, nevertheless delivered just as good outcomes as the counsellors, who encountered this level of depression more commonly in routine practice. Further research is needed into the patient perspective on the treatment of depression with co-morbidities, and specifically the value they place on the comorbid symptoms being addressed concurrently.

Our research raises some important questions about the clinical practice of acupuncturists and counsellors when treating a population with depression when combined with unmanaged drug and alcohol addictions. Further research might be useful to explore appropriate strategies, which might be about ensuring the availability of options, including the involvement of other agencies, and practical support.

Conclusions

Long-term change appears to be an important focus within the practices of both acupuncturists and counsellors. Practitioners of both interventions generally stressed that, for longer-term benefit, there needs to be an individualised approach with a focus on root causes. Acupuncturists more often emphasised the importance of addressing concurrent physical symptoms and highlighted the importance of relevant lifestyle change. Counsellors commonly stressed the importance of the therapeutic relationship and emphasised the need for appropriate "pacing" such that the timing of the counselling process is geared to the "readiness" to change.

Supporting Information

Text S1 Consolidated criteria for reporting qualitative studies (COREQ): 32-item checklist.
(DOCX)

Acknowledgments

We acknowledge with appreciation the contributions of the practitioners who were interviewed or who attended the focus group, Janet Eldred for providing support for the management of both the trial and the sub-study, and Anne Burton for undertaking the transcriptions. This research is supported by the National Institute for Health Research (NIHR) under Programme Grants for Applied Research (Grant No. RP-PG-0707-10186). The views expressed in this presentation are those of the author(s) and not necessarily those of the NHS, the NIHR or the Department of Health. The funders had no role in study design, data collection and analysis, decision to publish, or preparation of the manuscript.

Author Contributions

Conceived and designed the experiments: HM LN RC SR HL SP AH KS. Performed the experiments: LN RC. Analyzed the data: HM LN RC. Contributed reagents/materials/analysis tools: HM LN RC KS. Contributed to the writing of the manuscript: HM LN RC. Revision of the manuscript: HM LN RC SR HL SP AH KS.

References

1. Parker G (2009) Antidepressants on trial: how valid is the evidence? Br J Psychiatry: 1–3.
2. Kirsch I, Deacon BJ, Huedo-Medina TB, Scoboria A, Moore TJ, et al. (2008) Initial severity and antidepressant benefits: a meta-analysis of data submitted to the Food and Drug Administration. PLoS Med 5: e45.
3. Mind (2002) My Choice: A Survey. Available: http://www.mind.org.uk/News+policy+and+campaigns/Press+archive/Mind+launches+campaign+for+more+choice+of+mental+health+services+at+GP+level.htm. Accessed 13 January 2008.
4. MacPherson H, Richmond S, Bland M, Brealey S, Gabe R, et al. (2013) Acupuncture and Counselling for Depression in Primary Care: A Randomised Controlled Trial. PLoS Medicine 10: e1001518. doi:10.1371/journal.pmed.1001518.
5. Centre for Outcomes Research & Effectiveness (CORE) (n.d.) Humanistic Psychological Therapies Competences Framework. Available: http://www.ucl.ac.uk/clinical-psychology/CORE/humanistic_framework.htm#. Accessed 30 September 2013.
6. MacPherson H, Elliot B, Hopton A, Lansdown H, Richmond S (2013) Acupuncture for Depression: Patterns of Diagnosis and Treatment within a Randomised Controlled Trial. Evid Based Complement Alternat Med 2013: 286048. doi:10.1155/2013/286048.
7. MacPherson H, Richmond S, Bland J, Lansdown H, Hopton A, et al. (2012) Acupuncture, Counselling, and Usual care for Depression (ACUDep): study protocol for a randomized controlled trial. Trials 13: 209.
8. Perren S, Godfrey M, Rowland N (2009) The long-term effects of counselling: The process and mechanisms that contribute to ongoing change from a user perspective. Counselling and Psychotherapy Research 9: 241–249. doi:10.1080/14733140903150745.
9. Braun V, Clarke V (2006) Using thematic analysis in psychology. Qualitative Research in Psychology 3: 77–101.

10. Ritchie J, Lewis J (2003) Qualitative Research Practice: A Guide for Social Science Students and Researchers. London:Sage.
11. Roth A, Hill A, Pilling S (2009) The competences required to deliver effective Humanistic Psychological Therapies. London, UK: University College London.
12. Hannes K (2011) Chapter 4: Critical appraisal of qualitative research. Supplementary Guidance for Inclusion of Qualitative Research in Cochrane Systematic Reviews of Interventions. Cochrane Collaboration Qualitative Methods Group. Available: http://cqrmg.cochrane.org/supplemental-handbook-guidance. Accessed 31 March 2014.
13. Smith CA, Hay PP, MacPherson H (2010) Acupuncture for depression. Cochrane Database Syst Rev: CD004046.
14. Bower P, Knowles S, Coventry PA, Rowland N (2011) Counselling for mental health and psychosocial problems in primary care. Cochrane Database Syst Rev: CD001025.
15. Research on humanistic-experiential psychotherapies (2013) Bergin and Garfield's handbook of psychotherapy and behavior change. Hoboken, NJ: John Wiley & Sons. pp. 495–538.
16. MacPherson H, Thorpe L, Thomas KJ (2006) Beyond needling - therapeutic processes in acupuncture care: a qualitative study nested within a low-back pain trial. J Altern Complement Med 12: 873–880.
17. Simon GE, VonKorff M, Piccinelli M, Fullerton C, Ormel J (1999) An international study of the relation between somatic symptoms and depression. N Engl J Med 341: 1329–1335. doi:10.1056/NEJM199910283411801.
18. Katona C, Peveler R, Dowrick C, Wessely S, Feinmann C, et al. (2005) Pain symptoms in depression: definition and clinical significance. ClinMed 5(4): 390–395.

18

The Nijmegen Decision Tool for Chronic Low Back Pain. Development of a Clinical Decision Tool for Secondary or Tertiary Spine Care Specialists

Miranda L. van Hooff[1]*, Jan van Loon[2], Jacques van Limbeek[3], Marinus de Kleuver[2,4]

1 Sint Maartenskliniek, Department of Research, Nijmegen, The Netherlands, **2** Sint Maartenskliniek, Department of Orthopedics, Nijmegen, The Netherlands, **3** Achmea Health Insurance Company, Zeist, The Netherlands, **4** VU University Medical Center, Department of Orthopedics, Amsterdam, The Netherlands

Abstract

Background: In Western Europe, low back pain has the greatest burden of all diseases. When back pain persists, different medical specialists are involved and a lack of consensus exists among these specialists for medical decision-making in Chronic Low Back Pain (CLBP).

Objective: To develop a decision tool for secondary or tertiary spine care specialists to decide which patients with CLBP should be seen by a spine surgeon or by other non-surgical medical specialists.

Methods: A Delphi study was performed to identify indicators predicting the outcome of interventions. In the preparatory stage evidence from international guidelines and literature were summarized. Eligible studies were reviews and longitudinal studies. Inclusion criteria: surgical or non-surgical interventions and persistence of complaints, CLBP-patients aged 18–65 years, reported baseline measures of predictive indicators, and one or more reported outcomes had to assess functional status, quality of life, pain intensity, employment status or a composite score. Subsequently, a three-round Delphi procedure, to reach consensus on candidate indicators, was performed among a multidisciplinary panel of 29 CLBP-professionals (>five years CLBP-experience). The pre-set threshold for general agreement was ≥70%. The final indicator set was used to develop a clinical decision tool.

Results: A draft list with 53 candidate indicators (38 with conclusive evidence and 15 with inconclusive evidence) was included for the Delphi study. Consensus was reached to include 47 indicators. A first version of the decision tool was developed, consisting of a web-based screening questionnaire and a provisional decision algorithm.

Conclusions: This is the first clinical decision tool based on current scientific evidence and formal multidisciplinary consensus that helps referring the patient for consultation to a spine surgeon or a non-surgical spine care specialist. We expect that this tool considerably helps in clinical decision-making spine care, thereby improving efficient use of scarce sources and the outcomes of spinal interventions.

Editor: Dino Samartzis, University of Hong Kong, Hong Kong

Funding: The authors have no support or funding to report.

Competing Interests: At the time of this research project, Dr. Van Limbeek was Director of Research, Development and Education of Sint Maartenskliniek and was involved in the project as epidemiologist and statistician. He left Sint Maartenskliniek in 2012 and is currently affiliated with the Health Insurance Company Achmea, where he was appointed as manager research ad interim and medical advisor. He contributed to the work reported in this article during his time in the Sint Maartenskliniek (epidemiological guidance, methodology) and in the writing of the manuscript during his time at Achmea. There is no conflict of interest or any proprietary issue with Achmea health care insurance. The authors confirm that this does not alter their adherence to PLOS ONE policies on sharing data and materials.

* Email: m.vanhooff@maartenskliniek.nl

Introduction

In Western Europe, Low back pain (LBP) is considered to have the greatest burden of disease for society [1]. In this global burden of disease study LBP is ranked higher than for example cancer, heart disease, cerebrovascular disease, chronic obstructive pulmonary disease and asthma, osteoarthritis or diabetes. In the Netherlands, approximately 44% of the population experiences at least once an episode of LBP, with one in five reporting persistent back pain resulting in chronic low back pain (CLBP; LBP lasting for more than three months [2,3]) with substantial limitations in functional activities after one year [4,5]. As the prevalence of CLBP appears to be increasing [6], CLBP is not only a burden for the patient but the related healthcare costs and productivity due to absence of work have a high health and socioeconomic impact on western societies [7–9]. Not surprisingly, CLBP is among the most common complaints of patients visiting a medical specialist in secondary care, i.e. spine surgeons, physiatrists, rheumatologists, pain consultants. The high number of CLBP patients overwhelms these healthcare providers and a significant number of second opinions and re-interventions are evident. With the limited health care budgets and given the high prevalence of CLBP and its substantial socioeconomically impact, it is essential to use resources of healthcare providers efficiently and to triage CLBP patients adequately in order to make sure that these patients see the right care giver timely. However, as yet such a valid classification system or decision tool is lacking and secondary care medical specialists are failing to reliably identify which patients will benefit from which surgical or non-surgical intervention.

One challenge in the development of a decision tool is that the CLBP population is heterogeneous. Therefore, it is unlikely that one intervention benefits all [10]. A longstanding duration of complaints is the only one common defining feature. It makes CLBP a complex problem and in fact it is a symptom referring to the location of the problem rather than a specific diagnosis [11]. The term itself is non-diagnostic for an underlying pathology and lacks specificity. Many authors have emphasized the biospychosocial influences on the development CLBP and persistence of symptoms [12,13] and a broad multidimensional approach is widely recognised. However, the failure to differentiate between underlying causes is one of the reasons that various surgical and non-surgical interventions exist for the same problem [14]. Moreover, studies evaluating these interventions for CLBP have led to inconsistent results [3,15–19] and rarely show more than a small to moderate overall benefit [3,20,21].

It is suggested that several different CLBP patient profiles might be identified which are likely to benefit from different recommended interventions [1,18,19,22–25]. These profiles are based on indicators modifying the effects of interventions [26] and with that related to the outcomes [24]. The ultimate outcomes of spinal interventions are patients' improved quality of life, restored functional status and relieved pain [27]. However, due to methodological heterogeneity, the current evidence is inconclusive regarding predictive indicators for a successful treatment outcome. Even though it is recognized that CLBP 'without biological causes' has to be distinguished from other spinal disorders that respond reliably to surgery [25,28], a recently performed nationwide survey among Dutch spine surgeons showed that even in the group 'with presumed biological causes' a lack of consensus exists in surgical decision making [29]. To distinguish patient profiles several treatment outcome-based classifications for decision making exist. However, they are all developed and studied as a guide for non-surgical interventions applied in primary care [24]. As a challenge with probably the greatest potential for improving outcomes and efficiently guiding patients to the right secondary health care professional (e.g. spine surgeon, pain consultant, physiatrist, rheumatologist), it is recommended to develop a classification system to direct CLBP patients, presented in secondary or tertiary back care, to both surgical and non-surgical interventions, based on biomedical and psychosocial indicators [11,22–25,30,31].

Therefore, the purpose of this study is to develop a clinical decision tool for CLBP, based on evidence in international guidelines and literature, and expert panel consensus using indicators predicting a successful treatment outcome. The decision tool supports secondary or tertiary back care specialists to decide which patients should be considered for a surgical intervention and which patients for a non-surgical intervention and therefore, it aims to triage patients to the appropriate health care professional. The ultimate goal is to improve treatment outcomes and to reduce related costs for society.

Methods

This study aimed to identify indicators predicting the outcome of interventions and the persistence of CLBP complaints by two stages: a preparatory stage followed by a three-round Delphi study. The preparatory stage consisted of a literature review. As we expected inconclusive evidence in the literature, a formal consensus (Delphi) procedure among a heterogeneous panel of experts in the CLBP field was planned and performed. We used a Modified Delphi Technique in order to realise an optimal integration of research-based knowledge and the clinical experience of experts [32] on this topic. Having identified the predictive indicators, a clinical decision tool, including a screening questionnaire and a provisional decision algorithm, was compiled. In the flow diagram of Figure 1 the overall process of the development of the Nijmegen decision tool for CLBP is presented.

Preparatory stage: Evidence from literature

The indicator set from which a clinical decision tool can be constructed is based on evidence found in international guidelines and in the literature, as these guidelines are normative for evidence based daily practice. As a starting point, the clinical flag approach [33] for clinical decision-making in CLBP and the indicators as recommended in the guidelines [22,23,34], are used. We performed a literature review searching for indicators predicting outcome of invasive or non-invasive interventions and persistence of CLBP. Appropriate studies were traced using MedLine, EMBASE and the Cochrane Library. The most relevant used search terms were: 'back pain' [MesH], 'chronic', 'predict', 'prognosis' [MesH], 'persistent', 'treatment outcome' [MesH], 'rehabilitation' [MesH], 'surgery' [MesH]. The search was restricted to include systematic and narrative reviews, randomized controlled trials (RCT) and prospective cohort studies. Studies were included when 1) CLBP was the primary complaint; 2) published in the period 2000–2010; 3) involved either surgical interventions for CLBP or non-surgical interventions or persistence of CLBP complaints; 4) age between 18–65 years; 5) baseline measures of predictive indicators are reported, as the time of assessment may influence the prognostic value of treatment outcome [35,36]; 6) at least one of the reported outcome measures had to assess functional status, quality of life, pain intensity, employment status or a composite score. CLBP was defined as more than three months continual or recurrent episodes of LBP [2,3].

There were no language restrictions. Moreover, reference lists of included articles were scrutinized to identify articles not captured in the database search. When a systematic review was included, the original longitudinal studies (RCT or observational) of that systematic review were excluded from the current sample to avoid duplication or double use of the same data.

We used four international guidelines [22,23,31] and one national guideline [34]. The literature search revealed 33 relevant papers: eight systematic reviews [36–43], four narrative reviews [44–47], three randomized studies [48–50], and eighteen observational studies [51–68]. All potential predictive indicators were classified into five main domains: sociodemographic; pain; somatic; psychological; and functioning & quality of life. Of each paper, data of available evidence was extracted regarding the predictive values of measured baseline determinants (indicators). The evidence is weighed according to the Levels of Evidence as defined by the Oxford Centre for Evidence-Based Medicine [69]. Per indicator the evidence is categorized into four categories: 1) indicator with proven predictive value (PV; evidence found that the concerning indicator has predictive value), 2) indicator with

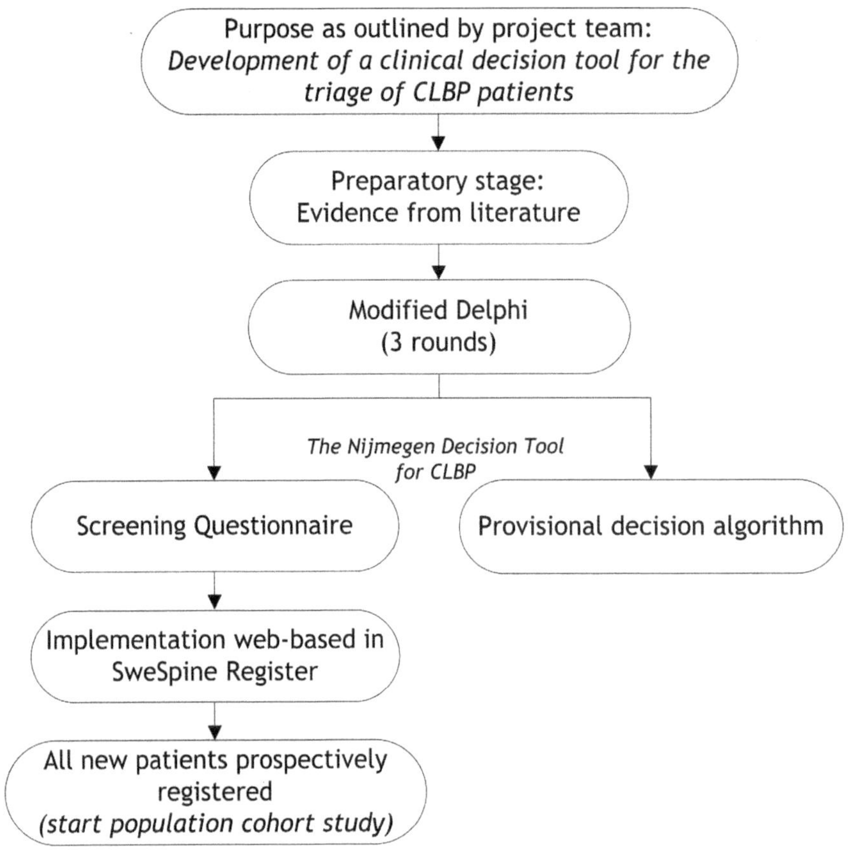

Figure 1. Flow diagram of the development of the Nijmegen Decision Tool for CLBP.

proven no predictive value (NP; evidence found that the concerning indicator has no predictive value), 3) indicator with inconclusive evidence (I; conflicting evidence found), and 4) indicator with no evidence found in literature (N). Subsequently, all indicators (PV, NP, and I) were selected and used for Phase 2 of this study (the Delphi Study). Indicators with non-predictive value and categorized NP were excluded from the sample as the evidence showed no predictive value for treatment outcome or for persistence of CLBP complaints. The included indicators are summarized in an evidence table, according to the design used in the related studies (data available in Table S1). Per indicator the evidence was summarized: the evidence is conclusive and of predictive value (C: PV) or the evidence is conclusive and of no predictive value (C: NP) or inconclusive evidence (I). These results are used in the Delphi study (Delphi-1 & 2).

Delphi Study

The Delphi technique is a commonly used method to develop clinical guidelines [70] and also used in healthcare indicator research [71]. The technique was originally developed in the 1950s by Dalkey and Helmer at the RAND Corporation as a method of eliciting and refining group judgements [72]. Delphi may be characterized as a systematic method for structuring a group communication process so that the process is effective in allowing a group of experts or 'expert panel', as a whole, to deal with a complex problem [73]. The method relies on three key features: 1) anonymous response to guarantee equality in experts opinions, 2) iteration and controlled feedback, and 3) statistical analysis of group responses [72]. The Delphi technique, as recently described [32,71], is a structured process that uses a recommended series of two or three rounds to gather expert opinions. When reaching consensus is difficult or consensus is unclear a physical panel meeting at the end is recommended, under the condition that the meeting should be well structured and should take place in favourable conditions (surrounding and environment) with a moderator (process leader), who is not one of the panellists, to contain the influence of dominant personalities (Modified Delphi Technique).

Project team. A project team was formed to conduct the process and the research and comprised a methodologist who is also a physician and who has a background in statistics (JvL), an orthopaedic spine surgeon (MdK) and a health scientist (MvH). The responsibilities of this project team were performing a review of clinical predictive indicators, weighing the evidence for each indicator, selecting a panel of experts, developing the questionnaires, organisation and conduct of email rounds and consensus meeting, analysing the responses, and compiling a draft version of the clinical decision tool.

Panellists. In the area of CLBP treatment different medical specialists are involved and knowledge gaps exist between different medical specialties [24]. Therefore, a heterogeneous group of experts was selected for the expert panel. Moreover, it is known that when exploring areas of uncertainty, a heterogeneous group is appropriate [70] and it is expected that heterogeneity in a decision-making group may lead to better performance [71]. Panellists were asked based on their willingness to participate, their intention to commit to the process, and their recognised knowledge of the topic. They were recruited in one hospital and were included in the panel when they met the following criteria: (1) professional background as a orthopaedic spine surgeon, anaesthesiologist & pain consultant, physiatrist, rheumatologist, psychologist, physical therapist, occupational therapist, psychomotor therapist, nurse practitioner; (2) CLBP care and cure is the main area of professional attention; (3) more than five years of clinical experience in the field; and (4) ability and willingness to respond to each email Delphi round within one week and to join the final Delphi consensus meeting.

Delphi procedure. The panellists were emailed explaining the purpose and the content of the study. To increase participation the panellists were asked to reply if they were willing to join and whether they intended to commit to the procedure. The whole procedure was performed in two months, April–May 2011. Two email Delphi rounds were planned to reach consensus. Consensus was defined as a 'general agreement of a substantial majority'. The threshold for general agreement was set at ≥70%. If an indicator reached a second time disagreement, the indicator is rejected. For the two email rounds participants were asked to respond and reply within one week. A third round, the final consensus meeting was performed to reach consensus about the included items and to construct a first draft clinical decision tool. During this meeting participants were allowed to discuss issues and exchange views supported by evidence, with the aim to resolve issues for indicators that had not passed the threshold for consensus. In each round the purpose and procedure of the current Delphi round and following Delphi rounds were explained.

Delphi-1. The initial draft list of indicators extracted from the literature review and arranged in a conceptual framework of domains was provided to the expert panel. They were asked to respond to three main sets of questions (Q). The Q1 set was based on international and national guidelines, which recommend an assessment of a minimal set of consistent prognostic indicators influencing the treatment outcome [22,23,31,74]. Compiled by the project team and supported by the literature review, this minimal set consisted of 32 indicators ('red' and 'yellow' flags, expectation of recovery, socio-economic status, sick leave, pain severity, prior episodes of LBP), for which agreement (YES or NO) was asked. The Q2 set was based on the results of the literature review and included 26 indicators with weighted evidence for which agreement for inclusion (YES or NO) was asked. Moreover, in Q3 the panellists were given the opportunity to suggest additional indicators for inclusion, based on scientific evidence and provided to the project team, and to write general comments. The items for which ≥70% agreement was reached were selected and included in the draft list for the final Consensus meeting (Delphi-3). The indicators for which consensus was not reached, were included in round 2 (Delphi-2).

Delphi-2. In the second round an anonymous feedback report with a summary of results of Delphi-1 was provided. In this summary an overview of results for each question and each indicator was given in count and percentages of agreement. Moreover, all suggested and newly formulated indicators, including the arguments and comments were presented. The Delphi-2 questionnaire contained both those indicators that did not reach the pre-set agreement level of ≥70% (Q1 and Q2; Delphi-1) and those that were newly formulated by the panellists (Q3; Delphi-1). In this round the panellists were requested to indicate with YES or NO which of the indicators of Q1 and Q2 absolutely needed to be included in the list? In Q3 a possibility was given to mention new indicators. The level of agreement was set at ≥70% among the panellists, i.e. these indicators were selected and included in the draft list for the following Consensus meeting (Delphi-3). A second time lack of consensus led to rejection of the concerning indicator.

Delphi-3 Consensus meeting. Before the meeting all panellists received a covering summary of results on both Delphi rounds which was similarly described and drafted as for the results of the first round. Moreover, a draft list was provided with indicators for which consensus (≥70%), no consensus (<70%) was reached, and the rejected indicators. During the meeting all indicators for which previously no consensus had been reached were reconsidered. Only if new arguments based on scientific or clinical evidence were provided, an attempt to reach a new consensus on that item was made. Moreover, the panellists were encouraged to consider alternative views when consensus could not be achieved [70]. The meeting had a formal character to ensure that all panellists had a chance to express their views, all indicators were considered, no discussion was allowed and only arguments could be provided, and the panellists made judgements individually. Consensus was reached by voting; raising hands. Only those indicators with ≥70% agreement were included in the final screening questionnaire, all others were rejected. A dedicated and independent process leader is a key element for a successful consensus meeting; this person facilitates the exchange of relevant information [70]. One of the project team members (JvL) is an experienced Delphi round facilitator, who was not one of the panellists, but who ensured that the process ran smoothly and that good-quality un-biased decisions were made. The project leader (MvH), not a member of the expert panel, assisted the process leader in process monitoring, ensured that all procedures ran according to the rules, counted the votes, compiled the minutes during the meeting and provided a full report after the meeting. The report included the followed procedures, the results of the voting rounds, the course of the discussions, the decisions made, and the final list of 'consensus indicators'. All panellists who joined the consensus meeting received a copy.

Development of the 'Nijmegen decision tool for CLBP'

The final list of 'consensus indicators' was used to compile a first version of the clinical decision tool. For the screening questionnaire existing international patient reported outcome measures (PROMs) were screened to identify whether the indicators are covered by these PROMs. The indicators were compared to existing questions used in the Swedish Spine Register (Swespine [www.4S.nu]). These questions were translated and screened for unambiguity and whether they measured the construct as intended by the indicator. The remaining indicators were converted to new questions. The screening questionnaire was built in the Dutch patient interface of Swespine. Based on the list of consensus indicators, international guidelines, and current practice a provisional decision algorithm was constructed.

Results

Preparatory stage: Evidence from literature

An initial draft list with 58 candidate indicators, categorized in five domains, and including the evidence was compiled. Table 1 shows the evidence summarized for all candidate indicators (the evidence and references per indicator are available in Table S1). For 38 (66%) candidate indicators conclusive evidence was found indicating a predictive value for treatment outcome or persistence of complaints (C: PV), 15 had inconclusive evidence for predicting outcome or persistence of pain complaints (I), and for five indicators conclusive evidence was found that the concerning indicator is of no predictive value (C: NP). These five indicators were removed from the initial draft list, leaving 53 candidate indicators and they were included in the Delphi study.

Table 1. Results Preparatory stage: Evidence from literature.

Domain	Category[1]	Study design[2]				Evidence[3]
		SR	*RCT*	*PC*	*NR*	
		n	n	n	n	
Sociodemographic	**Personal**					
	Age	4	-	8	4	I
	Gender	4	-	9	3	I
	Ethnicity	1	-	-	-	C: PV
	Body weight	3	-	1	-	I
	Marital status†	3	-	-	2	C: NP
	Health					
	Smoking	5	-	4	1	I
	Previous back surgery	1	-	2	-	C:PV
	Use of analgesics	1	-	1	1	I
	Social					
	Education	1	-	3	3	I
	Social status	1	-	-	1	I
	Functioning – leisure	1	-	1	-	I
	Social support	-	-	-	2	C: PV
	Work					
	Socio-economic status*	2	-	2	2	C: PV
	Work satisfaction	5	-	-	4	I
	Functioning – work	3	-	-	-	I
	Sick leave*	3	-	2	2	C: PV
	Compensation	3	-	3	-	I
	Litigation	-	-	-	1	C: PV
	Work ability	1	-	-	-	C: PV
	Work adjustment	1	-	-	-	C: PV
	Physical strenuousness	1	-	-	-	I
Pain	Duration	4	-	3	1	I
	Intensity*	5	1	11	3	C: PV
	Intensity – back	-	-	3	-	C: PV
	Intensity – leg	2	-	2	-	C: PV
	Interference daily activities	2	-	-	1	C: PV
	Frequency/preceding (prior) episodes*	1	-	1	2	I
Somatic	Diagnosis; co morbidities	1	-	2	1	C: PV
Physical & Biological	Bulging or protruded disc*	2	-	2	-	C: PV
	Loss of neurological function*	1	-	1	1	C: PV
	Red flags (n = 10)*#					C: PV
	Strength; endurance; mobility†	4	-	2	-	C: NP
	Central sensitisation†	1	-	-	-	C: NP
	Postural control; psychomotor speed†	1	-	-	-	C: NP
Psychologic	**Psychic affect**					
	Distress*	6	2	3	4	C: PV
	Anxiety*	3	2	2	4	C: PV
	Cognition					C: PV
	Catastrophizing*	5	3	7	3	C: PV
	Somatization*	4	-	1	1	C: PV
	Coping*	5	-	2	4	C: PV
	Intelligence†	1	-	-	-	C: NP
	Behaviour					

Table 1. Cont.

Domain	Category[1]	Study design[2]				Evidence[3]
		SR	*RCT*	*PC*	*NR*	
		n	n	n	n	
	Fear of movement/(re)Injury*	3	-	12	4	C: PV
	Expectations – work return*	1	-	3	2	C: PV
	Expectations – outcome/recovery*	2	-	1	2	C: PV
	Self-efficacy (incl. Readiness-to-change)	-	-	1	-	C: PV
	Pain avoidance & pain persistence	-	1	-	-	C: PV
Functioning & Quality of Life	Functioning in daily activities & walking	6	1	9	3	C: PV
	Health-related physical functioning	3	-	5	1	C: PV
	Health-related mental functioning	6	-	1	1	I
	General perceived health	1	-	2	1	C: PV

Initial draft list with indicators (n = 58) indicating a predictive value for treatment outcome or persistence of back pain, categorized in domains, including the number of studies found per study design and the resulting evidential value.
1. *Recommended in (inter-/) national guidelines;
#Pain started age <20 or >50 years, recent trauma, constant progressive pain, history of malignancies, prolonged use of corticosteroid use, HIV, recent unexplained weight loss, structural deformity, infectious disease (CBO 2010).
2. *SR* Systematic Review; *R* Randomized Clinical Trial; *PC* Prospective Cohort study; *NR* Narrative Review; *n* number of studies.
3. *I* Inconclusive evidence; *C* Conclusive evidence; *PV* Predictive Value; *NP* No Predictive value.
4. †Not included for phase 2 Delphi Study.

Delphi Study

Participants. A panel of 29 experts met the inclusion criteria and agreed to participate (orthopaedic spine surgeon [n = 7], anaesthesiologist & pain consultant [n = 3], physiatrist [n = 3], rheumatologist [n = 1], psychologist [n = 4], physical therapist [n = 7], occupational therapist [n = 1], psychomotor therapist [n = 1], nurse practitioner [n = 2]).

The response rate for the first Delphi round (Delphi-1) was 76% (n = 22) and for Delphi-2 69% (n = 20). The main reason for not responding in the first two rounds was due to absence from work and none of the approached panellists did not respond on both email rounds. All 29 panellists (100%) attended the final consensus meeting (Delphi-3).

Delphi-1. As shown in Figure 2, 48 indicators were selected in the first round based on consensus (≥70% agreement level). For five indicators consensus was not reached. Moreover, 26 indicators were newly formulated by the panel in the open end question (sociodemographic n = 9; pain n = 4; somatic n = 7; psychologic n = 3; functioning and quality of life n = 3) and these indicators were added to the Delphi-2 questionnaire. These 26 indicators consisted of:

A) six indicators mentioned in the Dutch guidelines for general practitioners: self-management of complaints, previous interventions, daily course of pain complaints, influence of rest, mobility and posture, previous episodes, and comorbidities (range and severity) [75]. The last two show overlap with previously identified indicators.
B) one indicator for inflammatory LBP (Calin criteria [76]).
C) ten newly formulated indicators with overlap with indicators of the initial draft list.
D) nine indicators with no predictive evidence and were rejected from the sample.

No further comments were made.

Delphi-2. As shown in Figure 2, 22 indicators were presented, including the 17 newly formulated and the five indicators for which no consensus was reached in Delphi-1. Of these, 14 reached the pre-set ≥70% agreement level for consensus. Five indicators were rejected as for the second time no consensus was reached. No new indicators were suggested and no further comments were made.

Delphi-3 Consensus meeting. All indicators on which consensus were reached in either Delphi-1 or 2 (62 indicators; 48+14) and those indicators no consensus was reached in Delphi-2 (3 indicators) were briefly discussed (Figure 2). After each indicator the panellists voted whether they still agreed or not. As shown in Table 2, at the meeting consensus was reached for 47 indicators (pre-set ≥70% agreement level), whereas eight indicators reached no consensus. These indicators were rejected, as well as ten indicators showing an overlap with the initial indicators.

Consensus was reached to re-formulate one indicator 'Body weight' into 'Body weight & BMI' and another indicator 'Pain-interference daily activities' switched domains from 'Pain' to the domain 'Functioning & Quality of Life'.

The remaining 47 indicators formed the backbone of the screenings questionnaire (36 with conclusive evidence for predictive value [77%] and 11 with inconclusive evidence; Table 2).

The 'Nijmegen decision tool for CLBP'

A first version of a clinical decision tool consisting of two parts was drafted by the project team: (1) A screening questionnaire, including all 47 indicators, and (2) a provisional decision algorithm.

1. The screening questionnaire. For the backbone of the screening questionnaire existing international patient reported outcome measures (PROMs) with well-established psychometric properties were screened to identify whether the 47 identified indicators were covered by these existing questionnaires (Table 3). Four of the 47 indicators are outcome indicators and adequately measured by the Oswestry Disability Index (ODI, version 2.1a) for

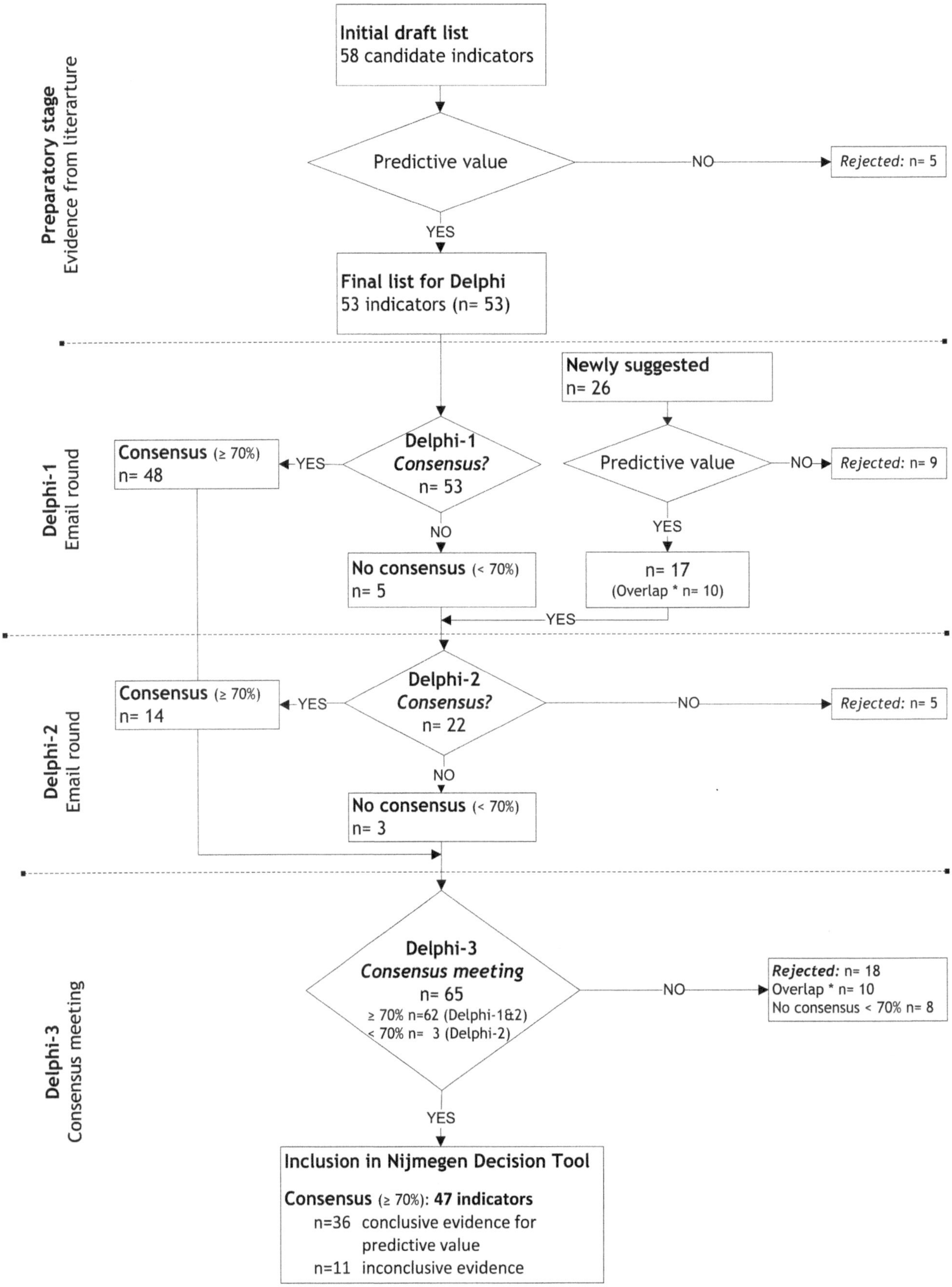

* *overlap* doublure in the definiton of indicators

Figure 2. Results of the Delphi Study. At each stage of the Delphi study the expert panel consensus for presented indicators is shown. To reach consensus the level of agreement was set at ≥70%. Indicators reaching full consensus were included in the Nijmegen Decision Tool.

functional status, the Short-Form 36 Health Survey Questionnaire (SF36) and the EuroQol (EQ-5D) for quality of life, and the Numeric Rating Scale (NRS) for back and leg pain. The STarT back is used as a screening tool for identifying the amount of risk for three psychological indicators (distress, catastrophizing, and fear of movement/(re)injury; i.e. 'yellow flags'). The remaining 40 indicators were compared to existing questions in the Swespine register. Analogous questions were translated and the remaining indicators were added as dichotomous or multiple choice questions in the final questionnaire. The complete screening questionnaire is available from the authors.

2. The provisional decision algorithm. The provisional decision algorithm is based on the flag approach and based on current practice. The red flag signs are thought to be associated with underlying pathology. Therefore, in the algorithm the presence of ≥1 red flag (e.g. previous history of malignancies, trauma) is indicative for a consultation by a spinal surgeon, whereas a high risk on yellow flags (i.e. distress, catastrophizing cognitions) is second most decisive as a high risk on yellow flags might be predictive for treatment failure.

Discussion

The purpose of this study was to develop a clinical decision tool for secondary or tertiary care specialists to decide which patients with chronic low back pain (CLBP) should be seen by a spine surgeon for consideration of a beneficial surgical intervention (including invasive pain management), and which patients in the future should best be seen by other medical specialists, e.g. physiatrists, rheumatologists or pain consultants. A study, consisting of a preparatory stage in which evidence from literature was summarized followed by a three-round Delphi study, contributed to the developed Nijmegen clinical decision tool for CLBP, which includes 1) a patient-based and web-based screening questionnaire and 2) a provisional decision algorithm.

In the preparatory stage of this study, we included in the literature review the evidence found in international guidelines [22,23,31] and the evidence from one national guideline [34], as these guidelines are normative for evidence based daily practice. However, studies included in these guidelines have led to inconsistent results and rarely show more than small to moderate overall benefit for different types of interventions, which makes it difficult to interpret which patient benefits from which intervention. Therefore, we performed a literature search covering the whole spectrum of CLBP ignoring specific medical specialties (explicit knowledge). This is supplemented by professional state-of-the-art knowledge derived from experiences in daily practice and collegial meetings and conferences, in a formal consensus (Delphi) study (implicit knowledge).

1. The screening questionnaire

The literature search revealed a large number of published studies (n = 33) related to the identification of predictive indicators for a successful treatment outcome or the prediction of persistence of CLBP complaints. As expected the result of this study is a long list of predictive indicators (n = 47), with most of them (77%) having scientific evidence for predictive value. To list and classify the indicators in Table 2 and 3 we used the conceptual model of patient outcomes (Poolman 2009) and identified five main domains: Sociodemographic, Pain, Somatic, Psychologic, and Functioning and Quality of Life. Overall, we found strong predictive evidence for successful outcome of spinal surgery for: previous back surgery and biological indicators (i.e. diagnosis; co-morbidities as diabetes, bulging or protruded disc, loss of neurological function, and 'red flags'). In this study consensus was reached to add BMI and smoking as indicators in the screening questionnaire and to evaluate their contribution to outcome of surgical interventions over time. Although the evidence is growing that high BMI [77] and smoking [63,64,78–80] are predictive for a poor outcome after surgery, the current scientific evidence is still inconclusive. Along with the predictive value of psychological indicators (yellow flags) [38,39,48] and expectations for treatment outcome [37,43,78] and work return [37,43,56], predictive indicators as high disability [36,38,39,48,80], being unemployed [37,43,64], and being involved in litigation and/or compensation claims [36,39,41,51,63,66,78] seem to lead to unfavourable outcome for all CLBP interventions.

2. The provisional decision algorithm

For this study we used the recommended clinical flag approach [33] for clinical decision-making in CLBP as a starting point [22,23,74]. A diagnostic triage based on 'red flag' signs is recommended [22,74,81] as red flag signs are features thought to be associated with a high risk of serious underlying disorders, such as infection, inflammatory disease, cancer or fracture [33,82] or nerve root disease [46]. The presence of a red flag alerts clinicians to the need for further examination and specific management [82–84]. In this study consensus was reached that the presence of one or more red flag signs is indicative for a consultation by a spinal surgeon, which was incorporated as a first step in the provisional decision algorithm. However, the guideline recommendations on diagnostic triage based on red flags are still not very strong [81]. Most of the patients with back pain show at least one positive red flag and do not have a serious underlying condition. Taking the guideline recommendations literally could cause harm. These harms include unnecessary diagnostics, unnecessary exposure to radiation, as well as unnecessary treatments, including surgery [85]. Moreover, a summary [86] of two recently published Cochrane reviews aiming to detect the diagnostic accuracy of red flags to screen for vertebral fracture [84] and malignancy [83] concluded that a lack of evidence exists that one red flag used in isolation can be used to aid a clinician's judgement. We expect that combinations of red flags and clinical features might appear more informative to assist clinical decision-making [83,84,86]. Even though it is recommended to assess the so-called yellow flags [22,23] as well, it remains unclear what these indicators contribute to actual clinical decision-making. Large prospective studies are needed to evaluate the contribution of these indicators to successful treatment outcome. In this study consensus was reached that a high risk on yellow flags is the second most decisive for surgical or non-surgical interventions. We currently perform further studies to examine multifactorial diagnostic models and with that, the scientific value of combinations of flags and indicators, collected by means of the screening questionnaire, in clinical decision-making for further diagnostics and/or treatment.

CLBP is a multifactorial health condition and therefore, it has been widely recommended to develop a classification system or a decision tool to direct CLBP patients to interventions based on

Table 2. Results of the Delphi Study.

Domain	Category	Evidence
Sociodemographic	**Personal**	
	Age	I
	Gender	I
	Body weight & BMI	I
	Health	
	Smoking	I
	Previous back surgery	C
	Use of analgesics	I
	Self-management of complaints	C
	Interventions in the past	C
	Social	
	Social status	I
	Functioning – leisure	I
	Social support	C
	Work	
	Socio-economic status*	C
	Work satisfaction	I
	Functioning – work	I
	Sick leave*	C
	Litigation	C
Pain	Duration	I
	Intensity*	C
	Intensity – back	C
	Intensity – leg	C
	Frequency/preceding (prior) episodes*	I
	Daily course of pain complaints	C
	Influence of rest, mobility, and posture	C
Somatic	Diagnosis; co morbidities (Red Flag)	C
Physical & Biological	Bulging or protruded disc* (Red Flag)	C
	Loss of neurological function* (Red Flag)	C
	Red flags (n = 11)*	C
	Pain started age <20 or >50 years	
	Significant trauma	
	Pain is constant and non-mechanical	
	Pain in thoracic spine	
	Deformities (i.e. scoliosis, lumbar kyphosis)	
	Previous history of malignities/cancer	
	History of intravenous drug use	
	AIDS/HIV	
	Currently steroid use	
	Recent unexplained weight loss	
	Calin criteria for axial spondylarthritis	C
Psychologic	**Psychic affect**	
	Distress*	C
	Anxiety*	C
	Cognition	
	Catastrophizing*	C
	Somatization*	C
	Coping*	C
	Behaviour	

Table 2. Cont.

Domain	Category	Evidence
	Fear of movement/(re)injury*	C
	Expectations – work return*	C
	Expectations – outcome/recovery*	C
Functioning &	Functioning in daily activities & walking	C
Quality of Life	Pain-interference daily activities	
	Health-related physical functioning	C

* Recommended in international guidelines.
Newly formulated indicators are printed in italics.
I Inconclusive evidence; *C* Conclusive evidence.
Final list with 'full consensus' indicators categorized in domains, including the resulting evidential value.

biomedical and psychosocial indicators [11,22–25,30,31]. To date we are not aware of any study covering the whole spectrum and to our knowledge the Nijmegen decision tool for CLBP is the first published patient screening questionnaire and provisional decision algorithm. The backbone of the screening questionnaire consists of Dutch versions of international validated PROMs. To be able to make our future study results comparable and to be able to perform benchmark studies in the future, we selected commonly used PROMs covering those indicators that are treatment outcome-related (functioning in daily activities with ODI, quality of life with SF36 and EQ5D, and pain intensity with NRS) [87]. These PROMs are also used in the Swedish Spine Register (Swespine [www.4S.nu]). To screen yellow flags and determine the risk of psychological influence on treatment outcome we implemented the Dutch version of the STarT back screening tool [88–90]. Although validated and useful in primary care [88,91–93] further research is needed to evaluate the validity and feasibility of prognostic screening with this tool in secondary or tertiary back care. To our knowledge, for the remaining indicators of the screening questionnaire no validated and reliable questionnaires exist. Large and methodological sound studies are needed for the feasibility and validity of these questions and whether (a combination of) these indicators contribute to successful treatment outcome.

In March 2012 the screening questionnaire was implemented in the Dutch patient interface of the Swespine. Swespine was chosen as it is one of the largest, oldest and most studied national registries, which covers both PROMs and clinical results [94], which allows benchmarking data in future. After pilot testing and some minor adjustments (e.g. grammatical and spelling mistakes, wording of questions, and technical issues related to the system), the web-based register started in May 2012. The registry is an ideal instrument to obtain meaningful data prospectively, to define normative values, to identify patient profiles, to confirm differences in treatment outcomes for subpopulations [25,95]. The results can be used for quality assurance, quality improvement and for research purposes [94]. To study the provisional clinical decision algorithm, since May 2012 all LBP patients referred to our clinic complete the screening questionnaire web-based and treated patients are systematically followed over time for two years by completing the same PROMs at predefined follow-up moments. With that, in future it should be possible to identify patient profiles (phenotypes} predicting a beneficial treatment outcome for each type of surgical or non-surgical intervention, for all the referred, treated and untreated patients. At the same time data of the individual patients are presented in PDF-format in the electronic medical record (EMR) of the patient and contributes to individual decision-making in the clinic.

Strengths and Weaknesses

Although for 36 of the 47 indicators conclusive evidence is available in the literature that they have predictive value for treatment outcome in patients with CLBP, for 11 indicators the

Table 3. Backbone screening questionnaire.

Domains	Flag approach [33]	Results Phase 2 *(current study)* Indicators (n = 47)	Questions
Sociodemographic	Blue & Black	13	Multiple choice
		3	Dichotomous
Pain	n.a.	5	Multiple choice
		2	NRS (0–10)*
Somatic	Red	14	Dichotomous
Psychosocial	Yellow	3	STarT back screening tool[88]
		4	Multiple choice
		1	Dichotomous
Functioning & Quality of Life	n.a.	2	ODI (v2.1a); SF36; EQ-5D*

* standard & agreed to implement in Swespine register www.4s.nu.

evidence was inconclusive. These indicators were included in the Delphi study, based on the expert opinion of a panel of LBP clinicians. However, the formal, structured, and systematic character of the Modified Delphi Technique is of great value in indicator research when scientific evidence for indicators is inconclusive or lacking [71]. Moreover, to overcome the knowledge gaps existing between different medical specialties in the CLBP field [24], we used this technique in a multidisciplinary panel of specialists as it is argued to successfully bring together and to synthesize the knowledge of the whole expert group [71]. All health professionals came from one hospital specialised in spine care and the generalisation to other secondary or tertiary spine practices in other countries and healthcare environments might be limited. Strength of this study is that the panel included diverse professionals covering the secondary surgical and non-surgical CLBP care. Moreover, the decision tool is based on international accepted guidelines and evidence published in literature, covering the whole spectrum of CLBP. We weighed the evidence in literature according to the Levels of Evidence [69]. By combining this explicit knowledge with the implicit knowledge of the expert panel in the three-round Delphi study, after refinement of the decision algorithm, and after validation of the tool in other settings, we expect that the Nijmegen Decision Tool for CLBP could be used in general secondary and tertiary spine care.

Conclusion

This study has provided the first clinical decision tool for CLBP patients, based on current scientific evidence and formal consensus, covering the whole spectrum of CLBP. We expect that this relatively simple tool will considerably help a daily spine practice in clinical decision-making 1) to select the right CLBP patients for the right interventions, thereby improving the outcomes of spinal interventions, and 2) lead to a reduction in healthcare costs by reducing the number of inappropriate referrals to spine care professionals.

Supporting Information

Table S1 Preparatory stage - Summarized evidence and References per indicator.
(PDF)

Author Contributions

Conceived and designed the experiments: MvH J. van Limbeek MdK. Performed the experiments: MvH J. van Loon J. van Limbeek MdK. Analyzed the data: MvH J. van Limbeek MdK. Contributed reagents/materials/analysis tools: MvH J. van Limbeek MdK. Contributed to the writing of the manuscript: MvH J. van Loon J. van Limbeek MdK.

References

1. Murray CJ, Vos T, Lozano R, Naghavi M, Flaxman AD, et al. (2012) Disability-adjusted life years (DALYs) for 291 diseases and injuries in 21 regions, 1990–2010: a systematic analysis for the Global Burden of Disease Study 2010. Lancet 380: 2197–2223
2. Frymoyer JW (1992) Predicting disability from low back pain. Clin Orthop Relat Res: 101–109
3. Henschke N, Kuijpers T, Rubinstein SM, van Middelkoop M, Ostelo R, et al. (2012) Trends over time in the size and quality of randomised controlled trials of interventions for chronic low-back pain. Eur Spine J 21: 375–381
4. Von Korff M, Saunders K (1996) The course of back pain in primary care. Spine (Phila Pa 1976.) 21: 2833–2837
5. Picavet HS, Schouten JS (2003) Musculoskeletal pain in the Netherlands: prevalences, consequences and risk groups, the DMC(3)-study. Pain 102: 167–178
6. Freburger JK, Holmes GM, Agans RP, Jackman AM, Darter JD, et al. (2009) The rising prevalence of chronic low back pain. Arch Intern Med 169: 251–258
7. Dagenais S, Caro J, Haldeman S (2008) A systematic review of low back pain cost of illness studies in the United States and internationally. Spine J 8: 8–20
8. Lambeek LC, van Tulder MW, Swinkels IC, Koppes LL, Anema JR, et al. (2011) The trend in total cost of back pain in The Netherlands in the period 2002 to 2007. Spine (Phila Pa 1976.) 36: 1050–1058
9. van Tulder MW (2011) Health technology assessment (HTA) increasingly important in spine research. Eur Spine J 20: 999–1000
10. Turk DC (2005) The potential of treatment matching for subgroups of patients with chronic pain: lumping versus splitting. Clin J Pain 21: 44–55
11. Bederman SS (2010) Predicting prognosis in sick-listed low back pain patients: sneaking a peak inside the black box. Spine J 10: 728–730
12. Truchon M (2001) Determinants of chronic disability related to low back pain: towards an integrative biopsychosocial model. Disabil Rehabil 23: 758–767
13. Weiner BK (2008) Spine update: the biopsychosocial model and spine care. Spine (Phila Pa 1976.) 33: 219–223
14. Haldeman S, Dagenais S (2008) A supermarket approach to the evidence-informed management of chronic low back pain. Spine J 8: 1–7
15. Fairbank J, Frost H, Wilson-MacDonald J, Yu LM, Barker K, et al. (2005) Randomised controlled trial to compare surgical stabilisation of the lumbar spine with an intensive rehabilitation programme for patients with chronic low back pain: the MRC spine stabilisation trial. BMJ 330: 1233
16. Mirza SK, Deyo RA (2007) Systematic review of randomized trials comparing lumbar fusion surgery to nonoperative care for treatment of chronic back pain. Spine (Phila Pa 1976.) 32: 816–823
17. Brox JI, Nygaard OP, Holm I, Keller A, Ingebrigtsen T, et al. (2010) Four-year follow-up of surgical versus non-surgical therapy for chronic low back pain. Ann Rheum Dis 69: 1643–1648
18. van Middelkoop M, Rubinstein SM, Kuijpers T, Verhagen AP, Ostelo R, et al. (2011) A systematic review on the effectiveness of physical and rehabilitation interventions for chronic non-specific low back pain. Eur Spine J 20: 19–39
19. Jacobs WC, Rubinstein SM, Koes B, van Tulder MW, Peul WC (2013) Evidence for surgery in degenerative lumbar spine disorders. Best Pract Res Clin Rheumatol 27: 673–684
20. Hall H, McIntosh G (2008) Low back pain (chronic). Clin Evid (Online) 2008
21. Wand BM, O'Connell NE (2008) Chronic non-specific low back pain - sub-groups or a single mechanism? BMC Musculoskelet Disord 9: 11
22. Airaksinen O, Brox JI, Cedraschi C, Hildebrandt J, Klaber-Moffett J, et al. (2006) Chapter 4. European guidelines for the management of chronic nonspecific low back pain. Eur Spine J 15 Suppl 2: S192–S300
23. NICE (National Institute for Health and Clinical Excellence) (2009) Low back pain: early management of persistent non-specific low back pain. NICE Clinical Guideline 88. Available: http://publications.nice.org.uk/low-back-pain-cg88. Accessed 2014 Mar 24.
24. Fairbank J, Gwilym SE, France JC, Daffner SD, Dettori J, et al. (2011) The role of classification of chronic low back pain. Spine (Phila Pa 1976.) 36: S19–S42
25. Fourney DR, Andersson G, Arnold PM, Dettori J, Cahana A, et al. (2011) Chronic low back pain: a heterogeneous condition with challenges for an evidence-based approach. Spine (Phila Pa 1976.) 36: S1–S9
26. Kamper SJ, Maher CG, Hancock MJ, Koes BW, Croft PR, et al. (2010) Treatment-based subgroups of low back pain: a guide to appraisal of research studies and a summary of current evidence. Best Pract Res Clin Rheumatol 24: 181–191
27. McCormick JD, Werner BC, Shimer AL (2013) Patient-reported outcome measures in spine surgery. J Am Acad Orthop Surg 21: 99–107
28. Glassman SD, Carreon LY, Anderson PA, Resnick DK (2011) A diagnostic classification for lumbar spine registry development. Spine J 11: 1108–1116
29. Willems PC, Staal JB, Walenkamp GH, de Bie RA (2013) Spinal fusion for chronic low back pain: systematic review on the accuracy of tests for patient selection. Spine J 13: 99–109
30. Koes BW, van Tulder MW, Thomas S (2006) Diagnosis and treatment of low back pain. BMJ 332: 1430–1434
31. Chou R, Loeser JD, Owens DK, Rosenquist RW, Atlas SJ, et al. (2009) Interventional therapies, surgery, and interdisciplinary rehabilitation for low back pain: an evidence-based clinical practice guideline from the American Pain Society. Spine (Phila Pa 1976.) 34: 1066–1077
32. Meijer R, Ihnenfeldt D, Vermeulen M, De HR, van Limbeek J (2003) The use of a modified Delphi procedure for the determination of 26 prognostic factors in the sub-acute stage of stroke. Int J Rehabil Res 26: 265–270
33. Main CJ, Williams AC (2002) Musculoskeletal pain. BMJ 325: 534–537
34. CBO Kwaliteitsinstituut voor de Gezondheidszorg (2009) Ketenzorgrichtlijn Aspecifiek Lage Rugpijn. Available: http://www.diliguide.nl/document/3272/ketenzorgrichtlijn-aspecifieke-lage-rugklachten.html. Accessed 2014 Mar 24.
35. Hasenbring M (1998) Predictors of efficacy in treatment of chronic low back pain. Curr Opin Anaesthesiol 11: 553–558
36. van der Hulst M, Vollenbroek-Hutten MM, Ijzerman MJ (2005) A systematic review of sociodemographic, physical, and psychological predictors of multidisciplinary rehabilitation-or, back school treatment outcome in patients with chronic low back pain. Spine (Phila Pa 1976.) 30: 813–825
37. Heitz CA, Hilfiker R, Bachmann LM, Joronen H, Lorenz T, et al. (2009) Comparison of risk factors predicting return to work between patients with subacute and chronic non-specific low back pain: systematic review. Eur Spine J 18: 1829–1835

38. den Boer JJ, Oostendorp RA, Beems T, Munneke M, Evers AW (2006) Continued disability and pain after lumbar disc surgery: the role of cognitive-behavioral factors. Pain 123: 45–52
39. Celestin J, Edwards RR, Jamison RN (2009) Pretreatment psychosocial variables as predictors of outcomes following lumbar surgery and spinal cord stimulation: a systematic review and literature synthesis. Pain Med 10: 639–653
40. Wessels T, van Tulder M, Sigl T, Ewert T, Limm H, et al. (2006) What predicts outcome in non-operative treatments of chronic low back pain? A systematic review. Eur Spine J 15: 1633–1644
41. Chou R, Shekelle P (2010) Will this patient develop persistent disabling low back pain? JAMA 303: 1295–1302
42. Pincus T, Burton AK, Vogel S, Field AP (2002) A systematic review of psychological factors as predictors of chronicity/disability in prospective cohorts of low back pain. Spine (Phila Pa 1976.) 27: E109–E120
43. Aalto TJ, Malmivaara A, Kovacs F, Herno A, Alen M, et al. (2006) Preoperative predictors for postoperative clinical outcome in lumbar spinal stenosis: systematic review. Spine (Phila Pa 1976.) 31: E648–E663
44. Melloh M, Elfering A, Egli PC, Roeder C, Barz T, et al. (2009) Identification of prognostic factors for chronicity in patients with low back pain: a review of screening instruments. Int Orthop 33: 301–313
45. Linton SJ (2000) A review of psychological risk factors in back and neck pain. Spine (Phila Pa 1976.) 25: 1148–1156
46. Cohen SP, Argoff CE, Carragee EJ (2008) Management of low back pain. BMJ 337: a2718
47. Grotle M, Foster NE, Dunn KM, Croft P (2010) Are prognostic indicators for poor outcome different for acute and chronic low back pain consulters in primary care? Pain 151: 790–797
48. Smeets RJ, Vlaeyen JW, Kester AD, Knottnerus JA (2006) Reduction of pain catastrophizing mediates the outcome of both physical and cognitive-behavioral treatment in chronic low back pain. J Pain 7: 261–271
49. Flink IK, Boersma K, Linton SJ (2010) Catastrophizing moderates the effect of exposure in vivo for back pain patients with pain-related fear. Eur J Pain 14: 887–892
50. Hasenbring MI, Hallner D, Rusu AC (2009) Fear-avoidance- and endurance-related responses to pain: development and validation of the Avoidance-Endurance Questionnaire (AEQ). Eur J Pain 13: 620–628
51. Trief PM, Ploutz-Snyder R, Fredrickson BE (2006) Emotional health predicts pain and function after fusion: a prospective multicenter study. Spine (Phila Pa 1976.) 31: 823–830
52. Swinkels-Meewisse IE, Roelofs J, Schouten EG, Verbeek AL, Oostendorp RA, et al. (2006) Fear of movement/(re)injury predicting chronic disabling low back pain: a prospective inception cohort study. Spine (Phila Pa 1976.) 31: 658–664
53. Costa LC, Maher CG, McAuley JH, Hancock MJ, Herbert RD, et al. (2009) Prognosis for patients with chronic low back pain: inception cohort study. BMJ 339: b3829
54. Picavet HS, Vlaeyen JW, Schouten JS (2002) Pain catastrophizing and kinesiophobia: predictors of chronic low back pain. Am J Epidemiol 156: 1028–1034
55. Hasenbring MI, Plaas H, Fischbein B, Willburger R (2006) The relationship between activity and pain in patients 6 months after lumbar disc surgery: do pain-related coping modes act as moderator variables? Eur J Pain 10: 701–709
56. Johansson AC, Linton SJ, Rosenblad A, Bergkvist L, Nilsson O (2010) A prospective study of cognitive behavioural factors as predictors of pain, disability and quality of life one year after lumbar disc surgery. Disabil Rehabil 32: 521–529
57. Gheldof EL, Crombez G, Van den Bussche E, Vinck J, Van Nieuwenhuyse A, et al. (2010) Pain-related fear predicts disability, but not pain severity: a path analytic approach of the fear-avoidance model. Eur J Pain 14: 870–879
58. Martel MO, Thibault P, Sullivan MJ (2010) The persistence of pain behaviors in patients with chronic back pain is independent of pain and psychological factors. Pain 151: 330–336
59. Costa LC, Maher CG, McAuley JH, Hancock MJ, Smeets RJ (2011) Self-efficacy is more important than fear of movement in mediating the relationship between pain and disability in chronic low back pain. Eur J Pain 15: 213–219
60. Woby SR, Watson PJ, Roach NK, Urmston M (2004) Are changes in fear-avoidance beliefs, catastrophizing, and appraisals of control, predictive of changes in chronic low back pain and disability? Eur J Pain 8: 201–210
61. Goubert L, Crombez G, van Damme S (2004) The role of neuroticism, pain catastrophizing and pain-related fear in vigilance to pain: a structural equations approach. Pain 107: 234–241
62. Wideman TH, Adams H, Sullivan MJ (2009) A prospective sequential analysis of the fear-avoidance model of pain. Pain 145: 45–51
63. Carreon LY, Glassman SD, Djurasovic M, Dimar JR, Johnson JR, et al. (2009) Are preoperative health-related quality of life scores predictive of clinical outcomes after lumbar fusion? Spine (Phila Pa 1976.) 34: 725–730
64. Atlas SJ, Keller RB, Wu YA, Deyo RA, Singer DE (2005) Long-term outcomes of surgical and nonsurgical management of lumbar spinal stenosis: 8 to 10 year results from the maine lumbar spine study. Spine (Phila Pa 1976.) 30: 936–943
65. Sinikallio S, Aalto T, Lehto SM, Airaksinen O, Herno A, et al. (2010) Depressive symptoms predict postoperative disability among patients with lumbar spinal stenosis: a two-year prospective study comparing two age groups. Disabil Rehabil 32: 462–468
66. Jensen OK, Nielsen CV, Stengaard-Pedersen K (2010) One-year prognosis in sick-listed low back pain patients with and without radiculopathy. Prognostic factors influencing pain and disability. Spine J 10: 659–675
67. Peters ML, Vlaeyen JW, Weber WE (2005) The joint contribution of physical pathology, pain-related fear and catastrophizing to chronic back pain disability. Pain 113: 45–50
68. Harms MC, Peers CE, Chase D (2010) Low back pain: what determines functional outcome at six months? An observational study. BMC Musculoskelet Disord 11: 236
69. Oxford Centre for Evidence-based Medicine Levels of Evidence (2009) Levels of Evidence. Online source. Available: www.cebm.net
70. Murphy MK, Black NA, Lamping DL, McKee CM, Sanderson CF, et al. (1998) Consensus development methods, and their use in clinical guideline development. Health Technol Assess 2: i–88
71. Boulkedid R, Abdoul H, Loustau M, Sibony O, Alberti C (2011) Using and reporting the Delphi method for selecting healthcare quality indicators: a systematic review. PLoS One 6: e20476
72. Dalkey NC (1969) The Delphi Method: An experimental study of group opinion. The Rand Corporation
73. Linstone AH, Turoff M (2002) The Delphi Method; Techniques and Applications.
74. CBO, Kwaliteitsinstituut voor de Gezondheidszorg (2009) Ketenzorgrichtlijn Aspecifiek Lage Rugpijn. Available: http://www.diliguide.nl/document/3272/ketenzorgrichtlijn-aspecifieke-lage-rugklachten.html. Accessed 2014 Mar 24.
75. Chavannes AW, Mens JMA, Koes BW, Lubbers WJ, Ostelo R, et al. (2005) NHG-Standaard Aspecifieke LageRugpijn. Huisarts en Wetenschap 48: 113–123
76. Rudwaleit M, Sieper J (2004) Diagnosis and early diagnosis of ankylosing spondylitis. Z Rheumatol 63: 193–202
77. Athiviraham A, Wali ZA, Yen D (2011) Predictive factors influencing clinical outcome with operative management of lumbar spinal stenosis. Spine J 11: 613–617
78. Soriano JC, Revuelta MS, Fuente MF, Diaz IC, Urena PM, et al. (2010) Predictors of outcome after decompressive lumbar surgery and instrumented posterolateral fusion. Eur Spine J 19: 1841–1848
79. Sanden B, Forsth P, Michaelsson K (2011) Smokers show less improvement than nonsmokers two years after surgery for lumbar spinal stenosis: a study of 4555 patients from the Swedish spine register. Spine (Phila Pa 1976.) 36: 1059–1064
80. Pearson A, Lurie J, Tosteson T, Zhao W, Abdu W, et al. (2012) Who should have surgery for spinal stenosis? Treatment effect predictors in SPORT. Spine (Phila Pa 1976.) 37: 1791–1802
81. Koes BW, van Tulder MW, Lin CW, Macedo LG, McAuley J, et al. (2010) An updated overview of clinical guidelines for the management of non-specific low back pain in primary care. Eur Spine J 19: 2075–2094
82. Centeno CJ, Elkins WL, Freeman M (2004) Waddell's signs revisited? Spine (Phila Pa 1976.) 29: 1392
83. Henschke N, Maher CG, Ostelo RW, de Vet HC, Macaskill P, et al. (2013) Red flags to screen for malignancy in patients with low-back pain. Cochrane Database Syst Rev 2: CD008686
84. Williams CM, Henschke N, Maher CG, van Tulder MW, Koes BW, et al. (2013) Red flags to screen for vertebral fracture in patients presenting with low-back pain. Cochrane Database Syst Rev 1: CD008643
85. Underwood M, Buchbinder R (2013) Red flags for back pain BMJ 347: f7432
86. Downie A, Williams CM, Henschke N, Hancock MJ, Ostelo RW, et al. (2013) Red flags to screen for malignancy and fracture in patients with low back pain: systematic review. BMJ 347: f7095
87. Rihn JA, Berven S, Allen T, Phillips FM, Currier BL, et al. (2009) Defining value in spine care. Am J Med Qual 24: 4S–14S
88. Hill JC, Whitehurst DG, Lewis M, Bryan S, Dunn KM, et al. (2011) Comparison of stratified primary care management for low back pain with current best practice (STarT Back): a randomised controlled trial. Lancet 378: 1560–1571
89. van Hooff ML, van Lankveld W, Anderson P, Apeldoorn A, van Hartingveld F, et al. (2011) The STarT Back Screening Tool: Dutch version. Available: http://www.keele.ac.uk/media/keeleuniversity/ri/primarycare/startbackmicro/Dutch_tool.pdf. Accessed 2014 Mar 24.
90. Apeldoorn A, van Hooff ML, Ostelo RWJG (2013) De STarT Back Screening Tool. FysioPraxis: 32–33
91. Morso L, Albert H, Kent P, Manniche C, Hill J (2011) Translation and discriminative validation of the STarT Back Screening Tool into Danish. Eur Spine J 20: 2166–2173
92. Kongsted A, Johannesen E, Leboeuf-Yde C (2011) Feasibility of the STarT back screening tool in chiropractic clinics: a cross-sectional study of patients with low back pain. Chiropr Man Therap 19: 10
93. Bruyere O, Demoulin M, Brereton C, Humblet F, Flynn D, et al. (2012) Translation validation of a new back pain screening questionnaire (the STarT Back Screening Tool) in French. Arch Public Health 70: 12
94. Stromqvist B, Fritzell P, Hagg O, Jonsson B, Sanden B (2013) Swespine: the Swedish spine register: the 2012 report. Eur Spine J 22: 953–974
95. Fritzell P, Stromqvist B, Hagg O (2006) A practical approach to spine registers in Europe: the Swedish experience. Eur Spine J 15 Suppl 1: S57–S63

Phantom Acupuncture: Dissociating Somatosensory and Cognitive/Affective Components of Acupuncture Stimulation with a Novel Form of Placebo Acupuncture

Jeungchan Lee[1], Vitaly Napadow[1,2], Jieun Kim[2], Seunggi Lee[3], Woojin Choi[3], Ted J. Kaptchuk[4], Kyungmo Park[1]*

1 Department of Biomedical Engineering, Kyung Hee University, Yongin, Gyeonggi, South Korea, **2** Martinos Center for Biomedical Imaging, Department of Radiology, Massachusetts General Hospital, Charlestown, Massachusetts, United States of America, **3** Department of Neuropsychiatry, College of Korean Medicine, Sangji University, Wonju, Gangwon, South Korea, **4** Program in Placebo Studies, Beth Israel Deaconess Medical Center, Harvard Medical School, Boston, Massachusetts, United States of America

Abstract

In a clinical setting, acupuncture treatment consists of multiple components including somatosensory stimulation, treatment context, and attention to needle-based procedures. In order to dissociate somatosensory versus contextual and attentional aspects of acupuncture, we devised a novel form of placebo acupuncture, a visual manipulation dubbed phantom acupuncture, which reproduces the acupuncture needling ritual without somatosensory tactile stimulation. Subjects (N = 20) received both real (REAL) and phantom (PHNT) acupuncture. Subjects were retrospectively classified into two groups based on PHNT credibility (PHNTc, who found phantom acupuncture credible; and PHNTnc, who did not). Autonomic and psychophysical responses were monitored. We found that PHNT can be delivered in a credible manner. Acupuncture needling, a complex, ritualistic somatosensory intervention, induces sympathetic activation (phasic skin conductance [SC] response), which may be specific to the somatosensory component of acupuncture. In contrast, contextual effects, such as needling credibility, are instead associated with a shift toward relative cardiovagal activation (decreased heart rate) during needling and sympathetic inhibition (decreased SC) and parasympathetic activation (decreased pupil size) following acupuncture needling. Visual stimulation characterizing the needling ritual is an important factor for phasic autonomic responses to acupuncture and may undelie the needling orienting response. Our study suggests that phantom acupuncture can be a viable sham control for acupuncture as it completely excludes the somatosensory component of real needling while maintaining the credibility of the acupuncture treatment context in many subjects.

Editor: Xi Luo, Brown University, United States of America

Funding: The authors would like to thank the Korean National Research Foundation funded by the Ministry of Science, ICT and Future Planning (NRF-2011-0028968, NRF-2009-0076345), and the Ministry of Health & Welfare and Seoul Metropolitan Government (Traditional Korean Medicine R&D Project, HI13C0700). The study was also supported by the National Center for Complementary and Alternative Medicine (NCCAM), at the United States of America National Institutes of Health (NIH) (P01-AT006663, R01-AT007550, R01-AT004714 to VN, K24-AT004095 to TJK). The content is the sole responsibility of the authors and does not necessarily represent the official views of our funding agencies. The funders had no role in study design, data collection and analysis, decision to publish, or preparation of the manuscript.

Competing Interests: The authors have declared that no competing interests exist.

* Email: saenim@khu.ac.kr

Introduction

While acupuncture has been shown to reduce pain in many previous clinical trials, statistically significant differences between real and sham acupuncture have not been consistently demonstrated [1,2,3,4]. This may be due to the fact that sham acupuncture commonly has included a somatosensory or tactile component. In fact, previous studies have not separated the complex acupuncture ritual into its constituent components, which could better determine the specific effects of this therapeutic intervention [1]. In this study, we propose an experimental design that allows for a separation of the acupuncture ritual into a somatosensory and contextual component, with autonomic outflow and psychophysical outcome metrics.

Sham acupuncture, which has been used as a control in many acupuncture studies, has been shown to produce a physiological effect [5,6], as it affects skin receptors, which are known to be even more dense than muscle and fascial somatosensory and nociceptors [7,8]. In fact, sham acupuncture can produce similar somatosensory or pain intensity even without skin penetration [9,10]. Acupuncture is a multi-dimensional intervention, and usage of sham acupuncture techniques as controls in clinical trials would be aided by a better understanding of the different components related to the therapeutic effect of acupuncture [11]. For instance, the tactile component in sham acupuncture is considered essential for credibility of the needling ritual. But this may not be the case. Because tactile stimulation produces a

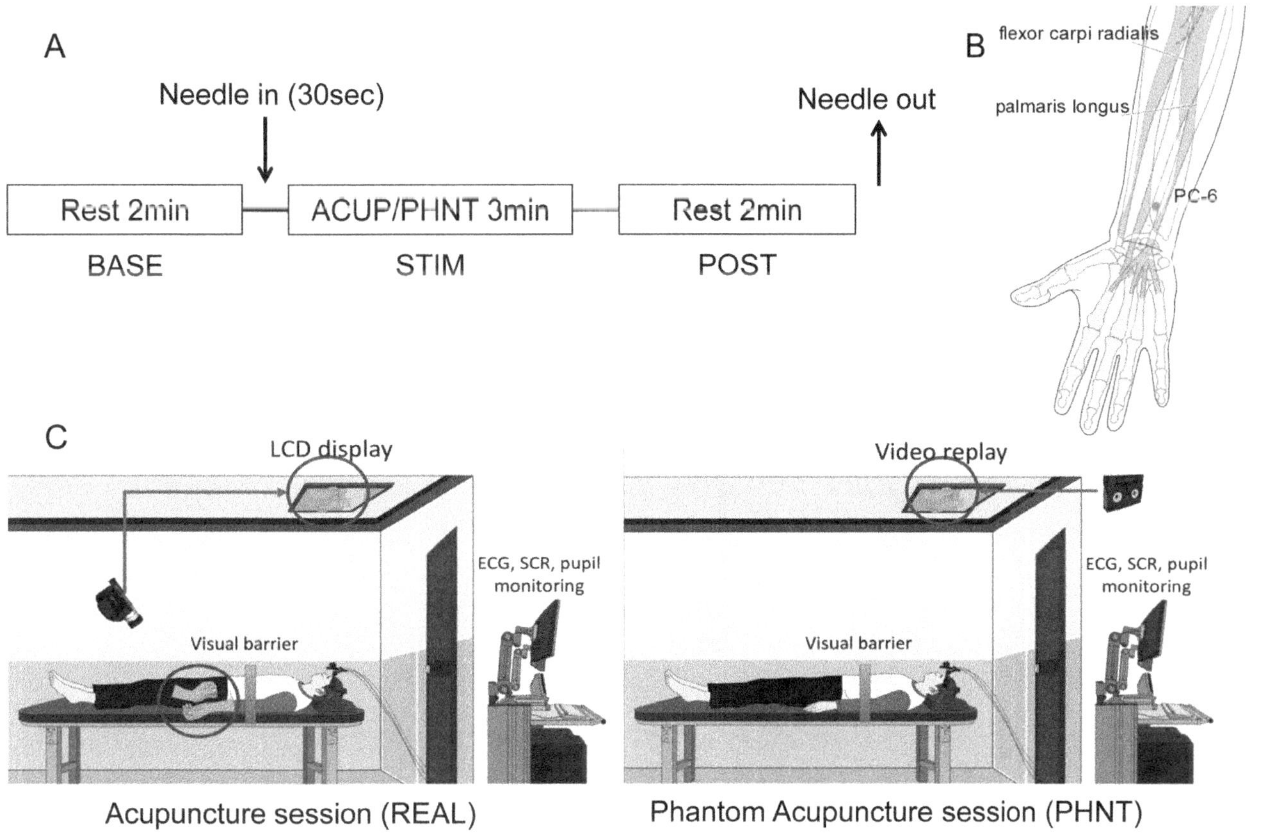

Figure 1. Experimental protocol. A. The paradigm consisted of 3-minute event-related stimulation (STIM, 3-second stimulation, ISI mean = 19.5 sec) surrounded by two 2-minute rest sessions (BASE and POST). **B.** Acupuncture stimulation location (PC6). **C.** Experimental setup for REAL and PHNT sessions. n.b. Figure in **B.** was modified from an image in 'WHO Regional Office for the Western Pacific, 2008, WHO Standard Acupuncture Point Locations in the Western Pacific Region, Manila'.

physiological response and may overlap therapeutic components of verum acupuncture, usage of sham acupuncture as a placebo control may be compromised, and there is great need for the development of a credible sham acupuncture procedure that does not include somatosensory (tactile) stimulation [12].

In this study we employed several outcome measures to assess different components of acupuncture. Physiological measures estimated autonomic nervous system (ANS) activity. ANS responses have been reported to have clinical relevance to many disease processes. For example, heart rate changes have been associated with clinical improvements for PTSD [13] and chronic pain [14], and have been linked with memory recall [15], somatosensory processing [16] and emotional memory processing [17]. Moreover, many studies have explored acupuncture's effects on ANS activity. Yao et al. showed that acupuncture induces a temporary increase in sympathetic tone, followed by a more prolonged depression [18]. Other investigators have also noted increased sympathetic tone during acupuncture stimulation [19] and increased parasympathetic tone after the stimulation [20,21]. Other studies have linked acupuncture-induced HR decrease, with immune system modulation [22]. However, Lee et al. [23] found no definitive evidence of association between heart rate variability and clinical outcomes, perhaps due to variability in stimulation methods (e.g. needling intensity, duration and frequency), experimental conditions (e.g. measurement timing), or between-subject variability. In fact, individual autonomic response is easily influenced by subtle changes of experimental setup, necessitating a well-controlled design. Our previous study measured concurrent autonomic and brain responses in a neuroimaging study [5]. We showed that, on average, acupuncture produced HR decrease and SCR increase after manual needle stimulation, though individual stimuli could produce both HR increase and decrease. These variable responses were modulated by distinct neural circuitries. In summary, acupuncture induced ANS response may vary based on needling location, needling technique, and needling dose as well as psychological factors and temporal variability.

In this study, we developed a novel form of sham acupuncture which was credible for many subjects, but did not include somatosensory stimulation. This allowed us to dissociate three different components of acupuncture. These included a tactile stimulation-specific component, an attentional shift component (due to visual/somatosensory stimulation), and a cognitive component related to a credibility of the needling procedure. Psychophysical and psychophysiological outcomes were used to dissociate these different components of acupuncture.

Materials and Methods

All research procedures were approved by the Institutional Review Board (IRB) committee of Sangji University (IRB approval number: SJ 2007-071201), and investigations were conducted in accordance with the principles of the Declaration of Helsinki. All participants in the study provided written informed consent.

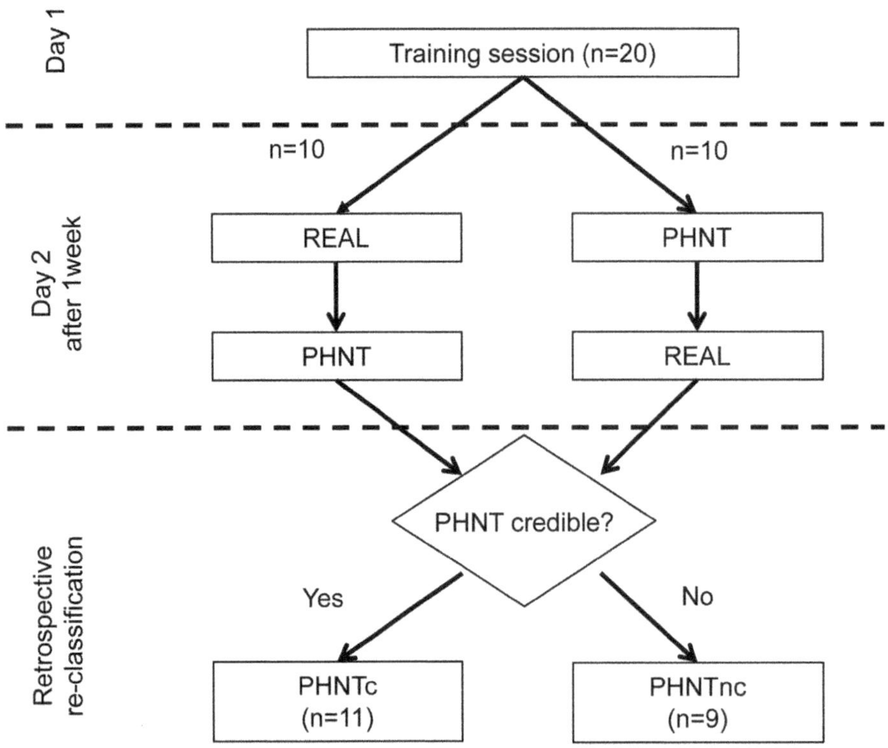

Figure 2. Study flow. Among twenty healthy subjects, ten received real acupuncture (REAL) first, while the rest received phantom acupuncture (PHNT) first, and they were re-classified into phantom credible (PHNTc) and phantom non-credible (PHNTnc) according to the needling credibility in phantom acupuncture (PHNT).

Subjects and Experimental Design

Twenty healthy, right handed female adults (21.8±2.6 years old) participated in both real acupuncture and sham control (phantom acupuncture) sessions in a crossover design. Subjects were recruited via fliers/webpage at the university and its neighborhood. Subjects were screened to exclude any autonomic dysfunction and asked not to take any pharmacological or autonomic modulating substance (e.g. caffeine) prior to testing.

A behavioral training session was completed 1 week prior to either experimental session, during which acupuncture stimulation was applied to the subjects in exactly the same way as during the real acupuncture (REAL) session to record a video clip of acupuncture needling prior to the actual acupuncture sessions. During this session, the acupuncture expectancy questionnaire was completed by study subjects to quantify individual variability in expectancy for acupuncture efficacy [24]. Subjects also completed the Edinburgh Handedness questionnaire [25]. The acupuncturist for this all subsequent sessions was an experienced practitioner (WC) with five years of clinical practice.

Real acupuncture (REAL) and phantom acupuncture (PHNT) sessions, separated by at least 40 min, were performed with pseudo-randomized order. For REAL, a 2-minute duration resting baseline (BASE) was followed by needle insertion (completed within 30 seconds, **Figure 1B**). The needle (0.3 mm*30 mm stainless steel needle, Dongbang Co., Korea) was inserted at left acupoint PC6 on the medial side of the right forearm and rotated manually at a rate of ~2 Hz. This acupoint is 2 cun (approximately 5 cm) proximal to the transverse wrist crease, between the tendons of the palmaris longus and flexor carpi radialis muscles, and is innervated by the median and antebrachial cutaneous nerves. This point is thought to be useful for cardiac conditions, as well as to control nausea and vomiting. It was chosen for this study because clinically, stimulation at this point has been used to modulate autonomic function and is known to induce robust acupuncture sensation [26].

The acupuncturist approached his hand to the acupoint and rotated the needle according to the stimulation timing that was implemented by computer (Psychtoolbox and Matlab, The MathWorks Inc., MA, USA) and relayed to the acupuncturist by auditory signals via headphones. Needle stimulation (STIM) comprised eight stimuli (3-second durations) at pseudo-randomized inter-stimulus interval ($\mu = 19.5$ second) over a duration of 3 minutes. Another 2 minute resting period (POST) followed this STIM period, where the acupuncture needle was retained in the arm (**Figure 1A**). The entire procedure (lasting ~7.5 minutes) was video-recorded and simultaneously displayed to the subject, who could not see the procedure directly due to a visual barrier.

For PHNT, the acupuncturist did not provide any tactile input to the subjects, and only approached his hand toward the acupoint. However, the video clip of prior acupuncture needling which was recorded at the previous REAL or training session was replayed to the subject, thus creating an illusion of needle insertion and stimulation (**Figure 1C**).

In order to perform the needle stimulation at the exact timing according to the experimental protocol, the acupuncturist followed auditory cues. After the stimulation timing signals were sent to the acupuncturist, the approaching time of acupuncturist's hand to the acupoint (PC6) in the video display were calculated retrospectively. The average time delay from onset of hand motion to reaching the acupoint was 0.77±0.26 second (mean±STD). Thus, actual acupuncture stimulations were applied about 0.8 second after the subject observed visual motion for the acupuncturist's hand.

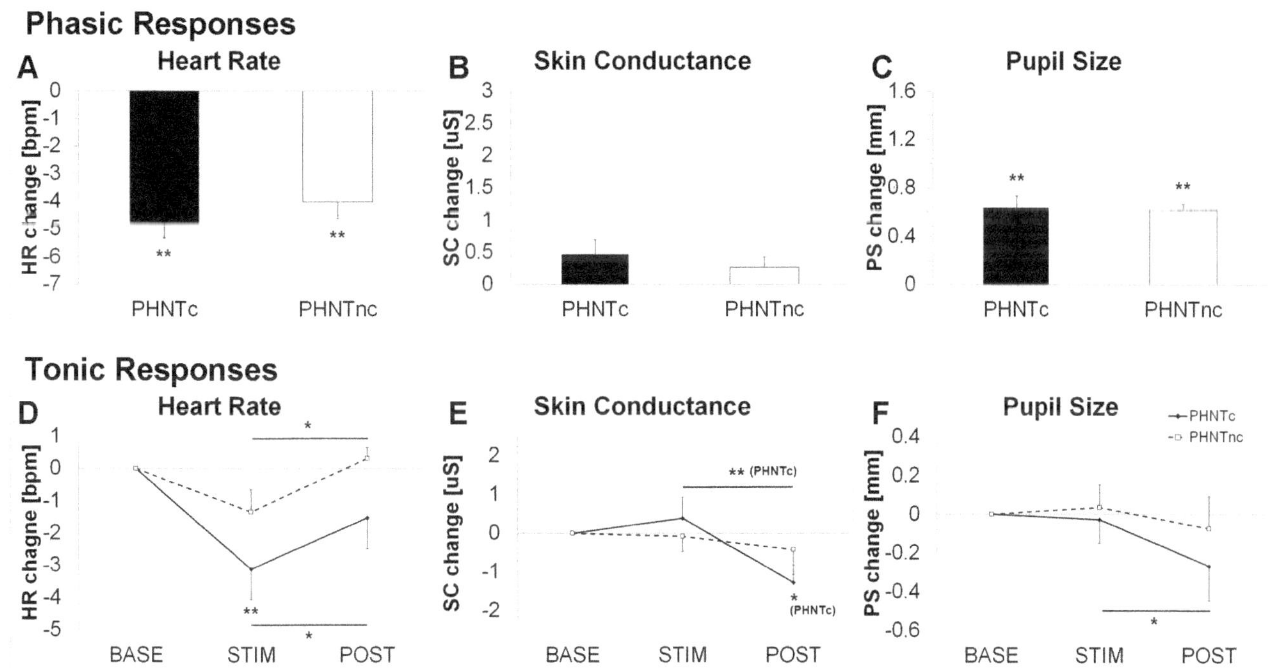

Figure 3. Influence of credibility on autonomic response modulation to phantom acupuncture. Phasic and tonic responses for heart rate (**A** and **D**), skin conductance (**B** and **E**), and pupil size (**C** and **F**) were contrasted between credible (PHNTc) and non-credible (PHNTnc) phantom acupuncture. n.b. *<0.05, **<0.01. Error bars represent standard error of the mean.

Subjects were either acupuncture-naïve (n = 2) or had only a few experiences with acupuncture treatment (n = 18, 6.0±6.7 times, mean±STD), and were informed that there would be two identical experimental acupuncture sessions. Subjects laid supine with their vision of distal body regions blocked by a barrier. They were told to look at the video display projected onto a monitor on the ceiling and were thus prevented from viewing the intervention occurring at the acupuncture point in their periphery (**Figure 1C**).

The PHNT session aimed to control for 'needling credibility,' but without somatosensory afference. In turn, the REAL session included both the 'somatosensory stimulation' as well as the needling credibility inherent to acupuncture.

Psychophysical Data Collection and Analysis

After each session, subjects were presented with a 10-point VAS and were asked to rate the intensity of different sensations they felt during the STIM period. We used an in-house Korean version of MGH Acupuncture Sensation Scale [27] comprising different "*deqi*" sensations (i.e. aching, soreness, pressure, heaviness, fullness, warmth, cool, numbness, tingling, and dull pain). In order to quantify the total intensity of acupuncture sensation experienced, we used the previously described MASS-Index [27]. This index attempts to balance breadth and depth of sensations as well as the number of different sensations chosen by the subject. The MASS index (MI) and individual sensation intensities were compared between stimulation groups using a paired *t*-test, significant at $p<0.05$.

Retrospective Re-classification According to Needling Credibility

After finishing both REAL and PHNT sessions, subjects were retrospectively separated into phantom credible (PHNTc, high needling credibility, n = 11) and phantom non-credible (PHNTnc, low needling credibility, n = 9) groups using a questionnaire and interview that evaluate the credibility of the procedure – e.g., whether or not they were able to differentiate the difference between real and phantom acupuncture, and if they believed they received real needle acupuncture in both sessions. Four subjects in the PHNTnc subgroup recognized the procedure as placebo when they noticed that the video clip of acupuncture needling was not synchronized with their hand's spontaneous movement. Five subjects in the PHNTnc subgroup had low credibility because they did not have any acupuncture sensation at the acupoint or surrounding region (**Figure 2**).

Multi-modal Physiological Data Collection and Analysis

To investigate any autonomic modulation specific to somatosensory afference or needling credibility following acupuncture, we recorded heart rate (HR), skin conductance (SC), and pupil size (PS) throughout the entire session (7.5 min). Subjects rested for at least 10 minutes prior to initiation of data collection. Electrocardiogram and electrical skin conductance were measured using commercial devices (PowerLab/800, ADinstruments, Australia) with a 1 kHz sampling rate. Pupil diameter was measured using a custom constructed pupilometry system that includes an image acquisition system (an IR camera and optical devices attached on a helmet) and analysis software enabling the estimation of precise pupil diameter for every image frame (30 frames/sec) using geometric correction, which compensate the errors induced by lens of the camera and by projection on two-dimensional image plane [28].

ANS outflow metrics (HR, SC, and PS) were computed for estimation of both a tonic response and a phasic event-related response. For the tonic response, the mean HR, SC and PS were calculated for three separate windows: BASE, STIM, and POST. For the phasic responses, the maximum change scores (typically decrease for HR, and increase for SC and PS) were calculated in a

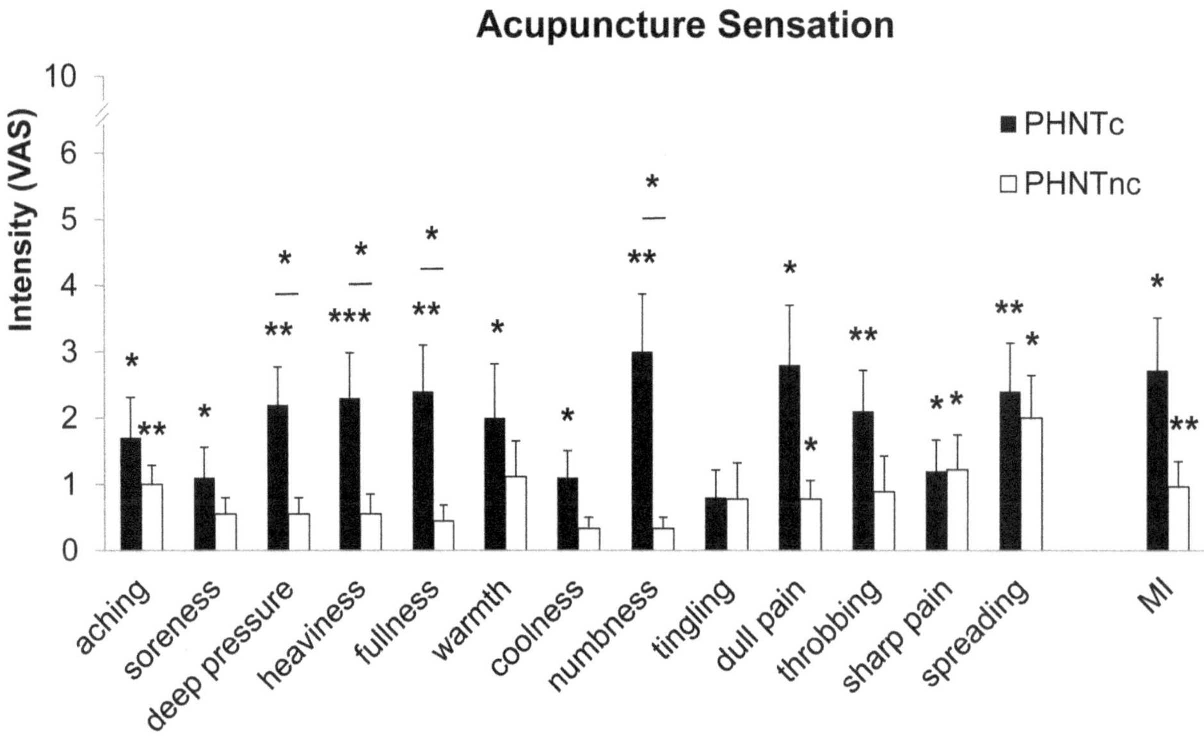

Figure 4. Influence of credibility on acupuncture sensations to phantom acupuncture. PHNTc reported significantly greater sensation intensity for numbness and dull pain (i.e. *deqi* sensations). n.b. *<0.05, **<0.01, ***<0.001. Error bars represent standard error of the mean.

6 second window (0~6 seconds after each stimulation onset), which was contrast to a baseline window (preceding 5 seconds, accounting for acupuncturist hand motion as previously mentioned; i.e., −5.8 to −0.8 sec, with −0.8 to 0 second excluded due to acupuncturist's reaction time).

Results

For the 20 subjects, order of REAL or PHNT session was pseudo-randomized such that 10 received real acupuncture first, while the rest received phantom acupuncture first. There was no significant difference in age (REAL first: 21.1±2.9 years old, PHNT first: 22.5±2.3 years old; mean±STD), handedness (REAL first: 73.4±28.9%, PHNT first: 68.3±54.7%; 100%: right handed, −100%: left handed), positive expectation about acupuncture efficacy (REAL first: 2.4±0.2, PHNT first: 2.3±0.5; out of 1 to 5 range) or state/trait anxiety (STAI-state: REAL first: 27.8±7.5, PHNT first: 26.8±5.6; STAI-trait: REAL first: 33.7±5.2, PHNT first: 31.8±8.3) between the two order groups. From retrospective credibility questionnaires, we classified our subjects into PHNTc (PHNT credible; who reported high needling credibility for PHNT, n = 11) and PHNTnc (PHNT non-credible; who reported low needling credibility, n = 9).

Needling credibility effects: PHNTc vs PHNTnc

For phasic ANS responses, regardless of needling credibility, we noted decreased HR (PHNTc = −4.75±0.58 BPM, P<0.001; PHNTnc = −4.01±0.62 BPM, P<0.001, mean±SEM) and increased PS (PHNTc = 0.64±0.10 mm, P<0.001; PHNTnc = 0.62±0.05 mm, P<0.001) in response to visual stimulation. We did not note a phasic SC response. No significant differences were noted between PHNTc and PHNTnc in terms of phasic ANS response (**Figure 3A–C**).

For tonic ANS responses, we noted significant decrease in tonic HR for PHNTc (Δ = −3.12±0.94 BPM, P<0.01) but not for PHNTnc (Δ = −1.33±0.68 BPM, P = 0.09) during STIM (compared to BASE). During POST, the tonic HR rebounded back to BASE levels. For SC and PS, only PHNTc showed significant tonic decreases during POST compared to STIM (SC response: Δ = −1.27±0.45 μS, P<0.001; PS response: Δ = −0.27±0.18 mm, P<0.05) (**Figure 3D–F**).

Interestingly, following PHNTc, subjects reported many different acupuncture sensations (e.g. aching = 1.7±0.6, P<0.05; soreness = 1.1±0.5, P<0.05; deep pressure = 2.2±0.6, P<0.01; heaviness = 2.3±0.7, P<0.001; fullness = 2.4±0.7, P<0.01; warmth = 2.0±0.8, P<0.05; coolness = 1.1±0.4, P<0.05; numbness = 3.0±0.9, P<0.01; dull pain = 2.8±0.9, P<0.05; throbbing = 2.1±0.6, P<0.01; sharp pain = 1.2±0.5, P<0.05; spreading = 2.4±0.7, P<0.01). For PHNTnc, reported sensations were more mild and fewer in number (i.e. aching = 1.0±0.3, P<0.01; dull pain = 0.8±0.3, P<0.05; sharp pain = 1.2±0.5, P<0.05; and spreading = 2.0±0.6, P<0.05). Significant differences between credible versus non-credible PHNT subgroups were noted for deep pressure (PHNTc = 2.2±0.6, PHNTnc = 0.6±0.2, P<0.05), heaviness (PHNTc = 2.3±0.7, PHNTnc = 0.6±0.3, P<0.05), fullness (PHNTc = 2.4±0.7, PHNTnc = 0.4±0.2, P<0.05), and numbness (PHNTc = 3.0±0.9, PHNTnc = 0.3±0.2, P<0.05) – all classic *deqi* sensations. Trending differences were noted for dull pain (PHNTc = 2.8±0.9, PHNTnc = 0.8±0.3, P = 0.06) and MI (PHNTc = 2.7±0.8, PHNTnc = 1.0±0.4, P = 0.08) (**Figure 4**).

Acupuncture somatosensory stimulation effects: REAL vs PHNTc

Comparisons between REAL and PHNTc were based on the data collected only from subjects who regarded phantom acupuncture as real (i.e., PHNTc) and was done using paired *t*-

tests. For phasic ANS response, there was significant phasic SC increase in response to somatosensory stimulation, for REAL (1.56±0.50 μS, P<0.001) but only trending response for PHNTc (0.47±0.23 μS, P = 0.07). We also noted significant phasic HR decreases (REAL = −5.07±0.87 BPM, P<0.001; PHNTc = −4.75±1.92 BPM, P<0.001) and PS increases (REAL = 0.70±0.10 mm, P<0.001; PHNTc = 0.64±0.10 mm, P<0.001) for both REAL and PHNTc sessions (**Figure 5A–C**).

We also noted significant tonic SC increase (STIM vs. BASE) for REAL (1.31±0.37 μS, P<0.01) but not PHNTc (0.39±0.54 μS, P = 0.49). Additionally, significant tonic SC decreases were noted from STIM to POST for both REAL (Δ = −1.67±1.15 μS, P<0.001) and PHNTc (Δ = −1.66±0.98 μS, P<0.001). For tonic HR response, significant decreases for STIM vs. BASE were noted for both REAL and PHNTc (PHNTc = −3.12±1.79 BPM, P<0.05; REAL = −2.24±1.35 BPM, P<0.01). Tonic HR rebounded back to baseline levels during POST (Δ = 1.60±0.98 BPM in PHNTc, P<0.05; Δ = 1.64±1.15 in REAL, P<0.001). Significant tonic PS decreases were found for POST (vs STIM) only in PHNTc (Δ = −0.31±0.66, P<0.05), but not in REAL (Δ = −0.24±0.48, P = 0.22) (**Figure 5D–F**).

Acupuncture sensations, such as aching, soreness, deep pressure, sharp pain etc., were reported following real acupuncture stimulation (REAL). Interestingly after PHNTc, even without any direct somatosensory stimulation, similar acupuncture sensation intensities as following REAL were also reported (aching pain: PHNTc = 1.7±0.6, REAL = 3.5±0.7, P = 0.07; deep pressure pain, PHNTc = 2.2±0.6, REAL = 2.9±0.7, P = 0.23; heaviness, PHNTc = 2.3±0.7, REAL = 2.6±0.7, P = 0.56; fullness, PHNTc = 2.4±0.7, REAL = 2.9±0.7, P = 0.43; numbness, PHNTc = 3.0±0.9, REAL = 2.3±0.7, P = 0.24; dull pain, PHNTc = 2.8±0.9, REAL = 2.5±0.6, P = 0.72). Greater sensation intensity was noted for REAL for a few other sensations, such as soreness (PHNTc = 1.1±0.5, REAL = 3.2±0.9, P<0.05), tingling pain (PHNTc = 0.8±0.4, REAL = 3.8±0.9, P<0.01) and sharp pain (PHNTc = 1.2±0.5, REAL = 4.1±0.7, P<0.01) (**Figure 6**).

Significant correlation between acupuncture sensation and autonomic response was found in PHNTc (deep pressure vs. phasic HR decrease: r = 0.73, P<0.05; deep pressure vs. phasic PS increase: r = −0.83, P<0.05; dull pain vs. phasic PS increase: r = −0.90, P<0.05) but not in REAL.

Temporal evolution of ANS response to REAL and PHNT

During the needle insertion, before the needle manipulation (1st–8th stim.), significant HR deceleration was observed in the three groups (REAL = −8.25±3.85 BPM, P<0.0001; PHNTc = −9.67±4.02, P<0.0001; PHNTnc = −9.25±4.59, P<0.0001). The amplitude of HR decrease, in subsequent needle manipulation, was then reduced but still significant compared to the baseline (P<0.05 for all events, **Figure 7A** for individual response, **Figure 3A** for average response of eight stimuli). No significant difference was found between groups at each event.

Pupil size also showed maximum increase at needle insertion in all groups (REAL = 1.57±0.74 mm, P<0.0001; PHNTc = 1.56±0.62 mm, P<0.0001; PHNTnc = 1.62±0.63 mm, P<0.0001), and maintained greater than the baseline (P<0.01 for all events, except the response from PHNTc at 8th stimulation; Δ = 0.48±0.79 mm, P = 0.09) (**Figure 7C** for individual response, **Figure 3C** for average response of eight stimuli). Significantly greater PS increase was observed at 8th needle manipulation in REAL than PHNTc (REAL = 0.64±0.35 mm, PHNTc = 0.36±0.28, P<0.05) (**Figure 7C**).

Significant SC increase was also produced by needle insertion (REAL = 4.81±3.56 μS, P<0.0001; PHNTc = 4.02±4.30 μS, P<0.05; PHNTnc = 3.01±1.78 μS, P<0.001), and the responses were reduced in subsequent manipulation but significantly

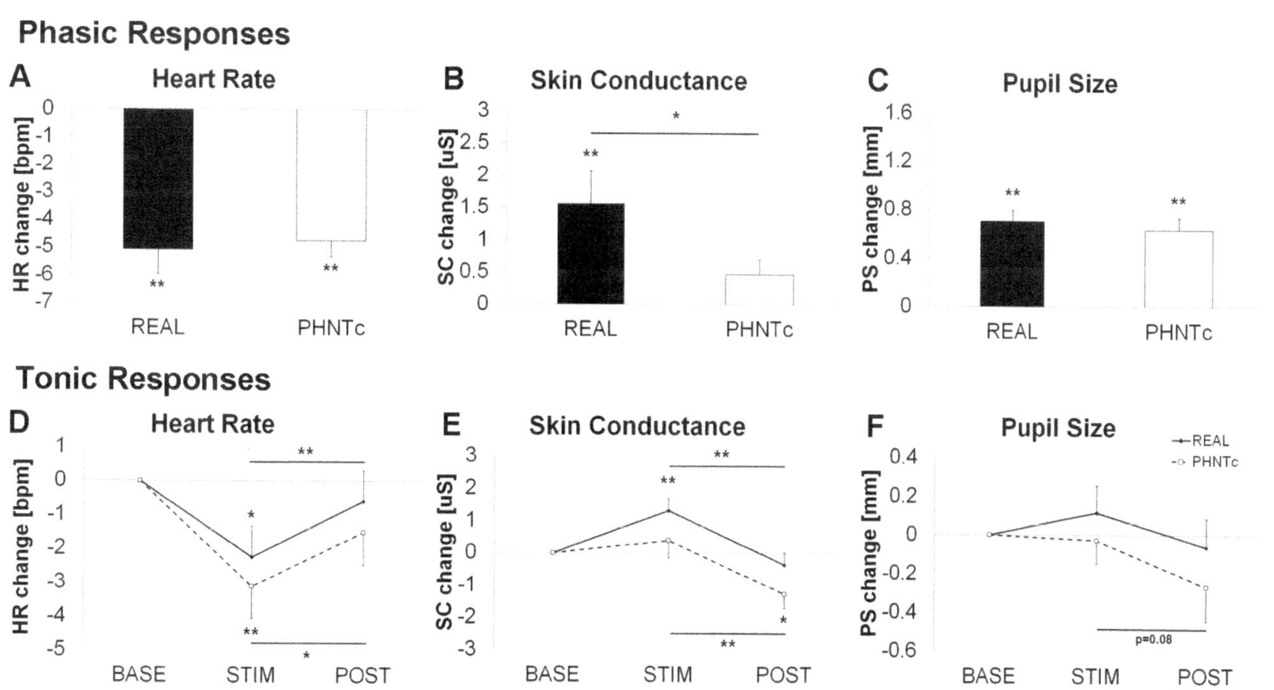

Figure 5. Influence of somatosensory needling on autonomic response modulation to real and phantom acupuncture. Phasic and tonic responses for heart rate (**A** and **D**), skin conductance (**B** and **E**), and pupil size (**C** and **F**) were contrasted between real (REAL) and credible (PHNTc) phantom acupuncture. Comparisons between REAL and PHNTc were based on the data collected only from subjects who regarded phantom acupuncture as real (i.e. PHNTc) and was done using paired *t*-tests. n.b. *<0.05, **<0.01. Error bars represent standard error of the mean.

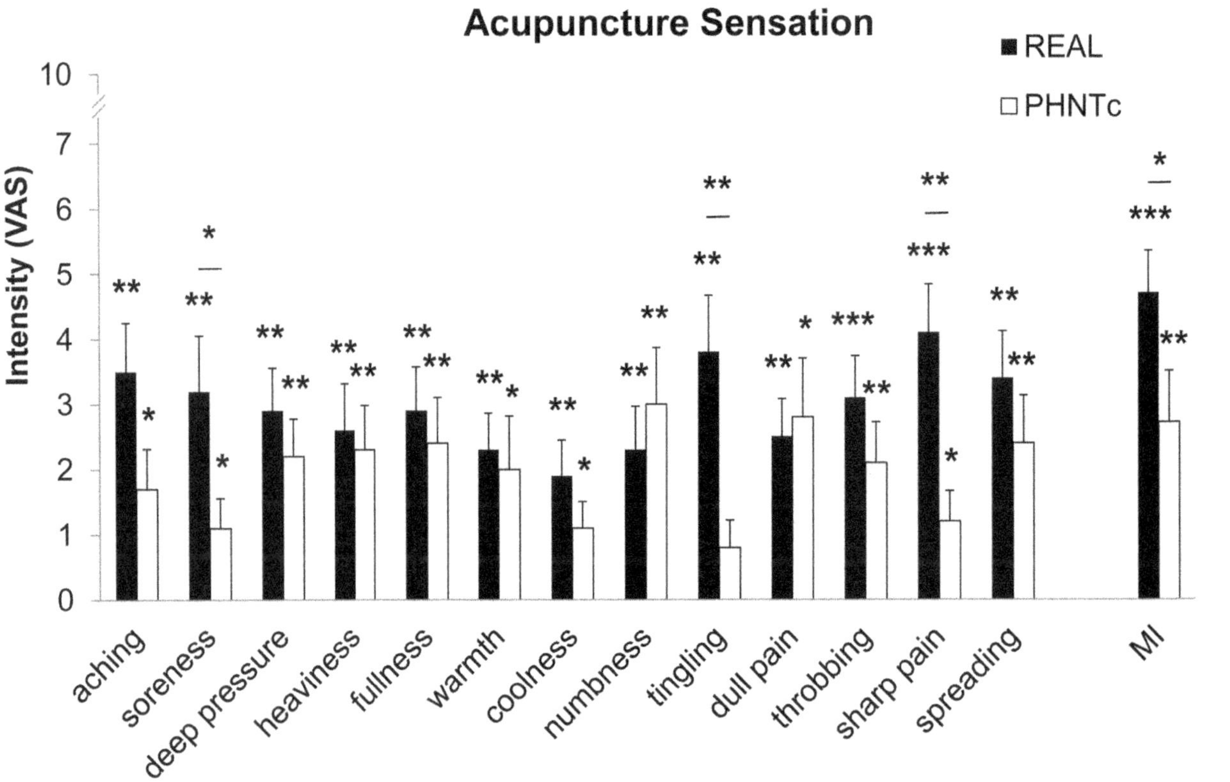

Figure 6. Influence of somatosensory needling on acupuncture sensations to real (REAL) and credible (PHNTc) phantom acupuncture. PHNTc reported similar sensation intensity as REAL for several *deqi*-related sensations (e.g., deep pressure, heaviness, fullness, numbness, dull pain). REAL produced greater sensation intensity for soreness, tingling, and sharp pain, as well as overall *deqi* sensation (i.e. MI). Comparisons between REAL and PHNTc were based on the data collected only from subjects who regarded phantom acupuncture as real (i.e. PHNTc) and was done using paired *t*-tests. n.b. *<0.05, **<0.01, ***<0.001. Error bars represent standard error of the mean.

maintained compared to the baseline in REAL ($P<0.05$ for all event) but not in PHNTc ($P>0.07$ for all events) and PHNTnc ($P>0.2$ for all events) (**Figure 7B** for individual response, **Figure 3B** for average response of eight stimuli).

Discussion

In this study, we have developed and tested a new form of placebo acupuncture, referred to as phantom acupuncture, which was characterized by an acupuncture needling intervention induced solely by visual display. We applied real (REAL) and phantom (PHNT) acupuncture and retrospectively re-classified subjects into two groups based on PHNT credibility (PHNTc, who found phantom acupuncture credible, $n = 11$; and PHNTnc, who did not find phantom acupuncture credible, $n = 9$). Physiological responses to REAL and PHNT were measured via autonomic response (heart rate, skin conductance, pupil size), while psychophysical responses were assessed by subjective ratings of needle sensation (Table 1). Real acupuncture induced greater skin conductance response, suggesting that the somatosensory component of acupuncture underlies the sympathetic outflow produced by acupuncture needle stimulation. We found that both real and phantom acupuncture (when credible) induced notable acupuncture sensation. The credibility of the ritual, a contextual component of acupuncture, was important for inducing robust *deqi* sensation, but was less important for autonomic response to purely visual phantom acupuncture, suggesting that some stimulus-associated autonomic response may be the result of subconscious processing that does not play a role in conscious cognitive re-evaluation of a ritual as credible or not.

Needling Credibility Effect: increased parasympathetic and decreased sympathetic activity

Physiological response to visual stimuli purporting to reflect needles entering the subject's skin, and being twisted, depended on whether or not the subjects believed the procedure to be credible. By contrasting PHNTc with PHNTnc, we were able to explore the acupuncture needling context independent from any somatosensory afference. Our data demonstrated that while phasic autonomic response to visual scenes of needle stimulation were not influenced by needling credibility (i.e. PHNTnc vs PHNTc), tonic autonomic responses were influenced. Specifically, compared to PHNTnc, PHNTc demonstrated HR deceleration during the stimulation period and decreased SCR/PS following stimulation (see **Figure 3**). Needling credibility may be associated with greater positive expectation of acupuncture efficacy and a generally more relaxed state, reflected in increased parasympathetic and decreased sympathetic activity, consistent with our data.

Our results showed that needling credibility influenced multi-organ autonomic response to needle-related stimuli. Previous studies have found that several brain regions implicated in placebo responses, such as pregenual anterior cingulate cortex, amygdala, and periaqueductal gray [29] are also associated with peripheral autonomic outflow and are components of a central autonomic network [30]. Other studies have noted that expectancy enhances heart rate change and sympathetic responses to deep brain

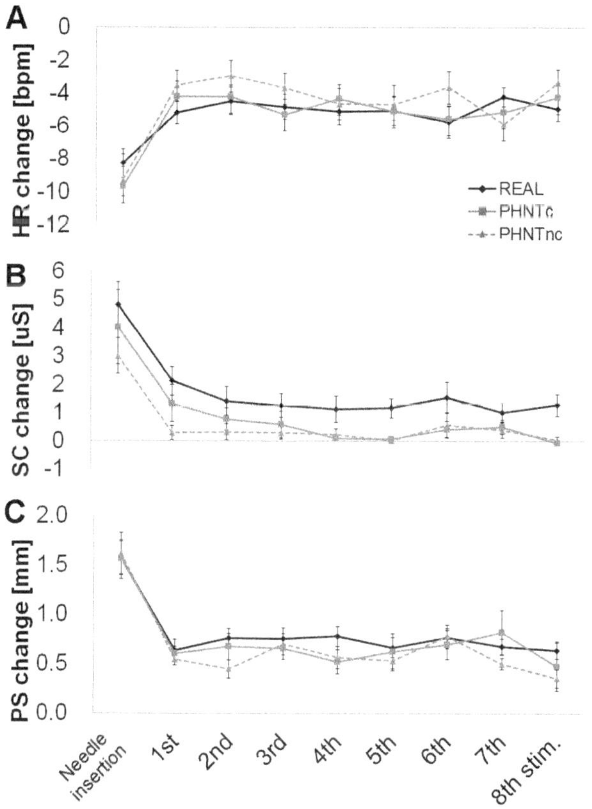

Figure 7. Temporal evolution of autonomic response to real (REAL) and phantom (credible, PHNTc; non-credible, PHNTnc) acupuncture. Needle insertion, whether real or phantom, produced significantly greater (A) HR decrease, (B) SC increase and (C) PS increase, compared to needle manipulation. ANS response to needle manipulation was relatively stable over all 8 manipulations for REAL (n = 20), PHNTc (n = 11), and PHNTnc (n = 9). SC increase was greater for REAL compared to PHNTc and especially PHNTnc, consistently over all stimuli. Error bars represent standard error of the mean.

stimulation of subthalamic limbic region in Parkinson patients [31]. In addition, placebo analgesia has been linked with reduced beta-adrenergic (not cardiovagal) heart response [32,33]. Thus, autonomic response may be an important factor in expectation and placebo-mediated outcomes. Phantom acupuncture clearly produces autonomic response and future studies should also link these multi-organ outflows with clinical outcomes in patient populations.

Interestingly, both phasic and tonic ANS response was evident for all three groups (REAL, PHNTc, PHNTnc), though more prominent in PHNT when the stimulus was judged to be credible. Visual feedback may be an important factor in augmenting a placebo intervention. Kaptchuk et al. have suggested that medical devices have an enhanced placebo effect and, specifically, that sham acupuncture is more effective than placebo pill on self-reported pain and symptom severity [34,35]. This hypothesis was recently corroborated in a systematic review of migraine prophylaxis [36]. Most prior sham acupuncture procedures include tactile (in addition to visual) stimulation, and can be characterized by adequate needling credibility. However, tactile stimulation may be an important component of a specific acupuncture effect, and some researchers have raised this point in questioning previous efficacy clinical trials which included both real and sham control acupuncture procedures [11,12]. While the visual component of acupuncture was found to also induce notable physiological response, particularly when phantom acupuncture was credible, our novel procedure was able to remove the somatosensory component and may be a viable procedure in future clinical trials aimed at dissociating the somatosensory versus visual components of acupuncture therapy.

Interestingly, the rated intensity of several acupuncture sensations (e.g. dull pain, heaviness, fullness, and numbness) associated with *deqi* sensation [27], were similar for PHNTc and REAL (see **Figure 6**). Hence, needling credibility leads to a mental rationalization of a perception anticipated by real needling (as all subjects experienced this at their initial session), even when a lack of somatosensory afference was incongruent to visual afference associated with needle insertion and stimulation. This effect may be similar to the rubber hand illusion, where body ownership is extended to an inanimate object, in this case a video recording [37]. Future studies should specifically explore if acupuncture sensation intensity can serve as a marker for needling credibility, and whether such sensations are closely linked to therapeutic efficacy in acupuncture trials. If sensation is the important variable for clinical outcomes, and if the sensation can be produced by needling credibility with no somatosensory afference, then this can be linked to the acupuncture placebo effect.

Somatosensory stimulation effect: sympathetic activation in SC response

To investigate the somatosensory stimulation effect, REAL and PHNTc were compared. Both REAL and PHNTc included a visual feedback component and were both credible acupuncture interventions, though PHNTc did not involve somatosensory afference. REAL showed significantly greater phasic and tonic SC responses, while PHNTc did not demonstrate significant SC response. This suggests that sudomotor activity is specifically driven by the tactile component of acupuncture needle stimulation. Somatosensory afference can be delivered by acupuncture

Table 1. Summarization of the physiological responses to real and phantom acupuncture stimulation.

	Parasympathetic tone	Sympathetic tone	Orienting response	Deqi sensation
REAL		↑ (SC-phasic/tonic)	↓ HR-phasic, ↑ PS-phasic	+++ (for most sensation items)
PHNTc	↑ (SC-tonic, PS-tonic)		↓ HR-phasic, ↑ PS-phasic	++ (for deep pressure, heaviness, fullness, numbness, dull pain, and spreading)
PHNTnc			↓ HR-phasic, ↑ PS-phasic	+ (for dull and sharp pain)

HR: Heart Rate, SC: Skin Conductance, PS: Pupil Szie, tonic: tonic response, phasic: phasic response, +++: around 2–4 out of 10 scale, ++: around 2–3 out of 10 scale, +: around 1 out of 10 scale.

through an ascending pathway, which carries information from spinal cord to reticular formation, PAG and thalamus, and then to ACC, SI/SII, insula and prefrontal cortex, where tactile input can have broader cognitive/affective influence [7]. In our study, SCR was mainly observed with REAL stimulation, which suggests that somatosensory afference specifically supports the previously noted sympathetic response to acupuncture [5,36] and may be similar to sympathetic modulation by other pain or pain-like stimuli [38].

Visual stimulus effects: the orienting response

As previously noted, the visual stimulus itself may induce physiological response regardless of needling credibility. In fact, PHNTc, PHNTnc, and REAL all shared the same visual stimulus and produced physiological activity consistent with an orienting response (OR). Physiologically, OR is characterized by parasympathetically driven HR deceleration, sympathetically driven SCR increase, and behavioral orienting toward novel stimuli [39]. OR is also associated with pupil dilation linked to emotional processing of stimuli [40,41]. These mixed autonomic responses likely reflect supra-spinal feedback and may be differentially associated with different aspects of cognitive and affective processing involved with attention distribution towards novel stimuli. Particularly for needle insertion, which was done before needle manipulation (see **Figure 7**), all three groups showed significant HR deceleration, SC increase, and PS dilation compared to the baseline, suggesting that the visual component of needle insertion (and perhaps needle manipulation) leads to a physiological OR. Subsequent needle manipulation events during the STIM period showed less robust ANS response compared to needle insertion, suggesting diminished salience to the subject leading to diminished physiological arousal. Importantly, lack of notable habituation across repeated needle manipulation stimuli for all three groups suggests that saliency was conserved and difference analyses using summary ANS outcome measures (pooled over all stimuli) were not confounded by preferential habituation in one or more groups.

The fact that all three groups demonstrated robust ANS response may have significant implications in terms of understanding the placebo effect. Most discussions of the placebo postulate that environmental learning cues mediated through either conscious expectations or classical conditioning are the principle psychological mechanism of placebo responses [42]. Recently there has been evidence that suggests that non-conscious and implicit framing may play a key role [43]. Our study found robust ANS outflow in response to phantom acupuncture, even when credibility was compromised. As sensation and autonomic response were likely to be classically conditioned from subjects' experience in the training session with real acupuncture, any ANS outflow following phantom acupuncture, whether credible or not, may feed back to the brain via afferent autonomic pathways and play an important role in subsequent sub-conscious placebo effects.

Psychophysical response to real and phantom acupuncture

Interestingly, while overall *deqi* sensation (i.e. MASS Index) was greater for REAL compared to PHNT, when the latter was credible, many key *deqi* sensations (e.g. dull pain, numbness, and deep pressure) were similar in intensity. This suggests that *deqi* sensations can be induced not only by somatosensory afference but also by visual suggestion of needle stimulation and needling credibility [37,44]. In fact, when PHNT was credible, greater *deqi* sensation intensity (e.g. deep pressure) was associated with greater phasic HR decrease and with smaller phasic PS increase, suggesting that credibility-mediated acupuncture sensation raised parasympathetic activity, and the increased activity may be linked with clinical outcomes in patients (i.e. placebo effect) as the parasympathetic shift or the sympathetic drop has been believed to be one of underlying mechanisms in clinical acupuncture efficacy.

Several limitations should be noted. Our study was performed in healthy subjects (i.e., young university students) and not patient populations, and sample size of this study was quite small. As acupuncture is a therapeutic intervention applied for various pathological states, these results may not extend to, for instance, chronic pain patients. Thus, further study on large sample of patients should be performed for clinical implication. Additionally, our outcomes included autonomic outflow and psychometric outcomes. More clinically-relevant outcomes such as evoked pain modulation, should also be explored. Other physiological outcomes, such as brain response measured by neuroimaging should also be investigated.

In conclusion, our study developed and tested a new form of placebo acupuncture, referred to as phantom acupuncture, which was characterized by an acupuncture needling intervention induced solely by visual display. We found that both real and phantom acupuncture (when credible) induced notable acupuncture sensation. Real acupuncture induced greater skin conductance response, suggesting that the somatosensory component of acupuncture underlies the sympathetic outflow produced by acupuncture needle stimulation. We also found that credibility of the ritual, a contextual component of acupuncture, was important for inducing robust *deqi* sensation, but was less important for autonomic response to purely visual phantom acupuncture, suggesting that some stimulus-associated autonomic response may be the result of sub-conscious processing that does not play a role in conscious cognitive re-evaluation of a ritual as credible or not.

Author Contributions

Conceived and designed the experiments: JL JK SL WC KP. Performed the experiments: JL JK SL WC KP. Analyzed the data: JL VN KP. Contributed to the writing of the manuscript: JL VN TJK KP.

References

1. Langevin HM, Wayne PM, Macpherson H, Schnyer R, Milley RM, et al. (2011) Paradoxes in acupuncture research: strategies for moving forward. Evid Based Complement Alternat Med. 2011: 180805.
2. Linde K, Streng A, Jürgens S, Hoppe A, Brinkhaus B, et al. (2005) Acupuncture for patients with migraine: a randomized controlled trial. JAMA. 293: 2118–2125.
3. Yao E, Gerritz PK, Henricson E, Abresch T, Kim J, et al. (2012) Randomized controlled trial comparing acupuncture with placebo acupuncture for the treatment of carpal tunnel syndrome. PM R. 4: 367–373.
4. Hempel S, Taylor SL, Solloway MR, Miake-Lye IM, Beroes JM, et al. (2014) Evidence Map of Acupuncture [Internet]. Washington (DC): Department of Veterans Affairs. Available: http://www.ncbi.nlm.nih.gov/books/NBK185072/.
5. Napadow V, Lee J, Kim J, Cina S, Maeda Y, et al. (2013). Brain correlates of phasic autonomic response to acupuncture stimulation: an event-related fMRI study. Hum Brain Mapp. 34: 2592–2606.
6. Madsen MV, Gøtzsche PC, Hróbjartsson A (2009) Acupuncture treatment for pain: systematic review of randomised clinical trials with acupuncture, placebo acupuncture, and no acupuncture groups. BMJ. 338: a3115. doi: 10.1136/bmj.a3115.
7. Almeida TF, Roizenblatt S, Tufik S (2004) Afferent pain pathways: a neuroanatomical review. Brain Res. 1000: 40–56.
8. McGlone F, Reilly D (2010) The cutaneous sensory system. Neurosci Biobehav Rev. 34: 148–159.

9. Streitberger K, Kleinhenz J (1998) Introducing a placebo needle into acupuncture research. Lancet. 25: 271–275.
10. Park J, White A, Lee H, Ernst E (1999) Development of a new sham needle. Acupunct Med. 17: 110–112.
11. White P, Lewith G, Hopwood V, Prescott P (2003) The placebo needle, is it a valid and convincing placebo for use in acupuncture trials? A randomised, single-blind, cross-over pilot trial. Pain. 106: 401–409.
12. Lundeberg T, Lund I, Näslund J (2012) The needling sensation: A factor contributing to the specific effects of acupuncture? Acupuncture and related Therapies. 1: 2–4.
13. Shalev AY, Sahar T, Freedman S, Peri T, Glick N, et al. (1998) A prospective study of heart rate response following trauma and the subsequent development of posttraumatic stress disorder. Arch Gen Psychiatry. 55: 553–559.
14. Sparrow K (2007) Analysis of heart rate variability in acupuncture practice: can it improve outcome? Medical Acupuncture. 19: 37–41.
15. Abercrombie HC, Chambers AS, Greischar L, Monticelli RM (2008) Orienting, emotion, and memory: phasic and tonic variation in heart rate predicts memory for emotional pictures in men. Neurobiol Learn Mem. 90: 644–650.
16. Critchley HD, Mathias CJ, Josephs O, O'Doherty J, Zanini S, et al. (2003) Human cingulate cortex and autonomic control: converging neuroimaging and clinical evidence. Brain. 126: 2139–2152.
17. Anderson AK, Yamaguchi Y, Grabski W, Lacka D (2006) Emotional memories are not all created equal: evidence for selective memory enhancement. Learn Mem. 13: 711–718.
18. Yao T, Andersson S, Thorén P (1982) Long-lasting cardiovascular depression induced by acupuncture-like stimulation of the sciatic nerve in unanaesthetized spontaneously hypertensive rats. Brain Res. 240: 77–85.
19. Knardahl S, Elam M, Olausson B, Wallin BG (1998) Sympathetic nerve activity after acupuncture in humans. Pain. 75: 19–25.
20. Cao XD, Xu SF, Lu WX (1983) Inhibition of sympathetic nervous system by acupuncture. Acupunct Electrother Res. 8: 25–35.
21. Haker E, Egekvist H, Bjerring P (2000) Effect of sensory stimulation (acupuncture) on sympathetic and parasympathetic activities in healthy subjects. J Auton Nerv Syst. 79: 52–59.
22. Mori H, Nishijo K, Kawamura H, Abo T (2002) Unique immunomodulation by electro-acupuncture in humans possibly via stimulation of the autonomic nervous system. Neurosci Lett. 320: 21–24.
23. Lee S, Lee MS, Choi JY, Lee SW, Jeong SY, et al. (2010) Acupuncture and heart rate variability: a systematic review. Auton Neurosci. 155: 5–13.
24. Dennehy EB, Webb A, Suppes T (2002) Assessment of beliefs in the effectiveness of acupuncture for treatment of psychiatric symptoms. J Altern Complement Med. 8: 421–425.
25. Oldfield RC (1971) The assessment and analysis of handedness: the Edinburgh inventory. Neuropsychologia. 9(1): 97–113.
26. Beissner F, Deichmann R, Henke C, Bär KJ (2012) Acupuncture–deep pain with an autonomic dimension? Neuroimage. 60: 653–660.
27. Kong J, Gollub R, Huang T, Polich G, Napadow V, et al. (2007) Acupuncture de qi, from qualitative history to quantitative measurement. J Altern Complement Med. 13: 1059–1070.
28. Kim J, Park K, Khang G (2004) A method for size estimation of amorphous pupil in 3-dimensional geometry. Conf Proc IEEE Eng Med Biol Soc. 2: 1451–1454.
29. Zubieta JK, Stohler CS (2009) Neurobiological mechanisms of placebo responses. Ann N Y Acad Sci. 1156: 198–210.
30. Beissner F, Meissner K, Bär KJ, Napadow V (2013) The autonomic brain: an activation likelihood estimation meta-analysis for central processing of autonomic function. J Neurosci. 33(25): 10503–10511.
31. Lanotte M, Lopiano L, Torre E, Bergamasco B, Colloca L, et al. (2005) Expectation enhances autonomic responses to stimulation of the human subthalamic limbic region. Brain Behav Immun. 19: 500–509.
32. Pollo A, Vighetti S, Rainero I, Benedetti F (2003) Placebo analgesia and the heart. Pain. 102: 125–133.
33. Meissner K (2011) The placebo effect and the autonomic nervous system: evidence for an intimate relationship. Philos Trans R Soc Lond B Biol Sci. 366(1572): 1808–1817.
34. Kaptchuk TJ, Goldman P, Stone DA, Stason WB (2000) Do medical devices have enhanced placebo effects? J Clin Epidemiol. 53: 786–792.
35. Kaptchuk TJ, Stason WB, Davis RB, Legedza AR, Schnyer RN, et al. (2006) Sham device v inert pill: randomised controlled trial of two placebo treatments. BMJ. 332: 391–397.
36. Knardahl S, Elam M, Olausson B, Wallin BG (1998) Sympathetic nerve activity after acupuncture in humans. Pain. 75(1): 19–25.
37. Botvinick M, Cohen J (1998) Rubber hands 'feel' touch that eyes see. Nature. 391: 756.
38. Piché M, Arsenault M, Rainville P (2010) Dissection of perceptual, motor and autonomic components of brain activity evoked by noxious stimulation. Pain. 149: 453–462.
39. Sokolov E, Cacioppo J (1997) Orienting and defense reflexes: Vector coding and cardiac response. In: Lang P, Simons R, Balaban M, editors. Attention and Orienting: Sensory and Motivational Processes. Mahwah, NJ: Lawrence Erlbaum Associates Publishers.
40. Bradley MM (2009) Natural selective attention: orienting and emotion. Psychophysiology. 46: 1–11.
41. Lang PJ, Bradley MM (2010) Emotion and the motivational brain. Biol Psychol. 84: 437–450.
42. Finniss DG, Kaptchuk TJ, Miller F, Benedetti F (2010) Biological, clinical, and ethical advances of placebo effects. Lancet. 375(9715): 686–695.
43. Jensen KB, Kaptchuk TJ, Kirsch I, Raicek J, Lindstrom KM, et al. (2012) Nonconscious activation of placebo and nocebo pain responses. Proc Natl Acad Sci U S A. 109(39): 15959–15964.
44. Beissner F, Marzolff I (2012) Investigation of Acupuncture Sensation Patterns under Sensory Deprivation Using a Geographic Information System. Evid Based Complement Alternat Med. 2012: 591304.

Effects of Aprepitant on the Pharmacokinetics of Controlled-Release Oral Oxycodone in Cancer Patients

Yutaka Fujiwara[1,3]*, Masanori Toyoda[1], Naoko Chayahara[1], Naomi Kiyota[1], Takanobu Shimada[1], Yoshinori Imamura[1], Toru Mukohara[1,2], Hironobu Minami[1,2]

1 Division of Medical Oncology/Hematology, Kobe University Graduate School of Medicine, Kobe, Japan, **2** Cancer Center, Kobe University Graduate School of Medicine, Kobe, Japan, **3** Division of Investigational Cancer Therapeutics, Exploratory Oncology Research & Clinical Trial Center, National Cancer Center Hospital, Chiba, Japan

Abstract

Purpose: Oxycodone is a μ-opioid receptor agonist widely used in the treatment of cancer pain. The predominant metabolic pathway of oxycodone is CYP3A4-mediated N-demethylation to noroxycodone, while a minor proportion undergoes 3-O-demethylation to oxymorphone by CYP2D6. The aim of this study was to investigate the effects of the mild CYP3A4 inhibitor aprepitant on the pharmacokinetics of orally administered controlled-release (CR) oxycodone.

Method: This study design was an open-label, single-sequence with two phases in cancer patients with pain who continued to be administered orally with multiple doses of CR oxycodone every 8 or 12 hours. Plasma concentration of oxycodone and its metabolites were measured up to 8 hours after administration as follows: on day 1, CR oxycodone was administered alone; on day 2, CR oxycodone was administered with aprepitant (125 mg, at the same time of oxycodone dosing in the morning). The steady-state trough concentrations (Css) were measured from day 1 to day 3.

Results: Aprepitant increased the area under the plasma concentration-time curve (AUC_{0-8}) of oxycodone by 25% ($p<0.001$) and of oxymorphone by 34% ($p<0.001$), as well as decreased the AUC_{0-8} of noroxycodone by 14% ($p<0.001$). Moreover, aprepitant increased Css of oxycodone by 57% ($p=0.001$) and of oxymorphone by 36% ($p<0.001$) and decreased Css of noroxycodone by 24% ($p=0.02$) at day 3 compared to day 1.

Conclusions: The clinical use of aprepitant in patients receiving multiple doses of CR oxycodone for cancer pain significantly altered plasma concentration levels, but would not appear to need modification of the CR oxycodone dose.

Trial Registration: UMIN.ac.jp UMIN000003580.

Editor: Emanuel F. Petricoin, George Mason University, United States of America

Funding: This study was supported by a grant for Research on Applying Health Technology from the Ministry of Health, Labour, and Welfare of Japan and Yokoyama-Rinsyo foundation. However, the funders had no role in study design, data collection and analysis, decision to publish, or preparation of the manuscript.

Competing Interests: The authors have declared that no competing interests exist.

* Email: yutakafu@ncc.go.jp

Introduction

Oxycodone is a μ-opioid receptor agonist which is widely used in the treatment of cancer pain and chronic pain [1]. It is a semi-synthetic form of morphine with similar analgesic properties and side effects such as nausea, vomiting, constipation, somnolence, dizziness and pruritus [2]. At high dose or overdoses, oxycodone can cause shallow respiratory depression, somnolence progressing to stupor or coma, skeletal muscle flaccidity, etc. The oral bioavailability of oxycodone is 60 to 87%, and is higher than that of morphine [3–5]. Only 10% of the oxycodone dose is excreted unchanged in the urine and it is extensively metabolized by duodenal and hepatic cytochrome P450 (CYP) isozymes [6] [7]. The predominant metabolic pathway of oxycodone is CYP3A4-mediated N-demethylation to noroxycodone, while a minor proportion undergoes 3-O-demethylation CYP2D6 to oxymorphone, which is the active metabolite. Further oxidation of these metabolites via CYP2D6 (and CYP3A4) yields noroxymorphine [6]. Both of these metabolites are further metabolized into noroxymorphine.

Aprepitant, an orally available, selective neurokinin-1 receptor agonist, is effective for both acute and delayed chemotherapy-induced nausea and vomiting (CINV) and is used in combination with a 5-hydroxytryptamine-3 ($5HT_3$) antagonist and a corticosteroid (e.g., dexamethasone) for the treatment of moderately and highly emetogenic chemotherapy. The recommended dose of aprepitant is 125 mg prior to chemotherapy on day 1 and 80 mg once daily on days 2 and 3 (125-mg/80-mg regimen).

Aprepitant is metabolized by CYP isozymes 1A2, 2C19, and 3A4, and was shown to be a moderate inhibitor of CYP3A4 (K_i of about 10 μM for 1′ and 4-hydroxylation of midazolam and N-demethylation of diltiazem, respectively) in vitro and a very weak inhibitor of CYP2C19 and CYP2C9 [8]. Moreover, drug-drug interaction studies have indicated that aprepitant can inhibit CYP3A4 enzyme activity. When the standard oral dexamethasone regimen for CINV (20 mg on day 1 and 8 mg on days 2 to 5) was given concomitantly with aprepitant, the dexamethasone area under the time-concentration curve (AUC) from 0 to 24 hours increased approximately 2-fold on both day 1 and day 5 compared with the standard oral dexamethasone regimen alone [9]. When the methylprednisolone regimen consisted of 125 mg intravenously on day 1 and 40 mg orally on days 2 to 3, aprepitant increased the AUC of intravenous methylprednisolone 1.3-fold on day 1 and of oral methylprednisolone 2.5-fold on day 3 [9]. Conversely, several studies have not demonstrated that aprepitant use mediated clinically relevant effects on the pharmacokinetics of intravenously administered docetaxel or vinorelbine [10] [11].

At the 125-mg/80-mg regimen used for oral aprepitant administration for CINV, the peak plasma concentrations (Cmax) of 1,600 ng/mL (around 3.0 μM) and 1,400 ng/mL (around 2.6 μM) were reached in approximately 4 hours (Tmax) on day 1 and day 3, respectively [12]. As the intestinal drug concentration following oral administration is even higher than the plasma concentration, it is expected that orally-administered aprepitant inhibits intestinal CYP3A4 greater than intravenously-administered aprepitant and that orally co-administered drug is affected to a greater extent by the inhibitory effect of intestinal CYP3A4 than intravenously co-administered drug [9,13].

Concomitant use of oxycodone and aprepitant is used in clinical practice for cancer patient care. However, aprepitant might have the potential to increase the plasma concentrations of oxycodone and its metabolites via inhibition of CYP3A-mediated metabolism of oxycodone. As a result, the side effects of oxycodone may increase. In this study, we have therefore investigated the possible effects of the mild CYP3A4 inhibitor aprepitant on the pharmacokinetics of orally administered CR oxycodone in patients with cancer pain.

Methods

The protocol for this trial and supporting TREND checklist are available as supporting information; see Checklist S1, Protocol S1 and S2.

Patient selection criteria

The subjects were enrolled in patients whom continued to be administered CR oxycodone twice or three times daily for cancer pain and were planned to receive chemotherapy with aprepitant for CINV. Within the last 3 or more days to reach steady state, the subjects had received a fixed dose of CR oxycodone. Additional eligibility criteria were age≥18 years, histologically confirmed malignant solid tumor, and adequate organ function [serum total bilirubin less than 1.5×upper limits of normal (ULN), aspartate aminotransferase (AST) less than 2.5×ULN, alanine aminotransferase (ALT) less than 2.5×ULN, and serum creatinine less than 1.5×ULN]. Patients were excluded if they had gastrointestinal disorders that could affect ingestion or absorption of either CR oxycodone or aprepitant, and if they were receiving or likely to receive drugs or food that could act as potent CYP3A4 or CYP2D6 inhibitors or inducers. All patients provided written informed consent and study approval was obtained from the Institutional Review Board of Kobe University Hospital.

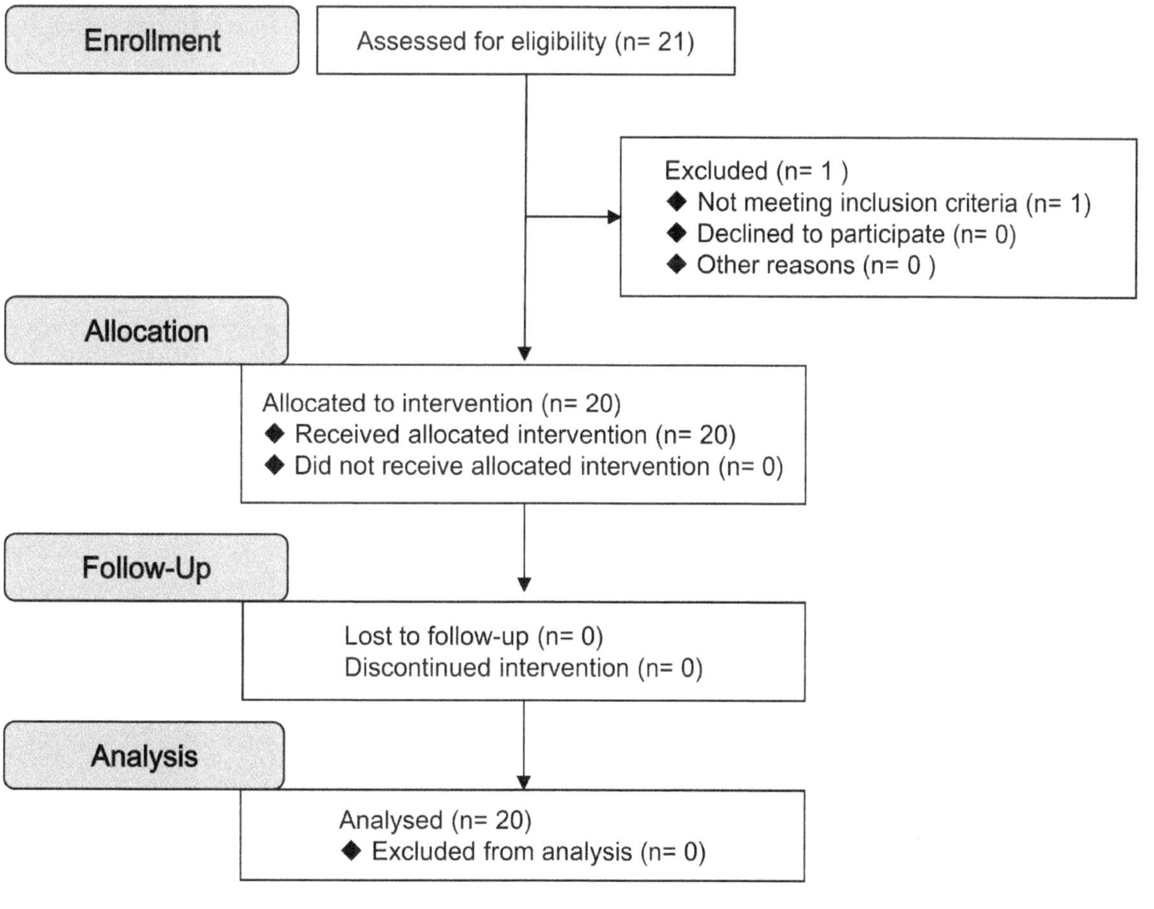

Figure 1. CONSORT flow diagram.

Table 1. Patient characteristics.

		Number of Patients (n = 20)
Gender	Male/female	17 (85%)/3 (15%)
Age	Median (range)	66.5 (44–77)
ECOG PS	1/2	13 (65%)/7 (35%)
Height (cm)	Median (range)	164.4 (138.5–177.1)
Weight (kg)	Median (range)	59.6 (37–77)
BSA (m^2)	Median (range)	1.64 (1.19–1.90)
Cancer type	Pancreatic cancer	8 (40%)
	Head and Neck cancer	4 (20%)
	NSCLC	2 (10%)
	CRC	2 (10%)
	CUP	2 (10%)
	Endometrial cancer	1 (5%)
	Cholangiocarcinoma	1 (5%)
Clinical stage	IV	20 (100%)
Anti-cancer agent	Platinum agent	8 (40%)
	Gemcitabine	7 (35%)
	Fluoropyrimidine	5 (25%)
	Taxanes	4 (20%)
	Anthracyclines	2 (10%)
	Irinotecan	2 (10%)
	Sunitinib	1 (5%)

Abbreviations: ECOG PS, Eastern Cooperative Oncology Group Performance Status; NSCLC, non-small cell lung cancer; CRC, colorectal cancer; CUP, cancer of unknown primary.

Study design

This study which was an open-label, two-period, single-sequence design was conducted at Kobe University Hospital. Patients were administered regularly with multiple-doses of oral CR oxycodone every 8 or 12 hours. Each patient was administered with the appropriate dose of oral CR oxycodone for their cancer pain. They received CR oxycodone alone (period A) on the previous day of planned chemotherapy and CR oxycodone with aprepitant (period B) on the day of chemotherapy. On the morning of period B, aprepitant was taken orally at the same time as CR oxycodone more than one hour prior to chemotherapy. Patients were participated in this study during blood sampling. Patients in hospital were given the dose of anticancer agents according to standard treatment schedule for their tumor types and were allowed to receive an antiemetic treatment with dexamethasone and a $5HT_3$ receptor antagonist where appropriate.

Outcome

The study objective was to investigate aprepitant might have the potential to increase the plasma concentrations of oxycodone and its metabolites via inhibition of CYP3A-mediated metabolism of oxycodone. The primary endpoint was pharmacokinetics of oxycodone and its metabolites with and without aprepitant administration. Secondary endpoints were safety and adverse event including nausea, vomiting, constipation, and somnolence. Patient characteristics and medication information were recorded

Table 2. Dose of Oxycodone.

Dose	Frequency of administration	Daily dosage	Number of patients
5 mg	every 12 hours	10 mg	6 (30%)
	every 8 hours	15 mg	2 (10%)
10 mg	every 12 hours	20 mg	6 (30%)
	every 8 hours	30 mg	3 (15%)
15 mg	every 12 hours	30 mg	1 (5%)
20 mg	every 12 hours	40 mg	1 (5%)
	every 8 hours	60 mg	1 (5%)

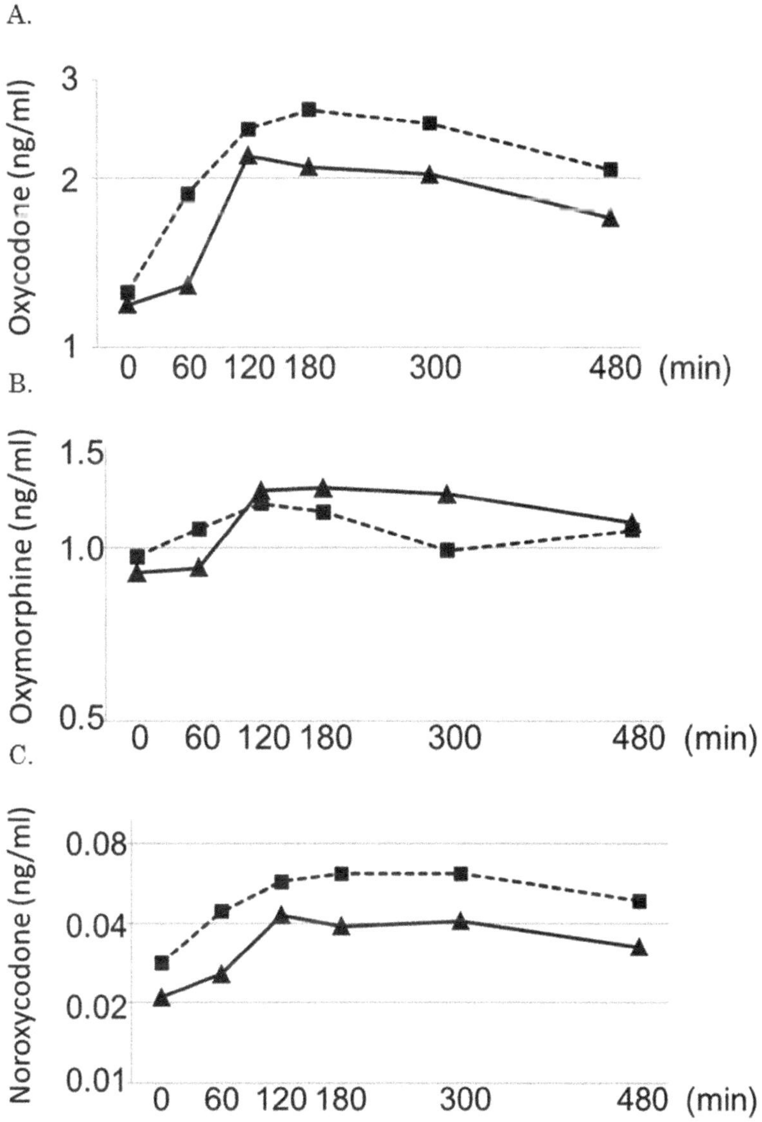

Figure 2. Mean plasma concentration curves of oxycodone, noroxycodone, and oxymorphone in patients (n = 6) who were administered with 10 mg of CR oxycodone every 12 hours alone (period A, triangles) or with aprepitant (period B, squares). ▲ without aprepitant, ■ with aprepitant.

throughout the study. Adverse events were evaluated using the CTCAE v4.0.

Blood sampling

Blood samples for pharmacokinetic analysis were collected immediately before and 1, 2, 3, 5, and 8 hour after administration of oxycodone in periods A and B. An additional sample was collected to allow for analysis of trough concentration before administration of oxycodone in the morning on the following day of period B. After blood was collected in lithium heparin-containing tubes, plasma was separated within 30 min by centrifugation at 1,500×g for 10 min at 4°C and stored at −80°C until analysis. Plasma concentrations of oxycodone, noroxycodone, and oxymorphone were determined using a liquid chromatography tandem mass spectrometric method. The lower limit of quantification was 0.1 ng/ml.

Pharmacokinetic analysis

Pharmacokinetic variables of oxycodone, noroxycodone, and oxymorphone were determined using the Pheoenix WinNonlin pharmacokinetic program (Pharsight, Mountain View, California). The Cmax and time to maximum concentration (Tmax) were observed directly from the data. The AUC with extrapolation to 8 hour (AUC_{0-8}) was calculated by the trapezoidal rule. The linear trapezoidal rule was used for successive increasing concentration values, and the logarithmic trapezoidal rule for decreasing concentration values. Metabolite-to-parent drug AUC ratios (AUCm/AUCp) were calculated to compare the relative abundance of each metabolite.

Statistical Analysis

This study was designed in order to exclude a clinically significant higher exposure to oxycodone and its metabolites. The null hypothesis was that coadministration of aprepitant would not

Table 3. Pharmacokinetic parameter of oxycodone and its metabolites.

	Oxycodone			Noroxycodone	Oxymorphone
	Cmax (ng/mL)	Tmax (hr)	$AUC_{0\to8}$ (ng*hr/mL)	$AUC_{0\to8}$ (ng*hr/mL)	$AUC_{0\to8}$ (ng*hr/mL)
Number of patients	20	20	20	20	15**
Without aprepitant	2.28	2.67	882	718	14.9
	(31.4%)	(57.7%)	(35.7%)	(45.2%)	(78.0%)
With aprepitant	2.79	3.62	1102	616	20.7
	(28.0%)	(32.1%)	(29.9%)	(51.6%)	(65.8%)
ratio	1.22		1.25	0.86	1.34
	(1.11–1.34)		(1.14–1.36)	(0.81–0.91)	(1.20–1.49)
p-value*	0.0002	0.07	0.00004	0.00005	0.00004

Abbreviations: Cmax, peak plasma concentration; Tmax, time to peak plasma concentration; $AUC_{0\to8}$, area under the time-concentration curve from 0 to 8 hours; ratio, the ratio of the geometric mean value of CR oxycodone with aprepitant to those without aprepitant.
Geometric mean (% coefficient variance).
Values were corrected for dose, assuming that all patients received 20 mg of oxycodone.
*Paired t-test for difference between logarithmic geometric means (two-sided).
**Five patients were excluded due to below lower limit of quantitation.

increase the plasma concentration of oxycodone to a clinically meaningful degree, i.e., the ratio of the geometric mean $AUC_{0\to8}$ for oxycodone between period A and period B would be <1.33. Package insert of oxycodone reports that the AUC of oxycodone in steady state was 216.2±97.4 ng.hr/ml [mean ± standard deviation, coefficient of variance (CV) was 45.1%] in patients with cancer pain (n = 32). We estimated that 20 subjects were needed to detect a 33% difference in the $AUC_{0\to8}$ for oxycodone at a power of 80% and level of significance $p<0.05$ (two-sided). The calculations used the sample size procedures in NCSS PASS 11 software. Data are expressed as the geometric mean ± SD. Statistical significance of logarithmic geometric means in AUC and Cmax was analyzed using a paired Student's t-test, with a probability level of 0.05 used as the criterion of significance. Tmax was analyzed using a Wilcoxon signed-rank test. All statistical analyses were performed with NCSS 2007 (NCSS, LLC. Kaysville, UT).

Results

Patient population

Twenty one patients were assessed for eligibility and 20 patients were allocated to intervention from September 2010 to December 2012 (Figure 1). Their characteristics are listed in Table 1. There were 17 men and 3 women with Eastern Cooperative Oncology Group performance status 1 to 2. The predominant tumor types were pancreatic cancer and head and neck cancer, with all patients having stage IV disease. Each patient was administered regularly with the appropriate dose of oral CR oxycodone every 8

Table 4. Trough concentrations of oxycodone and its metabolites.

	Oxycodone		Noroxycodone		Oxymorphone	
	N	(ng/mL)	N	(ng/mL)	N	(ng/mL)
Day 1 pre-dose	20	1.29	20	1.28	14	0.0243
Without aprepitant		(53.1%)		(46.2%)		(72.7%)
Day 2 pre-dose	20	1.22	20	1.23	14	0.0277
Without aprepitant		(49.3%)		(47.8%)		(68.8%)
Day 3 pre-dose	19	2.00	19	0.97	17	0.0321
With aprepitant		(49.2%)		(54.5%)		(78.8%)
Ratio (D3 to D1)	19	1.57	19	0.760	13	1.36
p-value*		0.001		0.00003		0.02
Ratio (D3 to D2)	19	1.65	19	0.796	13	1.32
p-value*		0.0001		0.00001		0.02

Abbreviations: N, number of patients; Ratio (D3 to D1), the ratio of the geometric mean trough concentration of CR oxycodone plus aprepitant on day 3 to those of CR oxycodone alone on day 1; Ratio (D3 to D2), the ratio of the geometric mean trough concentration of CR oxycodone plus aprepitant on day 3 to those of CR oxycodone alone on day 2.
Geometric mean (% coefficient variance).
Values were corrected for dose, assuming that all patients received 20 mg of oxycodone.
*Paired t-test for difference between logarithmic geometric means (two-sided).

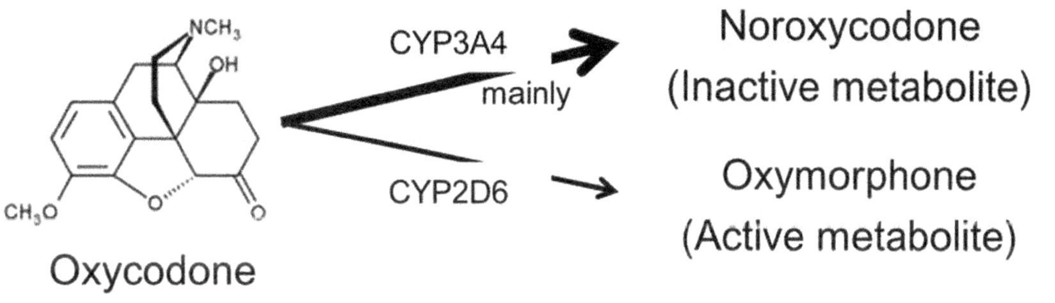

Figure 3. Metabolic pathway of Oxycodone.

or 12 hours (Table 2). The median daily dosage of oxycodone was 20 mg (range, 10–60 mg) and the mean was 21.5 mg, with the median for each dosage being 10 mg (range, 5–20 mg) and the mean being 9.25 mg.

Oxycodone and its metabolites pharmacokinetics

All 20 patients were assessed for pharmacokinetics of oxycodone and its metabolites with and without aprepitant administration. In five patients who were administered with 5 mg of oral CR oxycodone every 12 hours, the plasma oxymorphone concentration was below the limit of quantification. Table 3 and 4 summarize the pharmacokinetic parameters of oxycodone administered alone or with aprepitant. Figure 2 shows the geometric mean plasma concentrations of oxycodone and its metabolites in patients ($n = 6$) who were administered with 10 mg of CR oxycodone every 12 hours alone or with aprepitant. The ratio of the geometric mean AUC_{0-8} and Cmax of CR oxycodone plus aprepitant [1,102 ng*hr/ml (CV 29.9%) and 2.79 ng/ml (CV 28.0%), respectively] to those of CR oxycodone alone [882 ng*hr/ml (CV 35.7%) and 2.28 ng/ml (CV 31.4%), respectively] was 1.25 (95% CI 1.14, 1.36; CV 21.8%; $p = 0.00004$) and 1.22 (95% CI 1.11, 1.34; CV 20.6%; $p = 0.0002$), respectively. The ratio of the geometric mean AUC_{0-8} of noroxycodone and oxymorphone with aprepitant [616 ng*hr/ml (CV 51.6%) and 20.7 ng*hr/ml (CV 65.8%), respectively] to those without aprepitant [718 ng*hr/ml (CV 45.2%) and 14.9 ng*hr/ml (CV 78.0%), respectively] was 0.86 (95% CI 0.81, 0.91; $p = 0.00005$) and 1.34 (95% CI 1.20, 1.49; $p = 0.00004$), respectively. The plasma concentrations of oxycodone and its metabolites were affected significantly by presence or absence of aprepitant.

The trough concentration of oxycodone and its metabolite on day 1 were similar to those on day 2, because steady state was reached. However, these trough concentrations with aprepitant on day 3 were higher than those on day 1 and day 2. The ratio of the geometric mean trough concentration of CR oxycodone plus aprepitant on day 3 to those of CR oxycodone alone on day 2 was 1.65 in oxycodone ($p = 0.0001$), 0.796 in noroxycodone ($p = 0.00001$), and 1.32 in oxymorphone ($p = 0.02$), respectively.

In this study and clinical practice, there was no increased incidence in pharmacologic effect and side effects of oxycodone due to concomitant use of aprepitant.

Discussion

The predominant metabolic pathway of oxycodone is CYP3A4-mediated N-demethylation to noroxycodone, while a minor proportion undergoes 3-O-demethylation to oxymorphone by CYP2D6 (Figure 3). This study demonstrated that inhibition of CYP3A4-mediated N-demethylation by aprepitant significantly increased the AUC of oxycodone by 25% and decreased the AUC of noroxycodone by 14%, while subsequently increasing the AUC of oxymorphone by 34% through alternating CYP2D6 pathway. We estimated in advance that a clinical meaningful significant level of interaction between oxycodone and aprepitant would be a 33% increase in the ratio of the geometric mean $AUC_{0\rightarrow 8}$ under conditions where the CV was 45.1%. Essentially, the impact of aprepitant upon oxycodone was less than expected but the actual CV in the AUC of oxycodone was 30 and 35% in this study. Therefore, we consider that statistical significance was achieved as a result. In this study and clinical practice, there would be no increased incidence in pharmacologic effect and side effects of oxycodone due to concomitant use of aprepitant. We consider that a 25% increase (median 1.25; 95% CI 1.14, 1.36) in the ratio of the geometric mean $AUC_{0\rightarrow 8}$ is a statistically significant effect, but that, due to its less extent than expected, at this time there is no need to change the CR oxycodone dose in clinical use of aprepitant in cancer patients, with adequate attention. With regard to oxymorphone which is an active metabolite, because oxymorphone is a potent opioid that has a 4 to 6 times lower μ-opioid receptor affinity and lower concentration than oxycodone [6] [14], an increase of oxymorphone would be unlikely to have a significant impact on the clinical relevance. However, because the recommended dose of aprepitant is 125-mg/80-mg regimen over 3 days, it is important to further investigate the possible effects of the 125-mg/80-mg aprepitant regimen on the pharmacokinetics of orally administered CR oxycodone in patients with cancer pain.

Aprepitant had no detectable inhibitory effect on the pharmacokinetics of intravenously administered docetaxel or vinorelbine [10] [11] but resulted in increased plasma concentration of orally administered dexamethasone or CR oxycodone [9]. It is expected that an orally-coadministered drug is affected to a greater extent by an inhibitory effect of intestinal CYP3A4 than intravenously-administered drug due to the higher intestinal concentration of aprepitant as compared to the plasma concentration. Therefore, we consider that this result for CR oxycodone may not be applicable to intravenously administered oxycodone. In this study, our patients received individual dose and schedule of CR oxycodone and combined with various anti-cancer agents according to standard treatment for their tumor types. Additionally, we didn't conducted placebo-controlled trial, because the primary endpoint in this study is not pharmacodynamics of oxycodone and its metabolites but pharmacokinetics. These are limitations of study, because this study was conducted in subjects whom continued to be administered CR oxycodone routinely for cancer pain. Further study to validate effects of aprepitant on the pharmacokinetics and pharmacodynamics of controlled-release oral oxycodone pharmacokinetic is expected.

The trough concentration of oxycodone and its metabolite on day 1 pre-dose were similar to those on day 2 pre-dose, despite these trough concentrations with aprepitant on day 3 were higher than those on day1 and day 2. This indicated that the trough concentrations of CR oxycodone alone at steady state were not observed inter-day variability (Table 4). Meanwhile, the ratio of the geometric mean AUC_{0-8} and trough concentration of CR oxycodone plus aprepitant to those of CR oxycodone alone was 1.25 (range 0.98–1.96) and 1.65 (range 0.54–3.41), respectively, with wide inter-patient variability observed (Figures S1 and S2). A pharmacogenomics study showed that a CYP2D6 genotype had an impact on plasma concentrations of oxycodone and oxymorphone, and the metabolism of oxycodone [15]. First, we are now planning a further pharmacogenomics study. Secondly, we will analyze plasma concentrations of aprepitant and investigate the possible influence of aprepitant concentrations on the pharmacokinetics of orally administered CR oxycodone.

In conclusion, aprepitant increased the exposure of oxycodone by 25% due to inhibiting its CYP3A4-mediated N-demethylation. The clinical use of aprepitant in patients receiving multiple doses of CR oxycodone for cancer pain significantly altered plasma concentration levels, but would not appear to need modification of the CR oxycodone dose in clinical co-administration of aprepitant in cancer patients, with adequate attention.

Supporting Information

Figure S1 Individual value plot of AUC_{0-8} of (A) oxycodone (n = 20), (B) noroxycodone (n = 20), and (C) oxymorphone (n = 15) in patients who were administered with CR oxycodone alone or with aprepitant. Dose of CR oxycodone: circle (5 mg), triangle (10 mg), square (15 mg), and pentagon (20 mg).
(TIF)

Figure S2 Individual value plot of trough concentration of (a) oxycodone (n = 19), (b) noroxycodone (n = 19), and (c) oxymorphone (n = 13) in patients who were administered with CR oxycodone alone or with aprepitant. Dose of CR oxycodone: circle (5 mg), triangle (10 mg), square (15 mg), and pentagon (20 mg).
(TIF)

Checklist S1 TREND Statement Checklist.
(PDF)

Protocol S1 Clinical Study Protocol (Japanese version).
(PDF)

Protocol S2 Clinical Study Protocol (English version).
(DOCX)

Acknowledgments

We greatly appreciate all patients who participated in this study and their families; the assistance of the staff of the Division of Medical Oncology/ Hematology.

This work was supported by Yokoyama-Rinsyo foundation.

Author Contributions

Conceived and designed the experiments: YF, NC, HM. Performed the experiments: YF, MT, NC, NK, TS, YI, TM, HM. Analyzed the data: YF, MT, YI, HM. Contributed reagents/materials/analysis tools: YF, MT, HM. Wrote the paper: YF, MT, NC, YI, HM.

References

1. Kalso E (2005) Oxycodone. J Pain Symptom Manage 29: S47–56.
2. National Cancer Center. Cancer statistics in Japan 2010.
3. Leow KP, Smith MT, Williams B, Cramond T (1992) Single-dose and steady-state pharmacokinetics and pharmacodynamics of oxycodone in patients with cancer. Clin Pharmacol Ther 52: 487–495.
4. Poyhia R, Seppala T, Olkkola KT, Kalso E (1992) The pharmacokinetics and metabolism of oxycodone after intramuscular and oral administration to healthy subjects. Br J Clin Pharmacol 33: 617–621.
5. Leow KP, Cramond T, Smith MT (1995) Pharmacokinetics and pharmacodynamics of oxycodone when given intravenously and rectally to adult patients with cancer pain. Anesth Analg 80: 296–302.
6. Lalovic B, Phillips B, Risler LL, Howald W, Shen DD (2004) Quantitative contribution of CYP2D6 and CYP3A to oxycodone metabolism in human liver and intestinal microsomes. Drug Metab Dispos 32: 447–454.
7. Lalovic B, Kharasch E, Hoffer C, Risler L, Liu-Chen LY, et al. (2006) Pharmacokinetics and pharmacodynamics of oral oxycodone in healthy human subjects: role of circulating active metabolites. Clin Pharmacol Ther 79: 461–479.
8. Sanchez RI, Wang RW, Newton DJ, Bakhtiar R, Lu P, et al. (2004) Cytochrome P450 3A4 is the major enzyme involved in the metabolism of the substance P receptor antagonist aprepitant. Drug Metab Dispos 32: 1287–1292.
9. McCrea JB, Majumdar AK, Goldberg MR, Iwamoto M, Gargano C, et al. (2003) Effects of the neurokinin1 receptor antagonist aprepitant on the pharmacokinetics of dexamethasone and methylprednisolone. Clin Pharmacol Ther 74: 17–24.
10. Nygren P, Hande K, Petty KJ, Fedgchin M, van Dyck K, et al. (2005) Lack of effect of aprepitant on the pharmacokinetics of docetaxel in cancer patients. Cancer Chemother Pharmacol 55: 609–616.
11. Loos WJ, de Wit R, Freedman SJ, Van Dyck K, Gambale JJ, et al. (2007) Aprepitant when added to a standard antiemetic regimen consisting of ondansetron and dexamethasone does not affect vinorelbine pharmacokinetics in cancer patients. Cancer Chemother Pharmacol 59: 407–412.
12. Merck & Co I (2003) EMEND (aprepitant) capsules, for oral use. NJ, USA: Whitehouse Station.
13. Majumdar AK, McCrea JB, Panebianco DL, Hesney M, Dru J, et al. (2003) Effects of aprepitant on cytochrome P450 3A4 activity using midazolam as a probe. Clin Pharmacol Ther 74: 150–156.
14. Kalso E (2007) How different is oxycodone from morphine? Pain 132: 227–228.
15. Stamer UM, Zhang L, Book M, Lehmann LE, Stuber F, et al. (2013) CYP2D6 genotype dependent oxycodone metabolism in postoperative patients. PLoS One 8: e60239.

21

A Nation-Wide Study of Prevalence and Risk Factors for Fecal Impaction in Nursing Homes

Enrique Rey[1]*, Marta Barcelo[1], Maria Jose Jiménez Cebrián[2,3], Angel Alvarez-Sanchez[1], Manuel Diaz-Rubio[1], Alberto Lopez Rocha[3]

1 Division of Digestive Diseases, Hospital Clinico San Carlos, Universidad Complutense, Instituto de Investigacion Sanitaria San Carlos (IdISSC), Madrid, Spain, **2** Centro Valdeluz, Madrid, Spain, **3** Spanish Society of Nursing Homes Physicians (Sociedad Española de Medicos de Residencias - SEMER), Madrid, Spain

Abstract

Background: There are no existing studies that provide data regarding the epidemiology of, and risk factors for, fecal impaction, either in the general population or in any sub-group of people.

Objective: Estimate the prevalence of and factors associated with fecal impaction on a representative sample of the institutionalized elderly population.

Design: Two-phase study. Phase 1: pilot study validating the methodology in which all residents of a single nursing home participated. Phase 2: national multi-center cross-sectional study.

Setting: 34 randomly selected nursing homes.

Measurements: The presence of fecal impaction and associated factors were evaluated using three different tools: data collected from medical records; a self-completion questionnaire filled out by the subjects or a proxy; and a rectal examination.

Subjects: Older subjects living in nursing homes.

Results: The prevalence of chronic constipation was 70.7% (95%CI: 67.3–74.1%), of which 95.9% of patients were properly diagnosed and 43.1% were properly controlled. The prevalence of FI according to patient history was 47.3% (43.6–51.0%) and 6.6% (4.7–8.5%) according to rectal examination. Controlled constipation (OR: 9.8 [5.2–18.4]) and uncontrolled constipation (OR: 37.21 [19.7–70.1]), the number of medications (OR: 1.2 [1.1–1.3]), reduced functional capacity (OR: 0.98 [0.97–0.99]) and the occasional use of NSAIDs were independent risk factors for fecal impaction.

Conclusions: Constipation affects more than 70% of people living in nursing homes. Although it is properly diagnosed in more than 95% of cases, the disease is only controlled in less than 50%. Constipation, especially when not controlled, is the most significant risk factor leading to fecal impaction, which is prevalent in almost 50% of this population.

Editor: Antony Bayer, Cardiff University, United Kingdom

Funding: This project was funded by an unrestricted grant from Norgive Iberia. The funders has no role in study desing, data collection and analysis, decision to publish, or preparation of the manuscript.

Competing Interests: One of the authors are employed by a commercial company (Centro Valdeluz), but it does not alter the authors' adherence to PLOS ONE policies on sharing date and materials.

* Email: rey.enrique.spain@gmail.com

Background

The increase in life expectancy has led to a rise in the proportion of older people living in developed countries; in Europe, 17.1% of the population were over 65 years-old in 2008 and this is expected to rise to 23.5% in 2030 [1]. Older people require more assistance and care, which may be delivered at home, however sometimes a nursing home is necessary. In the USA, there were 17,000 nursing homes and 1.5 million residents in 2004 [2]. The need of long term care facilities has grown; according to a report from the Organisation for Economic Co-operation and Development (OECD), between 2000 and 2009 the number of beds in nursing homes grew in most countries, reaching an average of 44 per 1,000 inhabitants over 65 and this is expected to continue to grow [3].

Constipation is a condition characterized by infrequent or difficult defecation, and is one of the most common medical problems in institutionalized people. It is estimated to affect up to 80% of this population [4–6], given the multiple concurrent risk factors for constipation such as immobility, multiple medications, co-morbidity, and cognitive decline. The high prevalence of constipation in institutionalized elderly patients results in not only a reduced quality of life [7,8] and high economic burden [9–11], but it is also associated with the potentially serious complication of fecal impaction [12–14].

Table 1. Comparison between the pilot sample and the general sample.

	Pilot Sample (N = 199)	General Sample (N = 488)
Age		
≤80 years old	32 (16.1%)	130 (26.6%)
81–90 years old	113 (56.8%)	246 (50.4%)
>90 years old	54 (27.1%)	112 (23%)*
Gender [female N (%)]	144 (72.4%)	336 (68.9%)
Marital status [widow; N (%)]	127 (63.8%)	265 (56.5%)
Educational level [primary or less; N (%)]	139 (69.8%)	400 (81.9%)*
Time of stay in nursing home		
<1 year	8 (4%)	11 (2.3%)
1–10 years	76 (38.4%)	91 (18.8%)
>10 years	114 (57.6%)	382 (78.9%)*
Cognitive and Functional Status		
Functional disability (Barthel Index; score)	64.5±28.8 (0–100)	61.3±31.3 (0–100)
Cognitive impairment (Folstein Test; score)	23.0±8.4 (0–35)	22.1±8.6 (0–35)
Nutritional Status		
Body Mass Index (kg/m^2)	24.1±4.5 (14.9–43.3)	25.7±4.5 (14.7–41.5)*
Modified Ward Index (score)	5.5±5.7 (0–22)	3.6±4.9 (0–24)*
Fibre intake (g/day)	10.6±3.6 (3.9–21.9)	9.1±3.6 (2.5–24.4)*
Liquids intake (l/day)	1.5±0.3 (0.8–2.2)	1.6±0.5 (0.4–3.5)
Physical activity		
Immobility [bed-chair; N (%)]	56 (28.1%)	135 (28.7%)
Moderate or more [>60 min/day; N (%)]	31 (15.6%)	52 (12%)
Metodologic		
Needed proxy for completing [N (%)]	160 (80.4%)	384 (81.4%)
Understood every question [N (%)]	142 (71.4%)	364 (77.6%)
Co-Morbidity		
Diabetes [N (%)]	57 (28.6%)	129 (26.4%)
Thyroid disease [N (%)]	22 (11.1%)	55 (11.3%)
High blood pressure [N (%)]	132 (66.3%)	270 (55.3%)*
Cardiovascular diseases [N (%)]	100 (50.3%)	174 (35.6%)*
Respiratory diseases [N (%)]	50 (25.1%)	125 (25.6%)
Parkinson's disease [N (%)]	10 (5.0%)	36 (7.3%)
Stroke [N (%)]	37 (18.6%)	111 (23.1%)
Other Neurological diseases [N (%)]	78 (39.2%)	208 (42.6%)
Osteoarthritis [N (%)]	117 (58.8%)	302 (61.9%)
Renal/urinary disease [N (%)]	35 (17.6%)	66 (13.5%)
Depression [N (%)]	59 (29.6%)	200 (41.0%)*
Other psychiatric diseases [N (%)]	2 (1%)	44 (9.0%)*
Abdominal/abdominal wall Surgery [N (%)]	39 (19.6%)	110 (22.5%)
Number of Co-morbidities per subject	2.84±1.32 (0–7)	2.97±1.55 (0–8)
Drugs		
Antihypertensive drugs [N (%)]	147 (73.9%)	256 (52.4%)*
SSRIs [N (%)]	69 (34.7%)	176 (36.1%)
Tryciclic antidepressant drugs [N (%)]	7 (3.5%)	12 (2.5%)
Benzodiazepines [N (%)]	63 (31.7%)	130 (26.3%)
Hypolipemic drugs [N (%)]	53 (26.6%)	117 (24.0%)
PPIs [N (%)]	131 (65.8%)	277 (56.8%)
Calcium channel blockers [N (%)]	27 (13.6%)	53 (10.9%)
Nitrates [N (%)]	11 (5.5%)	48 (9.8%)
NSAIDs [N (%)]	26 (13.1%)	53 (10.9%)

Table 1. Cont.

	Pilot Sample (N = 199)	General Sample (N = 488)
ASA [N (%)]	68 (34.2%)	155 (31.8%)
Opiates [N (%)]	37 (18.6%)	25 (5.1%)*
Diuretics [N (%)]	84 (42.2%)	174 (35.6%)
Hypnotic drugs [N (%)]	52 (26.6%)	102 (20.9%)
Number of drugs per subject	4.56±2.29 (0–12)	4.02±2.20 (0–12)
Constipation		
Medical Diagnosis [N (%)]	119 (59.8%)	319 (65.4%)
Rome III Criteria [N (%)]	74 (37.2%)	183 (40.0%)
Regular laxatives		
Regular use of laxatives [N (%)]	114 (57.3%)	321 (65.8%)*
Regular use of enemas [N (%)]	4 (2.0%)	13 (2.7%)
Fecal Impaction		
Recurrent fecal impaction	62 (31.1%)	136 (27.8%)
Fecal impaction according to rectal examination	9 (4.5%)	35 (7.2%)

*p<0.05.

Although a definition of fecal impaction is elusive [15], it usually refers to the accumulation of hard feces in the rectum and colon that the subject cannot evacuate alone. There are no existing studies that provide data regarding the prevalence, incidence or risk factors for fecal impaction, either in the general population or in any subgroup of people. However, indirect data suggest that it is highly prevalent among institutionalized elderly patients, with 20% of those with fecal incontinence being diagnosed with the condition within a year [16], a prevalence of 25% in those with urinary dysfunction [17], 55% in those with diarrhea [18], and a description of stercoral ulcers (caused by fecal impaction) in autopsies of 1.3–5.7% of this population [19].

The following are considered risk factors for fecal impaction: certain medications including stimulant laxatives, immobility, neurological diseases such as Parkinson's or dementia, low fiber intake, chronic kidney failure, diabetes, or the existence of a malign neoplasm in any location [20], but there are no specific studies to support this.

The objective of this study is to estimate the prevalence of fecal impaction in a representative sample of the elderly institutionalized population, and to evaluate the risk factors associated with experiencing fecal impaction.

Materials and Methods

Design and population

The study was performed in two phases. The first phase consisted of a pilot study to validate the methodology, in which all residents of a single nursing home were invited to participate; the results of the validation have been published previously [21]. Once the first phase was complete and the methods were validated, the second phase was carried out: this was a national multi-center cross-sectional study. For the second phase, 34 nursing homes were selected at random from the SEMER (Sociedad Española de Médicos de Residencias [Spanish Society of Nursing Home Physicians]) members list, geographically proportional to the only estimation of the Spanish nursing home population [22]. For that purpose, physicians associated with the SEMER at the time of the study were classified into three geographical areas and chosen randomly by an officer (not related to SEMER) according to a prior specified geographical quota. When the physician either worked in the same nursing home of a previously selected physician, or was not reached (contact information not updated or impossibility to contact him/her directly after three calls on different days), an alternative physician was chosen in the same way.

Each nursing home physician was invited to include 25 residents in the study. Given that it was not possible to obtain lists of residents to form a purely random sample (due to national data protection laws), the residents of each nursing home were selected semi-randomly in accordance with pre-defined quotas according to the initial of the resident's surname and their year of birth (even/odd).

Ethical aspects

The study was approved by the Clinical Research Ethics Committee at Hospital Clinico San Carlos, and all of the study's participants or their legal representatives signed an informed consent document prior to their participation.

Protocol

The data gathering protocol included:

Clinical records abstraction. Clinical history (medical and nursing) data were gathered for each resident using a closed form that collected data on specific co-morbidities (detailed in Table 1), habitual or occasional use of several medications (detailed in Table 1), and the diagnosis of constipation. Specifically, data were gathered on diagnoses of fecal impaction in the last year, as well as its frequency and the treatment options used to resolve it.

Subject reported information. Each participating resident completed, with the help of a proxy if necessary, a questionnaire that included the items on abdominal and defecatory symptoms from the Rome III [23] questionnaire and on nutritional information, using the Spanish version of the Ward questionnaire [24]. For the analysis, the Ward score was modified, eliminating the item regarding the need for help with cooking, since there is a central dining room at each nursing home and none of the subjects cook for him or herself.

In addition, information was also collected on some lifestyle habits (liquid intake, fiber intake, physical exercise) with an ad-hoc questionnaire. All subjects were asked to record the average number of glasses or cups of liquid (including water, soda, soup, etc.) they drank daily during the morning, lunch, evening, dinner, and night. The daily intake of liquids was calculated as the sum of these amounts, estimating 0.2 liters per glass/cup. Fiber intake was calculated with a simplified food frequency questionnaire, including six questions referring to the usual weekly intake of fruits (1 question), vegetables (2 questions), cereals (1 question), legumes (1 question), and nuts (1 question). Answers were categorized as less than one ration weekly, 1 to 3 rations weekly, 3 to 6 rations weekly, one ration daily, and 2 or more rations daily. For the analyses, these categories were summarized as 0.5, 2, 4.5, 7 and 14 rations weekly, respectively. Total fiber intake was calculated assuming 2.5 g per ration of fruits, 3.5 g for vegetables, 1 g for cereals, 3 g for legumes and 1.5 g for nuts, and expressed as grams daily. To estimate physical activity, subjects were asked to describe their usual physical activity under one of the following items: "practice sports regularly", "walk long distances", "walk short distances (around my house)", "do not walk anywhere, or just a little bit", and classified for the analysis in three categories.

Objective measurements. All patients were evaluated in terms of functional capacity using the Barthel test [25] and cognitive capacity using the Lobo version of the Folstein mini-mental state exam [26,27]. Folstein's test is a widely used method to detect cognitive impairment. It is a questionnaire that evaluates temporal and spatial orientation, attention span, concentration and memory, capacity for abstraction (calculation), language ability, and visuospatial perception and ability to follow basic instructions. Validated Spanish Lobo's version provides a score ranging 0–35; 25 points or more indicates normal cognitive ability, 20 to 24 points a mild cognitive impairment, 15 to 19 a moderate impairment and 14 or less a severe cognitive impairment. Barthel's Index is a generic measure assessing the level of functional capacity independence) of the subjects for some basic activities of daily living, Each activity is evaluated by the physician with different prespecified scores according to the capacity of the examined subject to carry out these activities. The overall score ranges between 0 (completely dependent) to 100 points (completely independent). A score of 100 means complete functional capacity (independence), 90 to 99 good functional capacity (low dependence), 60 to 90 moderate functional capacity (moderate dependence), 20 to 60 low functional capacity (severe dependence), and 0 to 20 implies complete dependence.

In addition, the physician conducted a rectal examination (within two weeks of completion of the self-reported questionnaires), on all residents except those who did not consent to it. The physician was required to categorize the characteristics of the feces into one of the following categories: absence of feces, soft feces, non-impacted hard feces, and impacted feces. All physicians were provided with an information leaflet on the technique for carrying out a rectal examination and on the categorization to be used.

Definitions

A resident was considered to experience chronic constipation when he or she was diagnosed by the physician with constipation or, having not been diagnosed with chronic constipation in their clinical history, he or she complained of sufficient symptoms to meet the Rome III criteria for chronic constipation on the intestinal symptoms questionnaire. Constipation was further categorized as "uncontrolled constipation" when, on the Rome III intestinal symptoms questionnaire, the resident complained of sufficient symptoms to meet the Rome III criteria for chronic constipation, and as "controlled constipation" when the resident did not report sufficient symptoms to meet Rome III criteria despite having being diagnosed with constipation.

Fecal impaction was defined as the existence of a hard mass of feces in the rectum which the subject was unable expel. To estimate annual prevalence of fecal impaction we defined it as the medical diagnosis of fecal impaction as registered in the medical or nurse record of the subject in the last year, with recurring impaction being defined as a record of at least two episodes in the last year. Fecal impaction was defined on the rectal examination when the physician described the feces as hard and impacted. We applied these two definitions in the same population. Since fecal impaction is an intermittent event, the first definition was intended to estimate the annual prevalence of fecal impaction while the diagnosis through rectal examination was intended to estimate how many subjects are impacted at the same time.

Fecal incontinence was defined as the involuntary loss of liquid or solid stools occurring at least once monthly according to responses to a self-report questionnaire.

Analysis

Prevalences are reported as relative frequency accompanied by their 95% confidence interval. Quantitative variables are expressed as mean (standard deviation). Univariate analysis was used to evaluate possible risk factors associated with fecal impaction, and the factors associated with fecal impaction in that univariate analysis were subsequently included in a multivariate logistic regression (forward stepwise). Missing data were treated as missing.

Sample size

The sample size was set at 863 subjects, which allowed for the estimation of a prevalence of 10% with 2% precision.

Table 2. Association between the laxative treatment used and the constipation control level.

	N*	Controlled Constipation (N = 201)	Uncontrolled Constipation (N = 257)
No laxatives	23	6 (3%)	17 (6.6%)
Laxatives only occasionally	26	9 (4.5%)	17 (6.6%)
Bulk-forming laxatives	51	31 (15.4%)	20 (7.8%)
Osmotic laxatives**	293	128 (63.7%)	165 (64.2%)
Other laxatives or combinations	65	27 (13.4%)	38 (14.8%)

*28 subjects without symptomatic data to classify constipation control;
**260 (88.7%) were using lactulose and 33 (11.3%) were using PEG.

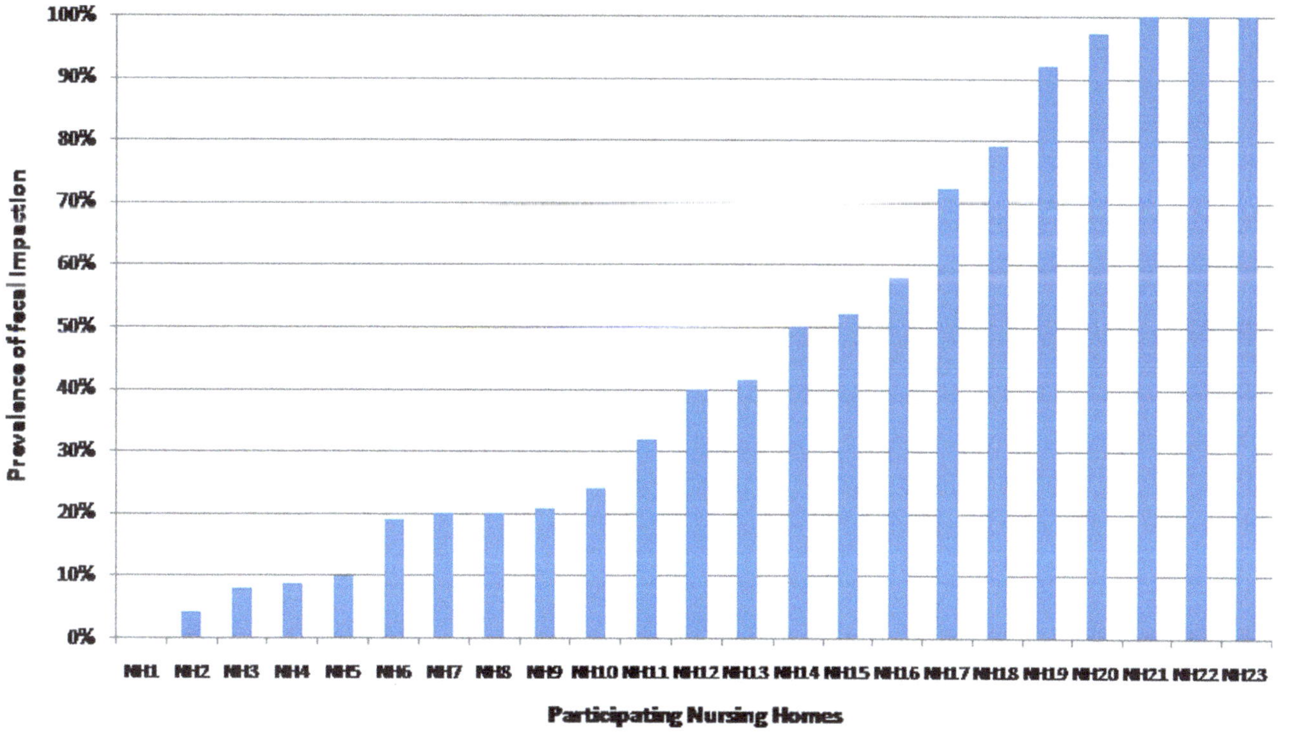

Figure 1. Annual prevalence of fecal impaction across the participating nursing hours.

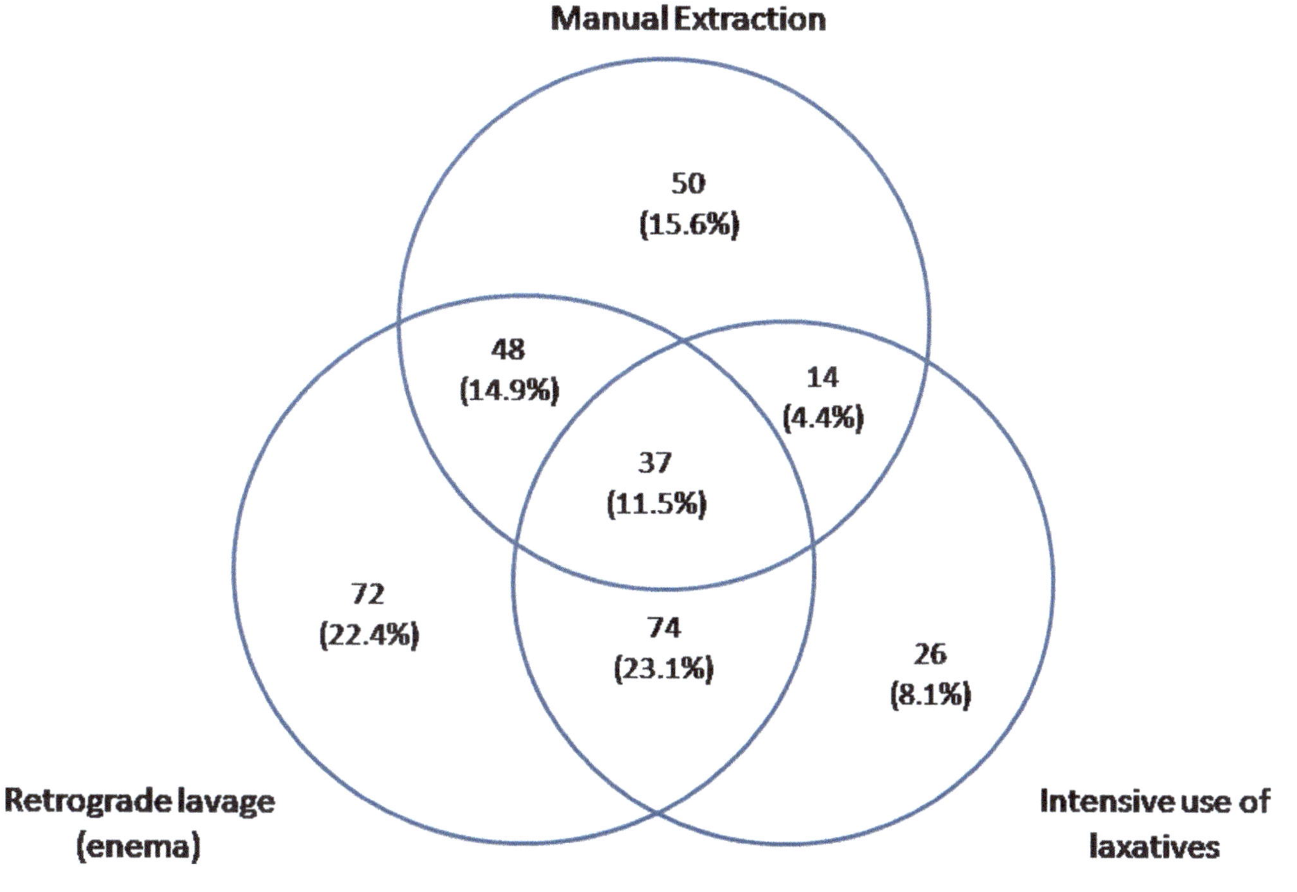

Figure 2. Methods used to solve fecal impaction in the population studied.

Table 3. Fecal Impaction and control of chronic constipation.

	Faecal impaction (medical records)	OR*	Faecal impaction (rectal examination)	OR*
No Constipation	15 (7.5%)	1	1 (0.5%)	1
Controlled constipation	96 (47.8%)	11.1 (6.1–20.1)	5 (2.5%)	4.9 (0.5–42.7)
Uncontrolled constipation	196 (76.3%)	39.2 (21.5–71.6)	35 (13.6%)	30.7 (4.2–226.4)

*adjusted by age and gender.

Results

Response rate

80% (N = 199) of the residents of a nursing home participated in the pilot study, and 21 of the 34 (61.7%; N = 488) invited nursing homes participated in the second phase, with an average of 25 subjects per site. There were no differences between the characteristics of the nursing homes that participated and those that did not. The participating nursing homes had capacity for 3302 residents (average: 157, range: 40–236) and 5 homes had a quality certificate issued because of the quality of their services. The 13 sites not participating had a total of 1736 residents (average: 134; range: 16–233) and one had a services quality certificate.

There were no relevant differences between the samples from the pilot study and from the general study, either in terms of the participants' socio-demographic, cognitive or functional traits, or in their medical characteristics (co-morbidities, use of medications), or in the prevalence of constipation, impaction, or the degree of control over constipation (Table 1). The proportion of subjects needing a proxy to complete a questionnaire was the same in both samples (80.4% vs 81.4%). We therefore believe that the general sample is representative of the nursing home population in Spain, and the samples were pooled for the final analysis, yielding a sample size of 687 subjects for analysis.

Prevalence of chronic constipation

The prevalence of chronic constipation was 70.7% (95%CI: 67.3–74.1%). In total, 466 subjects were diagnosed with constipation (67.8%; 95%CI: 64.3–71.3%) and 20 (2.9%; 95%CI: 1.7–4.2%) had symptoms of constipation sufficient to meet the Rome III criteria, although they had not been diagnosed with constipation in their medical history.

Of the residents with chronic constipation that filled out the symptoms questionnaire properly (N = 458), 201 (43.1%) were adequately controlled and 257 (52.9%) were not adequately controlled.

Prevalence of laxative consumption

63.3% (95%CI: 59.7–66.9%) of the subjects took laxatives on a regular basis. 53 (7.7%; 95%CI: 5.7–9.7%) subjects took bulk-producing laxatives, 313 (45.6%; 95%CI: 41.8–49.3%) took osmotic laxatives and 69 (10.0%; 95%CI: 7.8–12.3%) took other laxatives or combinations of laxatives. (Table 2) shows the relationship between the laxative guidelines followed and the control of constipation.

Prevalence of fecal impaction

According to their medical history, 325 subjects had experienced at least one episode of fecal impaction during the last year, which represents an annual prevalence of fecal impaction of 47.3% (95%CI: 43.6–51.0%). Variability of the prevalence of fecal impaction among participating nursing homes is shown in Figure 1. Of those with fecal impaction, 127 (18.5%) had experienced a single episode, 173 (25.2%) had experienced more than one episode but less than one per month, and 25 (3.6%) had experienced at least one episode per month. The prevalence of recurring fecal impaction was therefore 28.8% (95%CI: 25.4–32.2%).

Of the 665 (96.8%) residents that underwent rectal examination, 169 had non-impacted hard feces and 44 had impacted hard feces in the rectum, representing a prevalence of 6.6% (95%CI: 4.7–8.5%).

Methods to solve fecal impaction

Manual extraction was used in 151 persons, retrograde lavage was used in 236, and intensive use of laxatives in 155. Figure 2 shows how these therapeutic resources were used in the sample.

Chronic constipation and fecal impaction

The prevalence of fecal impaction, both according to the patient's medical history and present on rectal examination, was clearly related to constipation and the lack of adequate control of this ($p<0.001$; chi-squared test) (Table 3).

Fecal impaction and fecal incontinence

Prevalence of fecal incontinence was 16.4% (59 of 359) among those without history of fecal impaction and 28.2% (88 of 312) among those with history of fecal impaction ($p<0.001$; chi-2).

Factors associated with fecal impaction

In the univariate analysis, multiple factors (Table 4) were associated with the risk of having experienced fecal impaction in accordance with the diagnosis gathered from the medical history.

When the variables associated with fecal impaction in the univariate analysis were included in a final multivariate logistic regression model (forward stepwise), the factors independently associated with fecal impaction were controlled constipation (OR: 9.8 [5.2–18.4]) and uncontrolled constipation (OR: 37.21 [19.7–70.1]), the number of medications (OR: 1.2 [1.1–1.3]), reduced functional capacity (OR: 0.98 [0.97–0.99]) and the occasional use of NSAIDs (OR: 2.3 [1.2-4-5]) (Table 4).

Factors associated with fecal impaction in the rectal examination

In the univariate analysis, multiple factors (Table 5) were associated with the risk of having impacted feces in the rectum during the rectal examination.

Applying a multivariate model, without including constipation in its codification, because the existence of a single case in the reference category (no constipation) made calculations impossible, and including, in its place, two categories: (1) no constipation or

Table 4. Factors associated to Fecal Impaction.

	N	No Impaction	Impaction	OR not adjusted	OR adjusted*
Age (years)		83.6 (8.5)	85.1 (7.8)	**1.02 (1.00–1.04)**	
Gender					
Male	207	125 (60.4%)	82 (39.6%)	1	
Female	480	237 (49.4%)	243 (50.6%)	**1.56 (1.12–2.18)**	
Body Mass Index (kg/m2)		25.8 (4.4)	24.7 (4.5)	**0.94 (0.91–0.98)**	
Time of staying in nursing home (months)		38.4 (47.5)	43.9 (41.3)	1.00 (1.00–1.01)	
Functional Status (Barthel Index; score)		68.7 (29.0)	55.1 (30.7)	**0.99 (0.98–0.99)**	**0.98 (0.97–0.99)**
Cognitive Status (Folstein Test; score)		22.0 (8.9)	22.8 (8.2)	1.01 (0.99–1.03)	
Modified Ward Index (score)		3.3 (4.6)	5.2 (5.7)	**1.07 (1.04–1.11)**	
Fiber intake (g/day)		9.8 (3.9)	9.3 (3.3)	0.97 (0.93–1.01)	
Liquids intake (l/day)		1.6 (0.5)	1.5 (0.4)	0.90 (0.64–1.27)	
Physical activity					
Sport or long walks	71	53 (74.6%)	18 (25.4%)	1	
Light or moderate	407	230 (56.5%)	177 (43.5%)	**2.27 (1.28–4.00)**	
Minimum	191	76 (39.8%)	115 (60.2%)	**4.46 (2.43–8.18)**	
Number of co-morbidities		2.7+/−1.4	3.2+−1.5	**1.23 (1.11–1.36)**	
Diabetes					
No	501	256 (51.1%)	245 (48.9%)		
Yes	186	106 (57.0%)	80 (43.0%)	0.79 (0.56–1.11)	
Thyroid					
No	610	328 (53.8%)	282 (46.2%)		
Yes	77	34 (44.2%)	43 (55.8%)	1.47 (0.91–2.37)	
High blood pressure					
No	285	173 (60.7%)	112 (39.3%)		
Yes	402	189 (47.0%)	213 (53.0%)	**1.74 (1.28–2.37)**	
Cardiovascular diseases					
No	413	231 (55.9%)	182 (44.1%)		
Yes	274	131 (47.8%)	143 (52.2%)	**1.39 (1.02–1.88)**	
Respiratory diseases					
No	512	286 (55.9%)	226 (44.1%)		
Yes	175	76 (43.4%)	99 (56.6%)	**1.65 (1.17–2.33)**	
Parkinson's disease					
No	641	340 (53.0%)	301 (47.0%)		
Yes	46	22 (47.8%)	24 (52.2%)	1.23 (0.68–2.24)	
Stroke					
No	539	288 (53.4%)	251 (46.6%)		
Yes	148	74 (50.0%)	74 (50.0%)	1.15 (0.80–1.65)	
Other Neurological diseases					
No	400	212 (53.0%)	188 (47.0%)		
Yes	287	150 (52.3%)	137 (47.7%)	1.03 (0.76–1.40)	
Osteoarthritis					
No	268	168 (62.7%)	100 (37.3%)		
Yes	419	194 (46.3%)	225 (53.7%)	**1.95 (1.42–2.67)**	
Renal/Urinary diseases					
No	586	314 (53.6%)	272 (46.4%)		
Yes	101	48 (47.5%)	53 (52.5%)	1.27 (0.84–1.95)	
Constipation					
No	201	186 (92.5%)	15 (7.5%)	1	
Controlled	201	105 (52.2%)	96 (47.8%)	**11.33 (6.26–20.54)**	**9.8 (5.2–18.4)**
Uncontrolled	257	61 (23.7%)	196 (76.3%)	**39.84 (21.88–72.56)**	**37.21 (19.7–70.4)**

Table 4. Cont.

	N	No Impaction	Impaction	OR not adjusted	OR adjusted*
Depression					
No	428	242 (56.5%)	186 (43.5%)		
Yes	259	120 (46.3%)	139 (53.7%)	**1.51 (1.11–2.06)**	
Psychiatric-Other					
No	641	330 (51.5%)	311 (48.5%)		
Yes	46	32 (69.6%)	14 (30.4%)	**0.46 (0.24–0.89)**	
Abdominal Surgery					
No	548	292 (53.3%)	256 (46.7%)		
Yes	139	70 (50.4%)	69 (49.6%)	1.12 (0.77–1.63)	
Number of drugs		3.6+/−2.1	4.8+/−2.2	**1.29 (1.20–1.39)**	**1.2 (1.1–1.3)**
Antihypertensive					
No	281	168 (59.8%)	113 (40.2%)	1	
Regular	403	193 (47.9%)	210 (52.1%)	**1.62 (1.19–2.20)**	
Occasional	3	1 (33.3%)	2 (66.7%)	2.97 (0.27–33.18)	
SSRIs					
No	441	249 (56.5%)	192 (43.5%)	1	
Regular	245	113 (46.1%)	132 (53.9%)	**1.51 (1.11–2.07)**	
Occasional	1	0 (0.0%)	1 (100.0%)		
Tricyclic Antidepressant					
No	668	352 (52.7%)	316 (47.3%)	1	
Regular	19	10 (52.6%)	9 (47.4%)	1.00 (0.40–2.50)	
Benzodiazepine					
No	488	267 (54.7%)	221 (45.3%)	1	
Regular	193	94 (48.7%)	99 (51.3%)	1.27 (0.91–1.78)	
Occasional	6	1 (16.7%)	5 (83.3%)	6.04 (0.70–52.09)	
Hypolipemics					
No	515	276 (53.6%)	239 (46.4%)	1	
Regular	170	85 (50.0%)	85 (50.0%)	1.15 (0.82–1.63)	
Occasional	2	1 (50.0%)	1 (50.0%)	1.15 (0.07–18.56)	
PPIs					
No	258	159 (61.6%)	99 (38.4%)	1	
Regular	408	198 (48.5%)	210 (51.5%)	**1.70 (1.24–2.34)**	
Occasional	21	5 (23.8%)	16 (76.2%)	**5.14 (1.83–14.47)**	
Antacids					
No	655	350 (53.4%)	305 (46.6%)	1	
Regular	25	9 (36.0%)	16 (64.0%)	2.04 (0.89–4.68)	
Occasional	7	3 (42.9%)	4 (57.1%)	1.53 (0.34–6.89)	
Calcium channel blockers					
No	607	322 (53.0%)	285 (47.0%)	1	
Regular	80	40 (50.0%)	40 (50.0%)	1.13 (0.71–1.80)	
Nitrates					
No	627	346 (55.2%)	281 (44.8%)	1	
Regular	59	15 (25.4%)	44 (74.6%)	**3.61 (1.97–6.63)**	
Occasional	1	1 (100.0%)	0 (0.0%)		
NSAID					
No	517	297 (57.4%)	220 (42.6%)	1	
Regular	79	32 (40.5%)	47 (59.5%)	**1.98 (1.22–3.21)**	**1.7 (0.9–3.2)**
Occasional	91	33 (36.3%)	58 (63.7%)	**2.37 (1.50–3.76)**	**2.3 (1.2–4.5)**
ASA					

Table 4. Cont.

	N	No Impaction	Impaction	OR not adjusted	OR adjusted*
No	463	269 (58.1%)	194 (41.9%)	1	
Regular	223	93 (41.7%)	130 (58.3%)	**1.94 (1.40–2.68)**	
Occasional	1	0 (0.0%)	1 (100.0%)		
Opiates					
No	620	342 (55.2%)	278 (44.8%)	1	
Regular	62	18 (29.0%)	44 (71.0%)	**3.01 (1.70–5.32)**	
Occasional	5	2 (40.0%)	3 (60.0%)	1.85 (0.31–11.12)	
Antidiarrheals					
No	672	350 (52.1%)	322 (47.9%)	1	
Regular	5	4 (80.0%)	1 (20.0%)	0.27 (0.03–2.44)	
Occasional	10	8 (80.0%)	2 (20.0%)	0.27 (0.06–1.29)	
Anticholinergics					
No	628	332 (52.9%)	296 (47.1%)	1	
Habitual	59	30 (50.8%)	29 (49.2%)	1.08 (0.64–1.85)	
Diuretics					
No	406	236 (58.1%)	170 (41.9%)	1	
Regular	258	116 (45.0%)	142 (55.0%)	**1.70 (1.24–2.33)**	
Occasional	23	10 (43.5%)	13 (56.5%)	1.80 (0.77–4.21)	
Phenothiazines					
No	650	334 (51.4%)	316 (48.6%)	1	
Regular	37	28 (75.7%)	9 (24.3%)	**0.34 (0.16–0.73)**	
Hypnotics					
No	507	272 (53.6%)	235 (46.4%)	1	
Regular	155	80 (51.6%)	75 (48.4%)	1.09 (0.76–1.56)	
Occasional	25	10 (40.0%)	15 (60.0%)	1.74 (0.77–3.94)	

Nagelkerke $R^2 = 0.49$.

controlled constipation, (2) uncontrolled constipation, the factors independently associated with having impacted feces in the rectum during the rectal examination were the lack of control of constipation (OR: 11.84 [3.87–36.24]), the number of medications (OR: 1.26 [1.02–1.56]), reduced functional capacity (OR: 0.98 [0.97–0.99]), risk of malnutrition (OR: 1.14 [1.02–1.22]), the habitual use of ASA (OR: 3.12 [1.24–7.87]) and the occasional use of diuretics (OR: 18.94 [3.69–97.15]) (Table 6).

Discussion

This is the first study specifically designed to evaluate the prevalence of both constipation and fecal impaction in a sample representative of the nursing home population. The data available up until now came from studies that were not specifically designed for this objective, and were obtained from a single nursing home, which limits its interpretation in terms of representation, given the variation in standards of care and human and material resources among institutions.

Institutionalized elderly patients represent a very specific population, given that they can be expected to suffer constipation more frequently than the non-institutionalized elderly population due to the high prevalence of known risk factors for it [4,6,28–30], but they are under constant nursing and medical supervision. Our study provides information on the prevalence of the conditions studied, as well as on the outcome of care, and the known or supposed therapeutic and preventive measures taken against these.

Our study confirms that constipation in the nursing home population is very highly prevalent, affecting more than 70% of said population. Although there are no other studies on prevalence with which we can compare our results, this figure is similar to the one obtained in studies providing indirect data on the prevalence of constipation, such as the use of laxatives on at least an occasional basis by 93% of the residents of nursing homes [31], the daily use of laxatives by 50–74% of institutionalized persons [4–6,32], or the fact that more than 50% of institutionalized patients complain of straining or difficulty passing feces in more than 25% of bowel movements [33].

Moreover, in spite of the fact that constipation is well-known and is diagnosed correctly (95.9% of patients with constipation were correctly diagnosed in the study sample), treatment efforts to control it are generally insufficient, as shown by the fact that more than 50% of patients diagnosed with constipation continue to meet the Rome III criteria for constipation, in spite of the treatment prescribed by their physicians, and in spite of being surrounded by constant care. It may suggest that laxatives are less effective in this population; an alternative explanation is that the effectiveness of laxatives is not checked after prescription. Future studies should be focused on this relevant matter, since control of constipation is the main objective of treatment.

Table 5. Factors associated to Fecal Impaction in rectal examination.

	N	No Impaction	Impaction	OR not adjusted
Age (years)	687	84.2 (8.2)	86,3 (7.3)	1.04 (0.99–1.08)
Gender				
Male	207	195 (94.2%)	12 (5.8%)	1
Female	480	448 (93.3%)	32 (6.7%)	1.16 (0.59–2.30)
Body Mass Index (kg/m²)	643	25.2 (4.5)	26.0 (4.2)	1.04 (0.97–1.11)
Time of staying in nursing home (months)	682	40.3 (45.0)	50.6 (39.9)	**1.00 (1.00–1.01)**
Functional Status (Barthel Index; score)	642	63.3 (30.3)	46,4 (30.5)	**0.98 (0.97–0.99)**
Cognitive Status (Folstein Test; score)	673	22.3 (8.6)	23.6 (7.0)	1.02 (0.98–1.06)
Modified Ward Index (score)	687	3.9 (5.2)	7.8 (5.0)	**1.12 (1.07–1.17)**
Fibre intake (g/day)	665	9.6 (3.6)	8.3 (4.2)	**0.89 (0.80–0.98)**
Liquids intake (l/day)	664	1.6 (0.4)	1.3 (0.5)	**0.29 (0.13–0.63)**
Physical activity				
Sport or long walks	71	70 (98.6%)	1 (1.4%)	1
Light or moderate	407	378 (92.9%)	29 (7.1%)	5.37 (0.72–40.07)
Minimal	191	179 (93.7%)	12 (6.3%)	4.69 (0.60–36.77)
Number of co-morbidities	687	2.8 (1.4)	4.3 (18.8)	**1.77 (1.46–2.15)**
Diabetes				
No	501	476 (95.0%)	25 (5.0%)	1
Yes	186	167 (89.8%)	19 (10.2%)	**2.17 (1.16–4.04)**
Thyroid diseases				
No	610	575 (94.3%)	35 (5.7%)	1
Yes	77	68 (88.3%)	9 (11.7%)	**2.17 (1.00–4.72)**
High blood pressure				
No	285	274 (96.1%)	11 (3.9%)	1
Yes	402	369 (91.8%)	33 (8.2%)	**2.23 (1.11–4.49)**
Cardiovascular diseases				
No	413	399 (96.6%)	14 (3.4%)	1
Yes	274	244 (89.1%)	30 (10.9%)	**3.50 (1.82–6.74)**
Respiratory diseases				
No	512	496 (96.9%)	16 (3.1%)	1
Yes	175	147 (84.0%)	28 (16.0%)	**5.90 (3.11–11.21)**
Parkinson's Disease				
No	641	598 (93.3%)	43 (6,7%)	1
Yes	46	45 (97.8%)	1 (2.2%)	0.31 (0.04–2.30)
Stroke				
No	539	506 (93.9%)	33 (6.1%)	1
Yes	148	137 (92.6%)	11 (7.4%)	1.23 (0.61–2.50)
Other Neurological diseases				
No	400	372 (93.0%)	28 (7.0%)	1
Yes	287	271 (94.4%)	16 (5.6%)	0.78 (0.42–1.48)
Osteoarthritis				
No	268	259 (96.6%)	9 (3.4%)	1
Yes	419	384 (91.6%)	35 (8.4%)	**2.62 (1.24–5.55)**
Renal/Urinary Diseases				
No	586	551 (94.0%)	35 (6.0%)	1
Yes	101	92 (91.1%)	9 (8.9%)	1.54 (0.72–3.31)
Constipation				
No	201	200 (99.5%)	1 (0.5%)	1
Controlled	201	196 (97.5%)	5 (2.5%)	**5.10 (0.59–44.07)**
Uncontrolled	257	222 (86.4%)	35 (13.6%)	**31.53 (4.28–232.27)**

Table 5. Cont.

	N	No Impaction	Impaction	OR not adjusted
Anxiety Disorder				
No	492	469 (95.3%)	23 (4.7%)	1
Yes	195	174 (89.2%)	21 (10.8%)	**2.46 (1.33–4.56)**
Depression				
No	428	411 (96.0%)	17 (4.0%)	1
Yes	259	232 (89.6%)	27 (10.4%)	**2.81 (1.50–5.27)**
Other Psychiatric diseases				
No	641	600 (93.6%)	41 (6.4%)	1
Yes	46	43 (93.5%)	3 (6.5%)	1.02 (0.30–3.43)
Abdominal Surgery				
No	548	508 (92.7%)	40 (7.3%)	1
Yes	139	135 (97.1%)	4 (2.9%)	0.38 (0.13–1.07)
Number of drugs	687	4.0 (2.2)	6.2 (2.1)	**1.46 (1.28–1.67)**
Antihypertensive				
No	281	272 (96.8%)	9 (3.2%)	1
Regular	403	368 (91.3%)	35 (8.7%)	**2.87 (1.36–6.08)**
Occasional	3	3 (100.0%)	0 (0.0%)	
SSRIs				
No	441	422 (95.7%)	19 (4.3%)	1
Regular	245	220 (89.8%)	25 (10.2%)	**2.52 (1.36–4.68)**
Occasional	1	1 (100.0%)	0 (0.0%)	
Tricyclic Antidepressant				
No	668	625 (93.6%)	43 (6.4%)	1
Regular	19	18 (94.7%)	1 (5.3%)	0.81 (0.11–6.19)
Benzodiazepines				
No	488	460 (94.3%)	28 (5.7%)	1
Regular	193	177 (91.7%)	16 (8.3%)	1.49 (0.78–2.81)
Occasional	6	6 (100.0%)	0 (0.0%)	
Hypolipemics				
No	515	486 (94.4%)	29 (5.6%)	1
Regular	170	155 (91.2%)	15 (8.8%)	1.62 (0.85–3.10)
Occasional	2	2 (100.0%)	0 (0.0%)	
PPIs				
No	258	240 (93.0%)	18 (7.0%)	1
Regular	408	385 (94.4%)	23 (5.6%)	0.80 (0.42–1.51)
Occasional	21	18 (85.7%)	3 (14.3%)	2.22 (0.60–8.26)
Antiacids				
No	655	616 (94.0%)	39 (6.0%)	1
Regular	25	22 (88.0%)	3 (12.0%)	2.15 (0.62–7.51)
Occasional	7	5 (71.4%)	2 (28.6%)	**6.32 (1.19–33,61)**
Calcium channel blockers				
No	607	573 (94.4%)	34 (5.6%)	1
Regular	80	70 (87.5%)	10 (12.5%)	**2.41 (1.14–5.08)**
Nitrates				
No	627	595 (94.9%)	32 (5.1%)	1
Regular	59	47 (79.7%)	12 (20.3%)	**4.75 (2.29–9.82)**
NSAID				
No	517	492 (95.2%)	25 (4.8%)	1
Regular	79	68 (86.1%)	11 (13.9%)	**3.18 (1.50–6.76)**

Table 5. Cont.

	N	No Impaction	Impaction	OR not adjusted
Occasional	91	83 (91.2%)	8 (8.8%)	1.90 (0.83–4.35)
ASA				
No	463	449 (97.0%)	14 (3.0%)	1
Regular	223	193 (86.5%)	30 (13.5%)	**4.99 (2.59–9.61)**
Opiates				
No	620	581 (93.7%)	39 (6.3%)	1
Regular	62	59 (95.2%)	3 (4.8%)	0.76 (0.23–2.53)
Occasional	5	3 (60.0%)	2 (40.0%)	**9.93 (1.61–61.19)**
Antidiarrheals				
No	672	628 (93.5%)	44 (6.5%)	1
Regular	5	5 (100.0%)	0 (0.0%)	
Occasional	10	10 (100.0%)	0 (0.0%)	
Anticholinergics				
No	628	586 (93.3%)	42 (6.7%)	1
Regular	59	57 (96.6%)	2 (3.4%)	0.49 (0.12–2.08)
Diuretics				
No	406	396 (97.5%)	10 (2.5%)	1
Regular	258	230 (89.1%)	28 (10.9%)	**4.82 (2.30–10.11)**
Occasional	23	17 (73.9%)	6 (26.1%)	**13.98 (4.55–42.94)**
Phenothiazines				
No	650	607 (93.4%)	43 (6.6%)	1
Regular	37	36 (97.3%)	1 (2.7%)	0.39 (0.05–2.93)
Hypnotics				
No	507	474 (93.5%)	33 (6.5%)	1
Regular	155	147 (94.8%)	8 (5.2%)	0.78 (0.35–1.73)
Occasional	25	22 (88.0%)	3 (12.0%)	1.96 (0.56–6.88)

Our study provides, for the first time, figures on the prevalence of fecal impaction in the institutionalized population, revealing the enormous magnitude of the problem and its high recurrence rate. Around 50% of residents experienced fecal impaction at least once a year, 30% experienced recurring bouts, and 6.6% were impacted at any given time when a rectal examination was performed. This occurred despite them living in institutions that guarantee daily healthcare and that provide medical supervision, in many cases with procedures submitted for external evaluation and certification. Our figures for recurring fecal impaction align greatly with those obtained in a 1975 study, in which it was revealed that 39% of patients with fecal impaction had a prior history of impaction [34]. The fact that almost 40 years later the prevalence of recurring fecal impaction has not dropped to any

Table 6. Multivariate Model: factors associated with fecal impaction in rectal examination.

	P	OR adjusted*
Number of drugs	0,03	1.26 (1.02–1.56)
Functional Status (Barthel score)	0.02	0.98 (0.97–0.99)
Modified Ward index	<0.001	1.14 (1.02–1.22)
Uncontrolled constipation	<0.001	11.84 (3.87–36.24)
ASA	0.01	3.12 (1.24–7.87)
Diuretics		
No		
Regular	0.08	2.48 (0.90–6.81)
Occasional	<0.001	18.94 (3.69–97.15)

Nagelkerke R2 = 0.42.

significant extent clearly demonstrates that the measures currently being taken to prevent its occurrence are insufficient.

Of all the factors associated with fecal impaction, our study confirms that constipation is the most significant individual factor associated with the occurrence of fecal impaction. Moreover, the results reinforce the idea that the main risk factor, specifically, is the inability to control constipation, in spite of treatment. Other factors, such as a lack of activity, the risk of malnutrition, and medications taken, are additional factors that contribute to fecal impaction in a population with a high incidence of constipation.

Of all of the identified risk factors for fecal impaction, there is one that has not previously been described in the literature: the occasional use of NSAIDs. Although this is not one of the factors most strongly associated with fecal impaction, it is relevant due to the high prevalence of NSAID use in the institutionalized elderly population. Although we know that the use of NSAIDs is a risk factor for constipation in the general population [35], our study shows that it is also a risk factor for experiencing fecal impaction that is independent of the risk for constipation.

The fact that our study does not show an association with certain factors that have been related to fecal impaction in other studies, such as neurological co-morbidities [13], or low liquid intake [20], not even in the univariate analysis, is probably related to the nursing home healthcare staff's knowledge of these risk factors for constipation, and their thus paying special attention to them in these patients.

A notable limitation of our study is the semi-random selection of the patients at each nursing home, imposed by the data protection laws, which made it impossible for us to access the patient registry for each nursing home. Although some bias in the selection of the subjects may exist in some centers, it would have occurred in both directions towards the most well and the most unwell. Overall, we believe that the consequences of this limitation are minimal, since we were able to compare the semi-randomness at a single nursing home with 80% of the residents included with random selection of nursing homes. The nursing homes included in the study are representative of all of the nursing homes in Spain, in accordance with the nursing home physician's census from the SEMER. Moreover, the response rate was lower than expected, which allowed us to reach the pre-established sample size: nevertheless, the sample size reached allows for at least 4% accuracy for the prevalence of 47% observed for impaction.

The objectivity of the self-reported measures by this population may be considered another possible limitation to our study. Although the instruments used have been previously validated for this purpose, the study was controlled by categorizing the patients according to the degree of cognitive decline, and by including only the medically defined data as an outcome for the analysis. Although 100% self-reporting would be desirable, it is impossible in this population without the aid of a proxy. In fact, more than 80% needed a proxy to complete the questionnaire mainly for two reasons: functional limitation (visual or motor impairment), and cognitive limitations for self-completing the questionnaire. More than 70% of the participants were able to fully understand the questions included in the questionnaire; some required a proxy due to reading or writing difficulties. The remainder of subjects required a proxy for completing the questionnaire due to cognitive impairment, but in these subjects the usual caregiver is likely to provide more reliable answers than the subject. The pilot study was designed in part to address this limitation by evaluating if the project was affordable.

Another limitation that should be acknowledged is that estimates of food, fluid and fiber intake are approximate, but a more accurate measure, such as a 3-day diary, was unaffordable; in the pilot study we tested that approach and it was not possible to obtain complete and reliable information.

The final conclusions of our study from a practical and clinical point of view are that fecal impaction is a problem of significant magnitude and that constipation is the most relevant associated factor. In an environment of constant medical care such as a nursing home, particular attention should be paid to ensuring that treatment for constipation is effective, regardless of the patient's capacities, habits, medical characteristics, or co-treatments.

Author Contributions

Conceived and designed the experiments: ER MB. Performed the experiments: MJJC MB ER. Analyzed the data: ER MDR. Wrote the paper: ER MB MJJC AAS MDR ALR.

References

1. Konstantinos Giannakouris (2010) Regional population projections EUROPOP2008: Most EU regions face older population profile in 2030. Eurostat. Statistic in focus. http://epp.eurostat.ec.europa.eu/portal/page/portal/product_details/publication?p_product_code = KS-SF-10-001.
2. Jones AL, Dwyer LL, Bercovitz AR, Stahan G (2009) The National Nursing Home Survey: 2004 overview. National Center for Health Statistics Vital Health Stat;13(167). http://www.cdc.gov/nchs/data/nnhsd/nursinghomefacilities 2006.pdf
3. OECD (2011) "Long-term care beds in institutions and hospitals", in Health at a Glance 2011: OECD Indicators, OECD Publishing. http://dx.doi.org/10.1787/health_glance-2011-72-en.
4. Primrose WR, Capewell AE, Simpson GK, Smith RG (1987) Prescribing patterns observed in registered nursing homes and long-stay geriatric wards. Age Ageing January;16(1):25–8.
5. Kinnunen O (1991) Study of constipation in a geriatric hospital, day hospital, old people's home and at home. Aging (Milano) June;3(2):161–70.
6. Harari D, Gurwitz JH, Avorn J, Choodnovskiy I, Minaker KL (1994) Constipation: assessment and management in an institutionalized elderly population. J Am GeriatrSoc September;42(9):947–52.
7. O'Keefe EA, Talley NJ, Tangalos EG, Zinsmeister AR (1992) A bowel symptom questionnaire for the elderly. J Gerontol July;47(4):M116–M121.
8. Glia A, Lindberg G (1997) Quality of life in patients with different types of functional constipation. Scand J Gastroenterol November;32(11):1083–9.
9. Singh G, Lingala V, Wang H, Vadhavkar S, Kahler KH, et al. (2007) Use of health care resources and cost of care for adults with constipation. Clin Gastroenterol Hepatol September;5(9):1053–8.
10. Rao SS (2007) Constipation: evaluation and treatment of colonic and anorectal motility disorders. GastroenterolClin North Am September;36(3):687–711, x.
11. Dennison C, Prasad M, Lloyd A, Bhattacharyya SK, Dhawan R, et al. (2005) The health-related quality of life and economic burden of constipation. Pharmacoeconomics;23(5):461–76.
12. Kimberly BS (2007) Constipation in the elderly: implication in skilled nursing facilities. Director;15(3):20–3.
13. Gallagher P, O'Mahony D (2009) Constipation in old age. Best Pract Res ClinGastroenterol;23(6):875–87.
14. De Lillo AR, Rose S (2000) Functional bowel disorders in the geriatric patient: constipation, fecal impaction, and fecal incontinence. Am J Gastroenterol April;95(4):901–5.
15. Creason N, Sparks D (2000) Fecal impaction: a review. NursDiagn January;11(1):15–23.
16. Chassagne P, Landrin I, Neveu C, Czernichow P, Bouaniche M, et al. (1999) Fecal incontinence in the institutionalized elderly: incidence, risk factors, and prognosis. Am J Med February;106(2):185–90.
17. Starer P, Likourezos A, Dumapit G (2000) The association of fecal impaction and urinary retention in elderly nursing home patients. Arch GerontolGeriatr January;30(1):47–54.
18. Kinnunen O, Jauhonen P, Salokannel J, Kivela SL (1989) Diarrhea and fecal impaction in elderly long-stay patients. Z Gerontol November;22(6):321–3.
19. Lal S, Brown GN (1967) Some unusual complications of fecal impaction. Am J Proctol June;18(3):226–31.
20. Wrenn K (1989) Fecal impaction. N Engl J Med September 7;321(10):658–62.
21. Barcelo M, Jimenez-Cebrian MJ, Diaz-Rubio M, Rocha AL, Rey E (2013) Validation of a questionnaire for assessing fecal impaction in the elderly: impact of cognitive impairment, and using a proxy. BMC Geriatr;13:24.
22. Equipo Portal Mayores (2010) Estadisticas sobre residencias: distribucion de centros y plazas residenciales por provincia. Datos de octubre. Informes Portal

Mayores Núm 104 Pág: 19 p.ISSN: 1885-6780. Available: http://envejecimiento.csic.es/documentacion/biblioteca/registro.htm?id = 57572.
23. Morgan DR, Squella FE, Pena E, Mearin F, Rey E, et al. (2010) Multinational validation of the Spanish Rome III Adult diagnostic questionnaire: comparable sensitivity and specificity to English instrument (abstract). Gastroenterology;138(Suppl 1):S386.
24. Morillas J, Garcia-Talavera N, Martin-Pozuelo G, Reina AB, Zafrilla P (2006) [Detection of hyponutrition risk in non-institutionalised elderly]. NutrHosp November;21(6):650–6.
25. Mahoney FI, Barthel DW (1965) Functional evaluation: the Barthel index. Md State Med J February;14:61–5.
26. Lobo A, Ezquerra J, Gomez BF, Sala JM, Seva DA (1979) [Cognocitive mini-test (a simple practical test to detect intellectual changes in medical patients)]. Actas Luso EspNeurolPsiquiatrCienc Afines May;7(3):189–202.
27. Folstein MF, Folstein SE, McHugh PR (1975) "Mini-mental state". A practical method for grading the cognitive state of patients for the clinician. J Psychiatr Res November;12(3):189–98.
28. Bouras EP, Tangalos EG (2009) Chronic constipation in the elderly. GastroenterolClin North Am September;38(3):463–80.
29. Coyne KS, Cash B, Kopp Z, Gelhorn H, Milsom I, et al. (2011) The prevalence of chronic constipation and faecal incontinence among men and women with symptoms of overactive bladder. BJU Int Jan;107(2):254–61.
30. Talley NJ (2004) Definitions, epidemiology, and impact of chronic constipation. Rev GastroenterolDisord;4Suppl 2:S3–S10.
31. Frank L, Schmier J, Kleinman L, Siddique R, Beck C, et al. (2002) Time and economic cost of constipation care in nursing homes. J Am Med Dir Assoc July;3(4):215–23.
32. Wigzell FW (1969) The health of nonagenarians. GerontolClin (Basel) ;11(3):137–44.
33. Marfil C, Davies GJ, Dettmar PW (2005) Laxative use and its relationship with straining in a London elderly population: free-living versus institutionalised. J Nutr Health Aging ;9(3):185–7.
34. Gurll N, Steer M (1975) Diagnostic and therapeutic considerations for fecal impaction. Dis Colon Rectum September;18(6):507–11.
35. Chang JY, Locke GR, Schleck CD, Zinsmeister AR, Talley NJ (2007) Risk factors for chronic constipation and a possible role of analgesics. Neurogastroenterol Motil November;19(11):905–11.

Permissions

All chapters in this book were first published in PLOS ONE, by The Public Library of Science, hereby published with permission under the Creative Commons Attribution License or equivalent. Every chapter published in this book has been scrutinized by our experts. Their significance has been extensively debated. The topics covered herein carry significant findings which will fuel the growth of the discipline. They may even be implemented as practical applications or may be referred to as a beginning point for another development.

The contributors of this book come from diverse backgrounds, making this book a truly international effort. This book will bring forth new frontiers with its revolutionizing research information and detailed analysis of the nascent developments around the world.

We would like to thank all the contributing authors for lending their expertise to make the book truly unique. They have played a crucial role in the development of this book. Without their invaluable contributions this book wouldn't have been possible. They have made vital efforts to compile up to date information on the varied aspects of this subject to make this book a valuable addition to the collection of many professionals and students.

This book was conceptualized with the vision of imparting up-to-date information and advanced data in this field. To ensure the same, a matchless editorial board was set up. Every individual on the board went through rigorous rounds of assessment to prove their worth. After which they invested a large part of their time researching and compiling the most relevant data for our readers.

The editorial board has been involved in producing this book since its inception. They have spent rigorous hours researching and exploring the diverse topics which have resulted in the successful publishing of this book. They have passed on their knowledge of decades through this book. To expedite this challenging task, the publisher supported the team at every step. A small team of assistant editors was also appointed to further simplify the editing procedure and attain best results for the readers.

Apart from the editorial board, the designing team has also invested a significant amount of their time in understanding the subject and creating the most relevant covers. They scrutinized every image to scout for the most suitable representation of the subject and create an appropriate cover for the book.

The publishing team has been an ardent support to the editorial, designing and production team. Their endless efforts to recruit the best for this project, has resulted in the accomplishment of this book. They are a veteran in the field of academics and their pool of knowledge is as vast as their experience in printing. Their expertise and guidance has proved useful at every step. Their uncompromising quality standards have made this book an exceptional effort. Their encouragement from time to time has been an inspiration for everyone.

The publisher and the editorial board hope that this book will prove to be a valuable piece of knowledge for researchers, students, practitioners and scholars across the globe.

List of Contributors

Samantha Woo, Amy Walsh, Bruce W. S. Robinson, Anna K. Nowak and Richard A. Lake
National Centre for Asbestos Related Diseases, School of Medicine and Pharmacology, University of Western Australia, Harry Perkins Institute for Medical Research, Nedlands, Perth, Western Australia, Australia

Cleo Robinson
National Centre for Asbestos Related Diseases, School of Medicine and Pharmacology, University of Western Australia, Harry Perkins Institute for Medical Research, Nedlands, Perth, Western Australia, Australia
Anatomical Pathology, PathWest, Perth, Western Australia, Australia

Helman Alfonso
School of Public Health, Curtin University, Perth, Western Australia, Australia

Nola Olsen
Occupational Respiratory Epidemiology, School of Population Health, University of Western Australia, Perth, Western Australia, Australia

Arthur W. Musk
Occupational Respiratory Epidemiology, School of Population Health, University of Western Australia, Perth, Western Australia, Australia
Department of Respiratory Medicine, Sir Charles Gairdner Hospital, Perth, Western Australia, Australia

Kenneth Hsu, Yuen Ming Chung, Yasumi Endoh and Carolyn L. Geczy
Inflammation and Infection Research Centre, School of Medical Sciences, University of New South Wales, Sydney, New South Wales, Australia

Joanna Mika, Katarzyna Popiolek-Barczyk, Ewelina Rojewska, Wioletta Makuch, Katarzyna Starowicz, Barbara Przewlocka
Department of Pain Pharmacology, Institute of Pharmacology, Polish Academy of Sciences, Krakow, Poland

Juscimar C. Nunes, Jose R. C. Braz, Thais S. Oliveira, Yara M. M. Castiglia and
Leandro G. Braz
Department of Anesthesiology, Botucatu Medical School, UNESP - Univ Estadual Paulista, Botucatu, São Paulo, Brazil

Lidia R. de Carvalho
Department of Biostatistics, Institute of Biosciences, UNESP - Univ Estadual Paulista, Botucatu, São Paulo, Brazil

Anat Fisher and Colin R. Dormuth
Therapeutics Initiative, University of British Columbia, Vancouver, Canada
Department of Anesthesiology, Pharmacology & Therapeutics, University of British
Columbia, Vancouver, Canada

Ken Bassett
Therapeutics Initiative, University of British Columbia, Vancouver, Canada
Department of Anesthesiology, Pharmacology & Therapeutics, University of British
Columbia, Vancouver, Canada
Department of Family Practice, University of British Columbia, Vancouver, Canada

James M. Wright
Therapeutics Initiative, University of British Columbia, Vancouver, Canada Department of Anesthesiology, Pharmacology & Therapeutics, University of British
Columbia, Vancouver, Canada
Department of Medicine, University of British Columbia, Vancouver, Canada

Hugh Freeman
Department of Medicine, University of British Columbia, Vancouver, Canada

M. Alan Brookhart
Department of Epidemiology, Gillings School of Global Public Health, University of North Carolina, Chapel Hill, North Carolina, United States of America

Jakob M. Burgstaller, Boris F. Jenni, Johann Steurer and Ulrike Held
Horten Center for Patient Oriented Research and Knowledge Transfer, Department of Internal Medicine, University of Zurich, Zurich, Switzerland

Maria M. Wertli
Horten Center for Patient Oriented Research and Knowledge Transfer, Department of Internal Medicine, University of Zurich, Zurich, Switzerland
Cantonal Hospital Winterthur, Winterthur, Switzerland

Bo Huang, Wei-Xin Yuan and Guo-Dong Gao
Department of Neurosurgery, Tangdu Hospital of Fourth Military Medical University, Xi'an, Shaanxi, China

Li-Jun Heng and Peng Wang
Department of Neurosurgery, Tangdu Hospital of Fourth Military Medical University, Xi'an, Shaanxi, China
Department of Neurosurgery, Wuhan General Hospital of Guangzhou Military Command, Wuhan, Hubei, China

Lian-Ting Ma, Jian Song and Guo-Zheng Xu
Department of Neurosurgery, Wuhan General Hospital of Guangzhou Military Command, Wuhan, Hubei, China

Heng Guo
Department of Neurosurgery, PLA Chengdu General Hospital, Chengdu, Sichuan, China

Karim H. I. Abd-El-Maeboud, Mohamed A. M. F. Kortam, Mohamed S. Ali, Mostafa I. Ibrahim and Radwa M. M. Z. Mohamed
Department of Obstetrics and Gynecology, Faculty of Medicine, Ain Shams University, Cairo, Egypt

Yeong-Shiau Pu
Department of Urology, National Taiwan University Hospital, Taipei, Taiwan

Shuo-Meng Wang
Department of Urology, National Taiwan University Hospital, Taipei, Taiwan
Institute of Occupational Medicine and Industrial Hygiene, College of Public Health, National Taiwan University, Taipei, Taiwan

Ya-Yin Chen
Department of Urology, National Taiwan University Hospital, Taipei, Taiwan
Department of Statistics, Feng Chia University, Taichung, Taiwan

Ming-Nan Lai
Department of Statistics, Feng Chia University, Taichung, Taiwan

Alan Wei
School of Medicine, Stony Brook University, Stony Brook, New York, United States of America

Pau-Chung Chen
Institute of Occupational Medicine and Industrial Hygiene, College of Public Health, National Taiwan University, Taipei, Taiwan

Jung-Der Wang
Department of Public Health, National Cheng Kung University Medical College, Tainan City, Taiwan, 6 Departments of Internal Medicine and Occupational and Environmental Medicine, National Cheng Kung University Hospital, Tainan City, Taiwan

Shengai Li, Tracy Hu, Maria A. Beran and Sheng Li
Department of Physical Medicine and Rehabilitation, University of Texas Health Science Center at Houston, Houston, Texas, United States of America
Neurorehabilitation Research Laboratory TIRR Memorial Hermann Research Center, Houston, Texas, United States of America

Mark S. Gold1.
1 Department of Psychiatry and McKnight Brain Institute, University of Florida, College of Medicine, Gainesville, Florida, United States of America

Kenneth Blum
Department of Psychiatry and McKnight Brain Institute, University of Florida, College of Medicine, Gainesville, Florida, United States of America
Department of Clinical Neurology, PATH Foundation NY, New York, New York, United States of America
Dominion Diagnostics, LLC, North Kingstown, Rhode Island, United States of America
Human Integrated Services Unit University of Vermont Center for Clinical and Translational Science, and Department of Psychiatry, UVM College of Medicine, Burlington, Vermont, United States of America

David Han
Department of Management Science and Statistics, University of Texas at San Antonio, San Antonio, Texas, United States of America

John Femino
Meadows Edge Recovery Center, North Kingstown, Rhode Island, United States of America

David E. Smith
David Smith and Associates and Institute of Health and Aging, University of California San Francisco School of Medicine, San Francisco, California, United States of America

cott Saunders
Dominion Diagnostics, LLC, North Kingstown, Rhode Island, United States of America,

Thomas Simpatico
Human Integrated Services Unit University of Vermont Center for Clinical and Translational Science, and Department of Psychiatry, UVM College of Medicine, Burlington, Vermont, United States of America

Stephen J. Schoenthaler
Department of Sociology, California State University, Turlock, California, United States of America,

Marlene Oscar-Berman
Departments of Psychiatry, Neurology, and Anatomy and Neurobiology, Boston University School of Medicine, and Department of Veterans Affairs Healthcare System, Boston, Massachusetts, United States of America

Jason A. Miranda, Jamie Turner, Rebecca Dias and Huw Rees
Neusentis Research Unit, Pfizer, Cambridge, United Kingdom

Phil Stanley and Katrina Gore
Research Statistics, Clinical Research, Pfizer, Cambridge, United Kingdom

Chen Yu, Qing-Zhong Li and Hong-Juan Li
School of Pharmacy, Binzhou Medical University, Yantai, Shandong, China

Dong Qi
Department of Nephrology, Yantai Yu-Huang-Ding/Qingdao University Hospital, Yantai, Shandong, China

Wei Lian
Yantai Yan-Tai-Shan Hospital, Yantai, Shandong, China

Hua-Ying Fan
School of Pharmacy, Yantai University, Yantai, Shandong, China

Jianqiang Xiao, Yuriy Kotsurovskyy, Sarah P. Marshall and Eric J. Lang
Department of Neuroscience & Physiology, New York University School of Medicine, New York, New York, United States of America,

Nadia L. Cerminara Amelia Burroughs and Richard Apps
School of Physiology and Pharmacology, University of Bristol, Bristol, United Kingdom

Andrew K. Wise
The Bionics Institute, East Melbourne, Victoria, Australia

Hanako Aoki and Yuanjun Luo
Department of Systems Neurophysiology,
Graduate School of Medicine, Tokyo Medical and Dental University, Tokyo, Japan

Izumi Sugihara
Department of Systems Neurophysiology, Graduate School of Medicine, Tokyo Medical and Dental University, Tokyo, Japan
Center for Brain Integration Research, Tokyo Medical and Dental University, Tokyo, Japan

Stephan Wolff, Christian Riedel and Olav Jansen
Dept of Neuroradiology, University Hospital of Kiel, Arnold-Heller-Strasse 3, Haus 41, 24105 Kiel, Germany

Torge Rempe
Dept of Neuroradiology, University Hospital of Kiel, Arnold-Heller-Strasse 3, Haus 41, 24105 Kiel, Germany
Dept of Neurology, University Hospital of Kiel, Arnold-Heller- Strasse

Janne Gierthmühlen
Dept of Neuroradiology, University Hospital of Kiel, Arnold-Heller-Strasse 3, Haus 41, 24105 Kiel, Germany
Haus 41, 24105 Kiel, Germany, 3 Division of Neurological Pain Research and Therapy, University Hospital of Kiel, Arnold-Heller-Strasse 3, Haus 41, 24105 Kiel, Germany

Ralf Baron
Dept of Neurology, University Hospital of Kiel, Arnold-Heller- Strasse
Haus 41, 24105 Kiel, Germany, 3 Division of Neurological Pain Research and Therapy, University Hospital of Kiel, Arnold-Heller-Strasse 3, Haus 41, 24105 Kiel, Germany

Patrick W. Stroman
Centre for Neuroscience Studies, Dept of Diagnostic Radiology, Dept of Physics, 228 Botterell Hall, Queen's University, Kingston, Ontario, Canada

John V. Roughan, Claire A. Coulter and Paul A. Flecknell
Comparative Biology Centre, The Medical School, University of Newcastle, Newcastle upon Tyne, United Kingdom

Huw D. Thomas
Northern Institute for Cancer Research, The Medical School, University of Newcastle, Newcastle upon Tyne, United Kingdom

Kenneth J. Sufka
Research Institute of Pharmaceutical Sciences and Departments of Psychology and
Pharmacology, Peabody Building, University of Mississippi, Oxford, Mississippi, United States of America

Hugh MacPherson, Stewart J. Richmond, Harriet Lansdow, Sara Perren, Ann Hopton and Karen Spilsbury
Department of Health Sciences, University of York, York, United Kingdom

Liz Newbronner
Department of Health Sciences, University of York, York, United Kingdom
Firefly Research & Evaluation, North Yorkshire, United Kingdom

Ruth Chamberlain
Firefly Research & Evaluation, North Yorkshire, United Kingdom

Miranda L. van Hooff
Sint Maartenskliniek, Department of Research, Nijmegen, The Netherlands

Jan van Loon
Sint Maartenskliniek, Department of Orthopedics, Nijmegen, The Netherlands

Jacques van Limbeek
Achmea Health Insurance Company, Zeist, The Netherlands

Marinus de Kleuver
Sint Maartenskliniek, Department of Orthopedics, Nijmegen, The Netherlands
VU University Medical Center, Department of Orthopedics, Amsterdam, The Netherlands

Jeungchan Lee and Kyungmo Park
Department of Biomedical Engineering, Kyung Hee University, Yongin, Gyeonggi, South Korea

Vitaly Napadow
Department of Biomedical Engineering, Kyung Hee University, Yongin, Gyeonggi, South Korea
Martinos Center for Biomedical Imaging, Department of Radiology, Massachusetts General Hospital, Charlestown, Massachusetts, United States of America

Jieun Kim
Martinos Center for Biomedical Imaging, Department of Radiology, Massachusetts General Hospital, Charlestown, Massachusetts, United States of America

Seunggi Lee and Woojin Choi
Department of Neuropsychiatry, College of Korean Medicine, Sangji University,
Wonju, Gangwon, South Korea

Ted J. Kaptchuk
Program in Placebo Studies, Beth Israel Deaconess Medical Center, Harvard Medical School, Boston, Massachusetts, United States of nAmerica

Masanori Toyoda, Naoko Chayahara, Naomi Kiyota, Takanobu Shimada and Yoshinori Imamura
Division of Medical Oncology/Hematology, Kobe University Graduate School of Medicine, Kobe, Japan

Yutaka Fujiwara
Division of Medical Oncology/Hematology, Kobe University Graduate School of Medicine, Kobe, Japan
Division of Investigational Cancer Therapeutics, Exploratory Oncology Research & Clinical Trial Center, National Cancer Center Hospital, Chiba, Japan

Toru Mukohara and Hironobu Minami
Division of Medical Oncology/Hematology, Kobe University Graduate School of Medicine, Kobe, Japan
Cancer Center, Kobe University Graduate School of Medicine, Kobe, Japan

Enrique Rey, Marta Barcelo, Angel Alvarez-Sanchez and Manuel Diaz-Rubio
Division of Digestive Diseases, Hospital Clinico San Carlos, Universidad Complutense, Instituto de Investigacion Sanitaria San Carlos (IdISSC), Madrid, Spain

Maria Jose Jiménez Cebrián
Centro Valdeluz, Madrid, Spain
Spanish Society of Nursing Homes Physicians (Sociedad Española de Medicos de Residencias - SEMER), Madrid, Spain

Alberto Lopez Rocha
Spanish Society of Nursing Homes Physicians (Sociedad Española de Medicos de Residencias - SEMER), Madrid, Spain

Index

physical. Ed.

$ 144.95

(N)